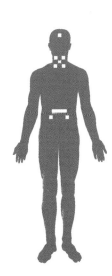

ATLAS
OF
ENDOCRINE
PATHOLOGY

ATLASES IN
DIAGNOSTIC SURGICAL PATHOLOGY

Consulting Editor

Gerald M. Bordin, M.D.
Department of Pathology
Scripps Clinic and Research Foundation

Published:

Wold, McLeod, Sim, and Unni:
ATLAS OF ORTHOPEDIC PATHOLOGY

Colby, Lombard, Yousem, and Kitaichi:
ATLAS OF PULMONARY SURGICAL PATHOLOGY

Kanel and Korula:
ATLAS OF LIVER PATHOLOGY

Owen and Kelly:
ATLAS OF GASTROINTESTINAL PATHOLOGY

Virmani:
ATLAS OF CARDIOVASCULAR PATHOLOGY

Ro, Grignon, Amin, and Ayala:
**ATLAS OF SURGICAL PATHOLOGY OF
THE MALE REPRODUCTIVE TRACT**

Wenig:
ATLAS OF HEAD AND NECK PATHOLOGY

Forthcoming Titles:

Ferry and Harris:
ATLAS OF LYMPHOID HYPERPLASIA AND LYMPHOMA

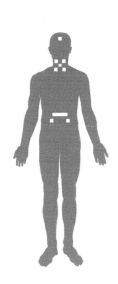

ATLAS
OF
ENDOCRINE
PATHOLOGY

Bruce M. Wenig, M.D.
Department of Otolaryngic and Endocrine Pathology
Armed Forces Institute of Pathology
Washington, D.C.

Clara S. Heffess, M.D.
Department of Otolaryngic and Endocrine Pathology
Armed Forces Institute of Pathology
Washington, D.C.

Carol F. Adair, M.D.
Department of Otolaryngic and Endocrine Pathology
Armed Forces Institute of Pathology
Washington, D.C.

W.B. SAUNDERS COMPANY
A Division of Harcourt Brace & Company

Philadelphia ■ London ■ Toronto ■ Montreal ■ Sydney ■ Tokyo

W.B. SAUNDERS COMPANY
A Division of Harcourt Brace & Company

The Curtis Center
Independence Square West
Philadelphia, Pennsylvania 19106

Library of Congress Cataloging-in-Publication Data

Wenig, Bruce M.
Atlas of endocrine pathology / Bruce M. Wenig, Clara S. Heffess,
Carol F. Adair.

p.   cm.

ISBN 0–7216–5917–9

1. Endocrine glands—Diseases—Atlases.   I. Heffess, Clara S.
II. Adair, Carol F.   III. Title.
[DNLM: 1. Endocrine Diseases—pathology—atlases.
2. Endocrine Glands—anatomy & histology—atlases.
WK 17 W75a 1997]

RC649.W46   1997   616.4—dc20

DNLM/DLC   96-29338

NOTICE

Medicine is an ever-changing field. Standard safety precautions must be followed, but as new research and clinical experience broaden our knowledge, changes in treatment and drug therapy become necessary or appropriate. Readers are advised to check the product information currently provided by the manufacturer of each drug to be administered to verify the recommended dose, the method and duration of administration, and contraindications. It is the responsibility of the treating physician relying on experience and knowledge of the patient to determine dosages and the best treatment for the patient. Neither the Publisher nor the editor assumes any responsibility for any injury and/or damage to persons or property.

THE PUBLISHER

DEDICATION

To my wife and best friend, Ana;
To our children, the loves of our life—Sarah Amelia, Eli Jonathan,
    and Jake Benjamin.
                                    Bruce M. Wenig

To my family, Luis, Alex, and Jessica, with love.
                                    Clara S. Heffess

To Bill and Martha Adair, the best of parents, with love;
To Dr. William J. Frable, with respect and sincere gratitude, for his
    example and for his teaching;
To all the Pathology Residents who have made my life and work
    ever so interesting.
                                    Carol F. Adair

To Dr. Clara S. Heffess for teaching us the finer details of Endocrine
    Pathology.
                                    Bruce M. Wenig and Carol F. Adair

PREFACE

The *Atlas of Endocrine Pathology* is organized into five major sections, including the pituitary gland, thyroid gland, parathyroid glands, pancreas (exocrine and endocrine), and adrenal glands. Each section begins with non-neoplastic lesions affecting that particular endocrine organ and is followed by sections of the neoplastic lesions (benign and malignant) of that organ. The format for each disease entity begins with its definition and any synonymous terms, which is then followed by the clinical details (incidence, demographic facts, signs and symptoms, etiology, and others), major radiographic features (if pertinent), pathologic features, differential diagnoses, treatment and behavior, and additional facts. Within each of these individual segments, only the major features are listed. As this Atlas is primarily pathology driven, we attempted to be as detailed and complete as possible in describing the pathologic features of each entity. The pathologic details primarily include the gross and microscopic features, and when applicable, the fine needle aspiration findings and histochemical, immunohistochemical, and electron microscopic features are also detailed. Unless specifically stated, the differential diagnosis section is a histopathologic differential diagnosis. Because of the limitation of space, the differential diagnosis lists only those diseases included in the differential diagnosis, but a cross reference to other sections of the book that detail the key entities included in the Differential Diagnosis is given. There are numerous tables included that succinctly list the key differentiating features of similar-appearing or diagnostically overlapping pathologic entities. The Additional Facts sections contain information that we felt was of practical importance to the surgical pathologist and/or clinician but that did not neatly "fit" within the previously detailed subdivisions.

The illustrations include clinical, radiographic, and gross pathology photographs when they significantly add to depiction of the disease state. The photomicrographs include the essential pathologic features for each disease. Illustrations of special stains (histochemistry and/or immunohistochemistry) or electron microscopy are included when helpful in illustrating an essential component of a given lesion. Key references for each disease entity are included, listing seminal articles and/or classic works and the current literature. We have also incorporated the anatomy, embryology, and histology of each organ in an appendix section of the book.

BRUCE M. WENIG
CLARA S. HEFFESS
CAROL F. ADAIR

ACKNOWLEDGMENTS

We would like to acknowledge the many pathologists who have submitted the interesting, challenging, and unusual endocrine cases to our division at the Armed Forces Institute of Pathology over the years; without their contributions this Atlas could not have been completed.

To Dr. Dennis K. Heffner, Chairman, Department of Otolaryngic and Endocrine Pathology, for his support, guidance, and friendship.

To Dr. Peter Buetow, Department of Radiologic Pathology, AFIP, and Dr. James L. Ownbey, Methodist Hospital, Department of Pathology, Lubbock, Texas, for kindly contributing various radiographs and gross photographs that appear in the book.

To the photographic staff at the AFIP, particularly George L. Jones and Luther Duckett, for their efforts to meet our needs and the superb quality of the photomicrographs that appear in this Atlas.

To the editorial staff of W.B. Saunders Company, including Lesley Day, Emily Byrne, Linda R. Garber, Sue Reilly, and Ruth Low, as well as the many other individuals with whom we did not deal on a frequent basis, for their assistance and professionalism.

CONTENTS

■ **CHAPTER 13**

■ **CHAPTER 14**

■ **CHAPTER 15**

■ **CHAPTER 16**

APPENDICES

■ **APPENDIX A**

■ **APPENDIX B**

■ **APPENDIX C**

■ **APPENDIX D**

■ **APPENDIX E**

CHAPTER 1

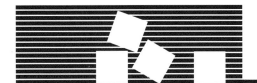

Non-Neoplastic Lesions of the Pituitary Gland

A. CLASSIFICATION OF NON-NEOPLASTIC LESIONS OF THE PITUITARY GLAND

Table 1–1
NON-NEOPLASTIC LESIONS
OF THE PITUITARY GLAND

Inflammatory Lesions

Abscess
Granulomatous inflammation
    Sarcoidosis
    Mycobacterial, Spirochetal, and fungal infection
Idiopathic
    Giant cell granuloma
Autoimmune
    Lymphocytic hypophysitis

Circulatory Disturbances

Hemorrhage and pituitary apoplexy
Infarction
Necrosis (Sheehan's syndrome)

Cysts

Dermoid cysts
Epidermoid cysts
Rathke's pouch cyst

Hyperplasia

Langerhans Cell Histiocytosis

Miscellaneous—Calcification and Abnormal Deposits

Amyloidosis and hemochromatosis
Empty sella syndrome

B. INFLAMMATORY LESIONS

1. Abscess

Definition: Acute (bacterial) infectious non-neoplastic collection of purulent material.

Clinical

- No gender predilection; occurs over a wide age range.
- Clinical presentation: bifrontal headache associated with visual disturbances, often bitemporal hemianopsia or meningitis, and pituitary dysfunction.
- Diseases predisposing to (secondary) development of pituitary abscess formation include:
  - Sepsis via hematogenous dissemination and extension from a purulent infection of adjacent structures (sinusitis, cavernous sinus osteomyelitis), and cavernous sinus thrombophlebitis.
  - Abscess superimposed on an intrasellar mass: pituitary adenoma, cyst, craniopharyngioma.
- Tissue cultures: may be helpful in establishing the causative microorganism.
- Common microorganisms implicated in acute infection of the pituitary gland: *Staphylococcus* and pneumococcus, among others.
- Laboratory findings: decreased hormone secretion, producing hypopituitarism.

Radiology

- Enlarged or eroded sella.

Pathology

Gross
- Necrotic tissue.

Histology
- Necrotic material associated with acute inflammatory infiltrate.
- *Histochemistry:* Special stains assist in identifying the causative microorganisms; however, the microorganisms are not always identifiable in tissue sections.

Differential Diagnosis

- Intrasellar cysts (Chapter 1D).
- Pituitary adenoma (Chapter 2B).
- Craniopharyngioma (Chapter 2D).
- Mycotic pituitary abscess.

Treatment and Prognosis

- Surgical drainage.
- Administration of appropriate antibiotics.
- Meningitis is a complication.
- Overall mortality is estimated to be 28% without meningitis and 45% with meningitis.

2. Granulomatous Inflammation

a. Sarcoidosis

Definition: Chronic granulomatous disease of unknown etiology with multiorgan involvement.

Clinical

- Systemic disease with generalized or focal organ involvement.
- Slightly more common in women than in men; occurs most often between the ages of 20 and 40 years.
- In the United States the majority of patients with sarcoidosis are black in a ratio of 10:1 to 17:1 (black to white).
- Clinical presentation is almost always referable to the respiratory system owing to preponderant pulmonary involvement. Respiratory signs include dyspnea, cough, and lymphadenopathy with involvement of intrathoracic nodes. Constitutional symptoms such as fever, malaise, anorexia, and weight loss occur; cutaneous lesions may also be seen. Occasionally, patients may be asymptomatic.
- Central nervous system involvement occurs in less than 10% of patients; in these patients, the hypothalamic-pituitary axis (posterior pituitary) is most commonly involved, causing diabetes insipidus.
- Involvement of the anterior pituitary is uncommon. When it does occur it causes dysfunction manifested by deficiency of one or more hormones or hyperprolactinemia.
- Laboratory findings are nonspecific depending on the organ involved.
- Pituitary involvement causes a decrease in secretion of one or more hormones.
- The diagnosis is made by a combination of clinical, radiographic, and histologic examinations; skin anergy is typical but nondiagnostic.

Radiology

- The sella is enlarged uncommonly owing to the fact that the anterior pituitary is usually not involved.
- In those cases with pituitary enlargement, imaging findings are nonspecific and resemble a macroadenoma or lymphocytic hypophysitis (enhancing intrasellar mass with suprasellar extension).

Pathology

Histology

- Multiple noncaseating granulomas composed of epithelioid histiocytes.
- Mixed inflammatory cell infiltrates with occasional Langhans' type giant cells.
- Intracytoplasmic asteroid and Schaumann's bodies may be present.
- All special stains for microorganisms are negative.

Differential Diagnosis

- Mycobacterial infection (Chapter 1B, #2b).
- Fungal infection (Chapter 1B, #2b).
- Giant cell granuloma (Chapter 1B, #3).

Treatment and Prognosis

- Treatment of choice is glucocorticoids.
- Overall prognosis is good.
- Approximately 50% of patients have some permanent organ dysfunction; in approximately 10% of patients, the disease remains active and recurs intermittently.

Additional Facts

- Although histologic evidence is necessary for diagnosis, the findings are not specific for the disease, and a definite diagnosis is rendered only on the basis of the clinical history, radiographs, blood tests, and lack of identification of an infectious agent. In this regard, a diagnosis of sarcoidosis is one of exclusion.

b. Mycobacterial, Spirochetal, and Fungal Infection

Definition: Infectious diseases caused by *Mycobacterium tuberculosis, Treponema pallidum,* and fungi.

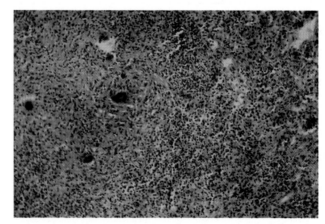

Figure 1–1. Tuberculosis. Epithelioid and multinucleated Langhans' type giant cells and inflammatory infiltrate involving the anterior pituitary gland.

Clinical

- Involvement of the anterior pituitary by these infectious agents is rare.
- Symptoms vary according to extent of involvement of the anterior pituitary gland, leading to hypopituitarism.
- Laboratory findings: decreased levels of one or more anterior pituitary hormones.
- Clinical work-up includes either radiographs, the tuberculin skin test, and microbiologic cultures, or serologic tests for evaluation of syphilis (nontreponemal or treponemal antibody tests).

Radiology

- Imaging findings are nonspecific; findings may resemble those of a macroadenoma or lymphocytic hypophysitis (enhancing intrasellar mass with suprasellar extension).

Pathology

Histology

- Noncaseating granulomas characterized by central necrosis surrounded by histiocytes and giant cells (tuberculosis).
- Inflammatory infiltrate with plasma cell predominance associated with scattered lymphocytes, histiocytes, and polymorphonuclear leukocytes (syphilis).
- Identification of microorganisms requires special stains. Acid-fast stains for tuberculosis may reveal beaded red or purple appearing microorganisms; tissue identification of acid-fast bacilli may be very difficult. The Warthin-Starry stain for syphilis reveals elongated, thin, rod-shaped structures.

Differential Diagnosis

- Other infectious agents.
- Giant cell granuloma (Chapter 1B, #3).

Treatment

- Antimicrobial therapy is the treatment of choice; it includes antituberculous agents, penicillin (for syphilis), and antimycotic agents.

3. Idiopathic

Giant Cell Granuloma

Definition: Idiopathic chronic inflammatory process of unknown etiology.

Clinical

- Localized disease causing destruction of the anterior hypophysis.
- Much more common in women than in men; occurs over a wide age range from 20 to 70 years.
- Symptoms vary from progressive hypopituitarism without visual disturbances to rare occurrences of hyperprolactinemia with amenorrhea and lactation as chief complaints.

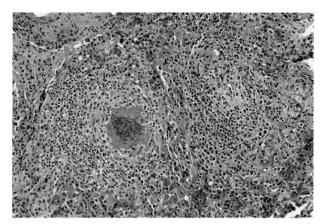

Figure 1–2. Giant cell granuloma. Noncaseating granulomatous inflammation with prominent multinucleated giant cells and lymphocytic infiltrate. No organisms were identified by special stains or culture.

- Occasionally, pituitary giant cell granuloma may be associated with similar granulomatous reactions in the thyroid, ovaries, and adrenal cortex.
- Destruction of the adenohypophysis with consequent hypopituitarism leads to atrophy of the thyroid and adrenal glands.
- Laboratory findings: decreased secretion of pituitary hormones or hyperprolactinemia.
- Etiology is obscure. An infectious or autoimmune cause is suggested; the latter is particularly likely in cases in which similar granulomatous reactions are present in other organ systems.

Radiology

- Enlargement of sella turcica.
- Computed tomographic (CT) scan and magnetic resonance imaging (MRI) may demonstrate a contrast-enhanced intrasellar mass with suprasellar extension; these radiographic features resemble those of a macroadenoma.

Pathology

Histology

- Noncaseating granulomas with multinucleated Langhans' giant cells and mild lymphocytic infiltration.
- Extensive fibrosis may occur with progression of disease.
- Microorganisms not identifiable by either special stains or culture (tuberculosis, fungi).

Differential Diagnosis

- Pituitary adenoma (Chapter 2B).
- Sarcoidosis (Chapter 1B, #2a).
- Mycobacterial infection (Chapter 1B, #2b).
- Fungal infection (Chapter 1B, #2B).

Treatment and Prognosis

- Surgery, using transsphenoidal approach.
- Histologic confirmation followed by long-term adequate hormone replacement.

Additional Facts

■ Giant cell granuloma is not associated with pregnancy.

4. Autoimmune

a. *Lymphocytic Hypophysitis*

Definition: Rare, destructive, inflammatory infiltration of the pituitary resulting in pituitary insufficiency, most often occurring in late pregnancy or the postpartum period.

Synonyms: Lymphocytic hypophysitis of pregnancy; pituitary insufficiency of pregnancy.

Clinical

■ Occurs predominantly in young females during late pregnancy or puerperium; occurs rarely in men.
■ Symptoms include headache and visual disturbances, amenorrhea, galactorrhea, and varying degrees of hypopituitarism.
■ May be associated with Hashimoto's thyroiditis, concomitant adrenalitis, and other endocrine organ dysfunctions.
■ Work-up includes radiographs, evaluation of pituitary hormones, and biopsy. The decrease in pituitary hormone secretion may vary from loss of one hormone to complete loss of pituitary endocrine function or hyperprolactinemia.
■ Laboratory findings: may also include detection of antipituitary antibodies, which are seen in up to 20% of patients.
■ Etiology is thought to have an autoimmune basis; this is supported by the association with other endocrine organ autoimmune disease and the presence of antipituitary antibodies.

Radiology

■ CT scan and MRI show pituitary enlargement and demonstrate a contrast-enhanced intrasellar mass with suprasellar extension.
■ Imaging findings simulate the appearance of a pituitary mass lesion (macroadenoma).

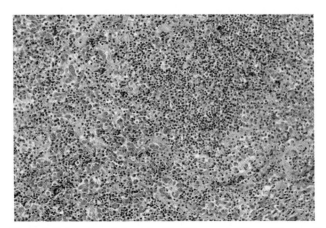

Figure 1–3. Lymphocytic hypophysitis. Effacement of the architecture of the pituitary gland by a lymphocytic infiltrate with residual endocrine cells. Granulomas and giant cells are not seen.

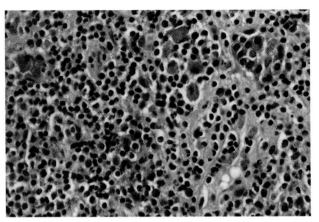

Figure 1–4. Lymphocytic hypophysitis. Higher magnification of Figure 1–3. Lymphocytic infiltrate with occasional plasma cells and scattered endocrine cells.

Pathology

Gross

■ Enlarged, yellow, firm gland.

Histology

■ Extensive cellular infiltrate composed of lymphocytes and plasma cells effaces the pituitary gland.
■ Lymphoid follicles with germinal centers may be evident.
■ Fibrosis, ranging from minimal to extensive, is present; complete replacement of the pituitary cells with only a few cells remaining may occur.
■ Well-formed granulomas are not present, although epithelioid histiocytes may be seen.

Differential Diagnosis

■ Granulomatous inflammation (Chapter 1B, #2).
■ Pituitary adenoma (Chapter 2B).
■ Nonspecific lymphocytic infiltrate in pituitary gland.

Treatment and Prognosis

■ Surgical decompression followed by supplemental hormone replacement is required.
■ If this diagnosis is suspected, a trial with steroids may be therapeutic.
■ The pituitary gland may regain normal size and endocrine function.

Additional Facts

■ In men, symptoms include headaches, impotence, and diminished libido with decreased serum testosterone levels.

C. CIRCULATORY DISTURBANCES

1. Hemorrhage and Pituitary Apoplexy

Definition: Pituitary apoplexy is a major hemorrhagic event that results from the rapid enlargement with hemorrhage and often with infarction, and complete destruction of a pituitary neoplasm (adenoma).

Clinical

- Acute hemorrhage is rare and is manifest by sudden development of neurologic symptoms due to rapid enlargement of a previously undiagnosed or diagnosed pituitary adenoma.
- Symptoms include sudden severe headache, nausea, vomiting, alterations in consciousness, meningism, visual disturbances, and ophthalmoplegia.
- Factors that may precipitate hemorrhage and are of etiologic importance include head trauma, anticoagulation, thrombosis, and therapy with bromocriptine or radiation.
- Pituitary apoplexy occurs mainly in patients with large nonfunctioning adenomas; approximately 10% of patients with adenomas present clinically with apoplexy.
- Patients may be previously asymptomatic or have a preexisting endocrinopathy; the latter may be ameliorated or improved after hemorrhagic infarction.

Pathology

Gross

- Specimen consists of necrotic tumor or blood.

Histology

- Necrotic tissue may obscure the presence of a neoplasm.
- The pattern obtained with a reticulin stain can help in identifying an adenoma.
- All immunophenotypes can be seen.

Treatment and Prognosis

- Pituitary apoplexy is considered a neurologic emergency that requires immediate surgical intervention.
- Sudden death can occur.

2. Infarction

- Infarction of the pituitary gland occurs with diabetes mellitus, sickle cell disease, increased intracranial pressure of any cause, cerebrovascular accidents, and transection of the pituitary stalk.
- Inadequate perfusion of the pituitary gland leads to ischemia with subsequent necrosis.
- Clinical pituitary insufficiency is not evident in patients who recover from small infarcts.
- Hypopituitarism develops after massive destruction of the anterior pituitary gland.

3. Necrosis (Sheehan's Syndrome)

Definition: Pituitary infarction associated with postpartum uterine hemorrhage resulting in permanent hypopituitarism.

Clinical

- Vasospasm in response to shock leading to pituitary ischemia and thrombosis has been postulated as a possible cause.
- The posterior lobe is usually spared because it does not depend on the portal system for its blood supply.

- The necrotic tissue is replaced by fibrosis, and atrophy of the anterior pituitary gland occurs, resulting in marked pituitary insufficiency.

D. CYSTS

1. Dermoid Cysts

Definition: Rare, slow-growing cystic lesions in the sellar region (suprasellar or intrasellar) resulting from inclusion of epithelial elements during closure of the neural tube.

Clinical

- Uncommon.
- No gender predilection; usually occur in childhood.
- Presentation: either asymptomatic or headache and visual disturbances.
- Typical site of occurrence: posterior cranial fossa. Usually occur in the midline in relation to the fontanelle or the fourth ventricle.

Radiology

- CT scan shows a low-density mass.
- MRI shows a heterogeneous signal intensity owing to the presence of sebaceous material and hair in association with the cyst, including a high signal intensity in T1-weighted images as a result of the increased lipid content.

Pathology

Gross

- Encapsulated, well-delineated mass with a thick wall and a yellowish, greasy content with or without matted hair; occasionally, calcifications may be present.

Histology

- Cyst is lined by stratified squamous epithelium that may include cutaneous adnexal structures (sebaceous glands or hair follicles) surrounded by a connective tissue capsule.
- Cyst content consists of desquamated epithelium and sebaceous secretion.
- A foreign body giant cell reaction (secondary to the cyst content) in the cyst wall can be seen; mature bone may be present.
- *Immunohistochemistry:* reactivity with epithelial markers (cytokeratin, epithelial membrane antigen) is present; adnexal structures demonstrate similar immunoreactivity to their cutaneous counterparts including a positive reaction to carcinoembryonic antigen (CEA).

Differential Diagnosis

- Epidermoid cysts (Chapter 1D, #2).
- Craniopharyngioma (Chapter 2D).

Treatment and Prognosis

- Surgical removal is the treatment of choice.
- Leakage of cyst content may result in chemical meningitis.

■ Incomplete resection results in recurrence; recurrence leads to an increased risk of infection.
■ Rare cases of malignant transformation of the cystic epithelium to squamous cell carcinoma have occurred.

2. Epidermoid Cysts

Synonyms: Pearly tumor, cholesteatoma.

Clinical

■ More common than dermoid cysts.
■ Equal gender predilection; peak incidence occurs in the fifth decade of life.
■ Presentation: either asymptomatic or with headache and visual disturbances.
■ Typical sites of occurrence: suprasellar and parasellar locations; most frequently seen in the cerebellopontine angle.
■ Presumed to be of developmental origin; rare examples have occurred iatrogenically with intracranial or intraspinal "implantation" of cutaneous epithelium secondary to lumbar puncture.

Radiology

■ CT scan shows a low-density mass.
■ MRI shows a variable signal intensity that depends on the cyst content:
  • High lipid content: bright (white) signal intensity on T1-weighted images.
  • Low lipid content: dark (black) signal intensity on T1-weighted images.

Pathology

Gross

■ Appears as either a unilocular cyst surrounded by a thin, smooth capsule or as a cystic structure with an irregular nodular surface and a glistening, whitish, flaky content; the latter is the origin of the term pearly tumor.
■ Can become larger than a dermoid cyst.

Histology

■ A capsule is present that varies in thickness but is generally thin.
■ The cyst lining is composed of stratified squamous epithelium, but, in contrast to the dermoid cyst, skin adnexal structures are not present.
■ The cyst content consists of desquamated epithelium, cholesterol crystals, and cellular debris.

Differential Diagnosis

■ Dermoid cyst (Chapter 1D, #1).
■ Craniopharyngioma (Chapter 2D).

Treatment and Prognosis

■ Surgical excision is the treatment of choice.
■ Leakage of cyst content may result in chemical meningitis.

■ Incomplete resection results in recurrence; recurrence leads to an increased risk of infection.
■ Rare examples of malignant transformation of the cystic epithelium to a squamous cell carcinoma have occurred.

3. Rathke's Pouch Cyst

Definition: Non-neoplastic intrasellar or suprasellar cystic mass derived from the remnants of Rathke's pouch lying between the developing anterior and intermediate lobes of the pituitary gland.

Clinical

■ Incidence at autopsy findings varies from 13% to 23%.
■ No gender predilection; occurs over a wide age range but is most common in adults.
■ Symptoms vary according to size and location:
  • Usually these lesions are asymptomatic and represent incidental findings seen on radiologic examination or at autopsy.
  • When these lesions are large enough (usually >1 cm), they may compress the optic chiasm, resulting in disturbances of the visual fields or hypothalamic-pituitary function.

Radiology

■ Sellar enlargement and erosion are seen on plain skull radiographs.
■ CT scans show an intrasellar cystic mass with or without suprasellar extension that does not enhance with contrast media.
■ MRI shows a well-circumscribed intrasellar or suprasellar mass; extrasellar extension can occur. Signal intensity may vary depending on the nature of the cyst lining or the cyst content:
  • Cysts lined by simple epithelium with clear fluid have the signal intensity of cerebrospinal fluid (CSF).
  • Cysts filled with mucus have a heterogeneous signal; those with high protein content appear hyperintense (white) on nonenhanced T1-weighted images.

Pathology

Gross

■ The cystic structure is generally small and thin walled and has a variable cyst content; usually measures from 0.5 to 1 cm in diameter.
■ An epithelial lining may be difficult to appreciate macroscopically; in some cases the cysts are almost entirely composed of mucin.

Histology

■ Characteristically, there is an epithelial lining that consists of a single layer of ciliated cuboidal or columnar epithelium with mucus secretory cells; squamous metaplasia can be seen and may predominate in any lesion, obscuring or completely replacing the ciliated cuboidal or columnar epithelium.

- Endocrine (pituitary) cells may be present in limited numbers.
- The cyst content usually includes thick mucus.
- *Immunohistochemistry:* The cyst lining is cytokeratin and epithelial membrane antigen positive; if endocrine (pituitary) cells are present, they will react with neuroendocrine markers (chromogranin, synaptophysin) and pituitary peptide hormone markers.

Differential Diagnosis

- Suprasellar craniopharyngiomas (Chapter 2D).
- Arachnoid cysts:
  - In contrast to Rathke's pouch cysts, the lining meningothelial cells of an arachnoid cyst are S-100 positive.
- Mucoceles originating in the paranasal sinuses:
  - Mucoceles are indistinguishable from Rathke's pouch cysts by histopathologic evaluation alone; the differentiation is predicated on radiographic observation of cystic extension from the paranasal sinuses into the intracranial cavity.

Treatment and Prognosis

- Surgical excision is the treatment of choice.
- These are benign lesions that are usually cured by surgical excision.

E. HYPERPLASIA

Definition: Nodular or diffuse, focal or multifocal abnormal increase in the number of cells; in general, only a single cell type predominates in pituitary hyperplasia.

Clinical

- Rare.
- No gender predilection; may occur over a wide age range.
- May be a primary disorder or may occur secondary to ectopic hormone-related substances produced by extrapituitary neoplasms or by loss of negative feedback to the pituitary gland in patients with various chronic hypofunctioning endocrine conditions:
  - Prolactin cell (PRL) hyperplasia may occur in women during pregnancy and lactation or in those taking estrogen, in patients with hypothyroidism, or in the pituitary adjacent to PRL cell adenomas.
  - Growth hormone (GH) cell hyperplasia is associated with ectopic production of growth hormone–releasing substances by extrapituitary (neuroendocrine) tumors.
  - Adrenocorticotrophic hormone (ACTH) cell hyperplasia is seen in patients with untreated Addison's disease and in those with ectopic production of ACTH-releasing substances by extrapituitary (neuroendocrine) tumors.
  - Thyrotrophic cell hyperplasia (due to thyroid-stimulating hormone [TSH]) can occur in patients with long-standing hypothyroidism.
  - Gonadotrophic cell hyperplasia may occur in patients with prolonged hypogonadism (Klinefelter's or

Turner's syndrome); in postmenopausal women the pituitary tends to be small without gonadotrophic cell hyperplasia despite the decreased production of follicle-stimulating hormone (FSH) or luteinizing hormone (LH) and increased secretion of FSH and LH by the pituitary gonadotrophic cells.

Pathology

Histology

- May be very difficult to diagnose in small biopsy specimens.
- The hyperplastic process may be a monofocal or multifocal nodular or diffuse proliferation of pituitary cells.
- In the nodular form the diagnosis is assisted by reticulin stains and immunohistochemistry:
  - Reticulin stain: acinar expansion with retention of the acinar configuration of the gland.
  - *Immunohistochemistry:* monohormonal pituitary peptide reactivity; less often, plurihormonal pituitary peptide reactivity is seen.
- The diffuse form of pituitary hyperplasia is difficult to diagnose and differentiate from a pituitary adenoma; differentiation may be assisted by reticulin stain, as follows:
  - Pituitary adenoma: evident by disruption of the reticulin pattern in which portions of the tumor appear devoid of reticulin fibers.
  - Hyperplasia: appears similar to the normal pituitary with retention of the delicate reticulin fibers throughout the cellular proliferation.

Differential Diagnosis

- Microadenoma (Chapter 2B).
- Adenoma (Chapter 2B).

Treatment and Prognosis

- Surgical resection can be performed in cases in which an intrasellar mass lesion is found.
- In cases of secondary pituitary hyperplasia, medical treatment of the underlying endocrine disorder (e.g., hypothyroidism or Addison's disease) or surgical removal of an extrapituitary (neuroendocrine) tumor is indicated.

Additional Facts

- Diagnosis can be made in autopsy cases if an intact pituitary gland is removed.
- Histologic diagnosis is difficult or impossible on small biopsy specimens because of insufficient material.

F. LANGERHANS CELL HISTIOCYTOSIS (LCH)

Definition: Rare systemic disease characterized by the proliferation of Langerhans cell.

Synonyms: Eosinophilic granuloma; histiocytosis X; Hand-Schüller-Christian disease; Letterer-Siwe disease; Langerhans cell granulomatosis.

Clinical

■ Involvement of the central nervous system is seen in up to 25% of cases; almost all such cases appear exclusively as intraosseous lesions.
■ Pituitary involvement by LCH is rare and occurs primarily as part of a systemic disease or by extension from one or more osseous foci; less often, unifocal or multifocal infiltrates occur in the hypothalamus or infundibulum.
■ There is no gender predilection; the disease occurs primarily in children and young adults.
■ LCH involves primarily the posterior lobe, the pituitary stalk, and the hypothalamus; the anterior lobe is usually not involved.
■ Clinical manifestations include diabetes insipidus and hypothalamic dysfunction.

Radiology

■ Findings on radiographs are nonspecific and resemble those of a macroadenoma or lymphocytic hypophysitis; they appear as an enhancing intrasellar mass with suprasellar extension. MRI may allow visualization of small lesions.

Pathology

Histology

■ Langerhans cells are characterized by the presence of enlarged cells containing vesicular nuclei with an indented, notched, grooved, vesicular, or "coffee-bean" shaped appearance, one or two nucleoli, and pale to eosinophilic finely vacuolated cytoplasm; intracytoplasmic phagocytosed cellular debris may be found.
■ Langerhans cells may grow in a diffuse pattern or may cluster to form granuloma-like foci.
■ A variable number of eosinophils, lymphocytes, plasma cells, and giant cells can be seen intermingled with the Langerhans cells.
■ Microglial cells and astrocytic reactions may be present.
■ Angiotropism is seen.
■ *Immunohistochemistry:* Langerhans cells react positively with S-100 protein, lysozyme, KP-1, and CD1a.
■ *Electron microscopy:* Intracytoplasmic rod-shaped granules (Birbeck's granules) are identified.

Differential Diagnosis

■ Infectious diseases (Chapter 1B, #2B).
■ Giant cell granuloma (Chapter 1B, #3).
■ Lymphoma (Chapter 2C, #2).

Treatment and Prognosis

■ Low-dose radiotherapy is used for solitary and multifocal LCH.
■ Systemic disease is treated by combination chemotherapy.

■ The prognosis for patients with limited disease is favorable, but systemic involvement generally, though not invariably, has a poor prognosis.

G. MISCELLANEOUS— CALCIFICATION AND ABNORMAL DEPOSITS

1. Amyloidosis and Hemochromatosis

■ Pituitary adenomas rarely show evidence of calcification on radiographs.
■ Prolactinomas show microscopic calcospherites.
■ Craniopharyngiomas produce evidence of calcification radiographically, strongly suggesting its diagnosis.
■ Amyloidosis can occur in prolactinomas.
■ Hemochromatosis appears in patients suffering from iron overload and may involve the adenohypophysis, in which abnormal amounts of hemosiderin pigment are found in all cell types; gonadotrophic cells are affected most frequently.

2. Empty Sella Syndrome

Definition: Reduction in the volume of sellar content due to the extension of the subarachnoid space into the sella turcica.

Clinical

■ The empty sella syndrome may be primary or secondary.
■ **Primary form**
  • Due to an incomplete or incompetent sellar diaphragm, the arachnoid membrane herniates downward (intrasel-

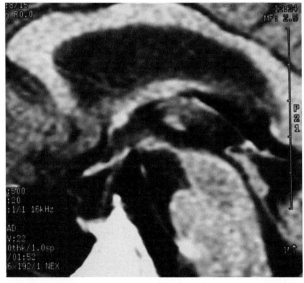

Figure 1–5. Empty sella syndrome. Sagittal T1-weighted MRI image demonstrates the sella being filled predominantly with cerebrospinal fluid. Note that the infundibular stalk follows a normal course and inserts in the midline of the flattened pituitary gland within the base of the sella.

lar arachnoidocele), causing chronic compression of the pituitary gland.
- Autopsy series have shown that nearly 50% of adults with the empty sella syndrome have a diaphragmatic defect (defined as a defect measuring 5 mm or more), but the incidence of primary empty sella syndrome is only 5%.
- Tends to occur in middle-aged women.
■ **Secondary form**
- The secondary form of empty sella syndrome is due to a variety of causes that allow herniation of the arachnoid membrane, including:
  - Surgical excision of sellar tumors.
  - Irradiation of the pituitary gland for sellar tumors.
  - Spontaneous infarction of the pituitary gland as in postpartum pituitary necrosis (Sheehan's syndrome).
  - Hemorrhagic infarction of an adenoma (pituitary apoplexy).
- This syndrome is most commonly seen in middle-aged obese women who are hypertensive.
■ Regardless of the cause, the empty sella syndrome may be characterized by:
- Headache of long-standing duration (the most common complaint); other complaints may include visual field defects or impaired pituitary function.
- Rhinorrhea of the CSF into the sphenoid sinuses through an eroded sellar floor due to increased intracranial pressure, which is considered the main etiologic factor. This is a striking clinical finding.
- Some degree of hypopituitarism in 30% of patients, although no clinical endocrine related symptoms are present.
- This syndrome is found incidentally on radiographic studies of the skull during investigation of complaints of headache.

Radiology

■ CT scans show an intrasellar low-density area consistent with empty sella syndrome.

Pathology

Histology

■ The surgical material may consist only of arachnoid membrane.
■ An adenoma may be present when this syndrome is associated with a pituitary adenoma.
■ *Immunohistochemistry:* All pituitary cell types can be identified.

Differential Diagnosis

■ Pituitary tumor (Chapter 2).

Treatment and Prognosis

■ Uncomplicated empty sella syndrome requires no treatment.

■ Spontaneous leakage of CSF is usually an indication for surgical management.

Bibliography

Abscess

Enzmann DR. Focal parenchymal infection. In: Enzmann DR, ed. Imaging of Infections and Inflammations of the Central Nervous System: Computed Tomography, Ultrasound, and Nuclear Magnetic Resonance. New York: Raven Press, 1984, pp. 53–54.

Lindholm J, Rasmussen P, Korsgaard O. Intrasellar or pituitary abscess. J Neurosurg 1973; 38:616–619.

Lloyd RV. Non-neoplastic pituitary lesions, including hyperplasia. In: Surgical Pathology of the Pituitary Gland: Major Problems in Pathology, Vol. 27. Philadelphia: W. B. Saunders, 1993, p. 28.

Tindall GT, Barrow L. Pituitary deficiency states. In: Disorders of the Pituitary. St. Louis: C. V. Mosby, 1986, p. 455.

Granulomas

Giampalmo A, Buffa D, Quaglia AC. AIDS pathology: Various critical considerations (especially regarding the brain, the heart, the lungs, the hypophysis and the adrenal glands). Pathologica (Italy) 1990; 82:663–677.

Lara Capellan JI, Cuellar Olmedo L, Martinez Martin J, et al. Intrasellar mass with hypopituitarism as a manifestation of sarcoidosis: Case report. J Neurosurg 1990; 73:283–286.

Missler U, Mack M, Nowack G, et al. Pituitary sarcoidosis. Klin Wochenschr 1990; 68:342–345.

Mosca L, Costanzy G, Antonacci C, et al. Hypophyseal pathology in AIDS. Histol Histopathol 1992; 7:291–300.

Tindall GT, Barrow L. Pituitary deficiency states. In: Tindall GT, Barrow L, eds. Disorders of the Pituitary. St. Louis: C. V. Mosby, 1986, pp. 455–456.

Winnacker JL, Becker KL, Katz S. Endocrine aspects of sarcoidosis. N Engl J Med 1968; 278:483–492.

Lymphocytic Hypophysitis

Abe T, Matsumoto K, Sanno N, Osamura Y. Lymphocytic hypophysitis: Case report. Neurosurgery 1995; 36:1016–1019.

Ahmadi J, Scott Meyers G, Segall HD, et al. Lymphocytic hypophysitis: Contrast-enhanced MR imaging in five cases. Radiology 1995; 195: 30–34.

Asa SL, Bilbao JM, Kovacs K, et al. Lymphocytic hypophysitis of pregnancy resulting in hypopituitarism: A distinct clinicopathologic entity. Ann Intern Med 1981; 95:166–171.

Beressi N, Cohen R, Beressi JP, et al. Pseudotumoral lymphocytic hypophysitis successfully treated by corticosteroid alone: First case report. Neurosurgery 1994; 35:505–508.

Bilton RN, Slavin M, Decker RE, et al. The course of lymphocytic hypophysitis (Comment). Surg Neurol 1992; 37:71 (source: Surg Neurol 1991; 36:40–43).

Case records of the Massachusetts General Hospital: Case 25-1995. N Engl J Med 1995; 333:441–447.

Lee JH, Laws ER Jr, Guthrie BL, et al. Lymphocytic hypophysitis: Occurrence in two men. Neurosurgery 1994; 34:159–163.

Nishioka H, Ito H, Miki T, Akada K. A case of lymphocytic hypophysitis with massive fibrosis and the role of surgical intervention. Surg Neurol 1994; 42:74–78.

Ozawa Y, Shishiba Y. Recovery from lymphocytic hypophysitis associated with painless thyroiditis: Clinical implications of circulatory antipituitary antibodies. Acta Endocrinol (Copenh) 1993; 128:493–498.

Paja M, Estrada J, Ojeda A, et al. Lymphocytic hypophysitis causing hypopituitarism and diabetes insipidus, and associated with autoimmune thyroiditis, in a non-pregnant woman. Postgrad Med J 1994; 70:220–224.

Pestell RG, Best JD, Alford FP. Lymphocytic hypophysitis: The clinical spectrum of the disorder and evidence for an autoimmune pathogenesis. Clin Endocrinol (Oxf) 1990; 33:457–466. Comment in: Clin Endocrinol (Oxf) 1991; 34:429–430.

Riedl M, Czech T, Slootweg J, et al. Lymphocytic hypophysitis presenting as a pituitary tumor in a 63-year-old man. Endocr Pathol 1995; 6: 159–166.

Circulatory Disturbances

Berthelot JL, Rey A. Apoplexie hypophysaire. Presse Med (Paris) 1995; 24:501–503.

Kovacs K. Necrosis of anterior pituitary in humans. Neuroendocrinology 1969; 4:170–199.

Lloyd RV. Non-neoplastic lesions, including hyperplasia. In: Surgical Pathology of the Pituitary Gland: Major Problems in Pathology, Vol. 27. Philadelphia: W. B. Saunders, 1993, pp. 26–28.

Masago A, Ueda Y, Kanai H, Nagai H, Umemura S. Pituitary apoplexy after pituitary function test: A report of two cases and review of the literature. Surg Neurol 1995; 43:158–165.

Plaut A. Pituitary necrosis in routine necropsies. Am J Pathol 1952; 25: 883–900.

Prager D, Braunstein GD. Pituitary disorders during pregnancy. Endocrinol Metab Clin North Am 1995; 24:1–14.

Sheehan HL, Davis JC. Pituitary necrosis. Br Med Bull 1968; 24:59–70.

Cysts

Barkovich AJ, Edwards MS, Cogan PH. MR evaluation of spinal dermal sinus tracts in children. AJNR 1991; 12:123–129.

Boggan JE, Davis RL, Zorman G, Wilson CB. Intrasellar epidermoid cyst: Case report. J Neurosurg 1983; 58:411–415.

Boyd HR. Iatrogenic intraspinal epidermoid: Report of a case. J Neurosurg 1966; 24:105–107.

Elster AD. Imaging of the sella: Anatomy and pathology. Semin Ultrasound CTMR 1993; 14:182–194.

Gluszcz A. A cancer arising in a dermoid cyst of the brain: A case report. J Neuropathol Exp Neurol 1962; 21:383–387.

Goldman SA, Gandy SE. Squamous cell carcinoma as a late complication of intracerebroventricular epidermoid cyst. J Neurosurg 1987; 66: 618–620.

Gutin PH, Boehm J, Bank WO, et al. Cerebral convexity epidermoid cyst subsequent to multiple percutaneous subdural aspiration. J Neurosurg 1980; 52:574–577.

Harrison MJ, Morgello S, Post KD. Epithelial cystic lesions of the sellar and parasellar region: A continuum of ectodermal derivatives? J Neurosurg 1994; 80:1018–1025.

Horowitz BL, Chari MV, James R, Bryan RN. MR of intracranial epidermoid tumors: Correlation of in vivo imaging with in vitro ^{13}C spectroscopy. AJNR 1990; 11:299–302.

Ikeda H, Yoshimoto T, Suzuki J. Immunohistochemical study of Rathke's cleft cyst. Acta Neuropathol (Berl) 1988; 77:33–38.

Ito H, Nishizaki T, Kajiwara K, Kin S. Pituitary nonadenomatous tumor (Rathke's cleft cyst). Nippon Rinsho (Jpn) 1993; 51:2711–2715.

Kucharczyk W, Peck WW, Kelly WM, et al. Rathke cleft cyst: CT, MR imaging, and pathologic features. Radiology 1987; 165:491–495.

Lewis AJ, Cooper PW, Kassel EE, Schwartz ML. Squamous cell carcinoma arising in a suprasellar epidermoid cyst: Case report. J Neurosurg 1983; 59:538–541.

Lunardi P, Missori P, Gagliardi FM, Firtuna A. Dermoid cysts of the posterior cranial fossa in children: Report of nine cases and review of the literature. Surg Neurol 1990; 34:39–42.

Miyagami M, Tsubokawa T. Histological and ultrastructural findings of benign intracranial cysts. Noshuyo Byori (Jpn) 1993; 10:151–160.

Ross DA, Norman D, Wilson CB. Radiologic characteristics and results of surgical management of Rathke's cysts in 43 patients. Neurosurgery 1992; 30:173–179.

Smith AS, Benson JE, Blaser SI, et al. Diagnosis of ruptured intracranial dermoid cyst: Value of MR over CT. AJNR 1991; 12:175–180.

Teramoto A, Hirakawa K, Sanno N, Osamura Y. Incidental pituitary lesions in 1,000 unselected autopsy specimens. Radiology 1994; 193:161–164.

Voelker JL, Campbell RL, Muller J. Clinical, radiographic, and pathological features of symptomatic Rathke's cleft cysts. J Neurosurg 1991; 74: 535–544.

Hyperplasia

Jay V, Kovacs K, Horvath E, et al. Idiopathic prolactin cell hyperplasia of the pituitary mimicking prolactin cell adenoma: A morphological study including immunocytochemistry, electron microscopy, and in situ hybridization. Acta Neuropathol (Berl) 1991; 82:147–151.

Kovacs K, Horvath E. Hyperplasia. In: Tumors of the Pituitary Gland. Atlas of Tumor Pathology, Fascicle 21, Second Series. Washington DC: Armed Forces Institute of Pathology, 1986, pp. 210–216.

Moran A, Asa SL, Kovacs K, et al. Gigantism due to pituitary mammosomatotroph hyperplasia. N Engl J Med 1990; 323:322–327.

Peillon F, Dupuy M, Li JY. Pituitary enlargement with suprasellar extension in functional hyperprolactinemia due to lactotroph hyperplasia: A pseudotumoral disease. J Clin Endocrinol Metab 1991; 73:1008–1015.

Scheithauer BW, Sano T, Kovacs K, et al. The pituitary gland in pregnancy: A clinicopathologic and immunohistochemical study of 69 cases. Mayo Clin Proc 1990; 65:461–474.

Takahashi Y, Negaki M, Shigemori M, et al. A case of pituitary adenoma and hyperplasia with primary hypothyroidism. No Shinkei Geka (Jpn) 1991; 19:741–745.

Langerhans Cell Histiocytosis

Kepes JJ, Kepes M. Predominantly cerebral forms of histiocytosis X: A reappraisal of (Gagel's hypothalamic granuloma), "granuloma infiltrans of the hypothalamus" and "Ayala's disease" with a report of four cases. Acta Neuropathol (Berl) 1969; 14:77–98.

Lieberman PH, Jones CR, Steinman RM, et al. Langerhans cell (eosinophilic) granulomatosis: A clinicopathologic study encompassing 50 years. Am J Surg Pathol 1996; 20:519–552.

Maghnie M, Arico M, Villa A, et al. MR of the hypothalamic-pituitary axis in Langerhans cell histiocytosis. AJNR 1992; 13:1365–1371.

Smolik EA, Devecerski M, Nelson JS, Smith KR Jr. Histiocytosis of the optic chiasm of an adult with hypopituitarism: Case report. J Neurosurg 1968; 29:290–295.

Tien RD, Newton TH, McDermott MW, et al. Thickened pituitary stalk on MR images in patient with diabetes insipidus and Langerhans cell histiocytosis. AJNR 1990; 11:703–708.

Deposits

Bononi PL, Martinez AJ, Nelson PB, Amico JA. Amyloid deposits in a prolactin-producing pituitary adenoma. J Endocrinol Invest 1993; 16: 339–443.

Hume Adams J, Duchen LW. Abnormal depositions in the pituitary gland. In: Greenfield's Neuropathology, 5th ed. New York: Oxford University Press, 1992, p. 1023.

Landolt AM, Kleihues P, Heitz PU. Amyloid deposits in pituitary adenomas: Differentiation of two types. Arch Pathol Lab Med 1987; 111: 453–458.

Lloyd RV. Non-neoplastic pituitary lesions, including hyperplasia. In: Surgical Pathology of the Pituitary Gland: Major Problems in Pathology, Vol 27. Philadelphia: W. B. Saunders, 1993, pp. 29–30.

Oerter KE, Kamp GA, Munson PJ, et al. Multiple hormone deficiencies in children with hemochromatosis. J Clin Endocrinol Metab 1993; 76: 357–361.

Smith LH Jr. Overview of hemochromatosis. West J Med 1990; 153: 296–308.

Empty Sella Syndrome

Asai JI, Fujimoto T, Fukushima Y. Empty sella as an intrasellar herniation of the third ventricle secondary to spontaneous degeneration of a prolactinoma. No Shinkei Geka (Jpn) 1994; 22:241–246.

Bakiri F, Bendib SE, Maoui R, et al. The sella turcica in Sheehan's syndrome: Computerized tomography study in 54 patients. J Endocrinol Invest 1991; 14:193–196.

Bergeron C, Kovacs K, Bilbao JM. Primary "empty sella": A histologic and immunologic study. Arch Intern Med 1979; 139:248–249.

Bergland RM, Ray BS, Torack RM. Anatomical variations in the pituitary gland and adjacent structures in 225 human autopsy cases. J Neurosurg 1968; 28:93–99.

Cacciari E, Zucchini S, Ambrosetto P, et al. Empty sella in children and adolescents with possible hypothalamic-pituitary disorders. J Clin Endocrinol Metab 1994; 78:767–771.

Gharib H, Frey HM, Laws ER Jr, et al. Co-existent primary empty sella syndrome and hyperprolactinemia: Report of 11 cases. Arch Intern Med 1983; 143:1383–1386.

Tindall GT, Barrow DL. The "empty sella" syndrome. In: Disorders of the Pituitary. St. Louis: C.V. Mosby, 1986, pp. 473–481.

CHAPTER 2

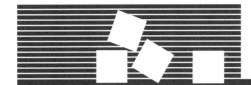

Neoplasms of the Pituitary Gland

A. CLASSIFICATION OF NEOPLASMS OF THE PITUITARY GLAND

Table 2–1
NEOPLASMS OF THE PITUITARY GLAND

A. Benign Neoplasms

1. Prolactin cell adenomas
2. Growth hormone–producing adenomas
   a. Densely granulated growth hormone cell adenoma
   b. Sparsely granulated growth hormone cell adenoma
   c. Mixed growth hormone cell and prolactin cell adenoma
   d. Mammosomatotrophic cell adenoma
   e. Acidophilic stem cell adenomas
3. Corticotrophic cell–producing adenomas
   a. Functioning corticotrophic cell adenomas, densely granulated
   b. Functioning corticotrophic cell adenoma, sparsely granulated
   c. Silent corticotrophic cell adenomas
   d. Nelson's syndrome
4. Glycoprotein hormone–producing adenomas
   a. Thyrotrophic cell adenoma
   b. Gonadotrophic cell adenoma
5. Adenomas with no hormone production
6. Plurihormonal adenoma
7. Ectopic pituitary adenomas
8. Invasive pituitary adenomas

B. Malignant Neoplasms

1. Pituitary carcinoma
2. Metastatic neoplasms to the pituitary gland

C. Neoplasms of the Sellar Region

   Craniopharyngioma

B. BENIGN NEOPLASMS

1. General Considerations

- Pituitary tumors represent 10% to 20% of all intracranial tumors.
- Pituitary neoplasms can be divided into three categories:
  - Benign and malignant.
  - Primary and secondary.
  - Epithelial and nonepithelial.

- The majority of pituitary tumors are adenomas and originate from the hormone-producing cells of the pituitary; pituitary adenomas include hormone-producing adenomas and inactive (nonhormone-producing) adenomas.
- Pituitary adenomas are classified according to the following features:
  - Size: microadenomas (measuring <1 cm in diameter) or macroadenomas (measuring >1 cm).
  - Function or immunophenotype: adenomas may be prolactin cell, somatotrophic (growth hormone-producing), corticotrophic cell (ACTH-producing), or thyrotrophic cell or gonadotrophic cell (glycoprotein hormone-producing); or they may have no hormone production or may be subclinical (null cell adenomas).
  - Cell type: chromophobic, basophilic, or acidophilic.
  - Quantity of hormone found functionally or immunophenotypically: monohormonal or plurihormonal.
  - Secretory granule content: sparsely granulated or densely granulated.
  - Location: within the pituitary gland proper or in ectopic (non-pituitary gland) sites.
  - Biologic behavior: benign (pituitary adenoma) or invasive and malignant (pituitary carcinoma).
  - Radiologic appearance (see later in this section).
- The majority of subclinical adenomas are null cell adenomas or prolactinomas; subclinical adenomas generally show no correlation between the clinical presentation and the tumor immunophenotype.
- A higher percentage of subclinical or small pituitary adenomas are now being diagnosed owing to the advent of more sophisticated radiographic imaging and better clinical laboratory (radioimmunoassay) testing.
- In general, adenomas are more common in women than in men, but this may depend on the cell type (prolactinomas and corticotrophic adenomas are more common in women, whereas growth hormone-secreting tumors are more common in men).
- Adenomas occur in all age ranges but are most common in the third to sixth decades of life. Fewer than 10% occur in children, but this too may depend on cell type because growth hormone-secreting tumors are often seen in children, whereas other cell types are more common in adults.

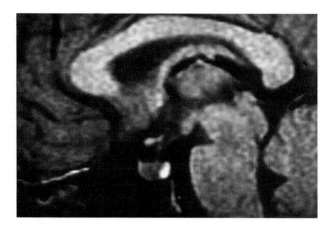

Figure 2–1. Normal sella. T1-weighted parasagittal MR demonstrates a normal pituitary and a pituitary stalk. The pituitary is centered in the base of the pituitary fossa.

Figure 2–2. Cross section of a normal pituitary gland.

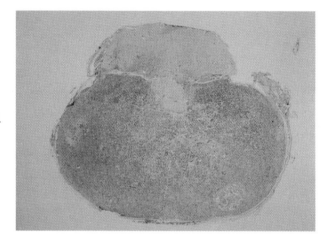

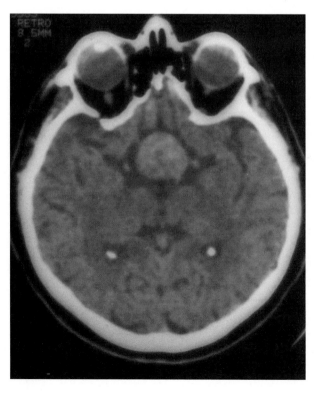

Figure 2–3. Pituitary adenoma. Axial contrast-enhanced CT scan (CECT) demonstrates a slightly hyperdense enhancing mass within the suprasellar cistern. There is a clear border of cerebrospinal fluid (CSF) between the tumor and the adjacent brain.

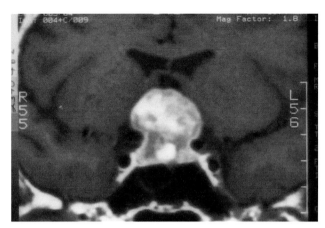

Figure 2–4. Pituitary adenoma. Coronal T1-weighted image post-contrast shows the mass enhancing intensely but somewhat heterogeneously. Note the clear border between the tumor and the adjacent brain.

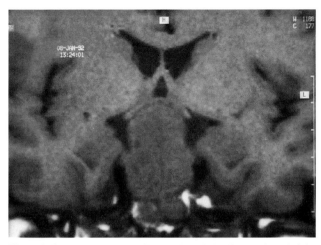

Figure 2–6. Pituitary adenoma. Coronal T1-weighted image after administration of gadolinium-diethylenetriamine pentaacetic acid (Gd-DTPA) demonstrates a heterogeneous but intense enhancement of the mass.

■ The clinical presentation associated with pituitary tumors varies and includes endocrinopathic manifestations that vary according to tumor cell type, headaches, and visual field disturbances resulting from compression of the optic chiasm.

■ Pituitary tumors in children may be more aggressive than those in adults.

■ Radiologic findings vary depending on the size of the tumor.

1. **Computed tomographic (CT) scan:**

   • Coronal sections are better than axial ones, but both may be necessary.

   • Microadenomas enhance less rapidly than the surrounding normal pituitary tissue and appear as hypodense areas on contrast-enhanced CT scans.

   • Unenhanced macroadenomas appear as isodense areas.

   • Enhanced macroadenomas have a modest uniform enhancement.

   • Hemorrhagic adenomas have an inhomogeneous hyperdense appearance.

2. **Magnetic resonance imaging (MRI):**

   • Pituitary lesions are better imaged by MRI than by CT scans because of the increased number of artifacts caused by the surrounding bone structures of the area.

   • Microadenomas enhance less rapidly than the surrounding normal pituitary tissue, appearing as hypointense areas on contrast-enhanced MRI images.

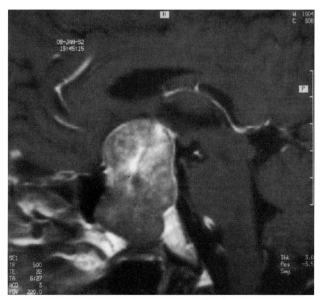

Figure 2–5. Pituitary adenoma. Coronal T1-weighted image demonstrates a mass arising from the sella and extending into the suprasellar cistern. There is an upward deviation of the optic chiasm and an impression on the third ventricle. There is no obvious invasion into the cavernous sinus.

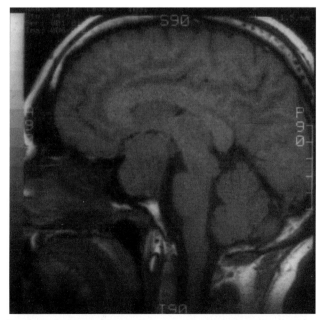

Figure 2–7. Pituitary adenoma. Coronal T1-weighted image demonstrates a large 3-cm mass arising from the pituitary and extending into the suprasellar cistern. The mass is isointense with the surrounding cortex.

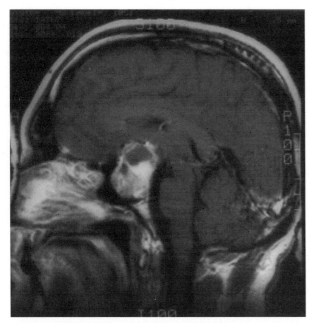

Figure 2–8. Pituitary adenoma. After administration of contrast agent there is an intense but heterogeneous enhancement. There are two dominant foci of nonenhancing tissue, compatible with necrosis or cyst formation.

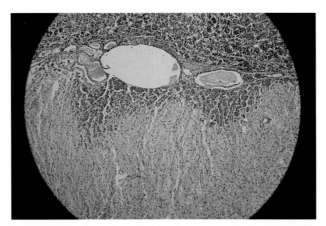

Figure 2–11. Pituitary gland. Ill-defined pars intermedia (vestige noted by the presence of colloid-filled follicles) and basophil invasion into the neurohypophysis.

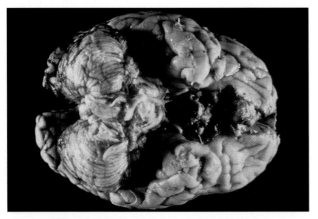

Figure 2–9. Pituitary adenoma. Autopsy specimen.

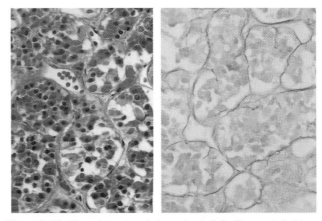

Figure 2–12. Normal anterior pituitary gland. *Left,* Characteristic histologic cordlike pattern, surrounded by capillaries. *Right,* The histologic appearance is accentuated by the reticulin stain showing the rich reticulin connective tissue framework.

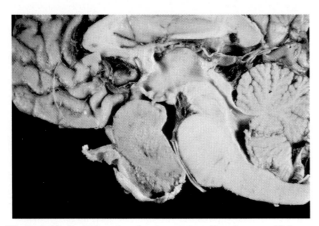

Figure 2–10. Sagittal section showing a suprasellar adenoma with homogeneous cut surface.

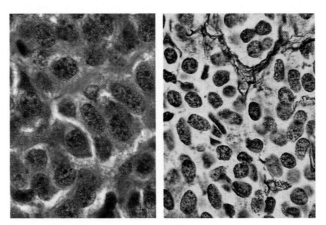

Figure 2–13. Pituitary adenoma. *Left,* Compared with the normal gland (see Fig. 2–12), the architectural pattern is disrupted. *Right,* Reticulin stain highlights the architectural disruption by the absence of the normal reticulin framework.

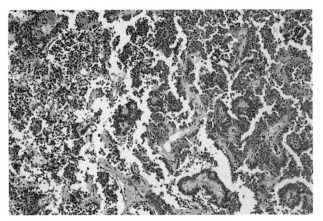

Figure 2–14. Pituitary adenoma. Histologic patterns. Pseudopapillary pattern.

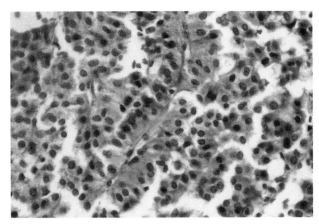

Figure 2–17. Pituitary adenoma. Perisinusoidal growth.

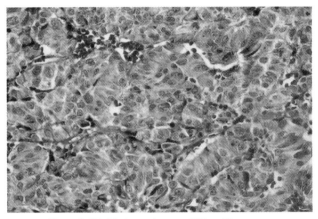

Figure 2–15. Pituitary adenoma. Ribbon-like pattern.

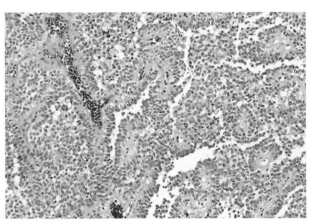

Figure 2–18. Pituitary adenoma. Rosette pattern.

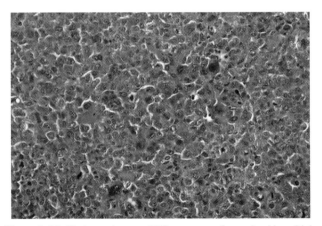

Figure 2–16. Pituitary adenoma. Diffuse pattern of growth with multiple mitoses.

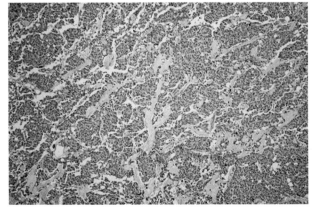

Figure 2–19. Pituitary adenoma. Diffuse pattern of growth with increased connective tissue stroma.

- Adenomas on T1-weighted images appear isotense and are strongly enhanced, sometimes inhomogenously.
- Hemorrhagic adenomas on T1-weighted images often produce a complex mixed signal.
- Pituitary adenomas are classified according to their radiologic findings as follows:
  - Grade I: Intrasellar adenoma measuring less than 1 cm (microadenoma) in which the sella is normal and shows only minimal configurational changes.

- Grade II: Intrasellar adenoma measuring more than 1 cm (macroadenoma) in which sellar enlargement is present but not bony destruction.
- Grade III: Diffuse adenoma with localized erosion of the sella; diffuse adenomas are defined as macroadenomas that fill the sella and compress the remaining pituitary into a thin membrane.
- Grade IV: Invasive adenoma with erosion of the sella.

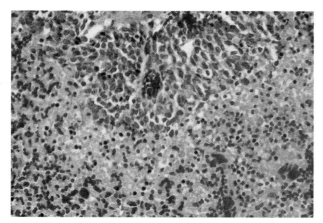

Figure 2–20. Pituitary adenoma. Hemorrhagic infarction.

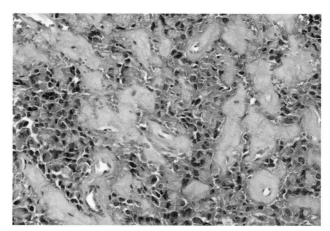

Figure 2–22. Pituitary adenoma. Radiation effect. Increased perivascular and intratumoral fibrosis. Cells display nuclear pleomorphism and hyperchromatism.

- Immunohistochemical features identified in all pituitary adenomas include reactivity with cytokeratin and various neuroendocrine markers (e.g., chromogranin, synaptophysin, and neuron-specific enolase); this immunoreactivity is not specific for the tumor but confirms the diagnosis in conjunction with the clinical, radiographic, and other pathologic (light microscopic) findings.
- The ultrastructural features of pituitary adenomas may vary according to cell type, but all pituitary adenomas include the presence of intracytoplasmic electron-dense neurosecretory granules that vary in size from 100 to more than 1000 nm in diameter.
- Options for treatment of an adenoma include the following modalities:
  • Surgery via the transsphenoidal approach.
  • Pharmacotherapy.
  • Radiotherapy.
- The most common malignant pituitary tumor is a metastatic tumor.
- Approximately 3% of pituitary adenomas are associated with the multiple endocrine neoplasia (MEN) syndrome.
- Treatment of pituitary tumors is by surgical excision.
- The majority of pituitary tumors are adenomas, which have an excellent prognosis.

2. Prolactin Cell–Producing Adenoma

Definition: Benign, well-differentiated neoplasm composed of prolactin or lactotrophic cells.

Synonyms: Prolactinoma, chromophobic adenoma; acidophilic adenoma.

Clinical

- Most common pituitary adenomas, accounting for approximately 30% of all pituitary adenomas.
- More common in women than in men; can occur at any age, but the peak incidence is between 20 and 30 years of age.
- Clinical symptoms may be related to endocrinopathy or mass effect.
- Clinical symptoms differ in the sexes:
  • In women, hyperprolactinemia causes:

1. Amenorrhea and galactorrhea; infertility may be present.
2. In 10% to 40% of women with amenorrhea prolactin levels are increased.

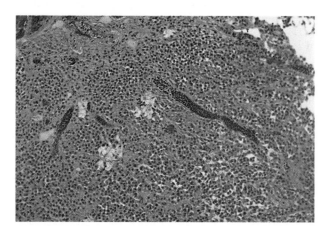

Figure 2–21. Infarcted pituitary adenoma. Patient with chronic lymphocytic leukemia.

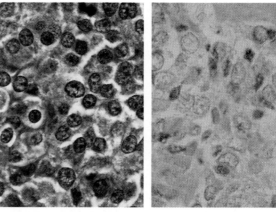

Figure 2–23. Prolactin-secreting adenoma. *Left,* Sparsely granulated prolactinoma. *Right,* Immunohistochemistry stain shows concentration of the prolactin granules in the Golgi's complex.

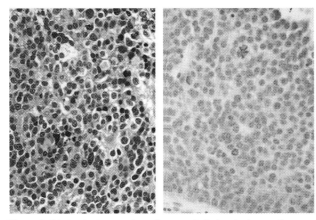

Figure 2–24. Prolactin-secreting adenoma. *Left,* Atypical sparsely granulated prolactinoma showing nuclear pleomorphism. *Right,* Prolactin immunoreactivity. Note the presence of increased mitoses, suggesting a potentially aggressive neoplasm.

3. In 30% of women with amenorrhea and galactorrhea a prolactin-secreting tumor is present.

   • In men, hyperprolactinemia causes:

1. Gonadal dysfunction with decreased libido and impotence.
2. Rarely is galactorrhea or gynecomastia present.

   • Microadenomas (<1 cm in size) are more frequent in women, and macroadenomas (>1 cm) are more frequent in men.

■ Macroadenomas tend to be more aggressive or invasive, and, because of the larger size, symptoms associated with macroadenomas include headache and visual defects produced by the mass effect of the tumor.
■ Laboratory studies
   • A serum prolactin level of over 300 μg/L is diagnostic of pituitary adenoma.
   • The concentration of prolactin is slightly higher in women (<20 μg/L) than in men. In pregnancy, the prolactin level reaches maximum values at term (from 100 to 300 μg/L), regaining normal levels 4 to 6 months postpartum. Serum prolactin levels of <150 μg/L may

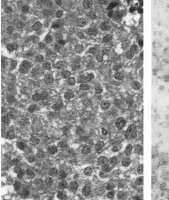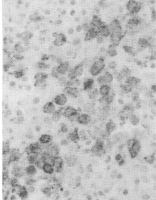

Figure 2–25. Prolactin-secreting adenoma. *Left,* Densely granulated prolactinoma. Note cytologic uniformity. *Right,* Diffusely intense prolactin immunoreactivity.

be due to pituitary stalk compression and are not diagnostic of a prolactinoma.
   • For diagnostic purposes, if basal or fasting levels of serum prolactin are elevated, it is prudent to obtain several serum prolactin samples before making the pathologic diagnosis.
   • Once pregnancy and hypothyroidism have been eliminated as etiologic factors and after a careful drug history has proved negative, a search for hypothalamic or pituitary disease is necessary.
   • One of the tests most widely used to differentiate hypothalamic from pituitary disease and to determine the presence of tumor is the administration of thyrotropin-releasing hormone (TRH) with measurement of the prolactin response. As a rule, most patients with a prolactin-secreting tumor have a diminished prolactin response to intravenous TRH; unfortunately, this response is not consistent enough to be of diagnostic value, and it is nonspecific in differentiating between hypothalamic and pituitary disease.
■ Causes of hyperprolactinemia include:

1. **Physiologic states:** pregnancy, nursing, and stress.
2. **Drugs:** dopamine receptor antagonists, antidepressants, antihypertensive medications, estrogen, and opiates.
3. **Primary hypothyroidism.**
4. **Pituitary tumors or lesions:** prolactinomas (microadenomas and macroadenomas), growth hormone-producing adenomas (acromegaly), corticotrophic cell-producing adenomas (Cushing's disease), hypothalamic lesions, and pituitary stalk section or compression.
5. **Other pituitary and nonpituitary lesions or tumors:** sarcoidosis, lymphocytic hypophysitis, empty sella syndrome, craniopharyngiomas, meningiomas, ectopic pinealomas, third ventricle tumors and aneurysms, and metastatic carcinomas.

Radiology

■ Radiographic evaluation is not always helpful in the diagnosis.
■ CT scans with contrast enhancement are suggested to assess gland homogeneity and the presence of focal lesions.
■ CT scans will establish the diagnosis of most adenomas with the exception of small adenomas that are difficult to delineate.
■ CT scans can determine not only the size of the tumor but also the degree of extension.

Pathology

Histology

■ Three patterns of growth can be seen: diffuse, papillary (microadenoma), and fibrotic with abundant connective tissue stroma (autopsy finding).
■ Histologically, the tumor is composed of large cells with irregular nuclei, prominent nucleoli, and a slightly basophilic cytoplasm.
■ Calcification is common and may be extensive in some cases. Psammoma bodies are seen in 15% to 20% of cases, and amyloid occurs in 5% to 10% of cases.

- Retrogressive changes with cyst formation are seen in fibrotic tumors.
- From the histologic standpoint, prolactinomas are classified as sparsely granulated prolactin cell adenomas and densely granulated prolactin cell adenomas (acidophilic adenomas) by light microscopy.
  - **Sparsely granulated prolactin cell adenoma (chromophobic adenomas)** is the most common form; they arise in the peripheral part of the lateral wings.
  - **Densely granulated prolactic cell adenoma (acidophilic adenomas)** is extremely rare and consists of nests of polyhedral cells with irregular ovoid nuclei separated by a vascular stroma.
- Approximately 50% of prolactinomas are invasive by the time of surgery; erosion of the bony sella as well as suprasellar growth has occurred. The incidence of invasion increases with the size of the tumor.
- *Immunohistochemistry:* conclusive diagnosis by immunoperoxidase-staining techniques has demonstrated a strong diffuse reaction with the antibody to prolactin. A characteristic strong reaction in the Golgi region (juxtanuclear stain) is seen in sparsely granulated adenomas. Unlike all other cellular types of pituitary adenomas, prolactin cell-producing adenomas show no reaction with the neuroendocrine cell marker chromogranin A; reaction with chromogranin B and synaptophysin is positive.
- *Electron microscopy:*
  - Cells similar to normal lactotrophs with numerous electron-dense secretory granules averaging 350 nm in diameter are seen.
  - Sparse, smaller, round or oval electron-dense granules averaging 200 to 300 nm in diameter are seen, as well as prominent rough endoplasmic reticulum forming concentric whorls (Neberkerns) and prominent Golgi complexes.
  - Misplaced granule exocytosis as opposed to the prolactin granule exocytosis that occurs in the normal pituitary is another diagnostic feature.

Differential Diagnosis

- Other types of pituitary adenomas.
- Sphenoidal, pharyngeal, or nasopharyngeal neoplasms.

Treatment and Prognosis

- Goals of treatment: suppression of excessive hormone production with a decrease in prolactin levels, a decrease in the size of any demonstrable tumor, with restoration of normal function and prevention of recurrence or progression of disease.
- Options for treatment of prolactinomas:

1. **Surgery**

- Success of transsphenoidal surgery depends on tumor size, preoperative serum prolactin values, and tumor extension.
- Surgery is curative most frequently in patients with microadenomas in which the preoperative level of prolactin is less than 250 μg/L; in patients with higher levels of serum prolactin preoperatively, the surgical results are poor and there is a significant risk of recurrence of disease.

2. **Pharmacotherapy**

- Bromocriptine, which was specifically developed as an inhibitor of prolactin secretion, has beneficial therapeutic effects.
- Administration of bromocriptine suppresses serum prolactin secretion in 47% to 96% of patients; bromocriptine decreases serum prolactin levels and provides symptomatic relief.
- The regressive changes (fibrosis) persist as long as the drug is taken on a regular daily basis; if the drug is withdrawn, the symptoms reappear, and tumor expansion and hyperprolactinemia recur.
- Common side effects of bromocriptine therapy are nausea and orthostatic hypotension at the beginning of therapy.

3. **Irradiation**

- Radiation therapy is recommended for recurrent or persistent disease or as adjuvant treatment with transsphenoidal surgery; it is not recommended as primary treatment.
- For microadenomas, the therapeutic approach includes observation, bromocriptine therapy, or transsphenoidal resection.

3. Growth Hormone–Producing Adenoma (Acromegaly)

Definition: Benign neoplasm composed of growth hormone (GH) cells or somatotrophs causing either acromegaly (if excessive hormone secretion occurs after or around the time of closure of the epiphysis) or gigantism (if the excessive secretion occurs prior to closure of the epiphysis of the long bones).

Synonym: Somatotrophic adenoma.

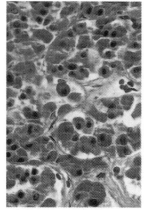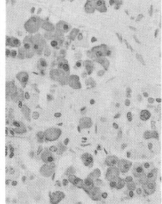

Figure 2–26. Growth hormone-producing adenoma. *Left,* Acidophilic cells with granular cytoplasm and round nuclei. *Right,* Diffusely intense growth hormone immunoreactivity.

Clinical

- GH-producing adenomas are the second most common type of pituitary adenoma and account for approximately 20% of all pituitary adenomas.
- Acromegaly is the second most common syndrome associated with pituitary hypersecretion and accounts for approximately 10% of all pituitary adenomas. Other conditions associated with increased GH secretion are hypothalamic lesions and ectopic hormone production by extrapituitary tumors.
- Affects primarily middle-aged women and men.
- Uncommon disease of insidious onset and slow progression.
- Clinical manifestations include enlargement of the bones, soft tissues, and cartilage overgrowth with increased hand, foot, and hat size.
- Other symptoms include:
  - Voice change and prognathism.
  - Neurologic and musculoskeletal manifestations with paresthesias of the hands, muscle weakness, joint pain, and headaches.
  - Hypertension, cardiovascular disease, sleep apnea, and diabetes mellitus.
  - Menstrual alterations with amenorrhea with or without prolactinemia in about 80% of women; depression is a relatively frequent manifestation.
  - Change in libido or impotence in men (occurs in about 50%).
- GH is under hypothalamic regulation; secretion is stimulated by growth hormone-releasing hormone (GHRH) and is inhibited by GH-releasing inhibitory factor (somatostatin, somatotropin-releasing inhibitory factor [SRIF]).
- Although GH is necessary for normal growth, it appears to act indirectly by stimulating the formation of other hormones synthesized in the liver, known as somatomedins (SM) or insulin-like growth factor (IGF).
- Diagnostic evaluation:
  - Serum or plasma level of GH is elevated and is not suppressed with administration of oral glucose.
  - Somatomedin C or insulin-like growth factor may be a more reliable index to hormonal activity in patients with acromegaly than is the level of GH in blood.
  - Serum prolactin may be normal or elevated.

Radiology

- Skull radiographs may show an abnormal sella, thickening of the skull with increased bone density, and enlargement of the sinuses.
- CT scans and MRI confirm the presence of a pituitary adenoma; small adenomas can be detected with the addition of contrast medium.

Pathology

Histology
- Five different types of adenomas have been associated with acromegaly.

a. Densely granulated GH cell adenoma.
b. Sparsely granulated GH cell adenoma.
c. Mixed GH cell and prolactin cell adenoma.
d. Mammosomatotrophic cell adenoma.
e. Acidophilic stem cell adenoma.

- These various adenomas differ in cellular and morphologic composition, hormonal production, and biologic behavior.
- Monohormonal variants are more common than bihormonal variants.
- *Immunohistochemistry:* confirms the presence of GH, but electron microscopy is necessary to determine the morphologic type.
- Densely granulated GH adenomas are slow growing tumors that have a better prognosis than the sparsely granulated tumors, which seem to be more aggressive.

a. Densely Granulated GH Cell Adenoma

Synonyms: Well-differentiated GH cell adenoma or acidophilic adenoma.

- This is a relatively vascular tumor. The cells have a diffuse, trabecular, or sinusoidal pattern of growth.
- Cells are polyhedral with round nuclei and granular acidophilic cytoplasm.
- *Immunohistochemistry:* diffuse strong cytoplasmic reaction with GH.
- *Electron microscopy:* cells are well differentiated and resemble normal cells.
  - Cytoplasm contains numerous round secretory granules or granules that are fusiform in shape due to crystallization of secretory material; these granules are specific for GH and range in size from 200 to 300 nm.
  - Cells have a prominent Golgi apparatus and a well-developed rough endoplasmic reticulum (RER).

b. Sparsely Granulated GH Cell Adenoma

Synonyms: Atypical GH cell adenoma; chromophobic cell adenoma.

- Composed of cells of various sizes with irregular, pleomorphic, eccentric, simple, or multiple nuclei.
- *Immunohistochemistry:* typical of this tumor is the demonstration of GH in the Golgi region and around the fibrous bodies. The latter are cytokeratin intermediate filaments that are hormone negative and are seen in almost all cells; this finding is diagnostic of this type of tumor.
- *Electron microscopy:* small, sparse secretory granules averaging 200 nm in diameter.

c. Mixed GH Cell and Prolactin Cell Adenoma

Synonyms: Acidophilic adenoma; chromophobic adenoma.

- Three of the five GH-producing adenomas are mixed cell types with two distinct cell populations of GH and prolactin cells.
- Among the group of mixed hormone-producing tumors, this is the most common one.

- Patients present with acromegaly and variable degrees and manifestations of hyperprolactinemia.
- Cell population consists of an admixture of cells.
- *Immunohistochemistry:* The staining pattern is also variable and depends on the proportions of densely or sparsely granulated cells of the two coexisting cell populations.
- *Electron microscopy:* The ultrastructural features of this neoplasm are characterized by the presence of both types of cell described in GH-producing adenomas and prolactinomas; the coexistence of the two populations of cells has been demonstrated by electron microscopy and double immunohistochemical techniques.

d. Mammosomatotrophic Cell Adenoma

Synonyms: Acidophilic adenoma; GH cell adenoma with extracellular GH deposits.

- Rare tumor derived from mammosomatotrophic cells present in the normal pituitary gland.
- Consists primarily of a GH-producing tumor with minimal prolactin elevation.
- Histology: Tumor has a diffuse pattern of growth.
- Immunohistochemistry: Tumor has a strong reaction with GH and a less intense reaction with prolactin.
- *Electron microscopy:*
  - Characteristic of this tumor type is the presence of a dual population of variable sized cytoplasmic secretory granules.
    - One population consists of smaller, round granules measuring up to 400 nm in diameter.
    - The second population consists of pleomorphic secretory granules that measure up to 2000 nm in diameter.
    - Both hormones are present in the same cell or in the same granule (immunogold–electron microscopic technique).
  - Electron microscopy is diagnostic for this tumor. The main distinguishing characteristic is the presence of electron-dense material in the intercellular spaces that originates from the extrusion of secretory granules and shows a negative reaction for prolactin and GH.

e. Acidophilic Stem Cell Adenoma

Synonyms: Chromophobic adenoma; invasive adenoma.

- Rare tumor; seems to be derived from a stem cell and is frequently invasive.
- This tumor produces prolactin predominantly and has a scanty reaction for GH.
- Recognition of this tumor is important because it appears to be more aggressive; it is larger, has a tendency to invade adjacent structures, and has relatively low hormonal activity.
- Histology: diffuse pattern of growth composed of chromophobic or acidophilic cells.
- Acidophilia is mainly due to increased mitochondria size and smooth endoplasmic reticulum (SER).
- *Immunohistochemistry:* prolactin and GH are detectable in the cells.

- Immunoelectron microscopy has revealed that the two hormones can be present in the same cell.
- Electron microscopy is diagnostic of this type of tumor; characteristic of this tumor are the presence of giant abnormal mitochondria visible on light microscopy as vacuoles; small, sparse secretory granules measuring less than 200 nm in diameter, misplaced exocytosis, and fibrous bodies.

Differential Diagnosis

- Cerebral gigantism: the sella and GH level are normal.
- Beckwith-Wiedemann's syndrome in children: GH level is normal.
- Paget's disease: radiographs of the head are diagnostic.
- Simple prognathism: GH level is normal.

Treatment and Prognosis

- Transsphenoidal microsurgery is the most widely used surgical approach to the treatment of acromegaly; it results in rapid regression of symptoms and is considered potentially curative.
- Postoperative complications include cerebrospinal fluid rhinorrhea, arterial injuries, hemorrhage, temporary visual loss, and infections.
- Irradiation:
  - Two modalities have been used–conventional radiation and heavy particle radiation. Radiation therapy should be considered one of the treatment choices in patients at risk or in those with incurable tumors.
  - Complications of radiotherapy: Sarcoma may develop in the radiation field.
- Pharmacotherapy:
  - Bromocriptine and related compounds have been used widely in patients with active acromegaly with good response and symptom improvement, but this treatment is not curative.
  - The amount of bromocriptine needed to achieve a good response is much higher than that needed in patients with hyperprolactinemic states; continuous treatment is required, and drug withdrawal is associated with return of elevated GH levels.

Additional Facts

- Cardiovascular disease is the most common cause of death.
- Patients with acromegaly are susceptible to colonic polyps and colon cancer.
- The presence of hypercalcemia suggests hyperparathyroidism as part of the MEN I syndrome.
- Ectopic production of GH hormone occurs in patients with islet cell tumors.

4. Corticotrophic Cell (ACTH)-Producing Adenoma (Cushing's Disease and Nelson's Syndrome)

Definition: Neoplastic and non-neoplastic proliferation of adrenocorticotropin-secreting cells.

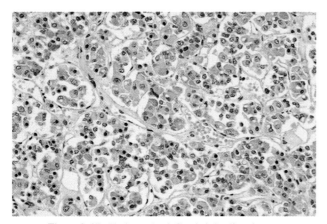

Figure 2–27. Pituitary gland. Crooke's hyaline change.

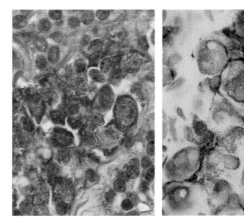

Figure 2–29. Pituitary gland. *Left,* Crooke's hyaline change. Periodic acid-Schiff (PAS) stain showing a purple granular reaction at the periphery of the cells and around the nuclei. The hyaline material is PAS negative. *Right,* Strong immunoreactivity demonstrated with cytokeratin.

Clinical

■ Constitutes the third most common cause of surgically removed pituitary tumors and accounts for approximately 15% of all pituitary adenomas.

■ All races and both sexes are affected; however, there is a female preponderance with a wide age distribution ranging from 20 to 60 years.

■ Most tumors are functioning adenomas; nonfunctioning adenomas have no biochemical or clinical evidence of excessive production of ACTH.

■ ACTH-producing adenomas fall into three categories:
  • Functioning corticotrophic adenomas associated with Cushing's syndrome (10%).
  • Functioning corticotrophic adenomas associated with Nelson's syndrome (2%).
  • Nonfunctioning or silent corticotrophic adenomas (3%).

■ Symptoms of functioning adenomas associated with Cushing's syndrome include obesity, hirsutism, purplish striae, muscle weakness, hypertension, amenorrhea, impotence in men, osteoporosis, fatigue, psychiatric abnormalities, diabetes mellitus, and hypokalemia.

■ Causes of hypercortisolism include pituitary adenomas or hyperplasia, adrenal tumors, ectopic sources of ACTH, and iatrogenic causes resulting from excess administration of exogenous corticosteroids.

■ Adrenocorticotropin is synthesized as part of a large precursor molecule termed proopiomelanocortin, which in the anterior pituitary is cleaved to yield ACTH, beta lipoprotein, and endorphins.

■ ACTH controls the release of cortisol from the adrenal cortex and is regulated by corticotrophin-releasing factor produced in the hypothalamus.

■ ACTH concentration is highest in the early morning and lowest in late evening.

■ Cortisol administration inhibits ACTH release.

■ In normal persons ACTH circulates in low concentrations (10 to 80 pg/ml).

■ Laboratory findings:
  • The presence of excess cortisol is established by finding increased urinary excretion of free cortisol and/or 17-hydroxycorticosteroids that fail to be suppressed after an overnight or 2-day trial with low-dose dexamethasone administration.
  • After a high dose of dexamethasone has been administered, patients with excessive ACTH secretion will

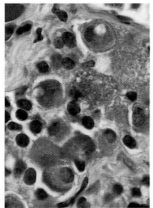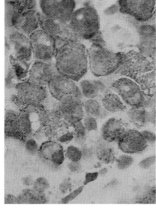

Figure 2–28. Pituitary gland. *Left,* Crooke's hyaline change in nontumorous parenchyma. *Right,* ACTH immunoreactivity showing displacement of the secretory granules toward the periphery of the cells.

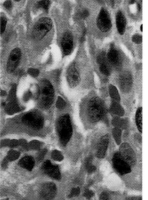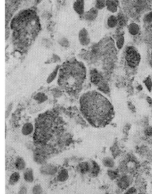

Figure 2–30. ACTH-producing adenoma. *Left,* Elongated basophilic cells with ovoid nuclei and conspicuous nucleoli. *Right,* Strong diffuse cytoplasmic ACTH immunoreactivity.

show a greater than 50% reduction in the 8:00 A.M. plasma cortisol level.
- In patients with Cushing's disease, urine 17-hydroxy-corticosteroids are increased after metyrapone administration.
- Cushing's disease is produced by microadenomas (3 to 6 mm in size) in 90% of patients and by macroadenomas in the remainder.
■ The location of the adenoma is the median portion of the anterior pituitary.

Radiology

■ Microadenomas may be difficult to detect on CT scans, even with the use of contrast-enhanced MRI.
■ At least 50% of patients with microadenomas have negative findings on CT scans owing to the small tumor size.

Pathology

Histology
a. Functioning Corticotrophic Cell Adenoma

(1) Densely Granulated Adenoma

Synonyms: Basophilic cell adenoma.

■ Composed of medium to large cells that are strongly basophilic with nuclei showing prominent nucleoli.
■ Cells are characteristically arranged to form follicles and rosette-like structures.
■ Nontumorous corticotrophic cells have a slightly acidophilic hyaline-like material in the cytoplasm (**Crooke's hyaline change**), which is diagnostic of hypercorticism.
■ Histochemistry: The secretory granules produce a strong periodic acid-Schiff (PAS)-positive reaction around the cell membrane.
■ *Immunohistochemistry:* The cells are positive for ACTH. In addition, α-endorphins and β-endorphins as well as β-lipotropin and α-melanocytic-stimulating hormone can be demonstrated.
■ *Electron microscopy:* The cells are densely granulated with pleomorphic secretory granules ranging from 250 to 700 nm in diameter and have an abundant RER and a prominent Golgi apparatus.
  - The hallmark of the corticotrophic cells is the presence of type 1 filaments arranged in bundles, as seen in Crooke's cells.

(2) Sparsely Granulated Adenoma

Synonyms: Chromophobic adenoma.

Clinical

■ Rare tumors; larger and more aggressive than densely granulated tumors.
■ Histology: diffuse pattern of growth.
■ Histochemistry: PAS negative.
■ *Immunohistochemistry:* faint reaction with ACTH.
■ *Electron microscopy:* secretory granules are sparse and smaller, measuring up to 200 nm in diameter.

Treatment and Prognosis

■ Transsphenoidal surgery is the most effective treatment; the cure rate is 75% to 93%.
■ Irradiation: Conventional radiation therapy will cure 15% of adults, and 30% of patients show improvement.
■ Pharmacotherapy: Drugs used for the treatment of Cushing's disease (with variable results) include mitotane, metyrapone, serotonin antagonists, and dopamine agonists.

Additional Facts

■ Corticotrophic cell hyperplasia is associated with Cushing's disease.
■ No evidence of adenoma is found during surgical exploration in 5% to 20% of patients.

b. Silent Corticotrophic Adenoma

Synonyms: Chromophobic or basophilic adenoma.

Clinical

■ This is a rare, endocrinologically inactive variant of an ACTH-producing tumor.
■ Despite the presence of immunoreactivity with ACTH, these tumors are not endocrinologically active and are not associated with signs or symptoms of excess ACTH production or laboratory evidence of elevated serum ACTH.
■ The absence of endocrinopathic manifestations despite the presence of ACTH may be due to:
  - The inability of the tumor to secrete ACTH.
  - The quantity of ACTH secretion may be too low to produce an effect.
  - ACTH is secreted into the serum but is degraded rapidly.
  - The ACTH produced by the tumor is an abnormal form that is undetectable or functionally inactive.
■ The tumor occurs in both sexes but has a slightly increased incidence in younger women.
■ These tumors are large (macroadenoma) and invasive and produce visual defects as the chief complaint.
■ These tumors tend to be aggressive and have a tendency to recur.
■ Infarction is common.
■ Occasionally associated with hyperprolactinemia of unknown mechanism.
■ Morphology and immunohistochemical features are similar to those of functioning tumors with α-endorphin and/or β-endorphin reactivity and a weak reaction for ACTH; scattered cells may react positively with GH and prolactin.
■ Ultrastructurally, three subtypes have been recognized:
  - Basophilic: indistinguishable from the typical functioning corticotrophic adenoma; PAS positive.
  - Chromophobic: small secretory granules are present and type I filaments are absent; PAS is weakly positive;
  - Acidophilic: increased amount of smooth endoplasmic reticulum, segmented Golgi apparatus, and small, peripherally located secretory granules. Cells have eccentrically located nuclei with prominent nucleoli; tumors

composed of these cells often are large and aggressive and have a tendency to recur.

c. Nelson's Syndrome

Definition: A condition characterized by the presence of hyperpigmentation due to a large ACTH-producing tumor following bilateral adrenalectomy for pre-existing Cushing's disease.

Clinical

- There are no distinctive clinical features associated with this syndrome.
- Patients with Cushing's disease treated by bilateral adrenalectomy develop progressive cutaneous pigmentation in overexposed areas of the body after surgery.
- Pituitary adenomas associated with Nelson's syndrome tend to be large (macroadenomas) and locally invasive in 25% of patients; symptoms related to mass effect such as visual disturbances and headaches may be present.
- Laboratory studies: plasma ACTH levels are elevated.
- Hyperpigmentation is related to increased plasma levels of β-melanocyte-stimulating hormone (β-MSH).
- Diagnosis is based on:
  - Previous history of Cushing's disease treated by bilateral adrenalectomy.
  - Progressive cutaneous pigmentation.
  - Elevated plasma ACTH.
  - Clinical evidence and CT scan confirmation of the presence of a pituitary adenoma.
- Results of treatment are relatively poor, and long-term cures are uncommon; symptomatic relief and control of the disease for a variable period of time can be achieved.
- Transsphenoidal surgery in tumors without evidence of local extension is an option.
- Radiation therapy as primary therapy or following surgery is effective in maintaining control of the disease for long periods of time.
- Pharmacotherapy: Cyproheptadine is used as adjunctive therapy.
- Approximately 20% of patients with Nelson's syndrome die from the disease; malignant transformation occurs in pituitary adenomas associated with Nelson's syndrome (pituitary carcinomas).

5. Glycoprotein Hormone–Producing Adenoma

- Glycoprotein hormone-producing adenomas are divided into two types:
  a. Thyrotrophic cell adenoma.
  b. Gonadotrophic cell adenoma.

a. Thyrotrophic Cell Adenoma

Synonyms: Thyroid-stimulating hormone (TSH)-secreting adenoma.

Clinical

- Extremely rare tumors representing the least common pituitary tumor type; they account for approximately 1% of all pituitary adenomas.
- Usually large (macroadenoma) and cause visual field defects.
- Most commonly associated with long-standing hypothyroidism.
- Occasionally associated with hyperthyroidism with autonomous TSH secretion and overproduction of the α subunit of the glycoprotein hormone.

Pathology

- Most are chromophobic and have weak PAS positivity.
- Immunohistochemistry: reactive with TSH markers.
- Electron microscopy: Sparse electron-dense secretory granules are present.

Treatment

- Surgery is recommended for large adenomas.
- Replacement treatment with thyroid hormone is used in hypothyroid patients.

b. Gonadotrophic Cell Adenoma

Synonyms: Follicle-stimulating hormone (FSH)–producing adenoma and luteinizing hormone (LH)–producing adenoma.

Clinical

- True incidence is unknown, but these tumors are believed to represent approximately 7% to 15% of all pituitary adenomas.
- Equal gender predilection; wide age range.
- Tumors are large (macroadenomas) and show suprasellar or parasellar extension.
- Presenting symptoms are related to visual abnormalities and hypopituitarism.
- Associated with amenorrhea and/or galactorrhea in women and decreased libido in men.
- From 20% to 25% of these tumors are considered to be nonfunctioning and are associated with no clinical syndromes; however, they produce gonadotropins.

Pathology

- The tumor cells are mostly chromophobic and have limited PAS positivity.
- The cells are polygonal or elongated and are often arranged in perivascular rosettes.
- *Immunohistochemistry:* reactive with FSH or LH or both.
- *Electron microscopy:* Scant numbers of secretory granules are present in a subplasmalemmal location.

Treatment

- Surgical excision

6. Adenomas with No Hormone Production

Definition: Pituitary adenoma with no clinical or immuno-histochemical evidence of hormone production.

Synonyms: Nonfunctioning adenoma; null cell adenoma; oncocytoma.

Clinical

- These tumors represent approximately 25% of nonfunctioning pituitary adenomas.
- They occur in both sexes and are most common in the fourth decade of life.
- They are usually large (macroadenomas) and produce visual disturbances as the chief complaint.
- Hypogonadism and hypothyroidism are frequently associated with this type of tumor or as a result of destruction of the pituitary parenchyma.

Pathology

- Most are either chromophobic (nononcocytic) or oncocytic.
- Oncocytomas are more common in older people and are characterized by the presence of abundant cytoplasmic mitochondria.
- Histochemistry: PAS negative.
- *Immunohistochemistry:* often negative; occasionally scattered cells react positively with FSH, LH, or TSH.
- *Electron microscopy:* sparse secretory granules.

Treatment

- Radical surgery followed by radiation therapy.

7. Plurihormonal Adenoma

Definition: (1) Pituitary tumor with multiple hormonal functions clinically; and/or (2) produces more than one hormone; and/or (3) cell type detected on immunohisto-chemistry and/or electron microscopy.

Clinical

- Plurihormonal adenomas are usually macroadenomas and may be invasive.
- Many of the adenomas associated with acromegaly are plurihormonal and include the presence of GH and one or more other hormones such as PRL or a glycoprotein hormone (TSH). Mixed adenomas producing GH and PRL represent well-defined tumor types. ACTH is a rare component in plurihormonal pituitary adenomas.
- Clinical symptoms related to the presence of immunoreactivity for more than one hormone are generally uncommon; low-grade hyperprolactinemia may occur, and hyperthyroidism is rare.

Pathology

Histology

- Plurihormonal adenomas may be monomorphous or polymorphous.

- Morphology of the cells does not always correspond to their functional differentiation (hormonal content).
- Immunohistochemistry: Immunoreactivity for more than one hormone is seen.
- *Electron microscopy:* The ultrastructural appearance is heterogeneous; some tumors are monomorphous, whereas others consist of two or more distinct cell types.

Treatment and Prognosis

- Similar to that for all other pituitary adenomas.

Additional Facts

- The reasons for the presence of more than one hormone are not completely understood; some possibilities include multidirectional differentiation or transdifferentiation (functional switch) of pituitary endocrine cells.

8. Ectopic Pituitary Adenoma

Definition: Benign extrasellar pituitary neoplasm arising from remnants of pituitary tissue (Rathke's pouch) along the pathway of embryologic development.

Clinical

- Equal gender predilection; occurs over a wide age range, usually between the fourth and eighth decades of life.
- Symptoms vary according to site and include airway obstruction, chronic sinusitis, visual field defects, and CSF leakage. Occasionally, symptoms may be associated with endocrine syndromes related to hormonal secretion (e.g., hirsutism).
- Most common sites of occurrence are the sphenoid sinus, followed by the nasopharynx and the suprasellar region (pars tuberalis); rarely, the tumors occur in the nasal cavity, ethmoid sinus, or temporal bone.

Radiology

- Among the diagnostic criteria is the presence of radiographic evidence of a normal pituitary gland and sella turcica.

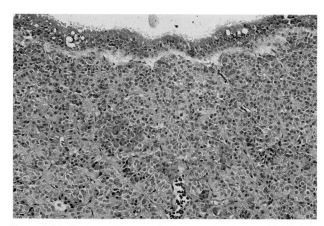

Figure 2–31. Ectopic pituitary plurihormonal adenoma: tumor beneath the lining ciliated epithelium of the sphenoid sinus.

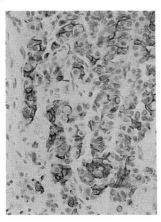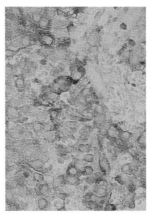

Figure 2–32. Ectopic pituitary plurihormal adenoma. Immunohistochemistry included *(left)* cytokeratin- and *(right)* chromogranin-positive reaction by the neoplastic cells.

■ A mass lesion with local invasive growth is seen in the site of involvement.

Pathology

Histology

■ These tumors are submucosal and show several patterns of growth, including a solid, organoid, and trabecular cellular arrangement with a fibrovascular stroma.
■ The cells include round nuclei with dispersed chromatin and granular eosinophilic cytoplasm.
■ Pleomorphism, necrosis, and mitotic activity are not seen.
■ *Immunohistochemistry:* chromogranin, synaptophysin, neuron-specific enolase (NSE), and cytokeratin reactivity. In addition, monohormonal, plurihormonal, or nonreactive results to pituitary-specific hormonal antibodies may be seen.

Differential Diagnosis

■ Neuroendocrine tumors (carcinoid, neuroendocrine carcinoma).
■ Site-specific primary malignant epithelial neoplasms.
■ Metastatic tumors.

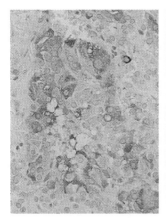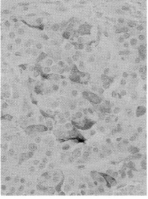

Figure 2–33. Ectopic pituitary plurihormonal adenoma. Immunohistochemistry included *(left)* thyroid-stimulating hormone (TSH) and *(right)* prolactin-positive reaction by the neoplastic cells.

Treatment and Prognosis

■ Surgical excision is considered the best treatment option.
■ Surgery is generally curative and prevents the tumor from recurring or progressing.
■ Good prognosis.

9. Invasive Pituitary Adenoma

Definition: Pituitary adenoma with a tendency to infiltrate or destroy adjacent structures (dura and bones); its biologic behavior is considered intermediate between that of adenomas and pituitary carcinomas.

Clinical

■ Overall incidence is approximately 35%, depending on the immunophenotype. Tumor occurs in younger population.
■ Signs and symptoms include visual disturbances, headache, cranial neuropathies, facial neuralgia, nausea, and dizziness resulting from increased intracranial pressure and endocrine dysfunction.
■ Estimated observed frequency of invasion is:
  • On radiographs: approximately 10%.
  • Intraoperatively: 40%.
  • On histologic sections on systematic examination of the dura: 90%.

Radiology

■ Radiologic examination shows destruction of the sella, bone erosion, invasion of the dura and cavernous sinus, and cranial nerve involvement.

Additional Facts

■ There is no correlation between the histologic appearance and the clinical behavior of the tumor.
■ Metastasis seldom develops.
■ There is a correlation between the size of the tumors and the degree of invasion; dural invasion is present in 60% of microadenomas, 80% of intrasellar adenomas, and 90% of tumors with suprasellar extension.
■ Most adenomas are chromophobic or sparsely granulated.
■ Immunoperoxidase staining of invasive adenomas has demonstrated increased expression of Ki-67 antigen and P105 proliferation–associated antigen.

C. MALIGNANT NEOPLASMS

1. Pituitary Carcinoma

Definition: A malignant neoplasm arising from the endocrine cells of the anterior pituitary that shows gross brain invasion or is capable of producing distant metastasis or both.

Clinical

■ Extremely rare.
■ Equal gender predilection.

- Age of occurrence:
  - In patients with evidence of cerebrospinal metastasis, age varies from 25 to 75 years; average, 43 years.
  - In patients with extracranial metastasis, age at presentation varies from 7 to 75 years; average, 44 years.
- Usually silent; patients generally do not present with evidence of clinical or biochemical endocrine activity or syndromes such as Cushing's disease, acromegaly, or hyperprolactinemia as a consequence of hormone secretion. Furthermore, patients do not present with headaches, visual disturbances, or nerve palsy related to mass effect.

Radiology

- Sellar enlargement and prominent extrasellar extension are seen in patients with carcinomas with craniospinal metastasis.
- Carcinomas with extracranial metastasis produce little or no sellar expansion but show evidence of erosion and destruction of the sellar floor.

Pathology

Histology

- Most pituitary carcinomas are chromophobic.
- Carcinomas of the anterior pituitary have a varied histologic appearance. Some are composed of cells with little nuclear pleomorphism and few or no mitotic figures; others have anaplastic features such as a marked increase in cellularity, bizarre nuclei, and increased mitotic activity.
- **The diagnosis of pituitary carcinoma cannot be based solely on the histologic appearance.**
- Confirmation of the diagnosis is based on the presence of brain invasion or of metastatic foci within the cerebrospinal space or extracranially that either resembles the pituitary tumor, has a hormonal phenotype that is similar to the primary tumor, or shows proof of endocrine differentiation by immunohistochemistry and electron microscopy.

Treatment and Prognosis

- Treatment options include surgery followed by radiation or pharmacotherapy in combination with surgery or radiotherapy.
- The most common sites of distant metastases are liver, lung, bone, and lymph nodes.
- Patients with cerebrospinal metastasis have a longer survival time than do patients with extracranial metastasis; the average survival time for the former is 8 years from onset of symptoms to death, whereas for the latter, the average survival time is 2½ years.

2. Metastatic Neoplasms to the Pituitary Gland

- Evidence of metastasis to the pituitary gland varies and depends mainly on an aggressive search for its presence.
- The incidence of metastasis to the pituitary gland ranges from less than 2% to 26% in autopsy series.

- The majority of patients have no clinical symptoms of pituitary involvement; panhypopituitarism is rare, but diabetes insipidus occurs in 6% to 33% of patients with metastatic tumor to the neurohypophysis.
- *In men,* the primary tumors that metastasize to the pituitary most frequently are lung, prostate, and stomach tumors.
- *In women,* breast, lung, and stomach tumors metastasize most frequently.
- Hematopoietic neoplasms such as leukemias and non-Hodgkin's lymphomas involve the pituitary gland in 23% of patients.
- Metastatic deposits via the systemic circulation are found most commonly in the posterior pituitary because of its extensive vascular supply, whereas the anterior lobe may be involved by direct extension of tumors in the vicinity or by extension from the posterior lobe to the anterior pituitary gland by the portal vessels.
- Metastasis occurs predominantly in normal glands; however, metastatic carcinomas to pituitary adenomas may occur.
- Survival time of patients with metastasis to the pituitary gland is short; death usually occurs in less than 1 year owing to the extent of carcinomatosis existing at the time of diagnosis.

D. NEOPLASM OF THE SELLAR REGION

Craniopharyngioma

Definition: Benign epithelial neoplasm arising from remnants of Rathke's pouch.

Synonyms: Rathke's pouch tumor, adamantinoma, ameloblastoma, epidermoid cyst, suprasellar cyst.

Clinical

- Represents from 3% to 5% of all intracranial neoplasms.
- Most common intracranial (nonglial) tumor of childhood and young adults; represents up to 9% of primary intracranial pediatric tumors.

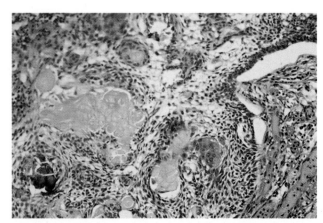

Figure 2–34. Craniopharyngioma. Note the characteristic histologic features of the tumor with palisading of the basal cells and stellate cells in a connective tissue stroma.

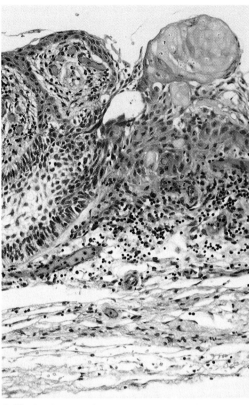

Figure 2–35. Craniopharyngioma. Prominent keratinization and lymphocytic infiltration of the stroma.

- No gender predilection.
- More than half of all craniopharyngiomas occur in children; the peak incidence in childhood (40% to 50%) is prior to age 20, but 45% of patients are over age 20; the tumor may also be detected in older patients.
- Most tumors are suprasellar (94%), and about 15% are intrasellar.
- Symptoms and signs are related to compression of sellar and suprasellar structures or endocrine abnormalities.
  - The most frequent complaint is headache owing to increased intracranial pressure and visual abnormalities with visual loss.
  - Less frequently, mental changes (deterioration and personality changes) and focal neurologic changes can occur.
  - Due to various degrees of hormonal deficiency, associated symptoms include delayed puberty, growth failure, and obesity; involvement of the hypothalamic-hypophyseal axis may be associated with diabetes insipidus and hyperprolactinemia.
  - Adults may present with visual field defects, papilledema, headache, mental deterioration, and hypogonadism.

Radiology

- Skull radiographs show sellar enlargement, calcifications, and signs of increased intracranial pressure.
- Suprasellar calcification and expansion of the sella in a child are highly suggestive of the presence of a craniopharyngioma.

- Nonenhanced CT scans show a heterogeneous, partially calcified suprasellar mass with cystic and solid components.
- Contrast-enhanced CT scans accentuate the density of the solid component.
- MRI shows a highly variable signal pattern; the most common appearance is a cyst that produces a hypointense signal on T1-weighted images and a hyperintense signal on T2-weighted images.

Pathology

Gross

- Size is variable, averaging 3 to 4 cm in diameter.
- Predominantly cystic with focal calcifications.
- External surface irregular and nodular.
- Appearance is multilocular or unilocular, microcystic or honeycomb pattern.
- Smooth cystic wall with occasional protruding papillae.

Histology

- Variable histologic features; histologic variants or patterns include
  - Adamantinomatous variant.
  - Papillary variant.
- Presence of more than one pattern in a given tumor is not uncommon.
- **Adamantinomatous ("classic") craniopharyngioma** consists of islands of epithelial cells, the center of which is composed of loosely arranged stellate cells with small nuclei and clear cytoplasm.
- Surrounding the stellate cells and separated by a thin connective tissue membrane is a row of basaloid-appearing columnar cells with polarized nuclei arranged in a palisade pattern; these features closely resemble the appearance of gnathic ameloblastomas.
- Another pattern consists of squamous cells exhibiting keratohyaline granules.
- The fibrovascular stroma shows degenerative changes resulting in the formation of cystic spaces rich in proteinaceous material and lined by columnar or pseudostratified epithelium containing cellular debris, colloid-like material, keratin debris, mononuclear cell infiltrates, foreign body giant cell reaction, cholesterol granulomas, gliosis, and psammoma bodies.
- Extensive fibrosis at the border adjacent to the brain may be mistaken for a glioma.
- Mitosis and cellular pleomorphism are infrequent.
- **Papillary craniopharyngioma** constitutes another variant. It represents approximately 10% of all cases, occurs predominantly in adulthood, and often involves the third ventricle.
- It differs from the classic tumor by the presence of papillae composed of squamous epithelium with little or no keratin, and it is without calcifications, palisading nuclei, foreign body giant cells, keratoid nodules, and cholesterol clefts.
- Malignant transformation may occur, characterized by nuclear pleomorphism, mitoses, prominent nucleoli, and foci of tumor necrosis.

Differential Diagnosis

- The clinical and histopathologic features of this tumor are diagnostic.

Treatment and Prognosis

- Treatment of craniopharyngiomas is generally unsatisfactory; a number of modalities have been employed.
- Complete surgical resection appears to be the treatment of choice.
- Incomplete removal of the tumor in patients with invasion of adjacent tissues is associated with a high incidence of recurrence.
- Adjuvant radiotherapy yields favorable results, prolongs survival, and delays recurrence but may induce postirradiation malignances (astrocytomas).
- Of the two histologic groups, the papillary type occurring in adults is associated with the worst prognosis and has a higher risk of recurrence.
- The 5-year survival rate varies from 21% to 82%.
- Endocrine deficiencies are permanent, and hormone substitution therapy is necessary.

Additional Facts

- Although these tumors are considered benign histologically, extension into the surrounding tissues may occur but is not indicative of malignancy, and clinical behavior cannot be predicted on the basis of the tumor's microscopic appearance.
- The histogenesis of this tumor type is still unresolved.
  - It is unlikely that craniopharyngiomas originate from squamous nests; these nests are more commonly found in adults, but the majority of these tumors occur in children, in whom such nests are uncommon.
  - Because of the histologic similarities of craniopharyngiomas with ameloblastomas of the jaw, it has been suggested that misplaced cells during embryologic development might give rise to craniopharyngiomas.

Bibliography

General Considerations

Bahn R, Scheithauer BW, Van Heerden JA, et al. Nonidentical expressions of multiple endocrine neoplasia, type I, in identical twins. Mayo Clin Proc 1986; 61:689–696.

Kanter SL, Mickle P, Hunter SB, et al. Pituitary adenomas in pediatric patients: Are they more invasive? Pediatr Neurosci 1985–1986; 12:202–204.

Kovacs K, Horvath E. Tumors of the pituitary gland. In: Armed Forces Institute of Pathology. Atlas of Tumor Pathology, Second series, Fascicle 21. Washington, D.C.: Armed Forces Institute of Pathology, 1986, pp. 57–69.

McComb DJ, Ryan N, Horvath E, et al. Subclinical adenomas of the human pituitary. Arch Pathol Lab Med 1983; 107:488–491.

Osborne AG. Brain tumors and tumorlike processes. In: Diagnostic Neuroradiology. St. Louis: CV Mosby, 1994, pp. 461–468.

Osborne AG. Miscellanous tumors, cysts and metastases. In: Diagnostic Neuroradiology. St. Louis: CV Mosby, 1994, pp. 649–654.

Scheithauer BW. The pituitary and sellar region. In: Sternberg SS, ed. Diagnostic Surgical Pathology. 2nd edition. New York: Raven Press, 1994, pp. 493–522.

Scheithauer BW, Laws ER Jr, Kovacs K, et al. Pituitary adenomas of the multiple endocrine neoplasia type I syndrome. Semin Diagn Pathol 1987; 4:205–211.

Pituitary Adenomas

Behncken A, Saeger W. Lectin-bindings in pituitary adenomas and normal pituitaries. Pathol Res Pract (Germany) 1991; 187:629–631.

Buckley N, Bates AS, Broome JC, et al. P53 protein accumulates in Cushing's adenomas and invasive non-functional adenomas. J Clin Endocrinol Metab 1995; 80:1513–1516.

Challa VR, Marshal RB, Hopkins MB, et al. Pathobiologic study of pituitary tumors: Report of 62 cases with a review of the recent literature. Hum Pathol 1985; 16:873–884.

Furuhata S, Kameya T, Otani M, Toya S. Prolactin presents in all pituitary tumors of acromegalic patients. Hum Pathol 1993; 24:10–15.

Gharib H, Carpenter PC, Scheithauer BW, Service FJ. The spectrum of inappropriate pituitary thyrotropin secretion associated with hyperthyroidism. Mayo Clin Proc 1982; 57:556–563.

Halliday WC, Asa SL, Kovacs K, Scheithauer BW. Intermediate filaments in the human pituitary gland: An immunohistochemical study. Can J Neurol Sci 1990; 17:131–136.

Horvath E. Ultrastructural markers in the pathologic diagnosis of pituitary adenomas. Ultrastruct Pathol 1994; 18:171–179.

Horvath E, Kovacs K. Ultrastructural diagnosis of pituitary adenomas. Microsc Res Tech 1992; 20:107–135.

Horvath E, Kovacs K. The adenohypophysis. In: Kovacs K, Asa SL, eds. Functional Endocrine Pathology. Vol. 1. 1991, pp. 245–281.

Inada K, Oda K, Utsunomiya H, Ito J, Osamura RY. Immunohistochemical analysis of GH-producing adenomas—with special emphasis on plurihormonality of individual tumor cells by double staining. Tokai J Exp Clin Med (Jpn) 1992; 17:213–222.

Kane LA, Leinung MC, Scheithauer BW, et al. Pituitary adenomas in childhood and adolescence. J Clin Endocrinol Metab 1994; 79:1135–1140.

Kontogeorgos G. Pituitary tumors. In: Polak JM, ed. Diagnostic Histopathology of Endocrine Tumors. Edinburgh: Churchill Livingstone, 1993, pp. 227–269.

Kontogeorgos G, Kovacs K, Horvath E, Scheithauer BW. Multiple adenomas of the human pituitary. A retrospective autopsy study with clinical implications. J Neurosurg 1991; 74:243–247.

Kovacs K, Horvath E. Tumors of the pituitary gland. In: Atlas of Tumor Pathology, Second series, Fascicle 21. Washington, D.C.: Armed Forces Institute of Pathology, 1986, pp. 1–264.

Lübke D, Saeger W, Lüdecke DK. Proliferation markers and EGF in ACTH-secreting adenomas and carcinomas of the pituitary. Endocr Pathol 1995; 6:45–55.

Matsuno A, Teramoto A, Takekoshi S, et al. HGH, PRL and ACTH gene expression in clinically nonfunctioning adenomas detected with nonisotopic in situ hybridization method. Endocr Pathol 1995; 6:13–20.

Minderman T, Wilson CB. Pediatric pituitary adenomas. Neurosurgery 1995; 36:259–269.

Nyquist P, Laws ER Jr, Elliot E. Novel features of tumors that secrete both growth hormone and prolactin in acromegaly. Neurosurgery 1994; 35:179–184.

Randall RV, Scheithauer BW, Laws ER Jr, et al. Pituitary adenomas associated with hyperprolactinemia: A clinical and immunohistochemical study of 97 patients operated on transsphenoidally. Mayo Clin Proc 1985; 60:753–762.

Riva C, Leutner M, Capella C, et al. Different expression of chromogranin A and chromogranin B in various types of pituitary adenomas. Zentralbl Pathol 1993; 139:165–170.

Röcken C, Uhlig H, Saeger W, et al. Amyloid deposits in pituitary adenomas: Immunohistochemistry and in situ hybridization. Endocr Pathol 1995; 6:135–143.

Salgado LR, Mendonca BB, Goldman J, et al. Failure of partial hypophysectomy as definitive treatment in Cushing's disease owing to nodular corticotrope hyperplasia: Report of four cases. Endocr Pathol 1995; 6:57–66.

Samuels MH, Ridgway EC. Glycoprotein-secreting pituitary adenoma. Baillieres Clin Endocrinol Metab 1995; 9:337–358.

Sanno N, Teramoto A, Matsuno A, et al. Clinical and immunohistochemical studies on TSH-secreting pituitary adenoma: Its multihormonality and expression of Pit-1. Mod Pathol 1994; 7:893–899.

Scheithauer BW. The pituitary and sellar region. In: Sternberg SS, ed. Diagnostic Surgical Pathology. 2nd edition. New York: Raven Press, 1994, pp. 493–522.

Scheithauer BW, Kovacs K, Stefaneanu L, et al. The pituitary in gigantism. Endocr Pathol 1995; 6:173–187.

Sirbelgeld DL, Mayberg MR, Berger MS, et al. Pituitary oncocytomas: Clinical features, characteristics in cell culture, and treatment recommendations. J Neurooncol 1993; 16:39–46.

Stefaneanu L, Kovacs K. Light microscopic, special stains and immunohistochemistry in the diagnosis of pituitary adenomas. In: Lloyd RV, ed. Surgical Pathology of the Pituitary Gland. Major Problems in Pathology, Vol. 27. Philadelphia: WB Saunders, 1993, pp. 34–51.

Terada T, Kovacs K, Stefaneanu L, Horvath E. Incidence, pathology and recurrence of pituitary adenomas: Study of 647 unselected surgical cases. Endocr Pathol 1995; 6:301–310.

Tindall GT, Barrow DL. Anatomy. In: Tindall GT, Barrow DL, eds. Disorders of the Pituitary. St. Louis: CV Mosby, 1986.

Yamada S, Aiba T, Sano T, et al. Growth hormone-producing adenomas: Correlations between clinical characteristics and morphology. Neurosurgery 1993; 33:20–27.

Plurihormonal Pituitary Adenomas

Corenblum B, Sirek AMT, Horvath E, et al. Human mixed somatotrophic and lactotrophic pituitary adenomas. J Clin Endocrinol Metab 1976; 42:857–863.

Guyda H, Robert F, Colle E, Hardy J. Histologic, ultrastructural, and hormonal characterization of a pituitary tumor secreting both hGH and prolactin. J Clin Endocrinol Metab 1973; 36:531–547.

Horvath E, Kovacs K. Fine structural cytology of the adenohypophysis in rat and man. J Electron Microsc Tech 1988; 8:401–432.

Horvath E, Kovacs K, Scheithauer BW, et al. Pituitary adenomas producing growth hormone, prolactin and one or more glycoprotein hormones. Ultrastruct Pathol 1984; 5:171–183.

Scheithauer BW, Horvath E, Kovacs K, et al. Plurihormonal pituitary adenomas. Semin Diagn Pathol 1986; 3:69–82.

Ectopic Pituitary Adenomas

Ciocca DR, Puy LA, Stati AO. Identification of seven hormone-producing cell types in the human pharyngeal hypophysis. J Clin Endocrinol Metab 1985; 60:212–216.

Langford L, Batsakis JG. Pituitary gland involvement of the sinonasal tract. Ann Otol Rhinol Laryngol 1995; 104:167–169.

Lloyd RV. Ectopic pituitary adenomas. In: Lloyd RV, ed. Surgical Pathology of the Pituitary Gland. Major Problems in Pathology, Vol. 27. Philadelphia: WB Saunders, 1993, pp. 116–120.

Lloyd RV, Chandler WF, Kovacs K, Ryan N. Ectopic pituitary adenomas with normal anterior pituitary glands. Am J Surg Pathol 1986; 10:546–552.

Tanaka T, Watanabe K, Nakasu S, Handa J. Suprasellar ectopic pituitary adenoma: Report of a case. No Shinkei Geka 1994; 22:1141–1145.

Wenig BM, Heffess CS, Adair CF, Thompson L, Heffner DK. Ectopic pituitary adenomas: A clinicopathologic study of 15 cases. Mod Pathol 1995; 8:56A.

Invasive Pituitary Adenomas

Daita G, Yonemasu Y, Nakai H, et al. Cavernous sinus invasion by pituitary adenomas—relationship between magnetic resonance imaging findings and histologically verified dural invasion. Neurol Med Chir (Tokyo) 1995; 35:17–21.

Gandour-Edwards R, Kapadia SB, Janecka IP, et al. Biologic markers of invasive pituitary adenomas involving the sphenoid sinus. Mod Pathol 1995; 8:160–164.

Ngu SL, Palmer FJ. Invasive pituitary adenoma mimicking meningioma. Australas Radiol 1995; 39:95–96.

Sautner D, Saeger W. Invasiveness of pituitary adenomas. Pathol Res Pract 1991; 187:632–636.

Scheithauer BW, Kovacs K, Laws ER Jr, Randall RV. Pathology of invasive pituitary tumors with special reference to functional classification. J Neurosurg 1986; 65:733–744.

Selman WR, Laws ER, Scheithauer BW, Carpenter SM. The occurrence of dural invasion in pituitary adenomas. J Neurosurg 1986; 64:402–407.

Pituitary Carcinoma

Atienza DM, Vigerski RJ, Lack EE, et al. Prolactin-producing pituitary carcinoma with pulmonary metastases. Cancer 1991; 68:1605–1610.

Frost AR, Tenner S, Tenner M, et al. ACTH-producing pituitary carcinoma presenting as the cauda equina syndrome. Arch Pathol Lab Med 1995; 119:93–96.

Jamjoom A, Moss T, Coakham H, et al. Cervical lymph node metastases from a pituitary carcinoma. Br J Neurosurg 1994; 8:87–92.

Levesque H, Freger P, Gancel A, et al. Primary carcinoma of the pituitary gland with Cushing's syndrome and metastases. Apropos of a case and review of the literature. Rev Med Interne 1991; 12:209–212.

Mixson AJ, Friedman TC, Katz DA, et al. Thyrotropin-secreting pituitary carcinoma. J Clin Endocrinol Metab 1993; 76:529–533.

O'Brian DP, Phillips JP, Rawluk DR, Farrell MA. Intracranial metastases from pituitary adenoma. Br J Neurosurg 1995; 9:211–218.

Pei L, Melmed S, Scheithauer B, et al. H-ras mutations in human pituitary carcinoma metastases. J Clin Endocrinol Metab 1994; 78:842–846.

Petterson T, MacFarlane IA, MacKenzie JM, Shaw MD. Prolactin secreting pituitary carcinoma. J Neurol Neurosurg Psychiat 1992; 55:1205–1206.

Popovic EA, Vatuone JR, Siu KH, et al. Malignant prolactinomas. Neurosurgery 1991; 29:127–130.

Sakamoto T, Itoh Y, Fushimi S, et al. Primary pituitary carcinoma with special cord metastasis—case report. Neurol Med Chir (Tokyo) 1990; 30:763–767.

Walker JD, Grossman A, Anderson JV, et al. Malignant prolactinoma with extracranial metastases: A report of three cases. Clin Endocrinol (Oxf) 1993; 38:411–419.

Metastasis to the Pituitary

Aaberg TM Jr, Kay M, Sternau L. Metastatic tumor to the pituitary. Am J Ophthalmol 1995; 119:779–785.

Nishio S, Tsukamoto H, Fukui M, Matsubara T. Hypophyseal metastatic hypernephroma mimicking a pituitary adenoma. Case report. Neurosurg Rev 1992; 15:319–322.

Verhels TJ, Vanden Broucke P, Dua G, et al. Pituitary metastasis mimicking a pituitary adenoma. A description of two cases. Acta Clin Belg 1995; 50:31–35.

Craniopharyngioma

Kornblith PL, Oldfield EH, Smith B. Tumors of the central nervous system. In: Calabresi P, Schein PS, eds. Medical Oncology. Basic Principles and Clinical Management of Cancer. 2nd edition. Section G: Neoplasms of the Central Nervous System and Supporting Structures. New York: McGraw-Hill, 1993, pp. 959–960.

Kovacs K, Horvath E. Tumors of the pituitary gland. In: Armed Forces Institute of Pathology. Atlas of Tumor Pathology, Second series, Fascicle 21. Washington, D.C.: Armed Forces Institute of Pathology, 1986, pp. 237–251.

Levin VA, Sheline GE, Gutin PH. Neoplasms of the central nervous system. In: DeVita VT, Hellman S, Rosenberg SA, eds. Cancer. Principles and Practice of Oncology. 3rd edition. Vol. 2. Philadelphia: JB Lippincott, 1989, pp. 1601–1602.

McKeever PE, Blaivas M, Sima AA. Neoplasms of the sellar region. In: Lloyd R, ed. Surgical Pathology of the Pituitary Gland. Major Problems in Pathology, Vol. 27. Philadelphia: WB Saunders, 1993, pp. 151–155.

Miller DC. Pathology of craniopharyngiomas: Clinical import of pathological findings. Pediatr Neurosurg 1994; 21:11–17.

Mincione GP, Mincione F, Mennonna P. Cytological features of craniopharyngioma. Pathologica 1991; 83:191–196.

Sklar CA. Craniopharyngioma: Endocrine abnormalities at presentation. Pediatr Neurosurg 1994; 21:18–20.

Szeifert GT, Sipos L, Horvath M, et al. Pathological characteristics of surgically removed craniopharyngiomas: Analysis of 131 cases. Acta Neurochir 1993; 124:139–143.

Tsunoda S, Sasaki T, Tsutsumi A, et al. Clinicopathologic study of craniopharyngioma with sebaceous differentiation. Noshuyo Byori 1993; 10:69–74.

Weiner HL, Wisoff JH, Rosenberg ME, et al. Craniopharyngiomas: A clinicopathological analysis of factors predictive of recurrence and functional outcome. Neurosurgery 1994; 35:1001–1011.

Yamada H, Haratake J, Narasaki T, Oda T. Embryonal craniopharyngioma: Case report of the morphogenesis of a craniopharyngioma. Cancer 1995; 75:2971–2977.

Zimmerman RA. Imaging of intrasellar, suprasellar and parasellar tumors. Semin Roentgenol 1990; 25:174–197.

CHAPTER 3

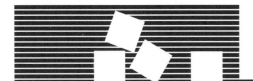

Non-Neoplastic Lesions of the Thyroid Gland

A. CLASSIFICATION OF NON-NEOPLASTIC LESIONS OF THE THYROID GLAND

- Table 3–1.

B. DEVELOPMENTAL

1. Heterotopia or Ectopic Thyroid Tissue

Definitions: *Heterotopia*—the presence of otherwise normal-appearing tissue in an abnormal location. *Ectopic thyroid tissue*—the presence of thyroid tissue in any location other than its normal anatomic position.

Synonyms: Aberrant rests; ectopia; choristoma.

- Ectopic thyroid tissue may be present in any location from the tongue (foramen cecum at the base of the tongue) to the suprasternal notch (site of the normal gland).
- Ectopic thyroid tissue may represent a failure of descent from the foramen cecum (median anlage) or, less likely, a differentiation of thyroid tissue in abnormal locations.
- Excluding thyroglossal duct cysts, the presence of ectopic thyroid tissue is rare and is almost exclusively seen in suprahyoid locations.
- The most common ectopic focus for thyroid tissue is the base of the tongue; such tissue is referred to as lingual thyroid.
- Normal thyroid tissue may be found within the soft tissue structures (fat and muscle) of the cervical neck; this reflects a developmental abnormality and should not be mistaken for malignancy. The absence of a tissue response such as fibrosis (desmoplasia) or the presence of architectural or cytomorphologic changes indicative of a neoplasm (i.e., papillary carcinoma) can be helpful in differentiating normal (ectopic) thyroid tissue from neoplastic thyroid tissue.
- Imaging with ^{123}I may establish the diagnosis noninvasively.
- Any thyroid tissue found lateral to the large neck vessels should be considered metastatic tumor rather than ectopia.

Table 3–1

CLASSIFICATION OF NON-NEOPLASTIC LESIONS OF THE THYROID

Developmental

Heterotopia or ectopia of thyroid tissue
Lingual thyroid
Thyroglossal duct cyst
Lateral aberrant thyroid, parasitic nodule, and mechanical implantation
Mediastinal thyroid and other sites of thyroid tissue
Intranodal thyroid inclusions
Struma ovarii and associated lesions
Follicular epithelial metaplasia: squamous metaplasia, oxyphilic metaplasia

"Inclusions" in the Thyroid

Intrathyroidal parathyroid tissue, thymic tissue, salivary gland tissue
Intrathyroidal epithelial (branchial cleftlike) cysts
Ultimobranchial apparatus rests
Intrathyroidal fat, muscle, and cartilage
Pigment and crystals in the thyroid
    Iron, lipofuscin, crystals
    Black thyroid (minocycline)

Nonautoimmune Thyroiditides (Inflammatory, Infectious and Noninfectious)

Acute inflammatory conditions
Infectious thyroiditis
Granulomatous thyroiditis (subacute thyroiditis, de Quervain's thyroiditis
Multifocal granulomatous thyroiditis (palpation thyroiditis)
Invasive fibrous thyroiditis (Reidel's disease)
Radiation thyroiditis
Drug-induced thyroiditis
Infectious granulomatous thyroiditis
Sarcoidosis of the thyroid gland

Autoimmune Thyroiditis

Chronic lymphocytic thyroiditis and Hashimoto's thyroiditis
Others
Autoimmune hyperthyroidism (diffuse hyperplasia or Graves' disease)

Goiters

Nodular goiter
Congenital inborn disorders (dyshormonogenetic goiter)
Amyloid goiter

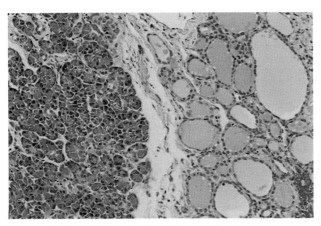

Figure 3–1. Ectopic thyroid tissue in the pancreas.

- Other sites in which ectopic thyroid tissue can occur include (moving in a cranial to a caudal direction):
  - Sella turcica, larynx, trachea, aortic arch, heart, pericardium, esophagus, hepatobiliary sites (liver, gallbladder, and common bile duct), pancreas, retroperitoneum, vagina, and inguinal region.
  - Histologically, ectopic foci of thyroid tissue should include the presence of thyroid tissue that appears normal with no features of thyroid papillary carcinoma and no evidence of bona fide thyroid malignant neoplasm that may be metastatic to these sites or directly extend to these sites.
  - In the presence of a malignant follicular-derived neoplasm within the thyroid gland proper, the presence of thyroid tissue in "ectopic" sites in all probability represents metastatic disease.
- In general, ectopic thyroid tissue is benign; however, different types of malignant neoplasms may arise within ectopic thyroid tissue, including papillary carcinoma and follicular carcinoma.
- Complete or partial agenesis of the thyroid gland is extremely rare.
- Rarely, familial thyroid ectopia may occur.

2. Lingual Thyroid

Clinical

- Affects women more than men; most often diagnosed in adolescence but may occur over a wide age range from birth to the seventh decade of life.
- Most frequently seen along the midline of the base of the tongue between the foramen cecum and the epiglottis; rarely, the body of the tongue may be affected.
- Most common symptom is dysphagia. Lingual thyroid may grow quite large, resulting in dyspnea, orthopnea, and severe respiratory distress. Other symptoms may include bleeding, voice changes, and a foreign body sensation.
- In more than 75% of patients cervical thyroid tissue is absent (total migration failure), and the lingual thyroid represents the only thyroid tissue present. Surgical removal of the lingual thyroid results in hypothyroidism.
- Appropriate preoperative clinical work-up for lingual thyroid includes scintigraphy studies with technetium or radioiodine in order to:
  - Determine whether normally placed thyroid tissue is present or absent.
  - Determine whether there are other ectopic foci of thyroid tissue (thyroid follicles may be found in the hyoid region).
  - Determine the functional activity of the lingual thyroid tissue.
- Seventy percent of patients with symptomatic lingual thyroid are hypothyroid, and 10% suffer from cretinism.

Radiology

- Computed tomographic (CT) scans show a mass at the base of the tongue that has a greater density than the tongue.

Pathology

Gross

- Lingual thyroid tissue generally is submucosal and varies in appearance from a smooth to a lobulated or nodular

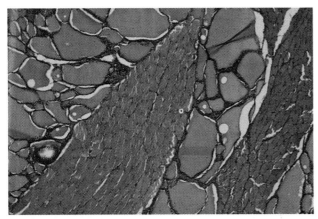

Figure 3–2. Thyroid tissue in skeletal muscle of the neck found near the isthmic portion of the thyroid. This thyroid tissue probably represents a developmental anomaly rather than ectopia.

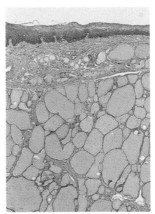 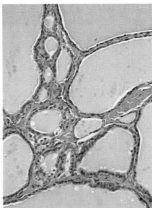

Figure 3–3. Lingual thyroid. *Left,* The lingual squamous epithelium overlies a submucosa that focally retains its seromucous glands but is replaced predominantly by unencapsulated benign thyroid tissue. *Right,* The thyroid follicular epithelium is essentially normal in appearance.

mass, red in color and with a soft to firm consistency; it ranges in size from 2 to 3 cm.
■ The overlying mucosa may be intact or ulcerated.

Histology

■ Ectopic thyroid tissue is submucosal and unencapsulated.
■ The thyroid tissue may be nodular and hypercellular; the thyroid follicular epithelium is essentially normal in appearance (i.e., without evidence of papillary carcinoma).
■ Thyroid tissue may extend into skeletal muscle.

Differential Diagnosis

■ Lymphoepithelial cyst of the oral cavity.

Treatment and Prognosis

■ Therapy for lingual thyroid varies:
  • For symptomatic patients, surgical excision (intraoral or by means of a pharyngotomy) is the treatment of choice; in patients without normally situated cervical thyroid tissue or other ectopic foci of thyroid tissue, autotransplantation of thyroid tissue into the neck muscles can be done.
  • Other modes of therapy include shrinking the mass through the use of thyroid hormones or radioactive iodine (^{131}I) to ablate the lingual thyroid. The use of radioactive iodine results in destruction of other thyroid tissue and may also cause sloughing of the gland and hemorrhage.
■ Prognosis is good.

Additional Facts

■ Malignant transformation of lingual thyroid tissue with metastasis to the cervical lymph nodes and lungs has been reported (limited to men who were older than 35 years of age), but this is rare, and not all of the reported cases are convincing.
■ Incisional biopsies must be performed with caution because they may cause sloughing of the gland, infection, necrosis, or hemorrhage.
■ The majority of patients who are symptomatic are women; contributing factors are thought to be related to puberty, pregnancy, and menopause.

3. Thyroglossal Duct Cyst

Definition: Persistence and cystic dilatation of the thyroglossal duct in the midline of the neck.

Clinical

■ No gender predilection; occurs over a wide age range, but the majority of patients present before the fourth decade of life.
■ Most of these cysts occur in the midline of the neck above the thyroid isthmus but below the level of the hyoid bone; thyroglossal duct cysts are nearly always connected to the hyoid bone. Uncommonly, they may occur lateral to the

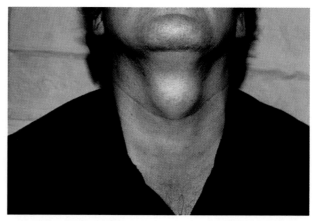

Figure 3–4. Thyroglossal duct cyst appearing as a midline neck mass at the level of the hyoid bone.

midline but not in the lateral portion of the neck (i.e., lateral to the jugular vein).
■ The clinical presentation of an uninfected thyroglossal duct cyst is usually that of an asymptomatic midline neck mass. The mass typically moves upward on swallowing. Inflamed or infected thyroglossal duct cysts may be associated with tenderness and pain.

Radiology

■ Midline round or elongated cystic lesion.
■ Expansion or destruction of the cartilaginous structure of the hyoid bone may be seen.
■ Seldom contains enough thyroid tissue to be seen on scintiscans.
■ The presence of nodular soft tissue excrescences in a midline cystic neck mass on CT scan may suggest the possibility of a papillary carcinoma arising in a thyroglossal duct cyst.

Pathology

Fine Needle Aspiration

■ Squamous or respiratory epithelium.
■ Inflammatory cells are frequently present (mature lymphocytes).

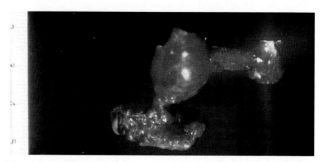

Figure 3–5. Thyroglossal duct cyst resection specimen (Sistrunk procedure) includes en bloc removal of the cyst, the middle third of the hyoid bone, and the suprahyoid tract.

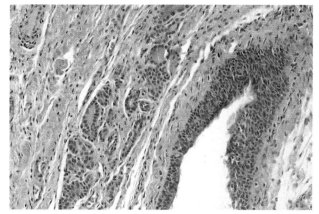

Figure 3–6. Thyroglossal duct cyst composed of a predominantly squamous epithelial lining with focal ciliated respiratory epithelium *(lower)* and benign thyroid tissue within the cyst wall.

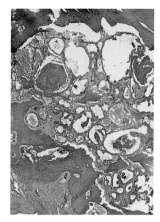
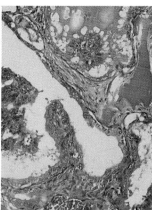

Figure 3–8. *Left,* This thyroid papillary carcinoma has arisen from a thyroglossal duct cyst within the hyoid bone (taken from the case shown in Fig. 3–7). *Right,* Papillary frond with fibrovascular core; the nuclear features are those of a papillary carcinoma.

Gross

- Thyroglossal duct cysts are smooth-walled cystic structures that usually measure less than 2 cm in diameter.
- The cystic content includes clear mucinous fluid; infected cysts contain purulent material.

Histology

- In noninflamed cysts, the cyst lining is composed of respiratory (columnar) epithelium, but it may also include squamous epithelium.
- In the presence of inflammation, the cyst lining undergoes metaplastic change and consists of squamous epithelium.
- The presence of thyroid tissue in the cyst wall varies and may depend on the extent of specimen sampling; in general, thyroid tissue is found in more than 60% of cases.
- The thyroid tissue may be normal, hyperplastic, and nodular, or neoplastic (see below).
- Fibrosis and a chronic inflammatory cell infiltrate are seen in the cyst wall.

Differential Diagnosis

- Thymic cyst.
- Metastatic (cystic) thyroid papillary carcinoma (Chapter 8D, #2).

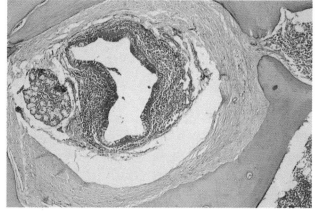

Figure 3–7. Thyroglossal duct cyst within the hyoid bone.

- Laryngocele.
- Branchial cleft cyst.

Treatment and Prognosis

- Surgery is the treatment of choice. En bloc surgical resection of the cyst, the middle third of the hyoid bone (Sistrunk procedure), and the suprahyoid tract up to the foramen cecum is recommended; this extended surgery will prevent recurrence.
- Adequate surgery results in cure with a low rate of recurrence, if any.

Additional Facts

- Both benign and malignant neoplasms may be associated with thyroglossal duct cysts.
- Benign tumors include follicular adenomas.
- Development of a carcinoma in a thyroglossal duct cyst is rare; most carcinomas that develop in this situation are papillary carcinomas, and there are rare examples of follicular carcinomas, squamous (epidermoid) carcinomas, and anaplastic carcinomas. Squamous or epidermoid carcinomas, in all probability, arise from the cyst lining rather than from the thyroid cell component.
- Papillary carcinomas arising from a thyroglossal duct cyst:
  - Occur more commonly in women than in men.
  - Occur over a wide age range (first to eighth decades of life).
  - Are of the usual morphologic type.
  - Are treated in the same way as benign thyroglossal duct cysts.
  - Have a similar (excellent) prognosis to that of thyroid papillary carcinomas.
  - May recur or metastasize and, rarely, may be lethal.
- C-cell related lesions, including medullary carcinomas, do not occur in thyroglossal duct cysts because of the different embryologic derivation of the C cells.

4. Lateral Aberrant Thyroid, Parasitic Nodule, and Mechanical Implantation

Definition: Thyroid tissue, normal or hyperplastic, located lateral to the jugular vein. Nodular hyperplasia of this "ectopic" tissue has been referred to as a parasitic nodule.

- Criteria for a diagnosis of lateral aberrant thyroid or parasitic nodule include the following:
  - The thyroid tissue is not identified in relation to a lymph node. If the thyroid tissue is seen in a lymph node, it should be considered a metastatic carcinoma. In cases of lateral aberrant thyroid with associated lymphocytic thyroiditis, the presence of a prominent lymphoid infiltrate gives the overall impression that the tissue is from a lymph node, leading to a mistaken diagnosis of metastatic carcinoma. However, nodal tissue has subcapsular sinuses, whereas thyroid tissue with lymphocytic thyroiditis does not.
  - The aberrant thyroid tissue should not demonstrate the histomorphologic features of a thyroid papillary carcinoma.
- The "aberrant" tissue may be connected to the thyroid by a thin fibrous strand that may or may not be appreciated by the surgeon or the pathologist, or there may be no discernible attachment to the thyroid gland proper.
- Mechanical implantation of thyroid tissue that is unattached to the thyroid gland may be the result of prior surgery or accidental trauma. In such instances, there is usually a prominent fibrotic reaction or suture material is associated with the thyroid tissue.

5. Mediastinal Thyroid (Substernal Goiter)

Definition: The presence of goitrous thyroid extending from the thyroid gland proper into the mediastinum (substernal or retrosternal).

- The clinical parameters including treatment of substernal goiter are similar to those described for goiters (adenomatoid nodules) situated within the normally located thyroid (see Chapter 7).
- As a multinodular goiter enlarges, it has a tendency to move inferiorly owing to fascial planes that favor this migration.
- When the thyroid gland enters the thoracic inlet, reduced pressure on inspiration may accelerate the migration; clinically, the inferior part of the gland cannot be determined owing to its location behind the manubrium.
- On chest x-rays, an anterior mediastinal mass may be seen. Thyroid scans (with ^{123}I) may show functional activity as well as the inferior extension of the thyroid gland.
- CT and magnetic resonance imaging (MRI) are extremely useful tools in the diagnosis of mediastinal goiters. Features of a mediastinal mass seen on CT scans that favor or suggest a thyroid origin (substernal goiter) include (1) anatomic continuity with the cervical thyroid; (2) CT density greater than that of muscle; (3) a rise in CT density and prolonged enhancement following contrast injection

($\geq$ 2 minutes); (4) multiple areas of calcification and proximity of the mass to the trachea.

- Most mediastinal goiters are benign (adenomatoid nodules), but thyroid malignancies may occur in mediastinal thyroid tissue, including follicular carcinomas, papillary carcinomas (microscopic, other), and anaplastic carcinoma.
- Mediastinal goiters generally do not respond to thyroid suppression treatment and require surgical removal; further, because of the risk of sudden enlargement with its accompanying possibility of airway compression or obstruction, intrathoracic goiters should be surgically removed.
- Mediastinal (substernal) thyroid tissue representing excessive migration of the thyroglossal duct can occur; however, in the presence of mediastinal goitrous tissue, it is probable that the hyperplastic thyroid extended into the mediastinum from its normal location.

6. Thyroid Inclusions in Lymph Nodes

- It is controversial whether benign thyroid inclusions in lymph nodes truly exist or whether *all* thyroid tissue located in lymph nodes, regardless of nodal site or degree of tumor differentiation, represents metastatic carcinoma from an occult primary thyroid tumor; we favor the latter interpretation.
- A diagnosis of metastatic thyroid papillary carcinoma can be made if the thyroid tissue is located in a lymph node. This is true irrespective of the architectural and/or cytomorphologic features. Thyroid follicular "inclusions" in lymph nodes should be considered as metastatic deposits. Certainly, the presence of abnormal thyroid tissue and/or psammoma bodies is indicative of a diagnosis of metastatic thyroid papillary carcinoma.
- Diagnostic confusion may occur when the thyroid is involved by chronic lymphocytic thyroiditis. This is particularly true when the lymphocytic thyroiditis is prominent

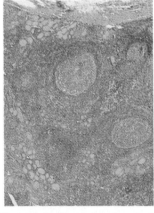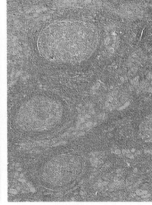

Figure 3–9. Chronic lymphocytic thyroiditis. The extent of lymphocytic thyroiditis, including numerous germinal centers, simulates the appearance of a lymph node. In this situation, the presence of thyroid tissue in particular, lying immediately beneath the thyroid capsule, may be misinterpreted as metastatic thyroid carcinoma to a lymph node. However, unlike a true lymph node, the tissue does not have subcapsular sinuses, and the thyroid tissue is dispersed relatively evenly throughout the tissue, a pattern that is not seen in metastatic papillary carcinoma.

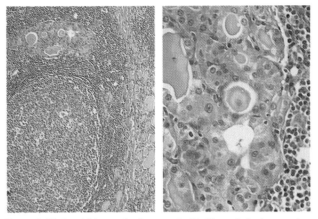

Figure 3–10. In addition to the features cited in Figure 3–9, changes characteristic of chronic lymphocytic thyroiditis include fibrosis and oxyphilic metaplasia of the thyroid follicular epithelium. Most important, the thyroid tissue does not show the cytomorphologic features of thyroid papillary carcinoma. The features shown overall in Figures 3–9 and 3–10 should help minimize potential diagnostic confusion with nodal metastatic thyroid carcinoma.

at the peripheral portion of the gland (subcapsular) or involves a nodule of displaced thyroid tissue located outside the main gland or within perithyroidal adipose tissue. In this situation, the lymphocytic thyroiditis, including germinal centers, could simulate the appearance of a lymph node, so that the thyroid tissue might be considered metastatic to a "lymph node." However, unlike genuine lymph nodes, this tissue does not have subcapsular spaces, and the thyroid follicular epithelium shows changes associated with lymphocytic (Hashimoto's) thyroiditis, including cytoplasmic oxyphilia and enlarged nuclei, but does not have the cytomorphologic features of papillary carcinoma.

7. Ovarian Thyroid Tissue

Definition: Thyroid tissue differentiation that occurs in the presence of an ovarian teratoma.

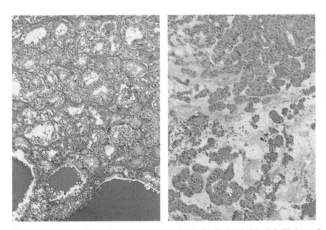

Figure 3–11. Proliferative struma ovarii. *Left,* Colloid-filled follicles of varying sizes. *Right,* Secondary degenerative changes such as fibrosis can be seen.

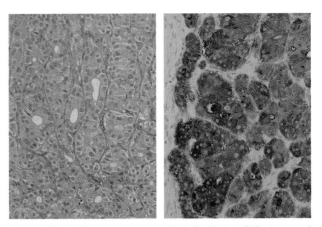

Figure 3–12. Proliferative struma ovarii. *Left,* Obvious follicular growth but minimal colloid (seen within the small follicles toward the lower end of the illustration). *Right,* Confirmation of thyroid follicular tissue is seen with thyroglobulin immunoreactivity.

a. Struma Ovarii

Definition: Ovarian teratomas in which at least 50% of the tissue component is composed of thyroid tissue.

Clinical

- The presence of thyroid tissue in ovarian teratomas varies and may be a function of adequate sampling; benign thyroid tissue occurs in from 5% to 15% of mature ovarian teratomas.
- May occur in a wide age range from the second to the ninth decades of life.
- Clinical presentation (of ovarian teratomas in general) is that of an abdominal mass with acute abdominal pain.
- Functional abnormalities including hyperthyroidism may occur. Patients may present with ascites that in the presence of an ovarian mass may suggest an ovarian carcinoma; ascites and hydrothorax ("pseudo-Meig's syndrome") may occur.
- Bilaterality may occur in up to 5% of cases.

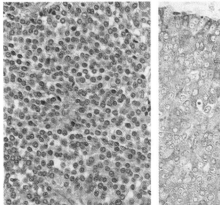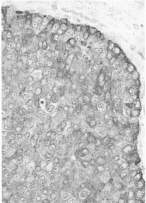

Figure 3–13. Strumal carcinoid. *Left,* The thyroid tissue within the ovary (not shown) was admixed with this cellular infiltrate composed of cells with round nuclei and a stippled chromatin. *Right,* These cells are chromogranin positive.

Pathology

Gross

■ Struma ovarii often resemble a nodular goiter, appearing as multiple glistening brown nodules.

Histology

■ Thyroid tissue may be only one of many tissue types of a teratoma and may represent only a minor component of an ovarian teratoma.
■ The histology of struma ovarii most often is that of normal-appearing thyroid tissue or a multinodular goiter with colloid-filled, variably sized follicles lined by flattened follicular epithelial cells. Papillary hyperplasia of the follicular epithelium may be seen. Secondary degenerative changes such as fibrosis, cyst formation, and hemorrhage may occur.
■ Discrete mass lesions composed of thyroid tissue with increased cellularity (without evidence of malignancy) may be seen and have been termed **proliferative struma ovarii.**
■ Clear cell and signet ring cell cytoplasmic changes may occur.
■ Changes characteristic of lymphocytic thyroiditis may occur in struma ovarii.
■ Thyroid neoplasms associated with struma ovarii are rare; in theory, any neoplasm affecting the thyroid follicular epithelium proper can occur in patients with struma ovarii, but the most common type of thyroid neoplasm occurring in this situation is papillary carcinoma (papillary and follicular variants).
■ The diagnosis of papillary carcinoma is based on the presence of architectural but especially cytomorphologic features; the presence of invasive growth (vascular or stromal) is not required for a diagnosis of papillary carcinoma.
■ Follicular carcinoma may occur in patients with struma ovarii. In contrast to a diagnosis of papillary carcinoma in this situation, a diagnosis of follicular carcinoma is based on the presence of capsular or vascular invasion and not on the cytologic features of the tumor.
■ Immunohistochemistry: Thyroglobulin reactivity is positive in struma ovarii as well as in thyroid follicular neoplasms (benign and malignant) associated with struma ovarii; reactivity with calcitonin and chromogranin is not present.

Treatment and Prognosis

■ The treatment for ovarian teratomas, including struma ovarii, is surgical excision; unilateral salpingo-oophorectomy or total abdominal hysterectomy and salpingo-oophorectomy (unilateral or bilateral) is recommended.
■ Surgical removal is curative.
■ In patients with benign struma ovarii, if the (cervical) thyroid gland is normal, it can be left alone.
■ Treatment for malignant struma ovarii is similar to benign struma ovarii.
■ Metastatic disease from a papillary carcinoma in patients with struma ovarii may occur to such sites as the contralateral ovary, peritoneum, regional lymph nodes, liver, or brain.

■ Treatment for metastatic thyroid (papillary) carcinoma in patients with struma ovarii may include surgical removal with or without supplemental radioactive iodine therapy. The use of radioactive iodine necessitates ablation of the cervical thyroid gland.
■ The overall prognosis associated with malignant thyroid tumors in struma ovarii has been good; although unusual, fatalities secondary to widespread metastatic disease have occurred.

Additional Facts

■ The term benign strumatosis has been used to describe the presence of thyroid follicular epithelium within the peritoneum; these foci should be considered as representative of metastatic thyroid carcinoma.
■ Rare instances of non-Hodgkin's malignant lymphomas have been reported in patients with struma ovarii.

b. Strumal Carcinoid

Definition: Ovarian tumor that includes the presence of thyroid tissue admixed with carcinoid tumor; in this tumor, other teratomatous elements are usually absent.

Clinical

■ The majority of women with strumal carcinoids are postmenopausal, but this tumor may occur over a wide age range from the third to the eighth decades of life.
■ The clinical presentation is similar to that of any ovarian teratoma (abdominal mass); rare instances of carcinoid syndrome have been reported.

Pathology

■ Histologically, strumal carcinoid is characterized by the presence of normal thyroid tissue admixed with the carcinoid tumor. The diagnosis is made as long as both components are present and is not based on whether one or the other predominates.
■ The carcinoid component has a trabecular growth pattern and is composed of cells with small, round to oval nuclei with dispersed ("salt and pepper") chromatin. Rarely, acellular eosinophilic extracellular material representing stromal amyloid deposition is present.
■ The carcinoid component will be argentaffin and argyrophilic positive. Immunohistochemical evaluation shows calcitonin and chromogranin reactivity but not thyroglobulin reactivity (but thyroglobulin is reactive in the noncarcinoid component of strumal carcinoid). Neurosecretory granules can be seen on ultrastructural analysis.
■ Treatment consists of surgical removal, comprising unilateral salpingo-oophorectomy in younger patients and bilateral oophorectomy and hysterectomy in older patients.
■ The prognosis is considered excellent following surgical removal even in the presence of metastatic tumor; however, fatalities have been reported.
■ The histogenesis of strumal carcinoid remains controversial. Most likely, both histologic elements of this tumor

arise from a common progenitor cell such as that giving rise to ovarian teratomas (an endodermal germ cell).

8. Metaplasia of Thyroid Follicular Epithelium

Definition: A benign process in which there is a phenotypic alteration from one cell type to another.

a. Squamous Metaplasia

- Squamous metaplasia of the thyroid is a benign process in which the normal follicular epithelium changes to one with squamous cell features.
- Squamous metaplasia of thyroid follicular epithelium can occur in a wide variety of situations (Table 3–2).
- The clinical features in which squamous metaplasia occurs is based on the pathologic process underlying it.
- Most often, squamous metaplasia of thyroid follicular epithelium is associated with lymphocytic thyroiditis and adenomatoid nodules with retrogressive changes; squamous metaplasia not infrequently is associated with thyroid papillary carcinoma (with or without lymphocytic thyroiditis).
- The histology of squamous metaplasia includes a bland appearance in which there are nests of round to oval cells (including "morule" formations) with no infiltrative growth. Keratinization and intercellular bridges can be seen, pleomorphism and atypia are absent, the nuclear to cytoplasmic ratio is low, and mitotic figures may be seen but are limited in number, and atypical mitoses are not present.
- Immunohistochemistry: Squamous metaplastic cells are cytokeratin positive, usually thyroglobulin negative, and show negative reactions with calcitonin, chromogranin, and carcinoembryonic antigen (CEA).
- Treatment and prognosis depend on the situation in which the squamous metaplasia occurs.

Additional Facts

- Primary thyroid squamous cell carcinoma and mucoepidermoid carcinoma are thought to arise from squamous metaplasia of thyroid follicular epithelial cells.

Table 3–2
THYROID LESIONS THAT MAY HAVE ASSOCIATED SQUAMOUS METAPLASIA

Non-Neoplastic

Nodular goiter (adenomatoid nodules)
Chronic lymphocytic thyroiditis (Hashimoto's thyroiditis) and variants
Following fine needle aspiration or biopsy
Developmental:
   Solid cell nests
   Thymic rests

Neoplasms

Papillary carcinoma
Diffuse sclerosing variant of papillary carcinoma
Primary squamous cell carcinoma
Primary mucoepidermoid carcinoma
Metastatic squamous cell carcinoma to the thyroid
Teratoma

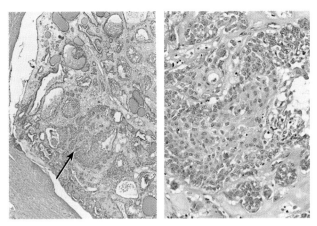

Figure 3–14. *Left,* Adenomatoid nodule with foci of squamous metaplasia *(arrow). Right,* At higher magnification, the metaplastic foci include individual cell keratinization.

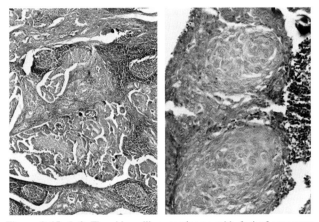

Figure 3–15. *Left,* Thyroid papillary carcinoma with foci of squamous metaplasia. *Right,* The metaplastic foci include squamous eddies or whorls.

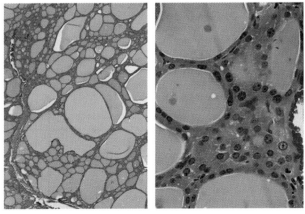

Figure 3–16. *Left,* Oxyphilic metaplasia occurring in an adenomatoid nodule. *Right,* Oxyphilic metaplasia is characterized by the presence of a brightly eosinophilic and granular cytoplasm. Cytoplasmic oxyphilia induces nuclear enlargement with pleomorphic changes. Prominent nucleoli are also seen. Despite the nuclear enlargement, the nuclei remain round and regular with a coarse chromatin pattern. These are not the features of a papillary carcinoma.

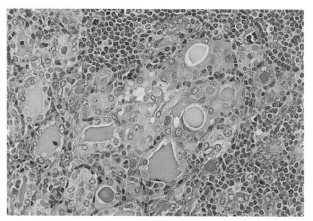

Figure 3–17. Oxyphilic metaplasia occurring in the presence of chronic lymphocytic thyroiditis. In this example, the nuclei are enlarged and have nuclear chromatin clearing, features that may raise the possibility of papillary carcinoma. In contrast to papillary carcinoma, the nuclei of cells in oxyphilic metaplasia remain round and regular. Additional cytomorphologic and architectural features of papillary carcinoma are not present.

- An alternative theory of the origin of squamous cells in the thyroid is that solid cell nests of ultimobranchial derivation are responsible for this change rather than follicular epithelial cells; however, there is much more evidence favoring a follicular epithelial cell origin for squamous cells in the thyroid gland.

b. Oxyphilic or Oncocytic Metaplasia

Definition: The word oncocyte is derived from the Greek word meaning "swollen" and results from an increase in the mitochondrial content of a cell. On light microscopy, an oxyphilic cell is one that has a prominent granular eosinophilic-appearing cell cytoplasm. Oxyphilia is not limited to the thyroid but occurs in many nonendocrine organs as well as in other endocrine organs (pituitary, parathyroid, adrenal gland).

Synonyms for oxyphilic cell: Oncocyte; Hürthle cell (the latter is restricted to the thyroid gland). In all other (extrathyroidal) sites, the use of the terms oxyphilic and oncocytic is interchangeable.

- Hürthle originally described the cell that is now thought to represent the parafollicular cell or C cell of ultimobranchial derivation and not the oncocyte; the latter was originally described by Askanazy.
- The use of the designation Hürthle, oxyphilic, or oncocytic in relation to thyroid lesions is purely descriptive and indicates a type of change in a cell; it does *not* indicate, in itself, a specific diagnosis or any specified biologic behavior. Too often, clinicians assume that a "Hürthle cell neoplasm" is malignant and is synonymous with a follicular carcinoma; this belief is erroneous because oxyphilic cell changes can be seen in both non-neoplastic and neoplastic (benign and malignant) thyroid lesions (Table 3–3).
- Histologically, an oxyphilic cell is characterized by the presence of an abundant eosinophilic, granular-appearing cytoplasm.

Table 3–3
THYROID LESIONS THAT MAY HAVE OXYPHILIC CELL CHANGES

Non-Neoplastic lesions

Nodular goiter (adenomatoid nodules)
Chronic lymphocytic thyroiditis (Hashimoto's thyroiditis)
Graves' disease
Postradiation
Aging

Neoplasms

Follicular adenoma variant
Follicular carcinoma variant
Papillary carcinoma variant
C-cell lesions

- Oxyphilia causes enlargement of the cell nucleus, which may lead to an erroneous diagnosis of papillary carcinoma. Diagnostic confusion may be minimized by evaluating the setting in which the oxyphilia occurs (e.g., the presence of a prominent lymphocytic cell infiltrate as seen in lymphocytic thyroiditis) as well as other changes that may support a diagnosis of papillary carcinoma (e.g., architectural and cytomorphologic features).
- In addition to the enlarged nuclei, central eosinophilic nucleoli often are a component of oxyphilic cells.
- Special stains for mitochondria include phosphotungstic acid-hematoxylin (PTAH) stain, in which the oxyphilic cell has a red granular appearance, and Novelli's stain, in which the oxyphilic cell has a dark purple and granular appearance.
- *Immunohistochemistry:* Thyroid oxyphilic cells are cytokeratin and vimentin positive and weakly thyroglobulin reactive; reactions with chromogranin and calcitonin are negative, and variable positive reactions with CEA may be seen.
- *Electron microscopy:* The cytoplasm is filled with mitochondria showing abnormalities in size, shape, and content.
- Oxyphilic cells, perhaps due to the oxygen-sensitive nature of mitochondria, may be easily traumatized, leading to marked degenerative changes following such events as fine needle aspiration. Degenerative changes in oxyphilic lesions may include pseudopapillary growth and infarction.
- Clear cell changes in follicular epithelial cells may be associated with, and perhaps arise from, oxyphilic metaplasia.
- There is no specific treatment for oxyphilic metaplasia of follicular epithelial cells; treatment and prognosis depend on the situation in which the oxyphilic cell changes are seen.

C. "INCLUSIONS" IN THE THYROID

The embryologic development of the thyroid in association with the branchial and pharyngeal pouches allows for incorporation of other branchial and pharyngeal pouch-derived endodermal and mesodermal structures within the thyroid gland.

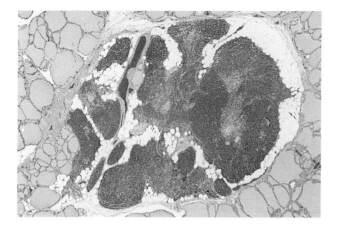

Figure 3–18. Intrathyroidal thymic tissue.

1. Intrathyroidal Parathyroid Tissue, Thymic Tissue, Salivary Gland Tissue

- Branchial and pharyngeal pouch endodermal structures in the thyroid gland include parathyroid tissue, thymic tissue, and salivary gland tissue.
- The presence of these heterotopic tissues generally is an incidental finding and is not cause for surgical removal of the gland.
- Heterotopic parathyroid tissues are found within the substance of the thyroid gland (intrathyroidal), not outside the thyroid gland (beyond the capsule). The presence of parathyroid tissue outside the gland reflects inadvertent surgical removal of parathyroid glands at the time of thyroid resection.
- In theory, any pathologic process that affects these tissues in their normal anatomic location may occur when they are located within the thyroid tissue; however, in general, the histologic appearance of heterotopic tissues is within normal limits, and pathologic changes of these tissues (i.e., hyperplasia, neoplasia) are rare.
  - Intrathyroidal hyperfunctioning parathyroid glands can occur; the hyperparathyroidism seen in these parathyroid glands is most often due to a parathyroid adenoma and less often to an intrathyroidal parathyroid carcinoma or hyperplasia.
  - Thymic-related neoplasms and salivary gland tumors are rare.
- At times, it may be difficult to differentiate thyroid from parathyroid tissues histologically.
  - Overlapping histomorphologic features of thyroid and parathyroid tissues may include:
1. Clear cell or oncocytic cytoplasmic changes.
2. The presence of follicle formations with luminal colloid-like material.

  - Features of parathyroid tissue that may help in differentiating it from thyroid follicular cells include:
1. Overall smaller cell size and hyperchromatic nuclei.
2. More pronounced nesting and/or trabecular growth pattern; distinct cell borders; intracytoplasmic PAS positivity.

3. More delicate vascular pattern.
4. Presence of chromogranin reactivity and absence of thyroglobulin immunoreactivity.

2. Intrathyroidal Epithelial/ Lymphoepithelial Cysts

- Considered uncommon; seen predominantly in adults.
- The majority of these cysts are found incidentally in thyroid glands removed for other reasons; occasionally, the cysts may become very large and present as a thyroid mass.
- Clinically detectable cysts may appear as "cold" nodules on thyroid scans; rarely as "hot" nodules.
- Histologically, the cysts vary in size from small indiscrete lesions to large dominant ones; a dense fibrous capsule separating the cystic lesion from the surrounding thyroid tissue may be present.
- The cysts are lined predominantly by a squamous epithelium consisting of one or more layers of cells; intermixed with the squamous epithelium is a columnar cell (respiratory-type) epithelium that may contain goblet cells that stain for mucin.
- A dense lymphocytic cell infiltrate is seen deep to the cystic epithelial lining; it may include lymphoid aggregates that have reactive germinal centers.
- These cysts almost invariably are associated with a chronic lymphocytic thyroiditis (Hashimoto's thyroiditis) in the thyroid gland.
- *Immunohistochemistry:* The cystic epithelial lining cells are reactive with cytokeratin and polyclonal CEA; no reactivity is present with thyroglobulin, calcitonin, or chromogranin.
- These cysts are of limited biologic concern.
- Because of their histologic similarities with branchial cleft cysts, these intrathyroidal cystic structures have been thought to be of branchial cleft derivation. However, the histogenesis of these cysts is not known; among the relevant considerations are the following possibilities:
  - These cysts are part of the spectrum of changes associated with chronic lymphocytic thyroiditis and represent secondary changes (squamous metaplastic foci with cystic changes). In support of this idea are the facts that

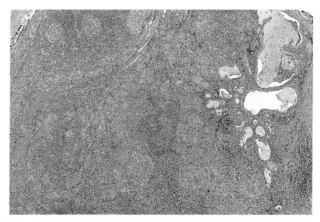

Figure 3–19. Chronic lymphocytic thyroiditis in which variably sized cystic structures filled with mucinous material are seen. These cysts may attain large sizes and represent the dominant pathologic process.

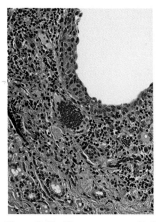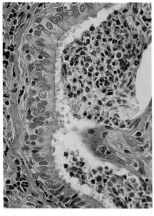

Figure 3–20. The cysts are usually lined by *(left)* squamous epithelium but may include *(right)* ciliated respiratory epithelium. The latter was photographed from cystic structures situated in a lateral thyroid lobe and not in more central (isthmic) portions of the gland, making a thyroglossal duct origin less likely.

(1) chronic lymphocytic thyroiditis is invariably present in the thyroid gland in which the intrathyroidal cysts are seen; (2) identical cysts are present as incidental findings in cases of lymphocytic thyroiditis, and (3) these cystic lesions often are multifocal and bilateral. We favor this interpretation.

- The cysts are acquired and represent cystic degenerative changes of a preexisting lesion (nodule or neoplasm).
- The cysts originate from developmental rests in the thyroid gland such as solid cell nests (SCN), which represent the vestiges of the branchial cleft-derived ultimobranchial apparatus. In support of this theory is the fact that other branchial cleft-derived structures (e.g., parathyroid glands, thymus) have been identified in the thyroid gland.

3. Ultimobranchial Apparatus Rests (Solid Cell Nests)

- Although solid cell nests (SCN) are the subject of debate, they are probably cellular remnants of the ultimobranchial apparatus.

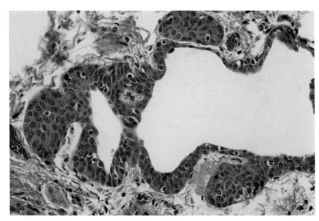

Figure 3–22. Higher magnification of the solid cell nests shows the cellular component composed predominantly of epidermoid-appearing cells with admixed clear-appearing cells.

- SCN within the thyroid tissue generally are found incidentally in thyroid glands removed for other reasons.
- When present, SCN are found to be localized to the lateral lobes (posterolateral and posteromedial aspects), reflecting the migration of ultimobranchial apparatus-derived thyroid cells exclusively to the lateral thyroid lobes.
- SCN, C-cell hyperplasia, and medullary carcinoma are not found and do not occur in the isthmic portion of the thyroid gland.
- SCN are not uncommon and can be found in over 25% of resected thyroid glands.
- SCN appear as small, discrete cell nests or cords composed of epithelial cells with a squamoid (epidermoid) appearance. Clear-appearing cells, cystic changes, and mucinous material are associated with SCN, but keratinization (horny pearl formations or individual cells) and intercellular bridges are not found.
- Mucicarminophilic material can be found in SCN. The presence of mucosubstances in SCN is thought to represent degenerative changes of the epidermoid cells and possibly represents true endodermal-derived C-cell conglomerates.

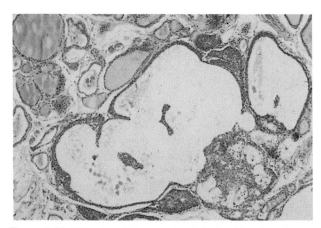

Figure 3–21. Ultimobranchial apparatus–derived solid cell nests composed of discrete foci of epidermoid-appearing cells. In this illustration, the solid cell nests have associated cystic changes.

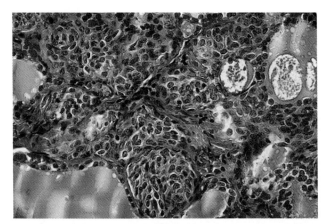

Figure 3–23. Solid cell nests composed of epithelial cells with a squamoid (epidermoid) appearance. Neither keratinization (horny pearl formation or individual cells) nor intercellular bridges are found.

- *Immunohistochemistry:* SCN react positively with calcitonin, chromogranin, synaptophysin, cytokeratin, and polyclonal CEA; they do not react with thyroglobulin.

4. Mesenchymal-Derived "Inclusions" in the Thyroid Gland

Like heterotopic endodermal structures in the thyroid gland, heterotopic mesodermal-derived structures such as fat, muscle, and cartilage can also be identified within the thyroid gland.

a. Fat in the Thyroid

Synonyms: Hamartomatous adiposity; adenolipomatosis.

- Rarely, mature adipose tissue is found within the thyroid gland under normal conditions.
- Mature adipose tissue in the thyroid is also associated with numerous pathologic conditions or lesions including:
  - Adenomatoid nodules, amyloid goiter, lymphocytic thyroiditis, thyroid atrophy, follicular adenoma (adenolipoma), papillary carcinoma, follicular carcinoma, and, rarely, diffuse hyperplasia and dyshormonogenetic goiter.
- The presence of (non-neoplastic) fatty tissue in the thyroid is an incidental finding on removal of the gland for other reasons.
- The amount and distribution of the mature fat varies from a few adipocytes present in a limited portion of the gland to substantial collections in multifocal sites.
- The adipose tissue is intimately admixed with the thyroid tissue and does not appear as a separate, solid mass lesion as it would in an adipose neoplasm.
- Mature adipocytes appear as fairly uniform cells with some variation in size and shape. They are characterized by the presence of a clear to vacuolated cytoplasm that compresses and eccentrically displaces the cell nucleus; the nuclei are hyperchromatic without pleomorphism.
- Rarely, foci of extramedullary hematopoiesis may be seen within the adipose tissue.
- The mechanism by which mature adipose tissue is found in the thyroid is not known; some possible explanations

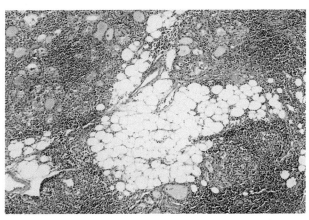

Figure 3–25. Lymphocytic thyroiditis with mature adipose tissue.

include embryologic rests, metaplasia from stromal fibroblasts, senile involution, and the presence of a true neoplastic component.
- Benign and malignant lipogenic tumors of the thyroid gland are extraordinarily uncommon.

b. Muscle in the Thyroid

- Like adipose tissue in the thyroid, skeletal muscle in the thyroid is an incidental finding and may be found in normal conditions as well as in a variety of pathologic conditions.
- The presence of non-neoplastic skeletal muscle in the thyroid is an incidental finding when the gland is removed for other reasons; it is typically found in association with the isthmic portion of the thyroid.
- The skeletal muscle is intimately admixed with the thyroid tissue and does not appear as a separate, solid mass lesion as it would in a myogenic neoplasm.
- Benign and malignant myogenic tumors of the thyroid gland are extraordinarily uncommon.

c. Cartilage in the Thyroid

- As with fat and skeletal muscle, mature cartilage may be found in the thyroid gland (adenochondroma); when

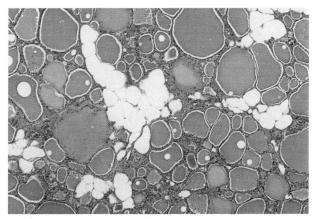

Figure 3–24. Mature adipose tissue in a normal thyroid.

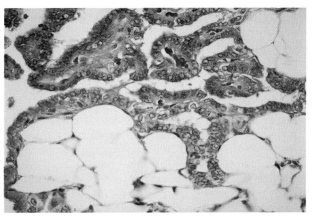

Figure 3–26. Thyroid papillary carcinoma with mature fat.

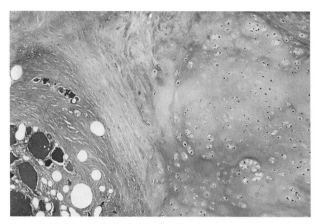

Figure 3–27. Chondroid foci occurring as a degenerative phenomenon in the setting of adenomatoid nodules.

found, it is an incidental finding in glands removed for other reasons.
■ Cartilage in the thyroid may also occur as a metaplastic process associated with some pathologic conditions of the thyroid (e.g., adenomatoid nodules).
■ Benign and malignant cartilaginous tumors of the thyroid gland are extraordinarily uncommon.

5. Pigment and Crystals in the Thyroid

a. Iron

■ Following hemorrhage with release of iron from the red blood cells, resorption takes place, and iron is converted to hemosiderin, which is stored in the cell cytoplasm of phagocytizing cells (macrophages).
■ In the thyroid, hemosiderin can be found in virtually all pathologic conditions and represents an incidental finding. It reflects a secondary phenomenon due to hemorrhage and can follow trauma (fine needle aspiration) and degenerative changes (adenomatoid nodules, neoplasms).
■ Hemosiderin can be found in macrophages, within the stromal tissues, or within the follicular epithelial cells. Hemosiderin is readily apparent in hematoxylin and eosin-stained slides and appears as a coarse brown to yellow pigment. If necessary, iron stains (Prussian blue, Mallory) can be used to identify iron and distinguish it from other pigments.
■ Rarely, iron may be stored in the thyroid as a component of a disorder of iron metabolism rather than as a secondary result of hemorrhage.

b. Lipofuscin

■ Lipofuscin pigment represents a degenerative (aging) phenomenon which consists of an intracytoplasmic accumulation of small yellow to light brown granular-appearing pigment. In the thyroid, lipofuscin pigment can be seen within the follicular epithelial cells.
■ The true nature of lipofuscin has yet to be determined, but it has been shown to react with lipid (Sudan IV) and lipofuscin stains and contains diastase-sensitive, periodic acid-Schiff (PAS)-positive intracytoplasmic material. It

also has lysosomes on electron microscopy and contains histidine and tryptophan; iron staining is absent.
■ Lipofuscin deposition in the thyroid gland is an incidental finding; it is more often seen in thyroid glands from older individuals.
■ There is no evidence that the presence of lipofuscin in any cell, including thyroid follicular cells, causes dysfunction or functional compromise of that cell.

c. Minocycline (Black Thyroid)

■ Minocycline, a tetracycline derivative that is administered to adults for the treatment of various conditions (infections, acne), may cause black pigmentation and discoloration of various sites including the skin and thyroid gland; the latter condition has been referred to as black thyroid.
■ The presence of minocycline-related pigmentation of the thyroid is, by and large, not associated with glandular enlargement (hyperplasia) or functional abnormalities of the gland. Rarely, hypothyroidism may be associated with minocycline pigmentation of the thyroid.
■ The minocycline pigment appears in the cytoplasm of follicular epithelial cells as black granules; it may also be seen within the follicle lumina as large black deposits admixed with colloid.
■ Minocycline shares histochemical, electron microscopic, and elemental analysis features with lipofuscin, including positive staining with PAS, lipid, and lipofuscin stains and the presence of lysosomes and autofluorescence. Argentaffin (Fontana) stains may be positive, and iron staining is negative.
■ The true composition of the minocycline pigment is still not fully known; possibilities include:
  • Degradation products of the drug combined with lipofuscin.
  • Oxidation degradation of the drug itself.
  • Drug interaction with and alteration of tyrosine metabolism.
  • Lysosomal dysfunction.
■ The localization of the pigment may vary from patient to patient such that in the presence of adenomatoid nodules or a follicular neoplasm the pigment may be seen:

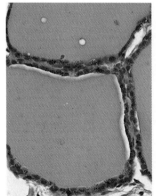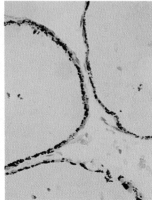

Figure 3–28. Minocycline pigment in follicular epithelial cells. *Left,* The pigment appears as granular and black on hematoxylin and eosin stain. *Right,* the pigment stains positively with argentaffin (Fontana) stains.

- In the pathologic component of the gland and not in the surrounding uninvolved thyroid.
- In the uninvolved thyroid but not in the pathologic component of the gland.
- In both the pathologic component of the gland and the surrounding uninvolved thyroid.
■ Antidepressant agents may be associated with red pigmentation of the thyroid; this is thought to be due to lysosomal accumulation of the drug itself.

d. Crystals

■ Intracolloidal crystals are found not infrequently in the thyroid gland under normal conditions as well as in pathologic conditions.
■ The finding of intracolloidal crystals is not associated with any specific diagnosis and may be present in virtually all thyroid abnormalities.
- The highest prevalence of crystals is associated with benign diseases, most commonly nodular goiters followed by follicular adenomas.
- Crystals may be associated with malignant tumors (follicular carcinomas, papillary carcinomas), but the prevalence is low.
- A low prevalence of crystals is associated with Graves' disease, lymphocytic thyroiditis, and subacute thyroiditis.
■ The frequency of crystal deposits within the thyroid gland appears to increase with age.
■ Intrathyroidal crystals are exclusively found in colloid and do not appear in the cytoplasm of the follicular epithelial cells or in stromal tissues.
■ The crystals are readily apparent by light microscopy; polarization enhances their detection.
■ The crystals vary in size and have a variety of geometric shapes.
■ Chemical analysis of the crystals indicates that they are composed of calcium oxalate.
■ The presence of intracolloidal crystals may be a function of increasing age or disease state; a separate population of patients who have an increased frequency of intracolloidal crystals are those undergoing hemodialysis for chronic renal failure.

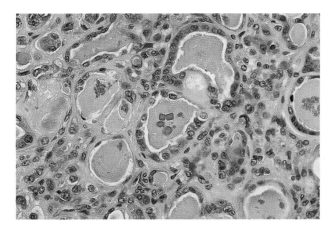

Figure 3–29. Intrafollicular crystals of varying sizes and geometric shapes.

■ The occurrence of crystals in the normal human thyroid is associated with a low-functional state of the thyroid follicles.

Bibliography

Heterotopia or Ectopic Thyroid Tissue

Guimaraes SB, Uceda JE, Lynn HB. Thyroglossal duct remnants in infants and children. Mayo Clin Proc 1972; 47:117–120.
Kaplan M, Kauli R, Lubin E, et al. Ectopic thyroid tissue. A clinical study of 30 children and review. J Pediatr 1978; 92:205–209.
Karelitz JR, Richards JB. Necessity of oblique views in evaluating the functional status of a thyroid nodule. J Nucl Med 1974; 15:782–785.
Kozol RA, Geelhoed GW, Flynn SD, Kinder B. Management of ectopic thyroid nodules. Surgery 1993; 114:1103–1107.
Larochelle D, Arcand P, Belzile M, Gagnon NB. Ectopic thyroid tissue—a review of the literature. J Otolaryngol 1979; 8:523–530.
LiVolsi V. Thyroid lesions in unusual locations. In: Surgical Pathology of the Thyroid. Major Problems in Pathology, Vol. 22. Philadelphia: WB Saunders, 1990, pp. 351–363.
Misaki T, Koh T, Shimbo S. Dual-site thyroid ectopy in a mother and son. Thyroid 1992; 2:325–327.
Salem MA. Ectopic thyroid mass adherent to the oesophagus. J Laryngol Otol 1992; 106:746–747.
Strohschneider T, Timm D, Worbes C. Ectopic thyroid gland tissue in the liver. Chirurg 1993; 64:751–753.

Lingual Thyroid

Alderson DJ, Lannigan FJ. Lingual thyroid presenting after previous thyroglossal cyst excision. J Laryngol Otolaryngol 1994; 108:341–343.
Baughman RA. Lingual thyroid and lingual thyroglossal tract remnants. A clinical and histopathologic study with a review of the literature. Oral Surg 1972; 34:781–799.
Kansal P, Sakati N, Rifai A, Woodhouse N. Lingual thyroid. Diagnosis and treatment. Arch Intern Med 1987; 147:2046–2048.
Katz AD, Zager WJ. The lingual thyroid. Its diagnosis and treatment. Arch Surg 1971; 102:582–585.
Nienas FW, Gorman CA, Devine KD, Woolner LB. Lingual thyroid. Clinical characteristics of 15 cases. Ann Intern Med 1973; 79:205–210.
Willinsky RA, Kassel EE, Cooper PW, et al. Computed tomography of lingual thyroid. J Comput Assist Tomogr 1987; 11:182–183.

Thyroglossal Duct Cyst

Allard RH. The thyroglossal cyst. Head Neck Surg 1982; 5:34–46.
Bourjat P, Cartier J, Woerther JP. Thyroglossal duct cyst in hyoid bone: CT confirmation. J Comput Assist Tomogr 1988; 12:871–873.
Fernandez JF, Ordoñez NG, Schultz PN, et al. Thyroglossal duct carcinoma. Surgery 1991; 110:928–934.
Jaques DA, Chambers RG, Oertel JE. Thyroglossal tract carcinoma. A review of the literature and addition of eighteen cases. Am J Surg 1970; 120:439–446.
LiVolsi VA, Perzin KH, Savetsky L. Carcinoma arising in median ectopic thyroid (including thyroglossal duct tissue). Cancer 1974; 34:1303–1315.
Maziak D, Borowy ZJ, Deitel M, et al. Management of papillary carcinoma arising in thyroglossal-duct anlage. Can J Surg 1992; 35:522–525.
Noyek AM, Friedberg J. Thyroglossal duct and ectopic thyroid disorders. Otolaryngol Clin North Am 1981; 14:187–201.
Silverman PM, Degesys GE, Ferguson BJ, Bierre AR. Papillary carcinoma in a thyroglossal cyst cyst: CT findings. J Comput Assist Tomogr 1985; 9:806–808.
Solomon JR, Rangecroft L. Thyroglossal-duct lesions in childhood. J Pediatr Surg 1984; 19:555–561.

Lateral Aberrant Thyroid, Parasitic Nodule, and Mechanical Implantation

Block MA, Wylie JA, Patton RB, Miller JM. Does benign thyroid tissue occur in the lateral part of the neck? Am J Surg 1966; 12:476–481.
Frantz VK, Forsythe R, Hanford JM, Rogers WM. Lateral aberrant thyroids. Ann Surg 1942; 115:161–183.
Hathaway BM. Innocuous accessory thyroid nodules. Arch Surg 1965; 90:222–227.

Klopp CT, Kirson SM. Therapeutic problems with ectopic non-cancerous follicular thyroid tissue in the neck: 18 case reports according to etiological factors. Ann Surg 1966; 163:653–664.

Kozol RA, Geelhoed GW, Flynn SD, Kinder B. Management of ectopic thyroid nodules. Surgery 1993; 114:1103–1107.

Moses DC, Thompson NW, Nishiyama RH, Sisson JC. Ectopic thyroid tissue in the neck. Benign or malignant. Cancer 1976; 38:361–365.

Sisson JC, Schmid RW, BeierWaltes WH. Sequestered nodular goiter. N Engl J Med 1964; 270:927–932.

Ward R. Relation of tumors of lateral aberrant thyroid tissue to malignant disease of the thyroid gland. Arch Surg 1940; 40:606–615.

Watson MG, Birchall JP, Soames JV. Is "lateral aberrant thyroid" always metastatic tumour? J Laryngol Otol 1992; 106:376–378.

Mediastinal Thyroid (Substernal Goiter)

Bashist B, Ellis K, Gold RP. Computed tomography of intrathoracic goiters. AJR 1983; 140:455–460.

Brown LR, Aughenbaugh GL. Masses of the anterior mediastinum: CT and MR imaging. AJR 1991; 157:1171–1180.

Glazer GM, Axel L, Moss AA. CT diagnosis of mediastinal thyroid. AJR 1982; 138:495–498.

Glikson M, Feigin RD, Libson E, Rubinow A. Anaplastic thyroid carcinoma in a retrosternal goiter presenting as fever of unknown origin. Am J Med 1990; 88:81–82.

Katlic MR, Wang CA, Grillo HC. Substernal goiter. Ann Thorac Surg 1985; 39:391–399.

Lawson VG. The management of airway involvement in thyroid tumors. Arch Otolaryngol 1983; 109:86–90.

LiVolsi V. Thyroid lesions in unusual locations. In: Surgical Pathology of the Thyroid. Major Problems in Pathology, Vol. 22. Philadelphia: W. B. Saunders, 1990, pp. 351–363.

Sand ME, Laws HL, McElvein RB. Substernal and intrathoracic goiter: Reconsideration of surgical approach. Am Surg 1983; 49:196–202.

Sanders LE, Rossi RL, Shahian DM, Williamson WA. Mediastinal goiters. The need for an aggressive approach. Arch Surg 1992; 127:609–613.

Wax MK, Briant TD. Management of substernal goitre. J Otolaryngol 1992; 21:165–170.

Wick MR. Mediastinal cysts and intrathoracic thyroid tumors. Semin Diagn Pathol 1990; 7:285–294.

Thyroid Inclusions in Lymph Nodes

Block MA, Wylie JA, Patton RB, Miller JM. Does benign thyroid tissue occur in the lateral part of the neck. Am J Surg 1966; 12:476–481.

Gerard-Marchant R, Caillou B. Thyroid inclusions in cervical lymph nodes. Clin Endocrinol Metab 1981; 10:337–349.

LiVolsi VA, Perzin KH, Savetsky L. Carcinoma arising in median ectopic thyroid (including thyroglossal duct tissue). Cancer 1974; 34:1303–1315.

Meyer JS, Steinberg JS. Microscopically benign thyroid follicles in cervical lymph nodes. Serial section study of lymph node inclusions and entire thyroid gland in 5 cases. Cancer 1969; 24:302–311.

Roth L. Inclusions of nonneoplastic thyroid tissue within cervical lymph nodes. Cancer 1965; 18:105–111.

Ovarian Thyroid Tissue and Strumal Carcinoid

Brunskill PJ, Rollason TP, Nicholson HO. Malignant follicular variant of papillary struma ovarii. Histopathology 1990; 17:574–576.

Caruso PA, Marsh MR, Minowitz S, Karten G. An intense clinicopathologic study of 305 teratomas of the ovary. Cancer 1971; 27:343–348.

Devaney K, Snyder R, Norris HJ, Tavassoli FA. Proliferative and histologically malignant struma ovarii: A clinicopathologic study of 54 cases. Int J Gynecol Pathol 1993; 12:333–343.

Kempers RD, Dockerty MB, Hoffman DL, Bartholomew LG. Struma ovarii—ascitic, hyperthyroid, and asymptomatic syndromes. Ann Intern Med 1970; 72:883–893.

Marcial-Rojas RA, Medina R. A clinical and pathologic analysis of 268 dermoid tumors. Arch Pathol 1958; 66:577–589.

Robboy SJ, Scully RE. Strumal carcinoid of the ovary: An analysis of 50 cases of a distinctive tumor composed of thyroid tissue and carcinoid. Cancer 1980; 46:2019–2034.

Rosenblum NG, LiVolsi VA, Edmonds PR, Mikuta JJ. Malignant struma ovarii. Gynecol Oncol 1989; 32:224–227.

Talerman A. Carcinoid tumors of the ovary. J Cancer Res Clin Oncol 1984; 107:125–135.

Woodruff JD, Rauh JT, Markley RL. Ovarian struma. Obstet Gynecol 1966; 27:194–202.

Metaplasia of Thyroid Follicular Epithelium

Squamous Metaplasia

Bullock WK, Hummer GJ, Kahler JE. Squamous metaplasia of the thyroid gland. Cancer 1952; 5:966–974.

Dube VE, Joyce TG. Extreme squamous metaplasia in Hashimoto's thyroiditis. Cancer 1971; 27:434–437.

Goldberg HM, Harvey P. Squamous cell cysts of the thyroid. With special reference to the aetiology of squamous epithelium in the human thyroid. Br J Surg 1956; 43:565–569.

LiVolsi VA: Squamous lesions of the thyroid. In: Surgical Pathology of the Thyroid. Major Problems in Pathology, Vol. 22. Philadelphia: W. B. Saunders, 1990, pp. 289–302.

LiVolsi VA, Merino MJ. Squamous cells in the human thyroid gland. Am J Surg Pathol 1978; 2:133–140.

Wenig BM, Adair CF, Heffess CS. Primary mucoepidermoid carcinoma of the thyroid gland: A report of six cases and a review of the literature of a follicular epithelial-derived tumor. Hum Pathol 1995; 26:1099–1108.

Oxyphilic Metaplasia

Bronner MP, LiVolsi VA. Oxyphilic (Askanazy/Hürthle cell) tumors of the thyroid: Microscopic features predict biologic behavior. Surg Pathol 1988; 1:137–150.

Flint A, Lloyd RV. Hürthle-cell neoplasms of the thyroid gland. Pathol Annu 1990; 25(Part 1):37–52.

Friedman NB. Cellular involution in thyroid gland: significance of Hürthle cells in myxedema, exhaustion atrophy, Hashimoto's disease and reaction to irradiation, thiouracil therapy and subtotal resection. J Clin Endocrinol 1949; 9:874–882.

Johnson TL, Lloyd RV, Burney RE, Thompson NW. Hürthle cell thyroid tumors: An immunohistochemical study. Cancer 1987; 59:107–112.

Kendall CH, McCluskey E, Naylor J. Oxyphil cells in thyroid disease: a uniform change? J Clin Pathol 1986; 39:908–912.

Nesland JM, Sobrinho-Simões MA, Holm R, et al. Hürthle cell lesions of the thyroid: A combined study using transmission electron microscopy, scanning electron microscopy, and immunocytochemistry. Ultrastruct Pathol 1985; 8:269–290.

Intrathyroidal Parathyroid Tissue, Thymic Tissue, and Salivary Gland Tissue

Cameselle-Teijeiro J, Varela-Durán J. Intrathyroid salivary gland-type tissue in multinodular goiter. Virchows Arch 1994; 425:331–334.

Carpenter GR, Emery JL. Inclusions in the human thyroid. J Anat 1976; 122:77–89.

Sawady J, Mendelsohn G, Sirota RL, Taxy JB. The intrathyroidal hyperfunctioning parathyroid gland. Mod Pathol 1989; 2:652–657.

Intrathyroidal Epithelial (Branchial Cleft-Like) Cysts

Apel RL, Asa SL, Chalvardjian A, LiVolsi VA. Intrathyroidal lymphoepithelial cysts of probable branchial origin. Hum Pathol 1994; 25:1238–1242.

Beckner ME, Shultz JJ, Richardson T. Solid and cystic ultimobranchial body remnants in the thyroid. Arch Pathol Lab Med 1990; 114:1049–1052.

Delabie J, De Wolf-Peters C, Cappelle L, et al. Branchial cleft like cysts of the thyroid. Am J Surg Pathol 1990; 14:1165–1167.

Dube VE, Joyce GT. Extreme squamous metaplasia in Hashimoto's thyroiditis. Cancer 1971; 27:434–437.

Louis DN, Vickery AL Jr, Rosai J, Wang CA. Multiple branchial-cleft cysts in Hashimoto's thyroiditis. Am J Surg Pathol 1989; 13:45–49.

Williams ED, Toyn CE, Harach HR. The ultimobranchial gland and congenital thyroid abnormalities in man. J Pathol 1989; 159:135–141.

Ultimobranchial Apparatus Rests (Solid Cell Nests)

Autelitano F, Santeusanio G, Tondo UD, et al. Immunohistochemical study of solid cell nests of the thyroid gland found from an autopsy study. Cancer 1987; 59:477–483.

Beckner ME, Shultz JJ, Richardson T. Solid and cystic ultimobranchial body remnants in the thyroid. Arch Pathol Lab Med 1990; 114:1049–1052.

Camaselle-Teijeiro J, Varela-Durán J, Sambade C, et al. Solid cell nests of the thyroid: Light microscopic and immunohistochemical profile. Hum Pathol 1994; 25:684–693.

Harach HR. Solid cell nests of the thyroid: An anatomical and immunohistochemical study for the presence of thyroglobulin. Acta Anat 1985; 122:249–253.

Harach HR. Mixed follicles of the human thyroid gland. Acta Anat 1987; 129:27–30.

Harach HR. Solid cell nests of the thyroid. J Pathol 1988; 155:191–200.

Harach HR, Vujanić GM, Jasani B. Ultimobranchial body nests in human fetal thyroid: An autopsy, histological, and immunohistochemical study in relation to solid cell nests and mucoepidermoid carcinoma. J Pathol 1993; 169:465–469.

Mizukami Y, Nonomura A, Michigishi T, et al. Solid cell nests of the thyroid: A histologic and immuno-histochemical study. Am J Clin Pathol 1994; 101:186–191.

Ozaki O, Ito K, Sugino K, et al. Solid cell nests of the thyroid gland. Virchows Arch [A] 1991; 418:201–205.

Vollenweider I, Hedinger C. Solid cell nests (SCN) in Hashimoto's thyroiditis. Virchows Arch [A] 1988; 412:357–363.

Williams ED, Toyn CE, Harach HR. The ultimobranchial gland and congenital thyroid abnormalities in man. J Pathol 1989; 159:135–141.

Mesenchymal-Derived "Inclusions" in the Thyroid Gland

Fat in the Thyroid

Chesky VE, Dreese WC, Hellwig CA. Adenolipomatosis of the thyroid. Surgery 1953; 34:38–45.

Fuller RH. Hamartomatous adiposity with superimposed amyloidosis of the thyroid gland. J Laryngol Otol 1963; 77:552–562.

Gnepp DR, Ogorzalek JM, Heffess CS. Fat-containing lesions of the thyroid gland. Am J Surg Pathol 1989; 13;605–612.

Hjorth L, Thomsen LB, Nielsen VT. Adenolipoma of the thyroid gland. Histopathology 1986; 10:91–96.

Schmidt C, Beham A, Sweeann HL. Extramedullary haematopoiesis in the thyroid gland. Histopathology 1989; 15:423–425.

Schröder S, Böcker W. Adenolipoma (thyrolipoma) of the thyroid gland: Report of two cases and review of the literature. Virchows Arch [A] 1984; 404:99–103.

Schröder S, Böcker W. Lipomatous lesions of the thyroid gland. Appl Pathol 1985; 3:140–149.

Muscle in the Thyroid

Carpenter GR, Emery JL. Inclusions in the human thyroid. J Anat 1976; 122:77–89.

Cartilage in the Thyroid

Finkle HL, Goldman RL. Heterotopic cartilage in the thyroid. Arch Pathol 1973; 95:48–49.

Visoña A, Pea M, Bozzola L, et al. Follicular adenoma of the thyroid gland with extensive chondroid metaplasia. Histopathology 1991; 18:278–279.

Weitaner S, Appenzeller J. Ectopic cartilage in thyroid. Oral Surg Oral Med Oral Pathol 1973; 36:241–242.

Wolvos TA, Chong FK, Razvi SA, Tully GL III. An unsual thyroid tumor: A comparison to a literature review of thyroid teratomas. Surgery 1985; 97:613–617.

Pigment and Crystals in the Thyroid

Alexander CB, Herrera GA, Jaffe K, Yu H. Black thyroid: Clinical manifestations, ultrastructural findings, and possible mechanisms. Hum Pathol 1985; 16:72–78.

Attwood HD, Dennett X. A black thyroid and minocycline treatment. Br Med J 1976; 2:1109–1110.

Borel DM, Reddy JK. Excessive lipofuscin accumulation in the thyroid gland in mucoviscidosis. Arch Pathol 1973; 96:269–271.

Gordon G, Sparano BM, Kramer AW, et al. Thyroid gland pigmentation and minocycline therapy. Am J Pathol 1984; 117:98–109.

Jennings TA, Shoehan CE, Chodos RB, Figge J. Follicular carcinoma associated with minocycline-induced black thyroid. Endocr Pathol 1996; 7:345–348.

Katoh R, Kawaoi A, Muramatsu A, et al. Birefringent (calcium oxalate) crystals in thyroid diseases. A clinico-pathological study with possible implications for differential diagnosis. Am J Surg Pathol 1993; 17:698–705.

Katoh R, Suzuki K, Hemmi A, Kawaoi A. Nature and significance of calcium oxalate crystals in normal human thyroid gland. A clinicopathological and immunohistochemical study. Virchows Arch [A] 1993; 422:301–306.

Landas SK, Schelper RL, Tio FO, Turner JW, Moore KC, Bennett-Gray J. Black thyroid syndrome: Exaggeration of a normal response? Am J Clin Pathol 1986; 85:411–418.

LiVolsi VA. Pigment, crystals, and infiltrative lesions of the thyroid. In: Surgical Pathology of the Thyroid. Major Problems in Pathology, Vol. 22. Philadelphia: WB Saunders, 1990, pp. 119–130.

MacMahon HE, Lee HY, Rivelis CF. Birefringent crystals in human thyroid. Acta Endocrinol 1968; 58:172–176.

Ohaki Y, Misugi K, Haesgawa H. "Black thyroid" associated with minocycline therapy. Acta Pathol Jpn 1986; 36:1367–1375.

Pastolero GC, Asa SL. Drug-related pigmentation of the thyroid associated with papillary carcinoma. Arch Pathol Lab Med 1994; 118:79–83.

Reid JD, Choi CH, Oldroyd NO. Calcium oxalate crystals in the thyroid: Their identification, prevalence, origin and possible significance. Am J Clin Pathol 1987; 87:443–454.

Richter MN, McCarty KS. Anisotropic crystals in the human thyroid gland. Am J Pathol 1954; 30:55–63.

CHAPTER 4

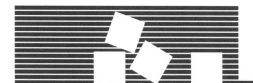

Hypothyroidism and Hyperthyroidism—General Considerations

A. HYPOTHYROIDISM

Definitions: *Primary hypothyroidism*—the clinical and pathologic state that results from decreased thyroidal thyroid hormone production. *Secondary hypothyroidism*—the result of decreased thyroid stimulation by thyroid-stimulating hormone (TSH) owing to pituitary disease. *Tertiary hypothyroidism*—the result of decreased thyroid stimulation by TSH due to decreased pituitary stimulation resulting from a deficiency of thyrotropin-releasing hormone (TRH).

Synonyms for secondary and tertiary hypothyroidism: Central or hypothyrotropic hypothyroidism. *Myxedema* is not synonymous with hypothyroidism but represents the accumulation of glycosaminoglycans in soft tissues (subcutaneous and other interstitial sites), resulting in the nonpitting edema characteristic of hypothyroid patients. Myxedema is most common in patients with severe (long-standing) primary hypothyroidism.

Clinical

- Hypothyroidism is the most common disorder of thyroid function.
- The causes of hypothyroidism are listed in Table 4–1.
- It has an equal gender predilection and may occur in all age groups but more commonly affects adults.
- It may be clinically overt or subclinical; subclinical hypothyroidism is defined as elevated serum TSH and normal thyroxine (T_4) and triiodothyronine (T_3) concentrations.
- The clinical features of hypothyroidism are independent of its cause; the clinical spectrum of severity may be broad even in patients with overt hypothyroidism, such that some patients may have very subtle manifestations of disease (few signs and symptoms), whereas others may have more extreme manifestations (myxedema coma).

Table 4–1
CAUSES OF HYPOTHYROIDISM

Primary Hypothyroidism

Chronic autoimmune thyroiditis
Surgery (total or subtotal thyroidectomy)
Radiation treatment (radioiodine, neck irradiation)
Iodine deficiency and excess
Drug-induced (antithyroidal medications)
Infiltrative diseases of the thyroid (neoplasms [primary and metastatic], fibrosing diseases [e.g., scleroderma], amyloidosis)
Inborn metabolic disorders (TSH unresponsiveness; iodide transport failure; defective peroxidase activity or production including *Pendred's syndrome* [familial deaf-mutism and goiter]; others)
Developmental abnormalities (thyroid agenesis)

Secondary Hypothyroidism

Pituitary disease (neoplasms, infarcts, trauma)

Tertiary Hypothyroidism

Hypothalamic disease (neoplasms, infectious disease, trauma)

Generalized Thyroid Hormone Resistance

Transient Hypothyroidism

Silent thyroiditis
Subacute thyroiditis

- Clinical signs and symptoms include (in no particular order): fatigue, lethargy, slow movements, slow speech, hoarseness, bradycardia, depression, cold intolerance, dry skin, decreased perspiration, nonpitting edema, anemia, decreased appetite, constipation, weight gain, arthralgia, hyporeflexia, paresthesia, menstrual abnormalities.
- Laboratory tests: Low serum free T_4 levels and elevated serum TSH levels confirm the presence of hypothyroidism.
- Factors potentially influencing the clinical features of hypothyroidism include:
  - Patient age: In children and adults, the effects are potentially reversible; in infants, hypothyroidism may result in irreversible mental and physical retardation (see later

46

section, Myxedematous Endemic Cretinism) unless treatment is initiated early.
- Presence of other diseases: If there is no generalized destruction of the gland, a compensatory increase in TSH secretion may maintain thyroid secretion at near-normal levels, causing the clinical manifestations of hypothyroidism to remain subclinical for years.
- Rate at which hypothyroidism develops: Patients with rapid onset of hypothyroidism have more symptoms than those who develop it gradually.
- Treatment of hypothyroidism may be as simple as replacing thyroxine (T_4). However, in some instances, hypothyroidism does not result from destruction of the gland but is due to another cause (see Table 4–1), which will not be remedied by thyroxine (T_4) replacement; in these instances, identification and treatment of the underlying cause is paramount in controlling the effects of the hypothyroidism.
- **Generalized myxedema**
  - Develops in patients with long-standing, severe generalized thyroid deficiency.
  - Clinical features result from glycosaminoglycan accumulation in soft tissues, resulting in a full face and nonpitting periorbital and cutaneous edema (most marked around the hands), which is not resorbed during recumbency (unlike cardiogenic edema).
  - The fluid accumulated in the soft tissues is composed of a mixture of mucopolysaccharides, hyaluronic acid, and chondroitin sulfate.
  - Fluid may accumulate in virtually every part of the body. Some of the resulting clinical signs and symptoms include:
    - Pulmonary signs: *Direct* pulmonary effects include altered pulmonary function test results, depressed ventilatory drive, pleural effusion, and decreased surfactant production in the neonate. *Indirect* pulmonary effects include phrenic nerve paralysis, congestive heart failure causing pulmonary edema, obesity causing atelectasis, and others.
    - Cardiovascular signs (myxedematous heart): The most common cardiovascular abnormality of hypothyroidism is pericardial effusion. Other changes relate to cardiac papillary muscle contractile abnormalities and electrical abnormalities resulting in sinus bradycardia (visible on electrocardiograms as prolonged QT intervals, flattening and inversion of T waves, and, in children, the so-called mosque sign, comprising a dome-shaped T wave and a partially obliterated ST segment). Radiographic findings include cardiomegaly. The incidence of atherosclerotic cardiovascular disease is increased in hypothyroid patients.
    - Renal signs: Alterations in renal hemodynamics and kidney function result in generalized fluid retention. Extravascular accumulation of protein-rich fluid (albumin and other proteins) results in weight gain, but there is a decrease in plasma volume and a fall in cardiac output.
    - Upper aerodigestive tract: Airway obstruction due to goiter, enlarged tongue, pharyngeal muscle dysfunction, myxoid polyps of the larynx.

- **Other manifestations of hypothyroidism**
  - Hematologic: Anemia is commonly seen in patients with hypothyroidism (up to 30% to 40%). It is most often normocytic or macrocytic and normochromic and represents a normal physiologic response. Thyroid hormone has a stimulatory effect on erythropoiesis via erythropoietin. A deficiency of thyroid hormone leads to a decrease in erythropoiesis owing to slowing of the metabolic rate, a decreased oxygen requirement, and a decrease in erythropoietin levels. A small percentage of hypothyroid patients (2% to 15%) have a microcytic anemia. There are few significant effects on white blood cells and platelets.
  - Neurologic: Manifestations of severe hypothyroidism include **myxedema coma:**
    - Rare syndrome representing extreme expression of hypothyroidism.
    - Most frequently occurs in winter, possibly associated with extreme cold.
    - Other possible precipitating factors: infection, drugs (anesthetics, sedatives, tranquilizers, narcotics, lithium), trauma, cerebrovascular accidents, congestive heart failure.
    - Cardinal features: hypothermia and unconsciousness.
    - High mortality rate in untreated patients; should be viewed as a medical emergency. Rapid diagnosis with immediate initiation of appropriate therapy is the key to preventing death. Therapy includes ventilatory support, control of water and electrolyte imbalances, temperature control, administration of hydrocortisone therapy in the presence of coexisting adrenal insufficiency, and initiation of thyroid hormone therapy.
- **Myxedematous endemic cretinism**
  - Associated with endemic goiter and severe iodine deficiency.
  - Most serious complication of endemic goiter. Irreversible abnormalities of intellect and physical development occur in a high percentage of patients with severe endemic goiter.
  - Clinical symptoms and signs include mental deficiency with defects in hearing and speech, disorders of standing and gait, and hypothyroidism and stunted growth.
  - Iodine deficiency is fundamental in the etiology of endemic cretinism; if severe enough, it may be the only causative factor. Other factors may include the presence of naturally occurring goitrogens, thyroid autoimmunity, a deficiency of trace elements (selenium, manganese), congenital infections, perinatal anoxia.
  - There is no specific therapy; rehabilitation is similar to that used for patients with cerebral palsy.
  - Prevention is accomplished by efficient iodine prophylaxis.

B. HYPERTHYROIDISM AND THYROTOXICOSIS

Definitions: *Hyperthyroidism*—sustained thyroid hyperfunction with sustained increase in production of thyroid hormones due to numerous causes (Table 4–2), resulting in systemic manifestations owing to unabated exposure to

Table 4–2
CAUSES OF HYPERTHYROIDISM

Primary Hyperthyroidism

Diffuse toxic goiter (Graves' disease)
Toxic nodular or multinodular goiter
Toxic adenoma
Subacute thyroiditis and other thyroiditides
Thyroid cancer
Iatrogenic/drug-induced
Ectopic thyroid tissue (e.g., struma ovarii)
Gestational trophoblastic disease (hydatidiform mole; choriocarcinoma)

Secondary Hyperthyroidism (excess TSH production)

Pituitary tumor
Inappropriate feedback response to thyroid hormone or end-organ
   resistance to thyroid hormone

thyroid hormones. *Thyrotoxicosis*—clinical syndrome resulting from increased serum concentration of thyroid hormones; may be associated with or independent of the causes of hyperthyroidism.

Clinical

- Hyperthyroidism is less common than hypothyroidism.
- The most common cause of spontaneous thyrotoxicosis is Graves' disease; the causes of hyperthyroidism with and without thyrotoxicosis are listed in Table 4–3.
- The clinical features of thyrotoxicosis are not specific, and there is marked variability in their severity. Among the factors that may determine the manifestations of disease are:

  (1) Age.
  (2) Presence or absence of a concomitant disease.

- Clinical signs and symptoms of thyrotoxicosis include nervousness, fatigue, weakness, heat intolerance, increased perspiration, hyperactivity, tachycardia, arrhythmias, palpitation, systolic hypertension, increased appetite, loss of weight, warm and moist skin, hyperreflexia, tremor, muscle weakness, and menstrual disturbances.
- Signs associated with specific causes of thyrotoxicosis include thyroid pain and tenderness with the presence of a goiter (diffuse or nodular). Ophthalmopathy and localized myxedema are both seen in Graves' disease.
- Biochemical confirmation of thyrotoxicosis can be determined by the presence of elevated levels of serum total

Table 4–3
DISEASES ASSOCIATED WITH THYROTOXICOSIS

Thyrotoxicosis-Associated Hyperthyroidism

Diffuse toxic goiter (Graves' disease)
Toxic nodular or multinodular goiter
Toxic adenoma
Thyroid cancer
Pituitary adenoma (thyrotrophic adenoma)

Thyrotoxicosis Not Associated with Hyperthyroidism

Subacute thyroiditis and other thyroiditides
Iatrogenic/drug-induced
Ectopic thyroid tissue (e.g., struma ovarii)

and free T_4 and T_3 and decreased serum TSH levels; biochemical confirmation of thyrotoxicosis does not include confirmation of the cause of disease.
- Most patients with thyrotoxicosis have overt clinical and biochemical disease, but thyrotoxicosis may also be subclinical (normal serum T_4 and T_3 and decreased TSH concentrations). Patients with subclinical hyperthyroidism may or may not have clinical evidence of disease; if present, it is generally mild.
- Elderly patients with thyrotoxicosis may present with predominant involvement of one organ system and without the classic signs and symptoms of thyrotoxicosis; this is referred to as apathetic thyrotoxicosis.
- Significant systemic manifestations of thyrotoxicosis

Cardiovascular
- The heart is a major target organ for thyroid hormone action.
- Hemodynamic changes: increased systolic (increased stroke volume and rapid heart rate) and diastolic (shortened circulation time and decreased cardiac indices) functions.
- Despite the presence of increased cardiac contractility and the high output state caused by thyrotoxicosis, cardiac failure may (paradoxically) occur, with decreased cardiac function resulting in evidence of congestive heart failure, including pitting edema and pulmonary congestion.
- Electrocardiographic signs include sinus tachycardia and atrial fibrillation.
- Mitral valve prolapse is a common abnormality found in patients with Graves' disease (the pathophysiologic mechanisms of mitral valve prolapse in these patients are not known).
- Exertional dyspnea exists even without evidence of heart failure.

Muscular
- Generalized weakness and muscular atrophy.
- Exophthalmic ophthalmoplegia (localized paralysis of ocular muscles) characterized by lid lag, lid retraction, and exophthalmos.
- Myasthenia gravis. The coexistence of myasthenia gravis and thyrotoxicosis is uncommon (occurring in <1% of patients); however, the incidence of thyrotoxicosis as a complication of myasthenia gravis is not as uncommon and occurs in up to 6% of myasthenia gravis patients.
- Periodic paralysis characterized by attacks of flaccid paralysis (affecting all extremities and the trunk) with areflexia and abolition of electrical excitability may be a rare complication of thyrotoxicosis.

Neurologic
- Neuropsychiatric disorders, characterized by nervousness, irritability, and tremulousness; anxiety disorders, depression, mania, and schizophreniform disorders may occur.
- Discrete neurologic syndromes: Chorea is an unusual manifestation of thyrotoxicosis.
- Severe acute systemic states with delirium, coma, and convulsions (thyrotoxicosis storm).

- **Thyrotoxicosis storm or crisis**
  - Relatively rare but represents a life-threatening syndrome characterized by exaggerated manifestations of thyrotoxicosis.
  - Cardinal manifestations include:

    Fever: usually >101.3°F (38.5°C).
    Tachycardia: out of proportion to the fever.
    Gastrointestinal dysfunction: nausea, vomiting, diarrhea, and jaundice (the last in severe cases).
    CNS-related symptoms: confusion, apathy, and, in extreme cases, coma.

  - These features in a patient with a goiter, Graves' disease ophthalmopathy, or a history of partially treated thyrotoxicosis may signal the diagnosis of thyrotoxicosis storm.
  - Laboratory findings: elevated serum total T_4 and T_3 levels, T_3-resin uptake, and 24-hour radioiodine uptake. These levels are above normal but are not substantially different from the levels seen in uncomplicated cases of thyrotoxicosis.
  - Among the causes of thyrotoxicosis storm are infection (most common), trauma (including vigorous palpation of the thyroid), surgery, hypoglycemia, stress, cessation of antithyroid drug medication, ^{131}I therapy, diabetic ketoacidosis, cerebrovascular accident, pulmonary ketoacidosis, and the use of iodinated contrast dyes.
  - The precise mechanism of thyrotoxicosis storm is not fully known and is probably multifactorial.
  - Therapy is directed against (1) the thyroid gland (inhibition of hormone synthesis and secretion); (2) the peripheral actions of thyroid hormone; and (3) the precipitating illness and aims to maintain normal homeostatic mechanisms (temperature, fluid and electrolyte balance, other).
- Treatment of thyrotoxicosis is directed at the cause of the hyperthyroid state. An underlying cause may not be readily established, rendering control of the disease difficult. Potential treatment modalities include the use of:
  - Antithyroid drugs (e.g., propylthiouracil, methimazole) in an attempt to make the patient euthyroid.
  - Other drugs, including iodide, potassium perchlorate, lithium, and β-adrenergic antagonistic drugs (e.g., propranolol, atenolol, metoprolol, nadolol).
  - Radioactive iodine.
  - Surgery: subtotal thyroidectomy.
- Prognosis depends on the cause of the thyrotoxicosis (see Table 4–3).

Bibliography

Hypothyroidism

Aber CP, Thompson GS. Factors associated with cardiac enlargement in myxedema. Br Heart J 1963; 25:421–424.

Braverman LE, Utiger RD. Introduction to hypothyroidism. In: Braverman LE, Utiger RD, eds. Werner and Ingbar's The Thyroid. A Fundamental and Clinical Text, 6th ed. Philadelphia: J.B. Lippincott, 1991, pp. 919–920.

Das KC, Mukherjee M, Sarkar TK, et al. Erythropoiesis and erythropoietin in hypo- and hyperthyroidism. J Clin Endocrinol Metab 1975; 40:211–220.

Delange F. Endemic cretinism. In: Braverman LE, Utiger RD, eds. Werner and Ingbar's The Thyroid. A Fundamental and Clinical Text, 6th ed. Philadelphia: J.B. Lippincott, 1991, pp. 942–955.

Dillmann WH. Biochemical basis of thyroid hormone action in the heart. Am J Med 1990; 88:626–630.

Fein HG, Rivlin RS. Anemia in thyroid diseases. Med Clin North Am 1975; 59:1133–1145.

Hall R, Scanlon MF. Hypothyroidism: Clinical features and complications. Clin Endocrinol Metab 1979; 8:29–38.

Kabakkaya Y, Bakan E, Yigitoglu MR, et al. Pendred's syndrome. Ann Otol Rhinol Laryngol 1993; 102:285–288.

Klein I. Thyroid hormone and the cardiovascular system. Am J Med 1990; 88:631–637.

Ladenson PW. Recognition and management of cardiovascular disease related to thyroid dysfunction. Am J Med 1990; 88:638–641.

Parving H-H, Hansen JM, Nielsen SL, et al. Mechanisms of edema formation in myxedema: Increased protein extravasation and relatively slow lymphatic drainage. N Engl J Med 1979; 301:460–465.

Sachdev Y, Hall R. Effusions into body cavities in hypothyroidism. Lancet 1975; 1:564–565.

Smith TJ. Connective tissue in hypothyroidism. In: Braverman LE, Utiger RD, eds. Werner and Ingbar's The Thyroid. A Fundamental and Clinical Text, 6th ed. Philadelphia: J.B. Lippincott, 1991, pp. 989–992.

Wartofsky L. Myxedema coma. In: Braverman LE, Utiger RD, eds. Werner and Ingbar's The Thyroid. A Fundamental and Clinical Text, 6th ed. Philadelphia: J.B. Lippincott, 1991, pp. 1084–1091.

Hyperthyroidism

Braverman LE, Utiger RD. Introduction to thyrotoxicosis. In: Werner and Ingbar's The Thyroid. A Fundamental and Clinical Text, 6th ed. Philadelphia: J.B. Lippincott, 1991, pp. 645–647.

Cooper DS. Treatment of thyrotoxicosis. In: Braverman LE, Utiger RD, eds. Werner and Ingbar's The Thyroid. A Fundamental and Clinical Text, 6th ed. Philadelphia: J.B. Lippincott, 1991, pp. 887–916.

DeLong GR, Adams RD. The neuromuscular system and brain in thyrotoxicosis. In: Braverman LE, Utiger RD, eds. Werner and Ingbar's The Thyroid. A Fundamental and Clinical Text, 6th ed. Philadelphia: J.B. Lippincott, 1991, pp. 793–802.

Devereux RB, Kramer-Fox R, Kligfield P. Mitral valve prolapse: Causes, clinical manifestations, and management. Ann Intern Med 1989; 111:305–317.

Dillmann WH. Biochemical basis of thyroid hormone action in the heart. Am J Med 1990; 88:626–630.

Friedman MJ, Okada RD, Ewy GA, Hellman DJ. Left ventricular systolic and diastolic function in hyperthyroidism. Am Heart J 1982; 104:1303–1308.

Klein I. Thyroid hormone and the cardiovascular system. Am J Med 1990; 88:631–637.

Ladenson PW. Recognition and management of cardiovascular disease related to thyroid dysfunction. Am J Med 1990; 88:638–641.

Merillon JP, Passa P, Chastre J, et al. Left ventricular function and hyperthyroidism. Br Heart J 1982; 46:137–143.

Trzepacz PT, Klein I, Robert M, et al. Graves' disease: An analysis of thyroid hormone levels and hyperthyroid signs and symptoms. Am J Med 1989; 87:558–561.

Wartofsky L. Thyrotoxic storm. In: Braverman LE, Utiger RD, eds. Werner and Ingbar's The Thyroid. A Fundamental and Clinical Text, 6th ed. Philadelphia: J.B. Lippincott, 1991, pp. 871–879.

CHAPTER 5

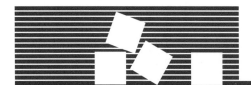

Nonautoimmune Thyroiditides

A. ACUTE (INFECTIOUS) THYROIDITIS

Definition: The presence of an inflammatory cell infiltrate dominated by polymorphonuclear leukocytes within the thyroid gland.

Synonyms: Acute suppurative or infectious thyroiditis.

Clinical

- Rare disease.
- No gender predilection; may occur in all age groups.
- Tends to develop in immunocompromised or malnourished patients; not infrequently it is associated with concomitant localized infections or is part of a systemic process (sepsis).
- The clinical presentation includes fever with swelling and pain in the neck region that may radiate or be referred to the jaw and ear region; additional signs and symptoms may include fatigue, dyspnea, dysphagia, and hoarseness.
- Thyroid glands are warm to hot on palpation.
- Patients are usually euthyroid, but both hyperthyroidism and hypothyroidism may occur.
- Etiologic agents may include bacteria, fungi, and, rarely, viruses.
- Cultures for microorganisms may be helpful in the diagnosis; microbiologic analysis can be performed on material obtained from fine needle aspiration.

Pathology

Fine Needle Aspiration

- Polymorphonuclear leukocytes are present.
- Microorganisms can be identified by histochemical analysis.

Gross

- Gross appearance varies and includes focal or diffuse enlargement; in some instances the thyroid appears normal.
- Abscess formation as shown by soft purulent areas can occur.

Histology

- Focal to diffuse acute inflammatory cell infiltrates (polymorphonuclear leukocytes) with destruction of follicular epithelial cells are present.
- Areas of abscess formation characterized by a dense pool of leukocytes may be seen.
- Areas of necrosis and leukocytic debris may be seen.
- Depending on the causative microorganism, the offending agent may or may not be identifiable on light microscopy. Special histochemical stains may assist in the identification of the microorganism.
- In severely immunocompromised patients, the typical granulomatous inflammatory process may not occur in the presence of mycobacterial or fungal infection; rather, changes characteristic of acute thyroiditis may be seen.

Treatment and Prognosis

- Treatment is predicated on the diagnosis and identification of the causative microbe; once the microorganism has been identified, appropriate antimicrobial therapy is initiated.
- Surgical intervention (drainage) may be required in the presence of abscess formation.
- The prognosis, especially for patients with bacteria-related acute thyroiditis, is excellent, and most patients experience recovery; rarely, recurrence and even death may occur.

B. GRANULOMATOUS THYROIDITIS

Definition: The presence of well-formed granulomas in the thyroid gland. The more common causes of granulomas in the thyroid are listed in Table 5–1.

Table 5–1
GRANULOMATOUS LESIONS OF THE THYROID GLAND

Infections (mycobacterial and fungal infections)
Sarcoidosis
Subacute thyroiditis (including silent thyroiditis)
Multifocal granulomatous thyroiditis (palpation thyroiditis)
Others

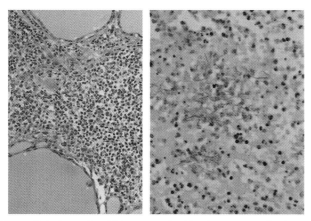

Figure 5–1. Acute thyroiditis characterized by the presence of polymorphonuclear leukocytes in the thyroid. In this case, filamentous gram-positive organisms consistent with *Nocardia* species were present (Brown and Brenn Gram stain).

1. Infectious Granulomatous Thyroiditis

Definition: Infectious thyroid disease caused by an identifiable microorganism that may or may not result in granulomatous inflammation.

Synonym: Acute mycotic thyroiditis.

Clinical

- Granulomatous inflammation of the thyroid caused by a microorganism is extremely uncommon.
- The typical clinical setting for this disease is an immunosuppressed or immunocompromised patient.
- The clinical presentation may be similar to that of acute thyroiditis and may include fever with swelling and pain in the neck region radiating or referred to the jaw and ear region.
- Thyroid glands are warm to hot on palpation.
- Patients are usually euthyroid, but both hyperthyroidism and hypothyroidism may occur.
- Etiologic agents may include various fungi and mycobacteria; mycobacterial infection of the thyroid is rare even in patients with miliary tuberculosis.

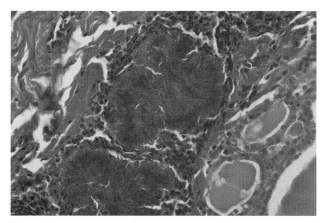

Figure 5–2. Actinomycotic thyroiditis characterized by the presence of "sulfur"granules typical of *Actinomyces* organisms.

- Cultures for microorganisms may be helpful in the diagnosis; microbiologic analysis can be performed on material obtained from fine needle aspiration.

Pathology

Gross

- Gross appearance varies but may include soft purulent (caseating) areas, abscess formation, and miliary tubercles.

Histology

- In immunocompromised patients the typical granulomatous inflammatory process may not occur in the presence of mycobacterial or fungal infection; rather, changes typical of acute thyroiditis are seen.
- Focal to diffuse acute inflammatory cell infiltrates (polymorphonuclear leukocytes) with destruction of the follicular epithelial cell architecture may be seen.
- Areas of abscess formation characterized by a dense pool of leukocytes can be seen.
- Areas of necrosis and leukocytic debris may be present.
- Classic caseating granulomas may be present in patients with either mycobacterial or fungal infections. These changes include foci of central necrosis surrounded by a histiocytic cell reaction with scattered associated multinucleated giant cells.
- Depending on the causative microorganism, the offending agent may or may not be identifiable on light microscopy. Special histochemical stains may assist in the identification of the microorganism.
  - Fungal infections: Gomori methenamine silver (GMS), periodic acid-Schiff (PAS), mucin stains.
  - Mycobacterial infections: Special stains based on the capability of the organism to form stable mycolate complexes with certain aryl methane dyes (referred to as acid-fast stains) may be used; depending on the stain, the organisms, when identified, may appear beaded or show a red or purple color. Organisms are often extremely difficult to identify and may defy detection despite all efforts.

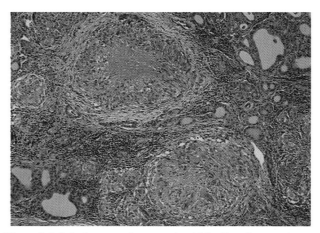

Figure 5–3. Infectious granulomatous thyroiditis. Caseating granulomas showing central necrosis surrounded by a histiocytic cell reaction including multinucleated giant cells. Although microorganisms were not found in the tissue, the patient did have tuberculosis.

Differential Diagnosis

■ Sarcoidosis (Chapter 5B, #2).

Treatment and Prognosis

■ Treatment is predicated on the diagnosis and identification of the causative microbe; once the organism has been identified, appropriate antimicrobial therapy is initiated.
■ Surgical intervention (drainage) may be required in patients with abscess formation.
■ The prognosis for patients with fungal infection of the thyroid is poor because it generally is a terminal event in immunocompromised patients.
■ The prognosis for mycobacterial infections of the thyroid correlates with the status of other organ system involvement.

Additional Facts

■ Regardless of the causative organism, the histologic picture of mycobacterial infections of the thyroid is the same.

2. Sarcoidosis of the Thyroid Gland

Definition: Sarcoidosis is a multisystem chronic granulomatous disease of unknown etiology; it may involve the thyroid as part of a systemic process or, rarely, may be localized to the thyroid.

Clinical (Limited to Thyroid Involvement)

■ Sarcoidosis of the thyroid gland is uncommon, and when it does occur it is more often part of a systemic disease rather than a disease isolated to the thyroid gland. In this setting, patients generally do not present with symptomatic thyroid disease, and the pathologic identification of thyroid involvement is made at autopsy or during resection of the thyroid gland for other reasons.
■ Isolated sarcoidosis of the thyroid gland is rare.

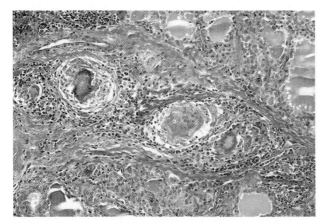

Figure 5–4. Sarcoidosis of the thyroid characterized by granulomatous inflammation. Typically, the granulomas associated with sarcoidosis do not have central necrotic material (caseation) but do have well-formed granulomas with a histiocytic cell infiltrate and multinucleated giant cells.

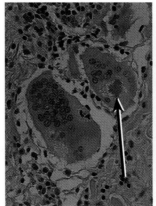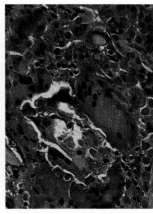

Figure 5–5. In sarcoidosis, the cytoplasm of the giant cells may include *(left)* star-shaped structures termed asteroid bodies *(arrow)* and/or *(right)* calcific laminated bodies called Schaumann's bodies.

■ There is no gender predilection; the disease occurs in all age groups but occurs most commonly in young adults.
■ The clinical presentation in patients with symptomatic thyroid disease includes a neck or thyroid mass that appears as a hypofunctioning "cold" nodule on thyroid scanning.
■ The clinical presentation in patients with a systemic disease includes fever, weight loss, and hilar adenopathy.
■ There are no laboratory findings specific for or diagnostic of sarcoidosis; cutaneous anergy to skin test antigens may be seen (Kveim test).
■ The diagnosis of sarcoidosis is generally one of exclusion and is made by correlation of the clinical, radiologic, and pathologic findings.

Pathology

Histology

■ Noncaseating granulomas consisting of epithelioid histiocytes surrounded by a mixed inflammatory infiltrate and multinucleated (Langhans' type) giant cells are seen.
■ Intracytoplasmic inclusions, including star-shaped or calcific laminated bodies called asteroid and Schaumann's bodies, respectively, can be seen.
■ All special stains for microorganisms (Brown and Hopps, GMS, Ziehl Neelsen [for acid-fast organisms]) are negative.
■ Immunohistochemistry: Thyroglobulin in the granulomatous foci is absent.

Differential Diagnosis

■ Mycobacterial infections (Chapter 5B, #1).
■ Fungal infections (Chapter 5B, #1).

Treatment and Prognosis

■ Patients presenting with a symptomatic thyroid nodule may undergo surgical resection of the mass; patients with systemic sarcoidosis are treated with corticosteroids.

- The prognosis for patients with systemic disease is generally good; up to 70% of patients improve or remain stable following therapy.
- Advanced multisystem disease leading to extensive pulmonary involvement and respiratory failure may occur but is seen in only a small percentage of cases.

Additional Facts

- The pathologic features of sarcoidosis are characteristic but are not specific; therefore, the histopathologic diagnosis of sarcoidosis can be considered only in the absence of identification of an infectious agent.

3. Subacute Thyroiditis (De Quervain's Thyroiditis)

Definition: A granulomatous inflammatory condition of the thyroid gland with characteristic clinical and pathologic findings.

Synonyms: Pseudogranulomatous or granulomatous thyroiditis; giant cell thyroiditis; acute simple thyroiditis; noninfectious thyroiditis; pseudotuberculous thyroiditis; migratory "creeping" thyroiditis; struma granulomatosa; thyroiditis acute simplex (as originally described by Mygind).

Clinical

- Less common than Graves' disease and chronic lymphocytic thyroiditis, representing <3% of all thyroid abnormalities.
- Affects women more than men (in a ratio of 3:1 to 6:1); occurs most commonly in the second to fifth decades of life but is uncommon in children and elderly persons.
- The clinical presentation is usually neck pain that may be localized to the thyroid (one lobe or the entire gland) or may radiate to the jaw, ears, face, and chest; general (systemic) manifestations may include malaise, fatigue, fever, chills, weight loss, anorexia, and myalgia.

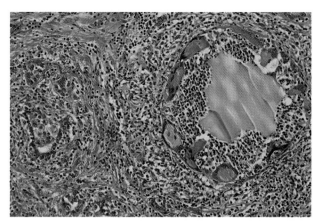

Figure 5–7. Subacute thyroiditis with destruction of the follicular epithelial cells, which are replaced by neutrophils and multinucleated giant cells. Colloid is still present and is seen "floating"within the neutrophilic cell infiltrate.

- On palpation, the gland is enlarged, exquisitely tender, and firm to hard; the enlargement is usually diffuse but may be asymmetrical with limited (unilateral) involvement.
- Laboratory findings change with the stage of disease:
  - *Early or hyperthyroid (thyrotoxic) phase:* Owing to damage to the thyroid follicular cells, a hyperthyroid condition results from elevated serum levels of thyroxine (T_4), triiodothyronine (T_3), and thyroglobulin. Serum and urine iodine levels are increased, and serum thyroid-stimulating hormone (TSH) levels are decreased.
  - *Later or hypothyroid phase:* With progression of disease, a hypothyroid state ensues owing to destruction of a larger portion of the gland and absence of hormone production and iodine uptake (decreased serum levels of T_4, T_3, and thyroglobulin, and increased serum TSH level). The hypothyroid phase in most patients lasts about 1 to 2 months, and an occasional patient remains permanently hypothyroid.
- The etiology of subacute thyroiditis is in all probability infectious, and there is strong evidence supporting a viral agent.
  - The clinical presentation may be preceded by an upper respiratory tract infection that may have a prodromal

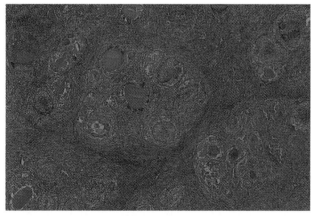

Figure 5–6. Subacute thyroiditis (de Quervain's thyroiditis). There is destruction of the follicular epithelial cells with colonization of the follicles by an inflammatory cell infiltrate that includes polymorphonuclear leukocytes and multinucleated giant cells. The gland has a lobular appearance with interlobular fibrosis.

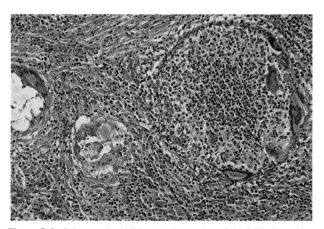

Figure 5–8. Subacute thyroiditis with destruction of the follicular epithelial cells with loss of colloid and colonization by neutrophils and multinucleated giant cells.

phase characterized by muscle aches and pains, malaise, and fatigue; concomitant elevation of the white blood cell count is not present as would be expected in a bacterial-related disease.
- This disorder is most often identified in the summer months, coinciding with summer enterovirus infections.
- Antibody studies (using acute and convalescent phase serum) have shown the presence of circulating antibodies to various viruses including mumps, measles, influenza, and Epstein-Barr viruses, coxsackievirus, adenovirus, and echovirus.
- Autoimmunity may play a role in the development of subacute thyroiditis. Thyroid antibodies are found in some patients with subacute thyroiditis; these antibodies are transiently present and disappear following resolution of the disease.
- An association between subacute thyroiditis and HLA-Bw35 supports a genetic predisposition to the development of this disease.

Radiology

- Radioisotopic scans in the early stages of disease show patchy and irregular uptake or no uptake at all.
- Ultrasound shows hypoechogenicity in the involved areas.

Pathology

Fine Needle Aspiration

- In the early stages of disease, acute inflammatory cells with microabscesses can be seen.
- As the disease progresses, a mixed inflammatory infiltrate is seen that includes lymphocytes, histiocytes, plasma cells, multinucleated giant cells, and polymorphonuclear leukocytes. Degenerative changes of follicular epithelial cells are present.
- If there is extensive fibrosis, aspirates may be acellular.

Gross

- On sectioning, the thyroid is found to be firm to hard and tan-white in color with one or more ill-defined nodules that vary in size from a few millimeters to several centimeters.

Histology

- The histologic appearance varies with the phase of disease.
  - *Early phase:*
    - Destruction of the follicular epithelial cells with extravasation and depletion of colloid occurs; the latter may be identifiable "floating" within the inflammatory cell infiltrate. Periodic acid-Schiff (PAS) is a simple and effective stain for the identification of colloid.
    - "Colonization" of the thyroid follicles by an inflammatory infiltrate consisting of polymorphonuclear leukocytes (including microabscesses) in the initial stages followed by mature lymphocytes, histiocytes, and multinucleated giant cells occurs. The inflammatory cells may involve the adjacent follicles.
  - *Later phase:*
    - Polymorphonuclear leukocytes are replaced by a chronic inflammatory infiltrate composed of lymphocytes, histiocytes, giant cells, and plasma cells.
    - Follicular epithelial cells are replaced by inflammatory cells.
    - Fibrosis is evident between follicles and between lobules.
  - *Regenerative phase:*
    - Follicular regeneration occurs.
    - Minimal residual irregular fibrosis is variably present.

Differential Diagnosis

- Multifocal granulomatous thyroiditis (palpation thyroiditis) (Chapter 5B, #5).
- Chronic lymphocytic thyroiditis (Chapter 6A and B).
- Mycobacterial infection (Chapter 5B, #1).
- Sarcoidosis (Chapter 5B, #2).
- Neoplastic proliferation (not usually a histologic problem but on the basis of the clinical appearance this may fall within the differential diagnosis).

Treatment and Prognosis

- The most effective therapy is corticosteroids, which result in resolution of symptoms in most patients. Therapeutic regimens are maintained for approximately 1 week and then are tapered over a period of about 1 month. Exacerbation of disease occurs in approximately 10% of patients when steroid therapy is reduced or stopped. In these patients readministration of steroids will resolve the symptoms, and ultimately the patients experience a full recovery.
- Salicylates and other nonsteroidal anti-inflammatory medications have been used with good results.
- Prognosis is excellent with complete resolution of disease; permanent hypothyroidism is rare but may occur in a limited number of patients.

Additional Facts

- The presence of antithyroid antibodies may represent a reaction to released antigens following follicular epithelial destruction rather than true autoimmunity.

4. Painless ("Silent") Subacute Thyroiditis

Clinical

- The incidence is not known but is estimated to be as high as 20% to 30% of all cases of subacute thyroiditis.
- Affects women more than men; most common in the third to sixth decades of life but may occur in all age ranges.
- Onset and severity of disease vary. The initial phase includes mild to moderate thyrotoxicosis lasting 1 to 2 months; this is followed by euthyroidism of several weeks duration, which in turn is followed by a hypothyroid phase lasting several months.
- Clinical presentation in the thyrotoxicosis phase is usual but may include in addition some of the more unusual

manifestations of thyrotoxicosis such as atrial fibrillation, diffuse myalgia, periodic paralysis, and lid lag and lid retraction. Exophthalmos, localized myxedema, and thyroid acropathy do not occur.

■ Approximately 50% of hypothyroid patients are symptomatic; however, supplemental T_4 therapy is not required.

■ Thyroid enlargement occurs in up to 60% of patients; enlargement may be asymmetrical (a dominant, firm mass is confined to one thyroid lobe). Pain and tenderness are rare and when present are mild.

■ Histologic changes are often those characteristic of subacute (granulomatous) thyroiditis.

■ The course of disease is similar to that seen in subacute thyroiditis.

5. Multifocal Granulomatous Thyroiditis (Palpation Thyroiditis)

Synonym: Martial arts thyroiditis.

■ Traumatically induced lesions are caused by vigorous clinical palpation of the thyroid.

■ No specific demographic or clinical parameters are associated.

■ Does not cause abnormalities in thyroid function (hypothyroidism or hyperthyroidism).

■ Incidental microscopic finding in thyroid glands resected for other reasons.

■ *Histology:*
  • Focal or multifocal lesion in which an isolated follicle or group of follicles show loss of follicular epithelial cells, and the presence of a mixed chronic inflammatory cell infiltrate composed predominantly of histiocytes as well as lymphocytes and plasma cells; multinucleated giant cells may be present as well.
  • Additional histologic changes include hemorrhage, hemosiderin deposition, and hemosiderin-laden macrophages.
  • The presence of colloid varies such that in some cases residual colloid is present and in others it is absent. PAS stain may be helpful in identifying residual colloid.

• Necrosis is generally not found but is occasionally present.

■ Diagnostic confusion may occur with C-cell hyperplasia. Differentiation can be assisted by immunohistochemistry findings as follows: Palpation thyroiditis—CD68 (KP1) and lysozyme positive; calcitonin and chromogranin negative. C-cell hyperplasia—calcitonin and chromogranin positive; thyroglobulin negative.

■ No specific treatment is required; in all probability, spontaneous regression of these histologic changes occurs.

■ These lesions are not associated with any untoward sequelae.

C. INVASIVE FIBROUS THYROIDITIS (RIEDEL'S DISEASE)

Definition: Idiopathic fibrosing process that is not per se an inflammatory thyroid disease (thyroiditis) of the thyroid gland.

Synonyms: Riedel's struma; ligneous thyroiditis.

Clinical

■ Uncommon.

■ Affects women slightly more often than men; primarily occurs in adults.

■ Clinical presentation includes painless neck mass and/or goiter, pressure in the anterior neck, dysphagia, dyspnea, stridor; rarely, vocal cord paralysis may occur.

■ The thyroid is enlarged, feels woody or stony hard on palpation, and is adherent or fixed to the surrounding structures in the neck. Involvement of the thyroid may be limited in extent, so that only one side is predominantly involved, but bilateral and complete involvement of the thyroid can also occur.

■ The presence of a hard and fixed thyroid mass clinically simulates the presentation of a neoplastic lesion, which is even more strongly suspected in cases in which there is cervical lymph node involvement.

■ Hypothyroidism occurs in 30% to 40% of these patients and is permanent; hypoparathyroidism may also occur.

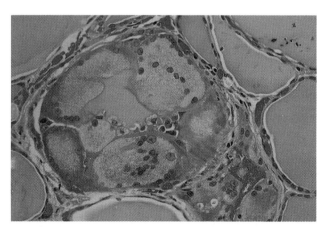

Figure 5–9. Palpation thyroiditis. This is a focal or multifocal process in which the thyroid follicular epithelial cells are replaced by histiocytes and multinucleated giant cells.

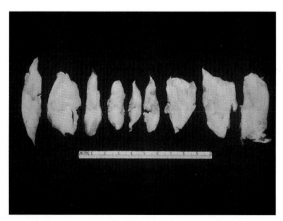

Figure 5–10. Invasive fibrous thyroiditis (Riedel's disease) characterized by replacement of the thyroid tissue by dense, firm to hard, tan-white fibrous tissue.

Figure 5–11. Invasive fibrous thyroiditis. Virtually all of the thyroid tissue is replaced by fibrous tissue with an associated chronic inflammatory cell infiltrate.

Figure 5–12. Invasive fibrous thyroiditis. Compared with Figure 5–11, the inflammatory cell infiltrate in this illustration is much less pronounced.

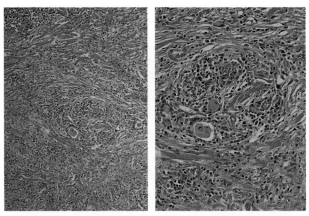

Figure 5–13. The inflammatory infiltrate in invasive fibrous thyroiditis includes an admixture of mature lymphocytes and plasma cells infiltrating throughout the thyroid gland. Remnants of colloid-filled thyroid follicles are seen surrounded by inflammatory cells, and there is an associated dense (keloid-like) fibrosis.

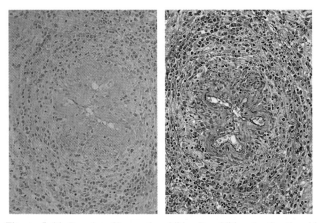

Figure 5–14. Invasive fibrous thyroiditis. In addition to the thyroid parenchyma, the inflammatory infiltrate also involves vascular spaces (vasculitis). *Left,* The inflammatory cells, composed of lymphocytes and plasma cells, infiltrates this blood vessel. *Right,* Elastic stain shows disruption with discontinuation of the black-staining elastic membranes by the inflammatory cell infiltrate that is present throughout the wall of this blood vessel.

- The presence of circulating antithyroid antibodies in a large proportion of patients favors an autoimmune pathogenesis.
- Riedel's disease may be a localized process, or it may be part of a systemic fibrosing disease; other possible sites of disease may include the retroperitoneum, mediastinum, retroorbital area, lung, sinonasal tract, and hepatobiliary tract. Only the retroperitoneal fibrosing process has been linked to a possible etiologic agent, the drug methysergide.

Pathology

Fine Needle Aspiration

- Typically, aspiration in patients with Riedel's disease generates a scanty amount of cellular material; this is referred to as a dry tap.

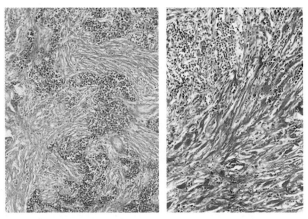

Figure 5–15. The fibrous and inflammatory process may involve extrathyroidal structures such as the soft tissue of the neck or, as seen here, the parathyroid glands *(left). Right,* trichrome stain highlighting the presence of dense fibrosis.

Gross

■ Thyroid tissue is replaced by a dense tan-white, firm to hard tissue.

Histology

■ Destruction and replacement of the thyroid parenchyma by dense collagen (keloid-like bands of fibrosis) occur. The fibrosing process is not confined to the thyroid but also involves extrathyroidal connective tissue structures such as muscle, adipose tissue, nerves, and vascular spaces; the parathyroid glands may also be involved.

■ In addition to fibrosis, a chronic inflammatory cell infiltrate composed of lymphocytes and plasma cells is present. Eosinophils may be present as well.

■ A vasculitis is present that involves primarily the veins (phlebitis); it is characterized by adventitial inflammation that may "invade" through the full thickness of the vessel wall that may create a thrombus-like effect.

■ Remnants of thyroid follicles may be present within the dense collagen, showing atrophic changes.

■ Riedel's disease is not associated with oxyphilic metaplasia of follicular epithelial cells (as seen in chronic lymphocytic thyroiditis) or granulomatous inflammation.

■ In some cases, preexisting or coexisting lesions, such as adenomatoid nodules or a follicular adenoma, may be present.

Differential Diagnosis

■ Hashimoto's thyroiditis, fibrosing variant (Chapter 6B).
■ Subacute thyroiditis (Chapter 5B, #3).

Treatment and Prognosis

■ Because of the extensive fibrosis involving the thyroid as well as the soft tissues of the neck, wide surgical resection is indicated; uninvolved thyroid need not be resected.

Additional Facts

■ The presence of antithyroid antibodies may represent a reaction to released antigens following follicular epithelial destruction (as in subacute thyroiditis) rather than an autoimmune condition.

D. RADIATION THYROIDITIS

Definition: Morphologic alterations of the thyroid due to external radiotherapy or radioiodine therapy resulting in a functional thyroid abnormality (hypothyroidism).

Clinical

External Radiotherapy

■ External irradiation of the neck is used to treat patients with mucosal tumors (typically, squamous cell carcinomas) of the upper aerodigestive tract, metastatic tumors in the neck (primarily those originating from the upper aerodigestive tract), and malignant lymphomas (Hodg-

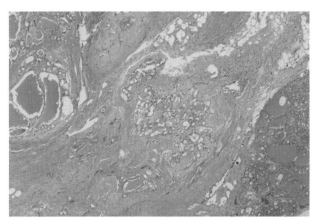

Figure 5–16. The radiation-induced changes of the thyroid gland may include nodular hyperplasia and prominent fibrosis.

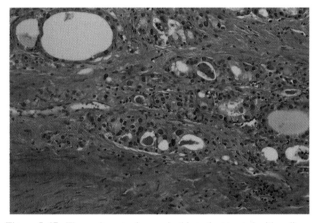

Figure 5–17. The nuclear atypia seen in this patient treated with radioactive iodine includes nucleomegaly with marked pleomorphism and hyperchromasia.

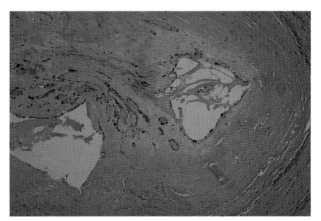

Figure 5–18. Marked parenchymal and vascular (not shown) sclerosis is another feature seen in radiation-associated changes of the thyroid. Follicular atrophy is present.

kin's and non-Hodgkin's lymphomas). In the past, external radiotherapy was used for the treatment of acne, enlarged tonsils and adenoids, thymic enlargement, benign cervical lymphadenopathy, pertussis, epilation, and benign tumors (hemangiomas).

- Hypothyroidism induced by external radiotherapy may occur in 25% to 50% of patients so treated.
- The time interval from the radiation treatment to the development of hypothyroidism usually ranges from 2 to 7 years; however, hypothyroidism may develop within 1 year from the time of radiation treatment.
- The effects (hypothyroidism) of external irradiation on the thyroid gland are dose related (i.e., the higher the dose, the higher the frequency of hypothyroidism).
- In most patients hypothyroidism is subclinical, but it may be overt. Patients with subclinical hypothyroidism may develop overt hypothyroidism later, whereas in other patients subclinical hypothyroidism is transient.
- The acute (i.e., weeks to months) effects of external irradiation (i.e., hypothyroidism) result in functional abnormalities (as determined by thyroid function testing) rather than any significant morphologic changes.
- The major effect of ionizing radiation on thyroid tissue is impairment of the reproductive capacity of the follicular cells.

Radioiodine Treatment (Iodine-131)

- Iodine-131 therapy is used in the treatment of hyperthyroidism, especially for patients with Graves' disease.
- The effects (hypothyroidism) of radioiodine therapy on the thyroid gland are less a function of dose than of time; in fact, virtually all patients eventually become hypothyroid after ^{131}I therapy, even 10 years or more after therapy.
- In patients who have received ^{131}I, overt hypothyroidism is usually preceded by subclinical hypothyroidism.

Pathology in Radiation Thyroiditis

- Externally irradiated thyroid glands are small and fibrotic.

Histology

- The morphologic changes seen in irradiation-induced hyperplastic thyroid glands include increased cellularity, papillary growth pattern, follicular atrophy, oxyphilic and/or squamous metaplasia, decreased or absent colloid, and severe cytologic atypia. The cytologic atypia is characterized by markedly enlarged and bizarrely shaped nuclei (nucleomegaly) with hyperchromasia, prominent nucleoli, and nuclear crowding. Cytologic atypia is randomly found and may be limited to one area or may be haphazardly found in several foci.
- In addition to the architectural and cytologic (nuclear) changes described earlier other changes include:
  • Parenchymal fibrosis.
  • Chronic (lymphocytic cell) inflammation.
  • Vascular sclerosis and intimal thickening (endarteritis obliterans); an associated inflammatory cell infiltrate cuffing the vessels can be seen.
- The atypical nuclear features seen in irradiated thyroid glands are not specific and may be seen in nonirradiated

thyroid glands; however, the vascular changes are fairly specific for irradiated tissues in general, including irradiated thyroid glands.

- Both benign and malignant tumors may develop secondary to external irradiation.
  • Nodules and follicular adenomas with atypical cytologic features including hypercellularity and markedly enlarged, hyperchromatic bizarre-appearing nuclei may be seen.
  • Papillary carcinoma is the most common malignant neoplasm to develop in this way; it is nearly always well differentiated.
  • Follicular carcinomas may develop; rarely, anaplastic carcinomas occur.

Differential Diagnosis

- Cellular adenomatoid nodules (Chapter 7A).
- Dyshormonogenetic goiter (Chapter 7B).
- Papillary carcinoma (Chapter 8D, #2).
- Follicular carcinoma (Chapter 8D, #1).

Treatment and Prognosis

- The hypothyroidism resulting from irradiation of the thyroid gland is treated by thyroid hormone therapy.
- Prophylactic thyroidectomy in patients who develop nodular hyperplasia following external irradiation can be considered.
- Complications of externally irradiated thyroid glands include the development of nodular hyperplasia and benign and malignant neoplasms.
- Papillary carcinoma is the most common malignant tumor to develop following external irradiation.
  • It may develop many years (decades) after radiotherapy.
  • The risk of developing postirradiation (papillary) carcinoma is small.
  • All ages of the population are at risk of developing postirradiation thyroid cancer.
  • These papillary carcinomas are of the usual type and do not behave in any unusual way.
  • Papillary carcinomas may be single or multifocal (within one lobe or distributed throughout the entire gland).
- The significance of radiation exposure in the genesis of thyroid medullary carcinoma is not known, although a small number of individual cases of medullary carcinoma have occurred in patients with a history of radiation exposure to the neck.
- There is no evidence that ^{131}I therapy causes thyroid neoplasms.

Additional Facts

- Radiation exposure from nuclear fallout induces the same morphologic changes as external beam irradiation, but the changes generally occur over a shorter period of time. Similarly, neoplastic lesions resulting from nuclear fallout exposure develop over much shorter periods of time than the same tumors developing after external beam radiotherapy.

E. DRUG-INDUCED THYROIDITIS

- Ingestion of certain medicines may be associated with the development of thyroiditis. However, prior to indicting any drug as the cause of thyroiditis, a detailed history and physical examination to exclude other possible causes of thyroiditis must be performed.
- Medicinal agents implicated in the development of thyroiditis include iodides, lithium salts, phenytoin, amiodarone, and bromide.

1. Iodide

- Iodide is used in the preparation of patients for surgery, for the management of thyrotoxic storm, and as an adjunct after radioiodine therapy.
- The action of iodide includes (1) decreased iodide transport; (2) decreased iodide oxidation and organification; (3) rapid blockage of the release of T_4 and T_3 from the thyroid.
- In patients with preexisting thyroid disease such as toxic nodular goiter, iodide may make the hyperthyroidism worse (**Jod-Basedow phenomenon** or iodine-induced hyperthyroidism). In patients with hyperthyroidism due to Graves' disease the hyperthyroid condition may be exacerbated with iodide therapy. In patients with goiter (endemic or sporadic), iodide added to the diet may induce hyperthyroidism.
- Iodine-induced goiter and hypothyroidism occur most often in individuals with preexisting thyroid disease (patients with chronic lymphocytic thyroiditis or treated Graves' disease) or thyroid ablative therapy (thyroidectomy or radioiodine). In these patients, hypothyroidism occurs with prolonged use of iodide or even following small doses of iodide, but the hypothyroidism is transient, and thyroid function returns to normal following cessation of iodide use. Iodine-induced goiter and hypothyroidism may occasionally occur in the fetus or neonate secondary to transplacental passage of iodine that was administered to the mother.
- Chronic iodide ingestion may lead to diffuse hyperplasia with papillary growth and lymphocytic cell infiltrate.

2. Lithium Salts

- Lithium is used in the treatment of manic-depressive disorders.
- The effects of lithium on the thyroid are similar to those of iodide and include (1) inhibition of thyroid hormone release; (2) inhibition of organification of iodine. The exact mechanisms of lithium's inhibitory action remain uncertain.
- In a small percentage of patients (5% to 15%), chronic lithium use (5 years or more) may be associated with:

  (1) Development of a goiter.
  (2) Development of hypothyroidism.
  (3) Both.

- Although the incidence of lithium-induced hypothyroidism is considered low, it is high enough to warrant monitoring patients who are receiving long-term lithium therapy.

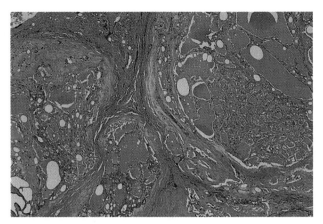

Figure 5–19. Lithium-associated changes of the thyroid gland are similar to the changes seen in radiation-treated glands including the presence of nodular hyperplasia with associated fibrosis.

- The histologic changes of lithium use include:
  - Diffuse hyperplasia with associated nuclear pleomorphism.
  - Lymphocytic cell infiltrates with or without germinal centers, follicular epithelial cell atrophy with or without oxyphilic metaplasia, and fibrosis. These changes are similar to those of chronic lymphocytic thyroiditis.
- The presence of antithyroid antibodies appears to be higher in patients with lithium-associated hypothyroidism (subclinical or overt) than in those without hypothyroidism.

3. Anticonvulsant Drugs

- Phenytoin and carbamazepine are used in the treatment of epilepsy.
- Their mode of action is to reduce serum total and free T_4 and, to a lesser extent, T_3 levels. Serum TSH concentrations are not elevated, but the addition of lithium to the therapy will raise serum TSH levels.
- Clinically significant hypothyroidism associated with these anticonvulsant drugs is uncommon.

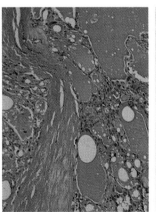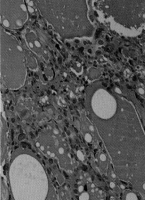

Figure 5–20. Like radiation-induced changes, the changes in the thyroid due to chronic lithium therapy include *(left)* the presence of atypical nodules characterized by increased cellularity and associated dense fibrosis. *Right,* The bizarre-appearing nuclei show nucleomegaly, pleomorphism, and hyperchromasia.

- Phenytoin is associated with systemic immune reactions, and an organ-specific reaction (i.e., thyroiditis) may represent a component of phenytoin-associated autoimmunity.

4. Amiodarone

- Amiodarone is used in the treatment of cardiac arrhythmias and angina.
- Amiodarone tablets contain a large percentage of iodine, and excess iodine release occurs during the metabolism of this drug.
- The effects of amiodarone on the thyroid include:
  - Iodide-related inhibition of thyroid hormone synthesis and secretion.
  - Impaired cellular uptake of thyroid hormones.
- Abnormal thyroid function occurs in nearly all patients receiving amiodarone.
- Amiodarone may cause hypothyroidism or hyperthyroidism.
- Symptomatic hypothyroidism usually occurs within the first year of treatment but may occur later; amiodarone-related (fatal) myxedema coma can occur.
- Amiodarone-induced hypothyroidism is associated with elevated circulating antithyroid antibodies, and this form of hypothyroidism may be related to an underlying autoimmune thyroiditis.
- Amiodarone-induced hyperthyroidism may be the result of follicular cell damage with subsequent thyroid antibody production (antithyroglobulin or antimicrosomal antibodies) or may induce a thyroid-specific autoimmunity.
- Histologic changes may include follicular epithelial cell degenerative changes with vacuolization and a lymphohistiocytic cell response.
- Discontinuing use will often reverse its adverse effects.

References

Acute (Infectious) Thyroiditis

Adler ME, Jordon G, Walter RM. Acute suppurative thyroiditis. West Med J 1978; 132:990–991.
Berger SA, Zonszein J, Villamena P, Mittman N. Infectious diseases of the thyroid gland. Rev Infect Dis 1983; 5:108–122.
Schubert MF, Kountz DS. Thyroiditis. A disease with many faces. Postgrad Med 1995; 98:101–103.
Singer PA. Thyroiditis. Acute, subacute and chronic. Med Clin North Am 1991; 75:61–77.
Sudar JM, Alleman MJ, Jonkers GJ, et al. Acute thyroiditis caused by *Moraxella nonliquefaciens*. Neth J Med 1994; 45:170–173.

Granulomatous Thyroiditis
Infectious Granulomatous Thyroiditis

Berger SA, Zonszein J, Villamena P, Mittman R. Infectious diseases of the thyroid gland. Rev Infect Dis 1983; 3:108–122.
Harach HR, Williams ED. The pathology of granulomatous diseases of the thyroid gland. Sarcoidosis 1990; 7:19–27.
Hizawa K, Okamura K, Sato K, et al. Tuberculous thyroiditis and miliary tuberculosis manifested postpartum in a patient with thyroid carcinoma. Endocrinol Jpn 1990; 37:571–576.
Kakudo K, Kanogoki M, Mitsunobu M, et al. Acute mycotic thyroiditis. Acta Pathol Jpn 1983; 33:147–151.
Sachs MK, Dickinson G, Amazon K. Tuberculous adenitis of the thyroid mimicking subacute thyroiditis. Am J Med 1988; 85:573–575.

Singer PA. Thyroiditis. Acute, subacute and chronic. Med Clin North Am 1991; 75:61–77.
Takami H, Kozakai M. Tuberculous thyroiditis: report of a case with a review of the literature. Endocr J 1994; 41:743–747.

Sarcoidosis of the Thyroid Gland

Cilley RE, Thompson NW, Lloyd RV, Shapiro B. Sarcoidosis of the thyroid presenting as a painful nodule. Thyroidology 1988; 1:61–62.
Harach HR, Williams ED. The pathology of granulomatous diseases of the thyroid gland. Sarcoidosis 1990; 7:19–27.
Sasaki H, Harada T, Eimoto T, et al. Case report: Comcomitant association of thyroid sarcoidosis and Hashimoto's thyroiditis. Am J Med Sci 1987; 294:441–443.
Vailati A, Marena C, Aristia L, et al. Sarcoidosis of the thyroid: Report of a case and a review of the literature. Sarcoidosis 1993; 10:66–68.
van Assendelft AHW, Kahlos T. Sarcoidosis of the thyroid gland. Sarcoidosis 1985; 2:154–156.

Subacute Thyroiditis

Greene JN. Subacute thyroiditis. Am J Med 1971; 51; 97–108.
Harach HR, Williams ED. The pathology of granulomatous diseases of the thyroid gland. Sarcoidosis 1990; 7:19–27.
Hay ID. Thyroiditis: a clinical update. Mayo Clin Proc 1985; 60:836–843.
Hazard JB. Thyroiditis: a review. Am J Clin Pathol 1955; 25:289–298.
Kitchener MI, Chapman IM. Subacute thyroiditis: a review of 105 cases. Clin Nucl Med 1989; 14:439–442.
Larsen PR. Serum triiodothyronine, thyroxine and thyrotropin during hyperthyroid, hypothyroid and recovery phases of subacute nonsuppurative thyroiditis. Metabolism 1974; 23:467–471.
Meachem G, Young MH. DeQuervain's subacute granulomatous thyroiditis: histological identification and incidence. J Clin Pathol 1963; 16:189–199.
Mizukami Y, Michigishi T, Kawato M, Matsubara F. Immunohistochemical and ultrastructural study of subacute thyroiditis, with special reference to multinucleated giant cells. Hum Pathol 1987; 18:929–935.
Nikolai TF. Silent thyroiditis and subacute thyroiditis. In: Braverman LE, Utiger RD, eds. Werner and Ingbar's The Thyroid. A fundamental and clinical text. Sixth edition. Philadelphia: J.B. Lippincott Co., 1991:710–727.
Reidbord HE, Fischer ER. Ultrastructural features of subacute granulomatous thyroiditis and Hashimoto's thyroiditis. Am J Clin Pathol 1973; 59:327–337.
Singer PA. Thyroiditis. Acute, subacute and chronic. Med Clin North Am 1991; 75:61–77.
Tikkanen MJ, Lamberg B-A. Hypothyroidism following subacute thyroiditis. Acta Endocrinol 1982; 101:348–353.
Volpé R. The pathology of thyroiditis. Hum Pathol 1978; 9:429–438.
Volpé R. Subacute (deQuervain's) thyroiditis. Clin Endocrinol Meb 1979; 8:81–95.
Volpé R. Subacute thyroiditis. Prog Clin Biol Res 1981; 74:115–134.
Wiehl AC, Daniels GH, Ridgeway, et al. Thyroid function tests during the early phase of subacute thyroiditis. J Clin Endocrinol Metab 1977; 44:1107–1114.
Woolner LB, McConahey WB, Beahrs OH. Granulomatous thyroiditis (deQuervain's thyroiditis). J Clin Endocrinol Metab 1957; 17:1202–1221.
Yoshida K, Sakurada T, Kaise N, et al. Serum free thyroxine and triiodothyronine concentrations in subacute thyroiditis. J Clin Endocrinol Metab 1982; 55:185–188.

Painless ("Silent") Subacute Thyroiditis

Nikolai TF. Silent thyroiditis and subacute thyroiditis. In: Braverman LE, Utiger RD, eds. Werner and Ingbar's The Thyroid. A fundamental and clinical text. Sixth edition. Philadelphia: J.B. Lippincott Co., 1991:710–727.

Multifocal Granulomatous Thyroiditis (Palpation Thyroiditis)

Blum M, Schloss MF. Martial-arts thyroiditis. N Engl J Med 1984; 311:199–200.
Carney JA, Moore SB, Northcutt RC, et al. Palpation thyroiditis (multifocal granulomatous thyroiditis). Am J Clin Pathol 1975; 64:639–647.
Harach HR. Palpation thyroiditis resembling C cell hyperplasia, Usefulness of immunohistochemistry in their differential diagnosis. Pathol Res Pract 1993; 189:488–490.

Invasive Fibrous Thyroiditis (Reidel's Disease)

Chopra D, Wool MS, Crosson A, Sawin CT. Reidel's struma associated with subacute thyroiditis, hypothyrodism, and hypoparathyrodism. J Clin Endocrin Metab 1978; 46:869–871.

De Lange WE, Freling NJM, Molenaar WM, Doorenbos H. Invasive fibrous thyroiditis (Reidel's struma): A manifestation of multifocal fibrosclerosis? A case report with review of the literature. Q J Med 1989; 72:709–717.

Davies D, Furness P. Reidel's disease with multiple organ fibrosis. Thorax 1984; 39:959–960.

Harach HR, Williams ED. Fibrous thyroiditis—an immunopathological study. Histopathology 1983; 7:739–751.

Heufelder AE, Hay ID. Evidence for autoimmune mechanisms in the evolution of invasive fibrous thyroiditis (Reidel's struma). Clin Investig 1994; 72:788–793.

Malotte MJ, Chonkich GD, Zuppan CW. Reidel's thyroiditis. Arch Otolaryngol Head Neck Surg 1991; 117:214–217.

Mitchison MJ. Retroperitoneal fibrosis revisited. Arch Pathol Lab Med 1986; 110:784–786.

Schwaegerle SM, Bauer TW, Esselstyn CB Jr. Reidel's thyroiditis. Am J Clin Pathol 1988; 90:715–722.

Woolner LB, McConahey WB, Beahrs OH. Invasive fibrous thyroiditis (Reidel's disease). J Clin Endocrinol Metab 1957; 17:201–220.

Zelmanovitz F, Zelmanovitz T, Beck M, et al. Reidel's thyroiditis associated with high titers of antimicrosomal and antithyroglobulin antibodies and hypothyrodism. J Endocrinol Invest 1994; 17:733–737.

Zimmermann-Belsing T, Feldt-Rasmussen U. Reidel's thyroiditis: an autoimmune or primary fibrotic disease? J Intern Med 1994; 235:271–274.

Radiation Thyroiditis

Carr RF, LiVolsi VA. Morphologic changes in the thyroid after irradiation for Hodgkin's and non-Hodgkin's lymphoma. Cancer 1990; 64: 825–829.

Constine LS, Donaldson SS, McDougall IR, et al. Thyroid dysfunction after radiotherapy in children with Hodgkin's disease. Cancer 1984; 53:878–883.

Cunnien AJ, Hay ID, Gorman CA, et al. Radioiodine-induced hypothyroidism in Graves' disease: factors associated with the increasing incidence. J Nucl Med 1982; 23:978–983.

Dunn EL, Nishiyama RH, Thompson NW. Medullary carcinoma of the thyroid gland. Surgery 1973; 73:848–858.

Fleming ID, Black TL, Thompson EI, et al. Thyroid dysfunction and neoplasia in children receiving neck irradiation for cancer. Cancer 1985; 55:1190–1194.

Fraker DL. Radiation exposure and other factors that predispose to human thyroid neoplasia. Surg Clin North Am 1995; 75:365–375.

Hancock SL, McDougall IR, Constine LS. Thyroid abnormalities after therapeutic external radiation. Int J Radiat Oncol Biol Phys 1995; 31:1165–1170.

Holm LE, Lundell G, Israelsson A, et al. Incidence of hypothyroidism occurring long after iodine-131 therapy for hyperthyroidism. J Nucl Med 1982; 23:103–107.

Holm LE. Changing annual incidence of hypothyroidism after iodine-131 therapy for hyperthyroidism, 1951–1975. J Nucl Med 1982; 23:108–112.

Kennedy JS, Thomson JA. The changes in the thyroid gland after irradiation with [131]-I or partial thyroidectomy for thyrotoxicosis. J Pathol 1974; 112:65–81.

Komorowski RA, Hanson GA. Morphologic changes in the thyroid following low-dose childhood radiation. Arch Pathol Lab Med 1977; 101:36–39.

Malone JF, Cullen MJ. Two mechanisms for hypothyrodism after [131]-I therapy. Lancet 1976; 2:73–75.

Nikiforov YE, Heffess CS, Korzenko AV, et al. Characteristics of follicular tumors and nonneoplastic thyroid lesions in children and adolescents exposed to radiation as a result of the Chernobyl disaster. Cancer 1995; 76:900–909.

Ron E, Lubin JH, Shore RE, et al. Thyroid cancer after exposure to external radiation: a pooled analysis of seven studies. Radiat Res 1995; 141:259–277.

Spitalnik PF, Straus FH, II. Patterns of human thyroid parenchymal reaction following low-dose childhood irradiation. Cancer 1978; 41:1098–1105.

Williams ED. Biologic effects of radiation on the thyroid. In: Braverman LE, Utiger RD, eds. Werner and Ingbar's The Thyroid. A fundamental and clinical text. Sixth edition. Philadelphia: J.B. Lippincott Co., 1991:421–436.

Drug-Induced Thyroiditis

Barsano CP. Other forms of primary hypothyroidism. In: Braverman LE, Utiger RD, eds. Werner and Ingbar's The Thyroid: A fundamental and clinical text. Sixth edition. Philadelphia: J.B. Lippincott Co., 1991:956–967.

Borowski GD, Garofano CD, Rose LI, et al. Effect of long term amiodarone therapy on thyroid hormone levels and thyroid function. Am J Med 1985; 78:443–450.

Emerson CH, Dyson WL, Utiger RD. Serum thyrotropin and thyroxine concentrations in patients receiving lithium carbonate. J Clin Endocrinol Metab 1973; 36:338–346.

Kaplan J, Ish-Shalom S. Goiter and hypothyroidism during re-treatment with amiodarone in a patient who previously experienced amiodarone-induced thyrotoxicosis. Am J Med 1991; 90:750–752.

Roti E, Vegenakis AG. Effect of excess iodide: clinical aspects. In: Braverman LE, Utiger RD, eds. Werner and Ingbar's The Thyroid. A fundamental and clinical text. Sixth edition. Philadelphia: J.B. Lippincott Co., 1991:390–402.

CHAPTER 6

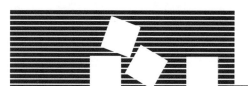

Autoimmune Thyroiditis

Definition: In the great majority of cases, the presence of lymphoid cells in the thyroid is an abnormal (probably autoimmune) phenomenon and can be placed in the general category of chronic lymphocytic thyroiditis. Lymphocytic infiltrates in the thyroid may be nonspecific (clinical or laboratory findings indicating thyroid disease is absent) and are often found in glands removed for other reasons, or they may represent a constellation of clinical and pathologic findings termed Hashimoto's thyroiditis. The causes of autoimmune thyroiditis are listed in Table 6–1.

A. CHRONIC (NONSPECIFIC) LYMPHOCYTIC THYROIDITIS

Clinical

- Affects women more than men; most common in older patients.
- No specific clinical findings (symptoms); clinical features are correlated with the dominant pathologic process (e.g., nodules, tumor, other) in which the lymphocytic thyroiditis is a secondary finding.
- Thyroid function, as determined by laboratory tests, is usually within normal limits (the patient is euthyroid); some patients may be hypothyroid, although clinical manifestations of hypothyroidism are absent.
- Laboratory evidence of autoimmune thyroiditis (presence of antithyroid antibodies) is usually absent.

Pathology

Gross

- In general, chronic nonspecific thyroiditis is an incidental finding and does not produce any mass lesions.

Histology

- Focal or multifocal aggregates of mature lymphocytes with or without germinal centers are seen.
- No quantitative parameters (total number of lymphocytes) are required for a diagnosis of lymphocytic thyroiditis; any lymphocytic cell infiltrate in the thyroid can be considered abnormal.

Table 6–1
AUTOIMMUNE THYROIDITIDES

Chronic (nonspecific) lymphocytic thyroiditis
Chronic lymphocytic thyroiditis or Hashimoto's thyroiditis
Fibrous variant of lymphocytic thyroiditis
Fibrous atrophy of the thyroid (idiopathic myxedema)
Juvenile type of lymphocytic thyroiditis
"Painless" thyroiditis with hyperthyroidism
"Hashitoxicosis"
Graves' disease (diffuse toxic hyperplasia)

- Associated fibrosis, oxyphilia of follicular cells, and follicular cell atrophy may be seen to a limited extent but are often not present.

Differential Diagnosis

- Malignant lymphoma (see next section, Chronic Lymphocytic Thyroiditis or Hashimoto's Thyroiditis)

Treatment and Prognosis

- No specific treatment requirements; treatment is directed at the main pathologic process to which lymphocytic thyroiditis is secondary.
- No specific prognostic parameters; by itself, lymphocytic thyroiditis has an excellent prognosis.

B. CHRONIC LYMPHOCYTIC THYROIDITIS OR HASHIMOTO'S THYROIDITIS

Synonyms: Struma lymphomatosa; classic form of autoimmune thyroiditis.

Clinical

- Much more common in women than men; occurs over a wide age range, and the frequency increases with age.
- Wide variation in the clinical features of autoimmune thyroiditis:
  - Many patients present with no signs or symptoms, and the diagnosis is made on the basis of laboratory tests of

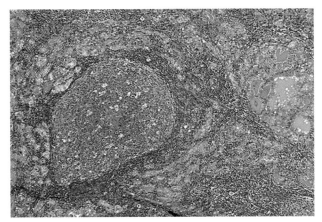

Figure 6–1. Lymphocytic thyroiditis. The lymphocytic cell infiltrate with germinal center is seen focally within the thyroid. The follicular epithelium is essentially unchanged and shows no features of Hashimoto's thyroiditis.

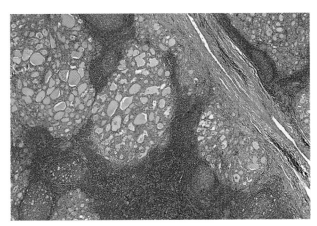

Figure 6–4. Chronic lymphocytic thyroiditis (Hashimoto's thyroiditis). Histologic characteristics include diffuse involvement of the thyroid gland in which mature lymphocytes, with or without germinal centers, are present. Additional changes include alterations of the thyroid follicular epithelium, including cytoplasmic oxyphilia and/or atrophy, and fibrosis.

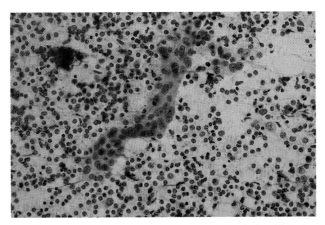

Figure 6–2. Fine needle aspiration (FNA) of Hashimoto's thyroiditis characterized by a prominent mixed lymphoplasmacytic infiltrate. Follicular epithelium is frequently scanty; the epithelium exhibits cytoplasmic oxyphilia, nuclear enlargement, and variable nuclear pleomorphism. The epithelium is usually arranged in sheetlike fragments. In more florid cases colloid is difficult to identify. Papanicolaou stain.

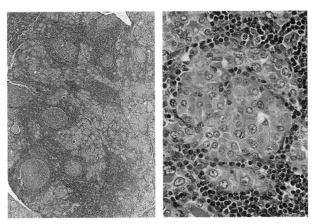

Figure 6–5. Chronic lymphocytic thyroiditis (Hashimoto's thyroiditis). *Left,* Diffuse involvement of the thyroid gland by a lymphocytic cell infiltrate with associated germinal centers, and oxyphilic changes of the follicular epithelial cells. *Right,* Higher magnification shows oxyphilic metaplasia characterized by a granular eosinophilic cytoplasm.

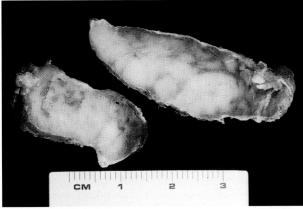

Figure 6–3. Chronic lymphocytic thyroiditis (Hashimoto's thyroiditis). Symmetrically enlarged thyroid gland characterized by a prominent multilobulated appearance; the lobules are tan-white and replace most of the thyroid tissue.

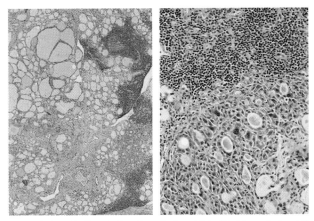

Figure 6–6. *Left,* Chronic lymphocytic thyroiditis (Hashimoto's thyroiditis) characterized by a mature lymphocytic cell infiltrate, germinal centers, follicular epithelial atrophy, oxyphilic metaplasia, and fibrosis. *Right,* Oxyphilic metaplasia with nuclear enlargement. The nuclei remain round and regular and do not have the irregularities seen in papillary carcinoma.

thyroid function, screening tests for thyroid antibodies, or incidental findings in thyroid glands that have been surgically excised for other reasons.
- In some patients, an enlarged thyroid is the only clinical manifestation of autoimmune thyroiditis.
- In many patients, there is clinical evidence of hypothyroidism. Patients present with a mass lesion (goiter) of the thyroid; typically, there is bilateral diffuse enlargement of the thyroid, but infrequently, a dominant mass lesion confined to one lobe of the thyroid and simulating a neoplastic proliferation may be seen.

■ Hashimoto's thyroiditis may occur in patients who are euthyroid and, rarely, in patients with hyperthyroidism; in patients who are not hypothyroid at presentation, evidence of hypothyroidism may develop with time.

■ Laboratory evidence of hypothyroidism may include decreased T_4 and possibly decreased T_3 levels (although the latter may be normal).

■ Laboratory evidence of autoimmune thyroiditis includes the presence of antithyroid antibodies (antithyroglobulin or antimicrosomal antibodies [antithyroid peroxidase]).

■ The precise antigen or antigens that cause autosensitization are unknown, but the presence of antithyroglobulin and antimicrosomal antibodies suggests that these antigens are involved. Thyroglobulin and thyroid peroxidase share epitopes, and it is possible that the initial antigen may result in a sequential response to the other antigen.

■ Unlike Graves' disease, in which thyroid-stimulating antibody is almost always present, this antibody is only occasionally present in Hashimoto's thyroiditis.

■ Patients with Hashimoto's thyroiditis have an increased incidence of different HLA-DR haplotypes (HLA-DR3, -DR4, and -DR5).

■ The incidence of Hashimoto's thyroiditis is higher in patients with Down's syndrome and Turner's syndrome.

■ Patients with Hashimoto's thyroiditis have a greater risk of other coexisting autoimmune diseases, including:
- Endocrine diseases: insulin-dependent diabetes mellitus, Addison's disease, autoimmune oophoritis, hypoparathyroidism, and hypophysitis.
- Nonendocrine diseases: Sjögren's syndrome, myasthenia gravis, pernicious anemia, thrombocytopenic purpura.
- Autoantibody: Patients with autoimmune thyroid disease (Hashimoto's thyroiditis, Graves' disease) have a higher prevalence of autoantibody not only against thyroid-specific antigens but also against nonthyroid-specific antigens (antibodies to nucleus, smooth muscle, and single-stranded DNA) than matched control patients.

■ Hashimoto's thyroiditis and Graves' disease share common features:
- Both conditions have been found in the same families or within the same thyroid gland.
- There are cases of identical twins in which one twin has Hashimoto's thyroiditis and the other has Graves' disease.
- Lymphocytic infiltration and various immunoglobulins have been found in the thyroid in both disorders.
- Thymic enlargement and thyroid autoantibodies are found in both diseases.

- Graves' disease may spontaneously culminate in Hashimoto's thyroiditis and hypothyroidism, and Hashimoto's thyroiditis (with or without hypothyroidism) may change into Graves' disease with hyperthyroidism.

■ Despite these shared features, there are sufficient differences (genetic, clinical, immunologic, and pathologic) to consider these diseases as distinct disorders and not the opposite ends of the spectrum of a single entity.

Pathology

Fine Needle Aspiration

■ There are mixed inflammatory cell infiltrates including mature lymphocytes and plasma cells. Multinucleated giant cells may be present. The presence of germinal centers may be reflected by a variety of lymphocytes and tingible body macrophages.

■ Follicular epithelial cells may show oxyphilic cytoplasmic changes, which usually appear in cohesive clusters but may appear singly.

■ Colloid is minimal to absent.

Gross

■ Symmetrically enlarged gland is firm and pale in color and is characterized by a prominent multilobulated appearance; the lobules tend to bulge from the cut surface and are separated by fibrous tissue.

■ The bilateral diffuse thyroid enlargement assists in decreasing clinical suspicion of a neoplastic proliferation, which usually appears as a single dominant mass.

■ The thyroid is not adherent to the surrounding structures.

Histology

■ At low magnification, lobules or nodules separated by thin fibrous tissue are seen.

■ The histologic hallmarks of Hashimoto's thyroiditis include:
- Diffuse involvement of the thyroid gland.
- Mature lymphocytic cell infiltrate with or without germinal centers.
- Follicular atrophy.
- Oxyphilic metaplasia of follicular epithelial cells.

■ In addition to lymphocytes, histiocytes, plasma cells, and giant cells may be present. The giant cells are seen within the follicles but are limited in extent and number, a neutrophilic infiltrate is not seen, and a granulomatous process is absent.

■ In contrast to the neoplastic lymphoid population of a malignant thyroid lymphoma, the lymphocytic cell infiltrate of chronic lymphocytic thyroiditis:
- Is confined to the thyroid gland and does not extend beyond the thyroid capsule into perithyroidal soft tissue.
- Usually shows no ''colonization'' of thyroid follicles (as in malignant lymphoma), although it may occur.

■ Thyroid atrophy is marked by the presence of small follicles with limited to absent colloid formation.

■ Fibrosis in and around the follicles can be seen; interlobular fibrosis gives the gland a nodular appearance.

■ Nuclear enlargement is associated with oxyphilic metaplasia; it may be accompanied by dispersed to optically clear-appearing nuclear chromatin. These changes may be confused with those of papillary carcinoma, but additional architectural or cytomorphologic features of papillary carcinoma are absent.

■ Additional changes that may be seen include squamous metaplasia of follicular epithelial cells (more common in the fibrous variant—see below) and intrathyroidal squamous-lined and ciliated respiratory epithelial-lined cysts; the latter may attain a fairly large size and may be mistaken for branchial cleft anomalies.

■ Immunohistochemistry: Lymphoid infiltrate shows both B-cell (CD20 [L26]) and T-cell (CD45RA [UCHL-1] or CD3) immunoreactivity. Light chain restriction is not present, although the B cells are most often of the IgG kappa type.

Differential Diagnosis

■ Non-Hodgkin's malignant lymphoma (Chapter 8F, #2).
■ Thyroid papillary carcinoma (Chapter 8D, #2).

Treatment and Prognosis

■ Thyroxine (T$_4$) therapy is the treatment of choice for all patients with hypothyroidism (overt or subclinical) resulting from autoimmune thyroiditis. Treatment generally is maintained lifelong because hypothyroidism will recur with cessation of T$_4$. Proper response to T$_4$ therapy includes a decrease in the levels of thyroid antibodies.

■ Immunosuppressive (corticosteroid) therapy may result in regression of thyroid enlargement and a decrease in thyroid antibody levels; however, because of the serious side effects of steroids and the efficacy of T$_4$ therapy, immunosuppressive therapy is not indicated.

■ Appropriate therapy for patients who are euthyroid but have enlarged glands (goiter) remains uncertain; T$_4$ administration may result in a decrease in size of the gland, but in other patients there is no diminution in size but rather a progressive enlargement of the thyroid. Further, up to 10% to 15% of patients may become hypothyroid.

■ Surgery can be recommended in patients who do not respond to T$_4$ therapy and have continued enlargement (with or without local symptoms) of the thyroid gland.

■ Patients with coexisting thyrotoxicosis should be treated accordingly.

■ The frequency of non-Hodgkin's malignant lymphoma is increased in patients with lymphocytic thyroiditis; however, patients with autoimmune thyroiditis are at no increased risk of developing a thyroid follicular epithelial or neuroendocrine neoplasm.

C. FIBROUS VARIANT OF HASHIMOTO'S THYROIDITIS

Synonym: Advanced lymphocytic thyroiditis.

■ This variant may occur in approximately 10% of cases of chronic lymphocytic thyroiditis.
■ Compared to the "classic type," the fibrous variant is
  • More common in men than in women.
  • Occurs in older patients.

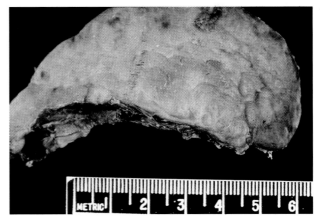

Figure 6–7. Advanced lymphocytic thyroiditis. The thyroid is diffusely enlarged and was firm to hard on palpation; fibrosis and a prominent lobulated appearance are seen.

Figure 6–8. Advanced lymphocytic thyroiditis. There is replacement of the thyroid tissue by a dense fibrous tissue, which replaces the follicular epithelium. The remnant of thyroid tissue showed the presence of follicular atrophy, squamous metaplasia, and lymphocytic cell infiltrate.

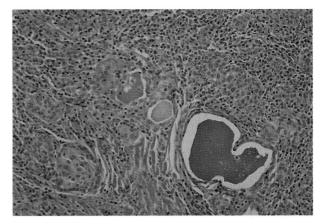

Figure 6–9. Higher magnification in advanced lymphocytic thyroiditis shows follicular atrophy, squamous metaplasia, fibrosis, lymphocytic cell infiltrate, and cystic changes of the thyroid follicles. The latter may attain a large size and be confused with branchial cleft cysts or other cystic proliferations.

- Patients present with symptoms of a large goiter that may produce dysphagia and dyspnea.
- Patients often present with severe hypothyroidism and have high titers of antithyroglobulin antibodies.

Pathology

Fine Needle Aspiration

- Due to marked fibrosis, aspiration generally yields very little material.

Gross

- Thyroid gland is diffusely enlarged, firm to hard, pale tan in color, and characterized by the presence of fibrosis and a prominent lobular appearance; the gland may weigh as much as 200 g or more.
- The thyroid is not adherent to the surrounding structures.

Histology

- At low power the characteristic features include the presence of an obvious nodular or lobular pattern of growth with associated dense fibrosis and a chronic inflammatory cell infiltrate.
- The fibrosis is keloid-like and has irregular broad bands of acellular fibrous tissue coursing in and around the remnant of the thyroid parenchymal tissue. The chronic inflammatory cell infiltrate can be seen within the fibrotic tissue.
- The remnant of thyroid tissue shows the changes characteristic of chronic lymphocytic thyroiditis including mature lymphocytic cell infiltrates with or without germinal centers, severe follicular atrophy, and oxyphilic metaplasia of the follicular epithelial cells.
- The inflammatory cell infiltrate includes mature lymphocytes as well as plasma cells.
- Squamous metaplasia may be prominently seen in this form of lymphocytic thyroiditis.

Differential Diagnosis

- Riedel's disease (Chapter 5C).

Treatment and Prognosis

- Surgical removal of the thyroid (total thyroidectomy) is indicated.
- Prognosis is considered good following removal of the gland, which relieves the symptoms.

D. FIBROUS ATROPHY OF THE THYROID (IDIOPATHIC MYXEDEMA)

- More common in women than in men; occurs in older patients.
- Aside from the enlarged goitrous thyroid, the clinical presentation and laboratory findings are similar to those described for the fibrous variant of lymphocytic thyroiditis, including severe hypothyroidism and high titers of antithyroglobulin antibodies.

- The thyroid gland is small and often weighs less than 5 g.
- The thyroid parenchyma is not recognizable and is replaced by a dense tan-white fibrous tissue.
- Histologically, the changes are similar to those of the fibrous variant of lymphocytic thyroiditis, including a prominent keloid-like fibrosis, chronic inflammatory cell infiltrates, and marked follicular atrophy with oncocytic and squamous metaplasia.
- Given the similarities in clinical findings and histopathologic appearance, fibrous atrophy of the thyroid and the fibrous variant of lymphocytic thyroiditis may be related, with the former representing the end stage of the clinical and morphologic continuum of the latter.

E. JUVENILE FORM OF LYMPHOCYTIC THYROIDITIS

- Much more common in females than in males; most common in adolescents and young adults.
- Most patients present with a small goiter with or without mild hypothyroidism.
- Some patients may present with signs and symptoms of thyrotoxicosis (tachycardia, nervousness, increased pulse pressure) rather than hypothyroidism.
- There may be a strong family history of thyroid disease (asymptomatic goiter, hypothyroidism, and Graves' hyperthyroidism.)
- Juvenile lymphocytic thyroiditis (Hashimoto's thyroiditis) most commonly occurs in the absence of abnormalities in another endocrine organ; however, it may be associated with deficiencies of the pancreas, adrenal glands, parathyroid glands, or gonads. The most common clinical entity is **Schmidt's syndrome,** characterized by a combination of Hashimoto's thyroiditis and adrenal insufficiency.
- Mild to marked elevated antithyroglobulin antibodies may be present. Thyroid autoantibodies have been found in 20% to 30% of children with type I diabetes mellitus, and elevated serum TSH levels have been found in around 10% of these children; therefore, it is recommended that all children with diabetes mellitus be screened for autoimmune thyroid disease.
- Histologically, this disease is characterized by a chronic lymphocytic infiltrate with only focal or absent follicular atrophy and metaplasia.
- Follicular epithelial hyperplasia may be present, correlating with a hyperthyroid state.
- Biologic behavior varies and includes spontaneous remission, progressive atrophy of the thyroid with progression to (severe) hypothyroidism, and recurrent hyperthyroidism.

F. PAINLESS THYROIDITIS WITH HYPERTHYROIDISM

- Initially, this entity was considered to be within the spectrum of subacute thyroiditis, but it is now recognized as a form of autoimmune thyroiditis.
- It primarily affects women in the younger age groups at the puerperium or postpartum.

- Patients present with episodic hyperthyroidism and elevated antithyroglobulin antibody levels.
- Histomorphologic changes are similar to those typical of the juvenile form of lymphocytic thyroiditis and include lymphocytic infiltration, oxyphilic metaplasia, and follicular hyperplasia.
- Biologic behavior varies and includes complete resolution, recurrent hyperthyroidism, and, rarely, progression to hypothyroidism.
- This entity differs from so-called **painless "silent" subacute thyroiditis** in that it:
  - Is an autoimmune disease.
  - Is associated with elevated levels of antithyroglobulin antibodies.
  - Lacks the histomorphologic features of subacute granulomatous thyroiditis; specifically, there is no granulomatous inflammation, and multinucleated giant cells are absent.
  - Is associated with a greater risk of permanent hypothyroidism and a higher recurrence rate.

G. HASHITOXICOSIS

Synonym: Hyperthyroiditis.

- This entity includes some of the categories listed earlier in this chapter, including the juvenile form of lymphocytic thyroiditis and painless thyroiditis with hyperthyroidism.
- These patients present with clinical evidence of Graves' disease (with or without laboratory confirmation of disease) and histologically demonstrate features of Hashimoto's thyroiditis, including lymphocytic infiltration, follicular atrophy, and metaplasia. In some cases, follicular hyperplasia is present with minimal or absent follicular atrophy and oxyphilic metaplasia.

H. AUTOIMMUNE HYPERTHYROIDISM (DIFFUSE TOXIC GOITER; GRAVES' DISEASE)

Definition: Organ-specific autoimmune disorder caused by the production of the autoantibodies (called thyrotropin receptor antibodies [TRA], thyroid-stimulating immunoglobulin (TSI), or thyroid-stimulating [auto]antibodies [TSAb]) that bind to TSH receptors on the thyroid follicular epithelial cells. This leads to overstimulation and enlargement of the thyroid gland with overproduction of thyroid hormones, suppression of TSH production from the pituitary gland, and clinical manifestations of hyperthyroidism. The TSH receptor antibody that stimulates the thyroid gland was originally called the long-acting thyroid stimulator (LATS).

Synonym: Basedow's disease.

Clinical

- Reported incidence in the United States ranges from 0.02% to 0.4% of the population.
- Represents the most common cause of hyperthyroidism and accounts for approximately 70% to 80% of all cases.

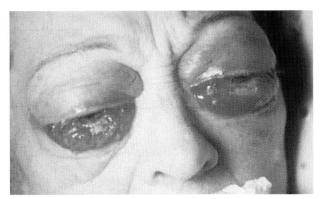

Figure 6–10. Diffuse hyperplasia (Graves' disease). Among the more obvious clinical manifestations of Graves' disease is the presence of ophthalmopathy.

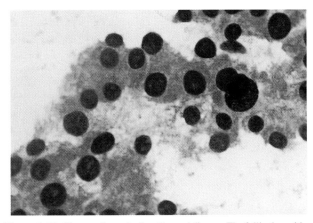

Figure 6–11. Fine needle aspiration, Graves' disease. The follicular epithelium in this fine needle aspirate of a patient with diffuse hyperplasia (Graves' disease) is arranged in orderly sheets with a honeycomb pattern, high cellularity, and lack of colloid. These features may suggest a follicular neoplasm with oxyphilia. The clinical history is most helpful in arriving at a correct interpretation. Note the prominent granularity of the cytoplasm, a common feature in Graves' disease. Diff-Quik stain.

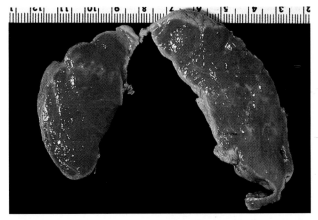

Figure 6–12. Total thyroidectomy specimen in Graves' disease showing diffuse and symmetric enlargement of the gland, which has a beefy red appearance.

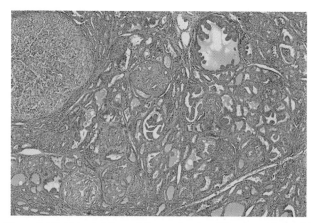

Figure 6–13. Untreated Graves' disease showing diffuse hyperplasia with prominent papillary architecture, increased cellularity, and relative absence of colloid.

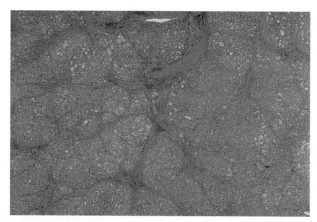

Figure 6–16. Prolonged radioiodine therapy in Graves' disease is associated with fibrosis, creating a nodular appearance.

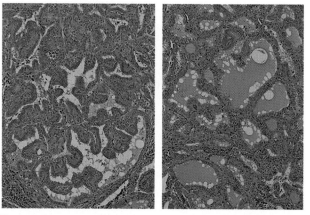

Figure 6–14. *Left,* Papillary hyperplasia in untreated Graves' disease. The papillae do not demonstrate the complexity of growth seen in papillary carcinoma. The nuclei are enlarged but lack the cytomorphologic characteristics of papillary carcinoma. *Right,* Focally, colloid can be seen. The colloid is artifactually distorted owing to fixation and has a "scalloped" appearance.

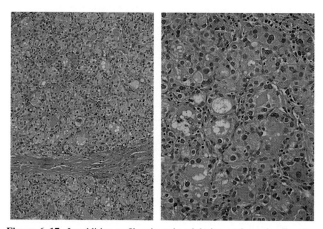

Figure 6–17. In addition to fibrosis and nodularity, prolonged radioactive iodine therapy may result in atypical nodules with increased cellularity and markedly bizarre nuclei (which show nucleomegaly, pleomorphism, and hyperchromasia).

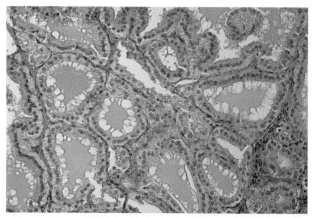

Figure 6–15. Treated Graves' disease. The involutional changes associated with radioiodine therapy include reversion of the follicular epithelial cells to their usual appearance (cuboidal to flat) and restoration of the colloid with no distortional changes.

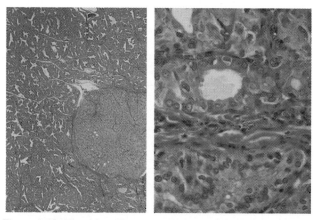

Figure 6–18. Thyroid papillary carcinoma is perhaps the most common malignant thyroid tumor seen in Graves' disease. *Left,* An incidentally identified focus of papillary carcinoma, appearing as a delineated nodule, stands out from the surrounding hyperplastic thyroid gland. *Right,* At higher magnification, the nuclei of papillary carcinoma *(top),* compared with those in the hyperplastic gland *(bottom),* are enlarged and show irregularities in size and shape, dispersed nuclear chromatin, and nuclear crowding or overlapping.

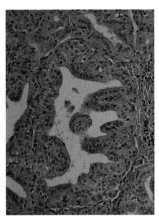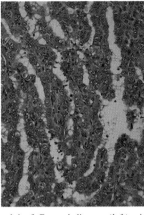

Figure 6–19. A comparison of the nuclei of Graves' disease *(left)* with those of papillary carcinoma *(right)* shows that in Graves' disease the nuclei are enlarged but do not display the array of changes that typify the nuclei of papillary carcinoma.

- Much more common in women than in men; may occur at any age but is most commonly seen in the third to sixth decades of life.
- Most patients with Graves' disease have both hyperthyroidism and goiter.
- Graves' disease causes the most florid signs and symptoms of thyrotoxicosis including nervousness, fatigue, muscle weakness, tremor, increased perspiration, warm and moist skin, nonpitting edematous changes of the skin, heat intolerance, palpitations, tachycardia, cardiac arrhythmias, systolic hypertension, hyperactivity, hyperreflexia, increased appetite, loss of weight, menstrual disturbances, stare, and eyelid retraction.
- The thyroid gland is enlarged. Characteristically, there is a diffuse, symmetrical bilateral enlargement, but asymmetrical enlargement is not uncommon. Lobulations or nodules can occur. The gland is generally not tender or painful, but these symptoms may be present.
- Continuous or systolic (palpable) thrills or (audible) bruits over one or both thyroid lobes are present in a minority of patients.
- Extrathyroidal manifestations of Graves' disease include the following:
  - **Ophthalmopathy:** Proptosis or a staring appearance (most common), blurred vision, diplopia, photophobia, lacrimation, retroocular pressure. Histologically, edema, lymphocytic cell infiltration, glycosaminoglycan deposition, and fibrosis of the extraocular muscles are found.
  - **Dermatologic:** (1) Localized (nonpitting) myxedema resulting from circumscribed accumulations of glycosaminoglycans. These changes are most frequently seen on the skin of the anterior lower legs (**pretibial myxedema**). Additional forms of Graves' dermopathies include (2) sharply circumscribed, tuberous, or nodular lesions, and (3) an elephantiasis form, also known as **thyroid acropachy,** which includes both edematous and nodular thickening of the extremities. Thyroid acropachy is the least common Graves' dermopathy, and most patients with this dermopathy

have clinically significant ophthalmopathy and localized myxedema.
- Laboratory findings
  - Thyroid function tests: Hyperthyroidism as seen by high serum total and free T_4 and T_3 concentrations with low serum TSH concentrations; in a patient with ophthalmopathy and a diffuse goiter, the presence of hyperthyroidism is diagnostic of Graves' disease, and measurements of thyroid-stimulating antibody are not needed for diagnostic purposes.
  - Pituitary-hypothalamic tests: Decreased to negligible levels of TSH and TRH (the tripeptide hypothalamic hormone).
- The autoimmune basis of this type of hyperthyroidism is suggested by:
  - The presence of elevated circulating TRA in these patients.
  - The higher incidence of a genetic predisposition to this and other autoimmune diseases.
  - The presence of HLA-DR type II antigen on follicular epithelial cell surfaces.
- Patients with autoimmune thyroid disease (Hashimoto's thyroiditis, Graves' disease) have a higher prevalence of autoantibody not only against thyroid-specific but also against nonthyroid-specific antigens (antibodies to nucleus, smooth muscle, and single-stranded DNA) than matched control patients.
- Stress has been implicated as an initiating factor in the clinical onset of Graves' disease. Some stress-related issues may include infection, psychological disturbances, or an accident.
- The initiating event or events leading to the production of TRA are unknown.

Radiology

- Most hyperthyroid patients have an increased (high) radioiodine uptake.
- In some hyperthyroid patients, radioiodine uptake is decreased (low); this includes patients with subacute thyroiditis, painless thyroiditis, and exogenous hyperthyroidism as well as those receiving iodide-containing drugs.

Pathology

Gross

- Diffuse and symmetric enlargement of the thyroid gland is the norm; however, asymmetric enlargement is not uncommon. Lobulations or (multi)nodules can occur.
- The gland appears beefy red and is rubbery to firm; it attains weights of 150 g or more.

Histology (Table 6–2)

a. Untreated Thyroid in Graves' Disease

NOTE: The following histologic changes are identified throughout the thyroid gland (i.e., the entire gland is af-

Table 6–2
HISTOLOGY OF GRAVES' DISEASE (UNTREATED AND TREATED) VERSUS PAPILLARY CARCINOMA

Features	Untreated Graves' Disease	Treated Graves' Disease	Papillary Carcinoma, Classic Type
Extent of disease	Diffuse; affects the entire thyroid gland with no residual normal (uninvolved) thyroid tissue seen	Diffuse; affects the entire thyroid gland with no residual normal (uninvolved) thyroid tissue seen	Limited; residual uninvolved thyroid tissue is present
Architecture	Diffuse hyperplasia	Variegated appearance; hyperplastic foci are haphazardly arrayed among areas in which hyperplastic changes are absent	Not a diffuse process; rather the neoplastic features are focally seen; non-neoplastic (normal) thyroid is identifiable
Papillae	Simple without complex branching	Simple without complex branching	Complex branching
Colloid	Minimal to absent; scalloping is present	Restored	Present; often the colloid in papillary carcinoma is darker than in the non-neoplastic thyroid
Cytomorphology	Columnar-appearing follicular epithelial cells with enlarged nuclei, amphophilic cytoplasm, and indistinct cell borders; nuclei are round and regular with coarse chromatin and are arranged along the basal aspect of the cell	In nonhyperplastic areas there are cuboidal to flattened follicular epithelial cells	Enlarged nuclei with irregularities in size and shape; dispersed to optically clear-appearing nuclear chromatin with margination of the chromatin along the nuclear membrane; nuclear grooves; nuclear inclusions, crowded and overlapping nuclei; loss of basal polarity of the nuclei

fected), and there is no histologic evidence of normal (unaffected) thyroid tissue.

■ Diffuse follicular hyperplasia with prominent papillary architecture; the overall lobular architecture of the gland is retained.
■ The follicular epithelial cells tend to be columnar in appearance with enlarged nuclei, amphophilic cytoplasm, and indistinct cell borders. Although nuclear enlargement with a clear appearance can be seen, in general the nuclei remain round and uniform with no irregularities in size and shape; they have a coarse and not optically clear or vesicular chromatin pattern and retain their orientation along the basal aspect of the cell. There is no crowding or overlapping and no haphazard arrangement.
■ The papillae in Graves' disease are simple and lack the complexity of growth (branching or arborization) seen in papillary carcinomas.
■ Colloid production is minimal to absent; the colloid that is present may be seen only focally and does not appear in all lumens. It is artifactually distorted owing to fixation, creating a "scalloped" appearance adjacent to the follicular epithelial cells.
■ Vascularity is prominent; minimal fibrosis or sclerosis is present.
■ Mature lymphocytic cell infiltrates, with or without germinal centers, are seen within the stroma.
■ Rarely, psammoma bodies can be seen in the absence of papillary carcinoma.

b. Treated Thyroid in Graves' Disease

NOTE: Iodine treatment results in involutional changes of the thyroid as a result of vascular ablation; medical therapy produces no changes in the histologic appearance of the thyroid in Graves' disease.

■ Follicular epithelial cells revert to their cuboidal or flat appearance.
■ Colloid is restored.

■ Papillary hyperplasia is reduced but is still seen.
■ With continued iodine treatment, follicular atrophy and fibrosis are seen; increased fibrosis results in a prominent nodular appearance of the thyroid gland.
■ These changes are variably apparent in the treated thyroid gland, so that remnants of hyperplastic-appearing thyroid may still be present even in a gland that shows treatment effects.
■ Additional changes that may be seen in long-standing cases of Graves' disease include fibrosis and cytologic atypia including enlarged, bizarre-appearing nuclei.

Differential Diagnosis

■ Thyroid papillary carcinoma (Chapter 8D, #2).
■ Dyshormonogenetic goiter (Chapter 7B).

Treatment and Prognosis

■ Medical therapy is the treatment of choice and may include:
 • Iodine therapy (potassium iodide) directed at the thyroid gland itself. This results in involutional changes of the thyroid gland secondary to vascular ablation.
 • Beta-blockers to control the peripheral manifestations of the disease. These drugs produce no changes in the pathologic appearance of the gland.
 • Thiouracil. This drug blocks the synthesis of thyroid hormones but produces minimal if any changes in the pathologic appearance of the thyroid gland.
■ Surgery (total thyroidectomy) is used for patients who are allergic to or noncompliant with medical therapy, pregnant women who are allergic to thionamides, patients with large goiters, and patients who prefer ablative (surgical) therapy to radioiodine therapy.
■ The course of hyperthyroidism in Graves' disease is variable.
 • Some patients have a course characterized by cycles of remission and relapse of variable duration.

- Some patients have an unremitting disease course.
- Some patients have only a single episode of disease.
■ Patients treated with antithyroid drugs are more apt to achieve remission; in about 10% to 15% of patients who have a remission, spontaneous hypothyroidism due to Hashimoto's thyroiditis ultimately occurs (decades later).
■ Thyroid cancer may develop in patients with Graves' disease. Most of these cancers are incidental papillary carcinomas, but some may be follicular carcinomas. A role for thyroid-stimulating antibodies in the development of thyroid cancer has been suggested, but there is no evidence to support this hypothesis.

Additional Facts

■ The pathogenesis of Graves' associated ophthalmopathy and localized myxedema remains unclear.

I. TOXIC NODULAR OR MULTINODULAR GOITER

Definition: The presence of thyrotoxicosis associated with a nodular or multinodular thyroid gland.

Synonym: Plummer's disease.

- Usually occurs in older patients, predominantly women, who have had a goiter for many years (a decade or more), but it can occur in younger individuals (in the fourth or fifth decade); there is no gender predilection.
- The nodules are usually benign, but there are rare examples of hyperfunctioning follicular carcinomas.
- The histomorphology is similar to that of diffuse toxic goiter (Graves' disease), except that the changes are limited to the nodular foci rather than involving the entire thyroid gland in a diffuse process.
- Surgery (partial or subtotal thyroidectomy) or radioiodine therapy is the treatment of choice. The goal of therapy is to remove the autonomous functioning nodule or nodules. Radioiodine is the preferred treatment for older patients who may be poor surgical candidates.
- The euthyroid state may be induced by antithyroid medication prior to surgery or radioiodine therapy.
- Recurrence of the toxic nodules may occur but is uncommon.

References

Chronic (Nonspecific) Lymphocytic Thyroiditis

Bastenie PA, Bonnyns M, Vanhaelst L. Grades of subclinical hypothyroidism in asymptomatic autoimmune thyroiditis revealed by thyrotropin-releasing hormone test. J Clin Endocrinol Metab 1980; 51:163–166.

Kurashima C, Hirokawa K. Focal lymphocytic infiltration of the thyroid in elderly people. Surv Synth Pathol Res 1985; 4:457–466.

Mizukami Y, Michigishi T, Kawato M, et al. Chronic thyroiditis: thyroid function and histologic correlation in 601 cases. Hum Pathol 1992; 23:980–988.

Singer PA. Thyroiditis. Acute, subacute and chronic. Med Clin North Am 1991; 75:61–77.

Chronic Lymphocytic Thyroiditis or Hashimoto's Thyroiditis

Aosaza K. Hashimoto's thyroiditis as a risk factor of thyroid lymphoma. Acta Pathol Jpn 1990; 407:459–468.

Aozasa K, Tajima K, Tominaga N, et al. Immunologic and immunohistochemical studies on chronic lymphocytic thyroiditis with or without thyroid lymphoma. Oncology 1991; 48:65–71.

Farid NR. Genetic factors in thyroid disease. In: Braverman LE, Utiger RD, eds. Werner and Ingbar's The Thyroid. A Fundamental and Clinical Text. 6th ed. Philadelphia: J.B. Lippincott, 1991, pp. 589–602.

Harach HR, Williams ED. Fibrous thyroiditis—an immunopathological study. Histopathology 1983; 7:739–751.

Hazard JB. Thyroiditis: A review. Part II. Am J Clin Pathol 1955; 25; 399–426.

Knecht H, Saremaslani P, Hedinger CE. Immunohistochemical findings in Hashimoto's thyroiditis and focal lymphocytic thyroiditis and thyroiditis de Quervain. Comparative study. Virchows Arch [A] 1981; 393:215–231.

Knecht H, Hedinger CE. Ultrastructural findings in Hashimoto's thyroiditis and focal lymphocytic thyroiditis with reference to giant cell formation. Histopathology 1982; 6:511–538.

Kohno Y, Naito N, Hiyama Y, et al. Thyroglobulin and thyroid peroxidase share common epitopes recognized by autoantibodies in patients with chronic autoimmune thyroiditis. J Clin Endocrinol Metab 1988; 67:899–907.

Louis DN, Vickery AL Jr, Rosai J, Wang CA. Multiple branchial-cleft cysts in Hashimoto's thyroiditis. Am J Surg Pathol 1989; 13:45–49.

Mizukami Y, Michigishi T, Kawato M, et al. Chronic thyroiditis: Thyroid function and histologic correlation in 601 cases. Hum Pathol 1992; 23:980–988.

Morita S, Arima T, Matsuda M. Prevalence of nonthyroid specific autoantibodies in autoimmune thyroid diseases. J Clin Endocrinol Metab 1995; 80:1203–1206.

Singer PA. Thyroiditis. Acute, subacute and chronic. Med Clin North Am 1991; 75:61–77.

Volpé R. The pathology of thyroiditis. Hum Pathol 1978; 9:429–438.

Volpé R. Autoimmune thyroiditis. In: Braverman LE, Utiger RD, eds. Werner and Ingbar's The Thyroid. A Fundamental and Clinical Text. 6th ed. Philadelphia: J.B. Lippincott, 1991, pp. 921–933.

Woolner LB, McConahey WM, Bearhs OH. Struma lymphomatosa (Hashimoto's thyroiditis) and related thyroid disorders. J Clin Endocrinol Metab 1959; 19:53–83.

Fibrous Variant of Hashimoto's Thyroiditis

Harach HR, Williams ED. Fibrous thyroiditis—an immunopathological study. Histopathology 1983; 7:739–751.

Katz SM, Vickery AL Jr. The fibrous variant of Hashimoto's thyroiditis. Hum Pathol 1974; 5:161–170.

Fibrous Atrophy of the Thyroid (Idiopathic Myxedema)

Bastenie PA, Bonnyns M, Vanhaelst L. Natural history of primary myxedema. Am J Med 1985; 79:91–100.

Katz SM, Vickery AL Jr. The fibrous variant of Hashimoto's thyroiditis. Hum Pathol 1974; 5:161–170.

Juvenile Form of Lymphocytic Thyroiditis

Fisher DA. Acquired juvenile hypothyroidism. In: Braverman LE, Utiger RD, eds. Werner and Ingbar's The Thyroid. A Fundamental and Clinical Text. 6th ed. Philadelphia: J.B. Lippincott, 1991, pp. 1228–1236.

Fisher DA, Pandian MR, Carlton E. Autoimmune thyroid disease: An expanding clinical spectrum. Pediatr Clin North Am 1987; 34:907–918.

Gilani BB, MacGillivray MH, Voorhees ML, et al. Thyroid hormone abnormalities at diagnosis of insulin-dependent diabetes mellitus in children. J Pediatr 1984; 105:218–222.

Mäenpää J, Raatikka M, Räsäänen J, et al. Natural course of juvenile autoimmune thyroiditis. J Pediatr 1985; 107:898–904.

Rallison ML, Dobyns BM, Keating FR, et al. Occurrence and natural history of chronic lymphocytic thyroiditis in childhood. J Pediatr 1975; 86:675–682.

Tung KSK, Ramos CV, Deodhar SD. Antithyroid antibodies in juvenile lymphocytic thyroiditis. Am J Clin Pathol 1974; 61:549–555.

Painless Thyroiditis with Hyperthyroidism

Ginsburg J, Walfish PG. Postpartum transient thyrotoxicosis with painless thyroiditis. Lancet 1977; 1; 1125–1127.

Mizukami Y, Michigishi T, Hashimoto T, et al. Silent thyroiditis: A histologic and immunohistochemical study. Hum Pathol 1988; 19:423–431.

Mizukami Y, Michigishi T, et al. Postpartum thyroiditis. A clinical, histologic and immunopathologic study of 15 cases. Am J Clin Pathol 1993;
100:200–205.

Nikolai TF, Coombs GJ, McKenzie AK, et al. Treatment of lymphocytic
thyroiditis with spontaneously resolving hyperthyroidism (silent thyroiditis). Arch Intern Med 1982; 142:2281–2283.

Nikolai TF, Turney SL, Roberts RC. Postpartum lymphocytic thyroiditis.
Arch Intern Med 1987; 147:221–224.

Vargas MT, Briones-Urbina R, Gladman D, et al. Antithyroid microsomal
autoantibodies and HLA-DR5 are associated with postpartum thyroid
dysfunction: Evidence supporting an autoimmune pathogenesis. J Clin
Endocrinol Metab 1988; 67:327–333.

Woolf PD. Transient painless thyroiditis with hyperthyroidism: a variant of
lymphocytic thyroiditis? Endocr Rev 1980; 1:411–420.

Woolf PD, Daly R. Thyrotoxicosis with painless thyroiditis. Am J Med
1976; 60:73–79.

Hashitoxicosis

Fatourechi V, McConahey WM, Woolner LB. Hyperthyroidism associated
with histologic Hashimoto's thyroiditis. Mayo Clin Proc 1971;
46:682–689.

Woolf PD. Transient painless thyroiditis with hyperthyroidism: A variant of
lymphocytic thyroiditis. Endocr Rev 1980; 4:411–420.

Autoimmune Hyperthyroidism

Adams DD, Purves HD. The role of thyrotropin in hyperthyroidism and exophthalmos. Metabolism 1957; 6:26–35.

Belfiore A, Garfalo MR, Giuffrida D, et al. Increased aggressiveness of thyroid cancer in patients with Graves' disease. J Clin Endocrinol Metab
1990; 70:830–835.

Cooper DS. Treatment of thyrotoxicosis. In: Braverman LE, Utiger RD,
eds. Werner and Ingbar's The Thyroid. A Fundamental and Clinical Text.
6th ed. Philadelphia: J.B. Lippincott, 1991, pp. 887–916.

Fatourechi V, Pajouhi M, Fransway AF. Dermopathy of Graves' disease
(pretibial myxedema). Review of 150 cases. Medicine 1994; 73:1–7.

Gossage AAR, Munro DS. The pathogenesis of Graves' disease. Clin Endocrinol Metab 1985; 14:299–330.

Livadas D, Psarras A, Koutras DA. Malignant cold thyroid nodules in hyperthyroidism. Br J Surg 1976; 63:726–728.

Morita S, Arima T, Matsuda M. Prevalence of nonthyroid specific autoantibodies in autoimmune thyroid diseases. J Clin Endocrinol Metab 1995;
80:1203–1206.

Ozaki O, Ito K, Mimura T, et al. Thyroid carcinoma after radioactive iodine
therapy for Graves' disease. World J Surg 1994; 18:518–521.

Schleusener H, Schwander J, Fisher C, et al. Prospective multicenter study
on the prediction of relapse after antithyroid drug treatment in patients
with Graves' disease. Acta Endocrinol 1989; 120:689–701.

Spaulding SW, Lippes H. Hyperthyroidism. Med Clin North Am 1985;
69:937–951.

Spjut HJ, Wareen WD, Ackerman LV. Clinical-pathologic study of 76 cases
of recurrent Graves' disease, toxic (nonexophthalmic) goiter, and nontoxic goiter. Arch Pathol Lab Med 1957; 27:367–392.

Strakosch CR, Wenzel BE, Row VV, et al. Immunology of autoimmune
thyroiditis. N Engl J Med 1982; 307:1499–1507.

Studer H, Gerber H. Toxic multinodular goiter. In: Braverman LE, Utiger
RD, eds. Werner and Ingbar's The Thyroid. A Fundamental and Clinical
Text. 6th ed. Philadelphia: J.B. Lippincott, 1991, pp. 692–697.

Tamai H, Kasagi K, Takaichi Y, et al. Development of spontaneous hypothyroidism in patients with Graves' disease treated with antithyroidal
drugs: Clinical, immunological and histologic findings in 26 patients. J
Clin Endocrinol Metab 1989; 69:49–53.

Volpé R. Graves' disease. In: Braverman LE, Utiger RD, eds. Werner and
Ingbar's The Thyroid. A Fundamental and Clinical Text. 6th ed. Philadelphia: J.B. Lippincott, 1991, pp. 648–657.

CHAPTER 7

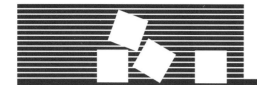

Goiters

Definition: Nodular or diffuse enlargement of the thyroid gland of any cause (Table 7–1). Presently, the term goiter is used to refer to benign (non-neoplastic) enlargement of the thyroid.

- In the presence of an intact hypothalamic-pituitary axis, any deficiency of circulating thyroid hormone will cause an increase in the production of thyroid-stimulating hormone (TSH or thyrotropin), which leads to increased activity of the thyroid follicular cells and results in glandular enlargement (hyperplasia). The same result will occur in the presence of circulating antibodies to thyroid follicular epithelial cells.
- The most common cause of deficiency of circulating thyroid hormone is a dietary deficiency of iodine.
- Other goitrogenic factors include dietary goitrogens (cyanoglucosides, cassava [manoic], naturally occurring goitrogens in groundwater and soybeans and in a specific plant genus *[Brassicae]*), goitrogenic drugs (lithium salts, iodides, aminoglutethimide, antithyroid drugs [propyl-thiouracil, methimazole, perchlorate, thiocyanate]), and physical agents (radiation).

Table 7–1
NON-NEOPLASTIC GOITROUS LESIONS

Endemic goiter
Dyshormonogenetic goiter or inborn error of thyroid metabolism
Amyloid goiter
Diffuse toxic goiter (Graves' disease)
Nodular toxic goiter

A. ADENOMATOID NODULES

Synonyms: Nodular goiter; multinodular goiter; simple nontoxic goiter; colloid goiter.

Clinical

- Clinically detectable nodules are found in less than 5% of the population; if thyroid nodules found at autopsy and on histologic examination of the thyroid are considered as

well, the incidence of adenomatoid nodules increases to 40% to 50% of the population.
- These nodules tend to be more common in women than in men; they occur over a wide age range but are seen predominantly in adults.
- Symptoms include nodular or diffuse enlargement of the thyroid gland. In patients with multinodular enlargement, there may be one or more dominant nodules. There is no site predilection. Nodules may reach large sizes, resulting in symptoms (e.g., dysphagia, airway obstruction) due to compression of adjacent structures.
- The majority of patients are euthyroid, but some patients may have hyperfunctioning nodules (elevated TSH levels). In a small percentage of patients, toxic or hyperfunctioning nodules may develop in the presence of multinodular goiter.
- There is no increased risk of cancer in patients with adenomatoid nodules.
- Etiology varies.

Radiology

- High-resolution ultrasound is the most sensitive method of detecting thyroid nodules; it may reveal nodules that are too small to be palpated.
- Multinodular adenomatoid thyroid glands appear as enlarged symmetric or asymmetric glands containing nodules of varying density. With contrast enhancement the nodules may appear uniformly enhanced, or enhancement may be poor owing to secondary degenerative changes such as hemorrhage, cyst formation, or necrosis.
- Areas of calcification are seen in a high percentage of cases.
- Large nodules may extend into the mediastinum (first the anterior mediastinum and then the posterior) or may compress adjacent structures such as the trachea, esophagus, and large vessels.

Pathology

Fine Needle Aspiration

- Abundant colloid, few follicles, and low cellularity; the amount of thyroid follicles, follicular epithelial cells, and colloid varies.

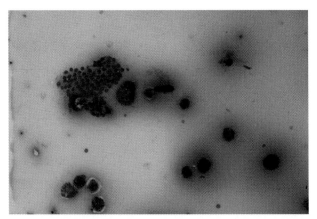

Figure 7–1. Fine needle aspiration (FNA) of adenomatoid nodules typically contain abundant colloid but only scant follicular epithelium. Hemosiderin-laden macrophages are common, particularly in lesions with cystic degeneration. Diff-Quik stain.

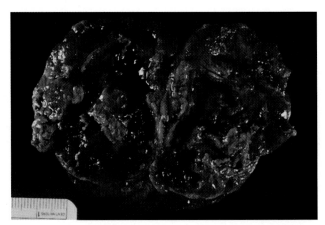

Figure 7–4. This adenomatoid nodule shows prominent degenerative changes, including hemorrhage and cyst formation.

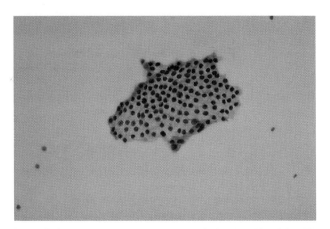

Figure 7–2. Fine needle aspiration (FNA) of adenomatoid nodules. Flat sheets of follicular epithelium, with cells arranged in an orderly honeycomb fashion and with distinct cell borders, predominate in fine needle aspirates of adenomatoid nodules. Cellularity is usually low. Papanicolaou stain.

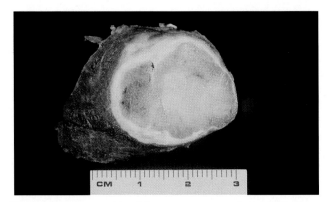

Figure 7–5. Adenomatoid nodules may present as a single mass lesion as seen here. This solid lesion appears to be encapsulated, suggesting the gross appearance of a true neoplastic growth (adenoma or carcinoma). In this case, the patient had received radiation therapy in childhood, and this nodule was cellular with associated fibrosis.

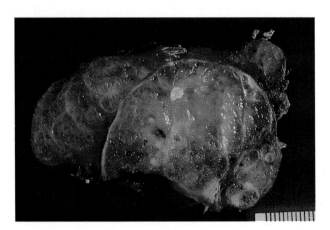

Figure 7–3. Multiple separate but similar-appearing, well-delineated colloid nodules. Intranodular and internodular fibrosis can be seen. Separate foci of calcification are present.

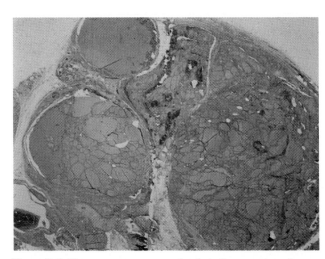

Figure 7–6. Three separate unencapsulated similar-appearing adenomatoid nodules.

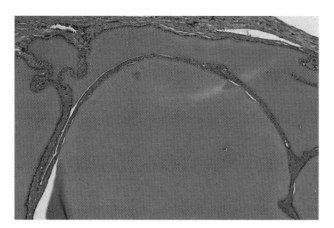

Figure 7–7. Markedly dilated colloid-filled follicles are seen in this adenomatoid nodule.

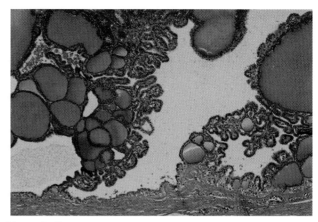

Figure 7–10. Additional degenerative changes in adenomatoid nodules may include the presence of a papillary growth.

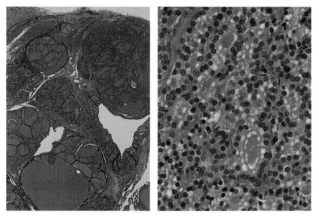

Figure 7–8. Cellular adenomatoid nodule. *Left,* This thyroid gland had multiple unencapsulated adenomatoid nodules including this one with cellular foci. *Right,* Higher magnification of the cellular areas shows cells with round and regular nuclei with a coarse chromatin pattern.

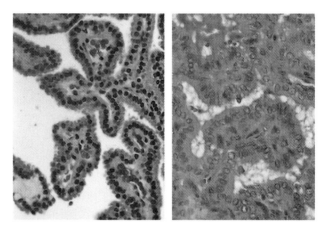

Figure 7–11. Comparison of an adenomatoid nodule with papillae *(left)* and a papillary carcinoma *(right)* shows the contrasting appearance of the nuclei. The stark differences in the nuclear morphology should limit any diagnostic confusion.

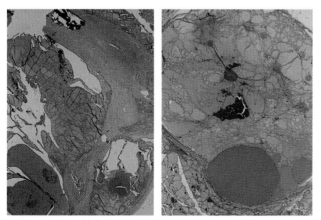

Figure 7–9. As shown here, secondary degenerative changes in adenomatoid nodules may include cyst formation, fibrosis, calcification, and hemorrhage.

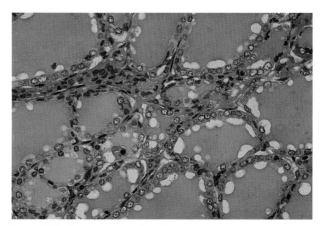

Figure 7–12. Due to poor fixation, the central aspects of an adenomatoid nodule (or, for that matter, a follicular adenoma or carcinoma) may have nuclear clearing, suggesting a diagnosis of papillary carcinoma. Despite the nuclear clearing, the nuclei retain their round and regular appearance and have a "clumpy" to coarse nuclear chromatin pattern, and the constellation of nuclear changes seen in papillary carcinoma is not present.

- Follicular cells are isolated or in sheets with a honeycomb pattern.
- Follicular epithelial nuclei are round, nucleoli are rare, and chromatin is opaque to coarsely granular.
- Secondary degenerative (retrogressive) changes may be present including reactive epithelial changes (cytoplasmic oxyphilia, prominent nucleoli, cytoplasmic hemosiderin), hemorrhage, macrophages (with or without hemosiderin), lymphocytes, giant cells, and calcific debris.
- In hyperplastic lesions, follicles predominate, and there is increased cellularity with scant colloid. Despite the increased cellularity, the epithelial cells are bland with no increase in nuclear size and no irregularities in size and shape.
- In involuted lesions, there is minimal cellularity and abundant colloid; the colloid appears as amorphous blue to orange material.

Gross

- Thyroid glands with adenomatoid nodules vary in appearance depending on the number and size of the nodules; generally, the gland is enlarged (slight to massive enlargement) and may achieve a weight of several hundred grams to a kilogram or more.
- Cut section may reveal one or multiple delineated nodules separated by a normal appearing parenchyma; the nodules appear brown and glistening.
- Secondary degenerative changes are common and may include cyst formation, fibrosis, calcification, hemorrhage, and necrosis.

Histology

- One or more nodules may be seen.
- The nodules may be unencapsulated or partly encapsulated, but complete encapsulation is not present.
- The follicles are dilated and filled with abundant colloid.
- Cellularity varies. In some nodules cellularity is not increased, and the follicular epithelial cells have a flattened (attenuated) appearance; other nodules may have increased cellularity (cellular nodules) with variable appearing cells including oncocytic and clear cells.
- The nuclei are round to oval with no irregularities in size and shape; they have a coarse nuclear chromatin (hyperchromatic) pattern and inconspicuous to small, centrally located nucleoli, and they retain a linear basal orientation in the cell.

- Nuclear changes that can be seen include grooves, crowding, and dispersed or vesicular appearing chromatin as well as intranuclear inclusions; the latter generally are not eosinophilic but are clear and "bubbly" in appearance and probably represent a processing artifact.
- The non-nodular thyroid is essentially normal (no hyperplastic changes). The thyroid parenchyma adjacent to the nodules is not compressed, and there is a comparable growth pattern in the adjacent gland.
- A lymphocytic and plasma cell infiltrate may be seen.
- Secondary (degenerative or retrogressive) changes may be seen, including coarse fibrosis, cyst formation, infarction, hemorrhage, hemosiderin-laden macrophages, and cholesterol granulomas. Squamous, osseous, and cartilaginous metaplasia may be present; thickened vascular spaces with associated calcifications (within the media) can be seen at the periphery.
- Additional changes may include the presence of papillary structures, oxyphilic metaplasia, and nuclear enlargement; these changes may suggest a diagnosis of papillary carcinoma.

Differential Diagnosis

- Follicular adenoma (Table 7–2) (Chapter 8C, #1).
- Papillary carcinoma, conventional type (Table 7–3) (Chapter 8D, #2).
- Papillary carcinoma, macrofollicular type (Chapter 8D, #2).

Treatment and Prognosis

- The treatment of choice for symptomatic adenomatoid nodules is surgical excision. Surgery should be as conservative as possible and should include resection of the mass lesion or lesions while sparing the remaining thyroid. A total thyroidectomy may be required in patients with multifocal, bilateral nodules.
- Radioiodine (^{131}I) therapy can be used for ablation of adenomatoid nodules; however, the nodules are relatively radioresistant, and higher doses of radioiodine are required for the treatment of adenomatoid nodules. Further, the larger the nodule, the higher the dose of radioiodine required for ablation. Risks associated with this form of treatment may include radiation exposure of the entire thyroid with a possibly increased risk of (1) cancer or (2) hypothyroidism.
- Prognosis in uncomplicated cases is excellent.

Table 7–2
ADENOMATOID NODULES VERSUS FOLLICULAR ADENOMA

Feature	Adenomatoid Nodules	Follicular Adenoma
Number	Multiple	Solitary
Capsule	Poor encapsulation; a capsule may be present but it does not completely encapsulate the mass	Well-developed, completely surrounding the mass
Adjacent thyroid gland	No compression of surrounding gland	Compression and/or atrophy of surrounding gland
Growth compared to remainder of thyroid gland	Comparable growth pattern in adjacent gland	Different growth pattern in adjacent gland
Appearance compared to remainder of thyroid gland	Dilated follicles and colloid nodules in gland are common	Remainder of gland without histopathologic abnormalities
Degenerative changes	Frequently present	Uncommon*

*An exception would be post–FNA degenerative changes in an adenoma with cytoplasmic oxyphilia.

Table 7–3
ADENOMATOID NODULES VERSUS PAPILLARY CARCINOMA

Features	Adenomatoid Nodules	Papillary Carcinoma
Papillae	Simple	Complex
Nuclei	1. Round and regular	1. Enlarged with irregularities in size and shape
	2. Dense chromatin (hyperchromatic)	2. Dispersed to optically clear chromatin pattern
	3. Linear polarity along basal aspect of cell	3. Disorganized orientation of nuclei with no linear polarity of the nuclei, which are haphazardly located within the cells
	4. Nuclei are not crowded or overlapping	4. Nuclear crowding and overlapping
	5. Nuclear grooves and "inclusions" may be present (the inclusions are not round and eosinophilic as in papillary carcinoma but clear and bubbly and are artifacts of tissue processing)	5. Nuclear grooves and intranuclear round and eosinophilic cytoplasmic inclusions
Fibrosis	Variable and irregular in appearance; may be markedly thickened in and around the follicles	Intratumoral and irregular in appearance
Calcifications	Dense deposits lacking any specific form (i.e., lamination or concentric rings), usually in fibrotic (acellular) foci and within the media of vessels	Laminated or concentric rings (psammoma bodies), seen in association with the neoplastic cellular infiltrate and in the connective tissue of the parenchyma

Additional Facts

■ There are no functional or morphologic features distinguishing sporadic from endemic goiter. The difference between these types of goiter is that endemic goiter is most often caused by an extrathyroidal growth-stimulating factor (e.g., iodine deficiency) leading to increased TSH secretion, whereas sporadically occurring goiter is not.

■ Thyrotoxicosis (hyperthyroidism) in people with multinodular goiters is called **Plummer's disease** (see Chapter 6I, Toxic Nodular Goiter).
  • It tends to affect older people with long-standing goiters.
  • It produces a "hot" nodule.

■ Occasionally, bona fide changes of papillary carcinoma may be identified in a limited portion of a nodular proliferation that otherwise demonstrates no histologic features of papillary carcinoma; in such cases, the diagnostic possibilities may include:

(1) The entire nodular lesion may be a papillary carcinoma, possibly representing the macrofollicular variant of papillary carcinoma.

(2) Some authorities advocate the possible development of a small focus of papillary carcinoma arising within an adenomatoid nodule. This has not been our experience. If an unequivocal focus of papillary carcinoma is seen within an adenomatoid nodule, then it probably falls within items (1) or (3).

(3) The papillary carcinoma focus represents intrathyroidal or intranodular spread from a separate focus of papillary carcinoma elsewhere in the gland.

■ In (1) above, the papillary carcinoma is confined to the nodular proliferation, is amenable to surgical removal, and has an excellent prognosis. The view that the entire nodule represents papillary carcinoma does not alter the treatment or prognosis as long as the lesion has been surgically removed.

B. DYSHORMONOGENETIC GOITER

Definition: Inherited or inborn errors of thyroid metabolism resulting in overstimulation (hyperplasia) of the thyroid gland. There are numerous causes of inborn errors of thyroid metabolism (Table 7–4), which result in impaired thyroid hormone synthesis, leading to a loss of negative feedback to the pituitary gland, which in turn leads to hypersecretion of TSH, causing continuous stimulation and hyperactivity of the thyroid.

Table 7–4
INHERITED METABOLIC DISORDERS OF THYROID METABOLISM RESULTING IN DYSHORMONOGENETIC GOITER

Unresponsiveness to TSH
Iodide transport failure
Defective peroxidase activity
Deficient hydrogen peroxide activity
  Receptor abnormality
  Inefficient iodide organification of *Pendred's syndrome* (familial deaf mutism and goiter)
Defective iodotyrosyl coupling and iodothyronine synthesis
Defective thyroglobulin
  Impaired synthesis (absence of synthesis of abnormal thyroglobulin)
  Defective transport
Defective iodotyrosine

Clinical

■ Inborn errors of thyroid metabolism are rare.

■ Too few cases have been reported to make any definitive statements about the mode of inheritance but, for those cases identified, it appears that autosomal recessive inheritance occurs more often than autosomal dominant inheritance.

■ There is no racial or ethnic predilection.

■ The thyroid abnormalities seen in disorders of thyroid hormonogenesis include goitrous thyroid and hypothyroidism; pituitary gland defects result in hypothyroidism but not a goiter.

■ The clinical presentation (signs and symptoms) depends on the severity of the error.
  • Severe defect: Presentation in early life (neonatal period) with (congenital) hypothyroidism, goiter, mental retardation, and growth abnormalities (cretinism).
  • Mild or less severe defect: presentation in adolescence or adult life with a goiter and minimal evidence of thyroid dysfunction; patients may be euthyroid.

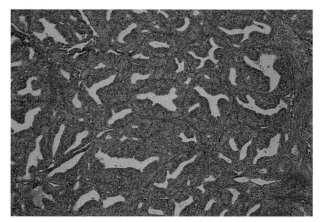

Figure 7–13. Dyshormonogenetic goiter. One of the histologic patterns of this lesion is the presence of papillary hyperplasia with minimal to absent colloid. Normal thyroid tissue is absent.

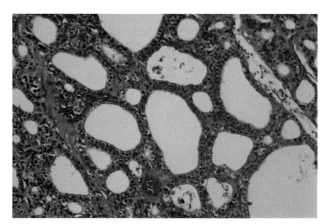

Figure 7–16. Dyshormonogenetic goiter with follicular growth. As in Figure 7–15, colloid is absent.

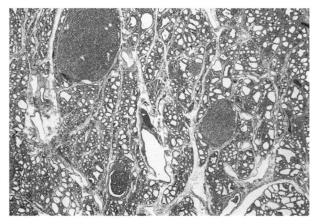

Figure 7–14. Dyshormonogenetic goiter is characterized by nodularity, fibrosis, and increased cellularity due to marked hyperplasia with decreased to absent colloid. A variegated cytomorphology can also be appreciated, with areas of relatively bland nuclei and other areas in which the nuclei are pleomorphic. Normal thyroid tissue is not present.

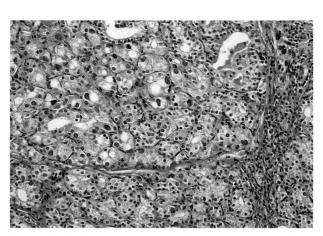

Figure 7–17. Dyshormonogenetic goiter. Nodular appearing thyroid with minimal to absent colloid formation, and with internodular fibrosis. The follicular epithelial cells within the nodules show marked nuclear atypia.

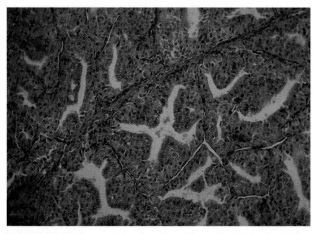

Figure 7–15. Dyshormonogenetic goiter with papillary hyperplasia. Note the absence of colloid.

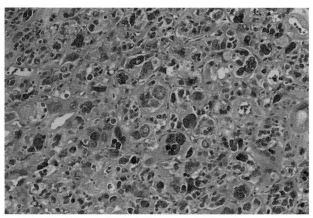

Figure 7–18. Dyshormonogenetic goiter. Higher magnification of Figure 7–17 shows the severe cytologic atypia, including hypercellularity with nucleomegaly, hyperchromasia, and intranuclear inclusions.

Table 7–5
DYSHORMONOGENETIC GOITER AND HISTOLOGIC SIMULATORS

	Dyshormonogenetic Goiter	Diffuse Hyperplasia (Untreated)	Papillary Carcinoma (Classic Type)	Adenomatoid Nodules (Nodular Goiter)
Gland involvement	Diffuse; thyroid is hyperplastic; no normal thyroid; multinodularity	Diffuse; thyroid is hyperplastic; no normal thyroid	Limited in extent; multifocal; intervening thyroid tissue is normal	Multiple nodules; intervening thyroid tissue is normal
Cellularity	Hypercellular throughout the gland	Hypercellular throughout the gland	Variable but typically more cellular than surrounding thyroid	Variable—ranges from hypocellular to hypercellular
Architecture	Multiple growth pattern, including solid, microfollicular, papillary, insular, and others. Papillae are usually simple in appearance but may be complex; they are often broad rather than narrow and have a fibrovascular stroma	Diffuse follicular hyperplasia. Prominent papillary architecture; lobular architecture is retained. Papillae are present, typically are simple in appearance but may be complex, and are often broad rather than narrow and have a fibrovascular stroma	Multiple growth patterns—papillary, follicular (microfollicular and macrofollicular), solid, trabecular. Papillary growth limited to neoplastic proliferation. Narrow papillae have a complex growth with fibrovascular stroma	Variably sized follicles widely dilated; retrogressive changes may include the presence of pseudopapillae within the follicular proliferation
Colloid	Scant to absent	Minimal to absent; scalloping is present	Present; darker (inspissated) appearing	Abundant; watery in appearance
Cytomorphology (follicular epithelial cells)	Variably appearing epithelial cells with round to oval nuclei, coarse chromatin, eosinophilic to clear cytoplasm; basal orientation of nuclei. Severe cytologic atypia is commonly present and includes bizarre nuclei with nucleomegaly and hyperchromasia in parenchyma and less often in nodules	Columnar cells; enlarged nuclei, amphophilic cytoplasm, indistinct cell borders. Nuclei are round and regular with coarse chromatin arranged along the basal aspect of the cell	Enlarged nuclei; irregularities in size and shape; haphazardly located in cell. Dispersed to optically clear chromatin; nuclear crowding and overlapping; nuclear grooves, and intranuclear round and eosinophilic inclusions; nondescript cytoplasm	Flattened cells, round and regular nuclei with a dense chromatin. Nuclei are linearly oriented along basal aspect of cell. Nuclear grooves; "inclusions" may be present, appearing clear and bubbly; they are artifacts of tissue processing
Fibrosis	Marked fibrosis; acellular fibrosis accentuates nodularity	Minimal to absent fibrosis in untreated patients or in patients without long-standing disease; when present, fibrosis is irregular and often creates a nodular appearing gland	Intratumoral; dense irregular bands	Variable and irregular in appearance; result of retrogressive changes

- There may be a family history of goiter.
- Laboratory evaluation for a patient in whom an inborn error of thyroid metabolism is suspected is complex and extensive. It follows a sequential flow chart depending on the findings of one or more test results. Among the tests that may be performed in patients being evaluated for thyroid dyshormonogenesis are:
  - T_4 and T_3 concentrations.
  - TSH levels.
  - Thyroxine-binding globulin (TBG) concentration.
  - Thyrotropin-releasing hormone (TRH) function and assessment of hypothalamic-pituitary function.
  - Radioiodine uptake and scanning.
  - Thyroglobulin antibodies (if present, the patient may have an autoimmune thyroiditis).
  - Hearing test (*sensorineural* deafness in the presence of a goiter and hypothyroidism is diagnostic of **Pendred's syndrome**).
  - Radioiodine kinetic studies for labeled urinary monoiodotyrosine (MIT) and diiodotyrosine (DIT). Defective iodotyrosine deiodination is characterized by release of

MIT and DIT in the degradation of thyroglobulin in the process of recovery of its thyroid hormones.
  - Surgical excision for histologic analysis.
- Diagnosis of an inborn error of thyroid metabolism can be made in utero by ultrasonography and measurement of TSH in amniotic fluid.

Pathology

NOTE: Regardless of the underlying cause, the pathologic changes (gross and microscopic) seen in the affected gland are essentially the same.

Gross

- The gland is enlarged and is multinodular with associated fibrosis; fibrosis may encapsulate individual nodules.

Histology

- Any normal appearing thyroid tissue is absent.
- The thyroid is characterized by nodularity, fibrosis, and marked follicular hyperplasia with prominent papillarity

(simple, not complex), hypercellularity, and DECREASED TO ABSENT COLLOID; microfollicular, trabecular, as well as other solid growth patterns can be seen.

- All of the above features may be present in any one gland, creating a variegated appearance at low magnification.
- The follicular epithelial cells vary in appearance and include cells with round to oval nuclei, a coarse chromatin pattern, eosinophilic to clear cytoplasm, and a basal orientation of the nuclei within the cell.
- Severe cytologic atypia is commonly present, including bizarre nuclei with nucleomegaly and hyperchromasia. These nuclear changes appear in the internodular thyroid tissue and occasionally at the periphery of the nodules.
- Mitoses can occasionally be found but are generally absent or low in number.
- Fibrosis consisting of thick acellular bands is seen throughout the gland; it may completely encircle ("encapsulate") the nodules.
- In contrast to diffuse hyperplasia (Graves' disease), a lymphocytic cell infiltrate is not present in dyshormonogenetic goiter.
- The presence of nodules surrounded by fibrosis may suggest a follicular neoplasm (adenoma or carcinoma); however, the fact that the entire thyroid gland is histologically abnormal may help in the diagnosis and in excluding a follicular adenoma or carcinoma from consideration.
- Despite the presence of prominent papillarity, the nuclear features do not conform to those seen in papillary carcinoma.
- Malignant thyroid tumors (papillary carcinoma or follicular carcinoma) may develop in patients with a dyshormonogenetic goiter. Features that may assist in the diagnosis include the following:
  - For papillary carcinoma: Characteristic architectural and cytomorphologic features need to be present (Table 7–5).
  - For follicular carcinoma: Diagnosis is somewhat more problematic in that "encapsulated" nodules of dyshormonogenetic goiter may appear to have foci of "invasive" growth into the capsule. The presence of vascular space invasion or metastatic follicular carcinoma would be diagnostic of a follicular carcinoma; however, there are no definitive cytologic features that can be used.
- *Histochemistry:* Periodic acid–Schiff (PAS) stain can be used to identify colloid.
- *Immunohistochemistry:* Thyroglobulin reactivity; absence of calcitonin or neuroendocrine markers (e.g., chromogranin, synaptophysin).

Differential Diagnosis (Table 7–5)

- Diffuse hyperplasia (Graves' disease) (Chapter 6).
- Adenomatoid nodules (Chapter 7A).
- Papillary carcinoma (Chapter 8D, #2).
- Follicular carcinoma (Chapter 8D, #1).
- Medullary carcinoma (Chapter 8D, #3).

Treatment and Prognosis

- Nonsurgical (medical) treatment is the same as that for any hypothyroid patient and includes thyroid hormone replacement.

- Surgery (partial or total thyroidectomy) may be necessary in patients with obstructive or pressure symptoms or in those in whom a malignant neoplasm is suspected.
- Patients with hypothyroidism due to generalized pituitary insufficiency may develop adrenal crisis if unmonitored medical treatment is given.
- Prognosis, especially for patients with mild disease, is excellent.
- In patients with severe forms of disease (congenital goiters or cretinism), mental and growth retardation may occur. In these patients, early detection with early medical management is essential to allow normal development of the nervous system and prevent permanent mental retardation.

Additional Facts

- The origin of the congenital nerve deafness seen in Pendred's syndrome is unknown.

C. AMYLOID GOITER

Definition: Symptomatic mass or clinically detectable thyroid enlargement due to amyloid deposition. Amyloid deposits represent an extracellular accumulation of fibrillar proteins that are associated with a variety of clinical settings and occur in a variety of tissue sites. Amyloidosis may become manifest in several forms including systemic amyloidosis (primary and secondary), multiple myeloma–associated amyloidosis, localized or solitary amyloidosis, and familial amyloidosis.

Clinical

- Very rare; more commonly, when amyloid is seen in the thyroid it is associated with medullary carcinoma.
- Amyloid deposition in the thyroid can occur as part of either primary or secondary systemic amyloidosis. It is more commonly seen as part of secondary systemic amyloidosis, in which setting the amyloid is usually found at autopsy rather than producing a symptomatic mass.
- Predisposing disorders associated with secondary systemic amyloidosis involving the thyroid include:
  - Chronic inflammatory diseases: infections (chronic osteomyelitis, pulmonary tuberculosis, chronic bronchitis with bronchiectasis, chronic peritonitis), rheumatoid arthritis, familial Mediterranean fever.
  - Neoplasms: Hodgkin's disease; other.
- In symptomatic amyloid goiter, the clinical presentation includes a nontender, rapidly enlarging neck mass that may be associated with dysphagia, dyspnea, and hoarseness.
- Patients are euthyroid, and thyroid dysfunction is not generally present. However, the amyloid deposition may be so extensive that it results in hypothyroidism.

Pathology

Gross

- The thyroid gland is diffusely enlarged and occasionally has a nodular appearance; it weighs from 25 to 300 g.
- The cut surface is white to tan and has a rubbery to firm consistency.

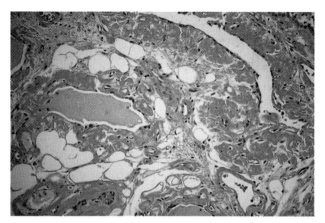

Figure 7–19. Amyloid goiter. The amyloid deposition is eosinophilic, acellular, and amorphous in appearance and almost completely replaces the thyroid parenchyma. Elongated thyroid follicles lined by attenuated follicular epithelial cells are seen, one of which still retains colloid material.

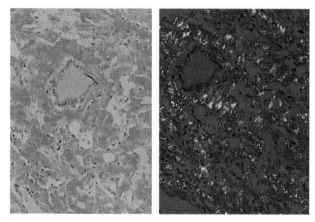

Figure 7–20. *Left,* Congo red stain showing the typical appearance of amyloid. *Right,* Congo red stain with polarization shows the characteristic apple-green birefringence that characterizes amyloid deposits.

Histology

- Diffuse amyloid deposition is usually seen, but focal (nodular) deposits may occur.
- The amyloid appears as extracellular eosinophilic, acellular, and amorphous material.
- In diffuse deposits, the amyloid is evenly distributed throughout the gland and replaces the thyroid parenchyma.
- In nodular deposits, the amyloid is focally distributed, and the remainder of the gland is essentially unremarkable.
- The degree of amyloid deposition may vary from moderate to extensive; amyloid is seen in both perifollicular and interfollicular locations, compressing the follicles.
- In the areas of amyloid deposition the residual follicles vary in appearance from elongated with normal colloid content to slitlike atrophic follicles without colloid. The follicular epithelial cells generally appear as flat single cells. Squamous metaplasia may be seen.
- Amyloid deposition is seen around vascular spaces ("angiocentric") and, less often, within the vessel walls. Vascular-related amyloid does not result in any functional compromise of the involved blood vessel.
- Additional associated findings may include a lymphocytic cell infiltrate, multinucleated giant cells and mature fat.
- *Histochemistry:* Stains for amyloid (Congo red, crystal violet, thioflavin-T) are positive. Apple-green birefringence is seen under polarized light with Congo red staining.
- *Immunohistochemistry:* Positive reaction with amyloid (AA) antibody is seen; reactions with calcitonin and chromogranin are not seen.
- *Electron microscopy:* Nonbranching fibrils varying in size from 50 Å to 150 Å in diameter are seen.

Differential Diagnosis

- Amyloid stroma in medullary carcinoma (Chapter 8E, #3).
- The amyloid may be mistaken for fibrous tissue; the latter may be associated with many thyroid diseases.

Treatment and Prognosis

- Treatment in symptomatic patients consists of thyroidectomy (partial or total).
- The prognosis in relation to thyroid amyloid deposition is excellent; however, the prognosis correlates with the patient's clinical condition and death may result from specific organ failure secondary to amyloid deposition in other organs (heart, kidney, or liver).
- The prognosis in relation to amyloid deposition in patients with medullary carcinoma correlates with the status of the medullary carcinoma.

References

Adenomatoid Nodules

Alter CA, Moshang T Jr. Diagnostic dilemma. The goiter. Pediatr Clin North Am 1991; 38:567–578.

Greenspan FS. The problem of nodular goiter. Med Clin North Am 1991; 75:195–209.

Ramelli F, Studer H, Bruggisser D. Pathogenesis of thyroid nodules in multinodular goiter. Am J Pathol 1982; 109:215–223.

Kini SR. Nodular goiter. In: Guides to Clinical Aspiration Biopsy. Thyroid. New York: Igaku-Shoin, 1996, pp. 41–57.

Studer H, Gerber H. Pathogenesis of nontoxic diffuse and nodular goiter. In: Braverman LE, Utiger RD, eds. Werner and Ingbar's The Thyroid. A Fundamental and Clinical Text, 6th ed. Philadelphia: J.B. Lippincott, 1991, pp. 1107–1113.

Studer H, Gerber H. Clinical manifestations and management of nontoxic diffuse and nodular goiter. In: Braverman LE, Utiger RD, eds. Werner and Ingbar's The Thyroid. A Fundamental and Clinical Text, 6th ed. Philadelphia: J.B. Lippincott, 1991, pp. 1114–1118.

Dyshormonogenetic Goiter

Abs R, Verheist J, Schoofs E, De Somer E. Hyperfunctioning follicular thyroid carcinoma in Pendred's syndrome. Cancer 1991; 67:2191–2193.

Farid NR. Genetic factors in thyroid disease. In: Braverman LE, Utiger RD, eds. Werner and Ingbar's The Thyroid. A Fundamental and Clinical Text, 6th ed. Philadelphia: J.B. Lippincott, 1991, pp. 588–602.

Kennedy JS. The pathology of dyshormonogenetic goitre. J Pathol 1969; 99:251–264.

Matos PS, Bisi H, Medeiros-Neto G. Dyshormonogenetic goiter. A morphological and immunohistochemical study. Endocr Pathol 1994; 5:49–58.

Medeiros-Neto GA, Billerbeck AE, Wajchenberg BL, Targovnik HM. Defective organification of iodide causing hereditary goitrous hypothyroidism. Thyroid 1993; 3:143–159.

Moore GH. The thyroid in sporadic goitrous cretinism: a report of three new cases, description of the pathologic anatomy of the thyroid glands, and a review of the literature. Arch Pathol Lab Med 1962; 74:35–58.

Vickery AL Jr. The diagnosis of malignancy in dyshormonogenetic goiter. Clin Endocrinol Metab 1981; 10:317–335.

Amyloid Goiter

Alvarez-Sala R, Prados C, Sastre Marcos J, et al. Amyloid goitre and hypothyroidism secondary to cystic fibrosis. Postgrad Med J 1995; 7:307–308.

Hamed G, Heffess CS, Shmookler BM, Wenig BM. Amyloid goiter. A clinicopathologic study of 14 cases and review of the literature. Am J Clin Pathol 1995; 104:306–312.

Kennedy JS, Thomson JA, Buchanan WM. Amyloid in the thyroid. Q J Med 1974; 43:127–143.

Rich MW. Hypothyroidism in association with systemic amyloidosis. Head Neck 1995; 17:343–345.

CHAPTER 8

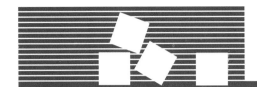

Thyroid Neoplasms

A. CLASSIFICATION OF NEOPLASMS OF THE THYROID GLAND

Table 8–1
CLASSIFICATION OF NEOPLASMS OF THE THYROID GLAND

Epithelial

Benign

Follicular adenoma and its variants

Malignant

Follicular carcinoma and its variants
Papillary carcinoma and its variants
Medullary carcinoma and its variants
Undifferentiated (anaplastic) carcinoma
Others:
    Squamous cell carcinoma
    Mucoepidermoid carcinoma

Nonepithelial

Benign

Paraganglioma
Teratomas
Mesenchymal tumors
    Vascular
    Myogenic
    Neural

Malignant

Malignant lymphoproliferative lesions
    Non-Hodgkin's malignant lymphoma
    Plasmacytoma
    Hodgkin's lymphoma
    Others
Sarcomas

Secondary Tumors (Metastases) to the Thyroid

Thymic-Related Lesions

Other Unusual Neoplasms and Neoplastic-like Lesions

Salivary gland-type tumors
Rosai-Dorfman disease
Eosinophilic granuloma
Inflammatory pseudotumors: plasma cell granuloma

B. THYROID NEOPLASMS— GENERAL CONSIDERATIONS

- Thyroid cancer is the most common endocrine malignancy but represents less than 2% of all human cancers diagnosed in the United States.
- The percentage of cancer deaths (mortality rate) due to thyroid carcinoma is low (0.4%).
- Clinically apparent thyroid nodules occur in a fairly large percentage of the population (up to 10%); although many of these nodules are probably benign, the differential diagnosis of any thyroid nodule includes a malignant thyroid neoplasm.
- The great majority of thyroid tumors are of follicular epithelial cell origin, a category that includes follicular adenoma, follicular carcinoma, papillary carcinoma, and all their variants; less common is the thyroid medullary carcinoma derived from the thyroid C cells.
- In general, thyroid tumors are more common in women than in men and occur in people of all ages, including children in the 1st and 2nd decades and elderly people.
- The classification of thyroid tumors is detailed at the beginning of this chapter (see Table 8–1).
- Radiation exposure is the only factor that has been shown unequivocally to cause thyroid cancer.
- Other factors that have been linked to but not definitively proved to be potential causes of thyroid cancer include:
  - Dietary iodine deficiency and iodine excess.
  - Pre-existing thyroid disease (adenomatoid nodules, lymphocytic thyroiditis, Graves' disease).
  - Hormonal factors (thyroid neoplasms occur more commonly in women than in men).
  - Drugs (lithium and phenobarbital).
  - Genetic predisposition: (1) familial pattern of non-medullary thyroid cancers has been noted; (2) follicular-derived thyroid cancers have been associated with HLA-DR7; (3) Gardner's syndrome—autosomal dominant inheritance of multiple adenomatous polyps of the large intestine, multiple osteomas of the skull and mandible, cutaneous keratinous cysts, and soft tissue tumors (e.g., fibromatosis)—is associated with an increased risk of thyroid papillary carcinoma; (4) Cowden disease (multiple hamartoma syndrome)—autosomal

dominant inheritance of multiple hamartomas, mucocutaneous lesions, including trichilemmomas, acral keratoses, and oral mucosal papillomas—is associated with an increased risk of follicular epithelial cell tumors (adenomatoid nodules, tumors); (3) multiple endocrine neoplasia (MEN) syndrome is linked to the development of C-cell–related lesions or neoplasms.

- Cellular oncogene abnormalities including activation, point mutations, somatic rearrangements, and decreased or increased expression of various proto-oncogenes (e.g., *ras, ret, trk, myc*).

■ **Clinical evaluation** of thyroid tumors includes the following factors:

- *Age:* Patients who are very young (<14 years) or older (>65 years) have a higher incidence of malignant thyroid tumors.
- *Gender:* Men are more apt to have malignant thyroid tumors than are women.
- *Family history:* Inheritance is linked with the development of medullary carcinoma and, less often, with follicular tumors.
- *History of radiation exposure or Hashimoto's thyroiditis:* These factors have been associated with the development of malignant thyroid tumors.
- *Clinical presentation:* Rapid enlargement of the thyroid or of long-standing thyroid nodule or nodules is the hallmark presentation of thyroid malignant tumors; hoarseness and/or vocal cord paralysis in the presence of a thyroid mass may indicate a malignant thyroid tumor.
- *Physical examination:* (1) Although not always true, multiple nodules are more likely to be benign, whereas solitary nodules are more likely to be malignant. (2) A hard and fixed thyroid mass is more likely to be malignant. (3) Ipsilateral cervical adenopathy may indicate metastasis from an identifiable or occult thyroid malignant tumor.
- **Radiologic findings:** (1) On radioactive iodine scans (^{131}I) the incidence of carcinoma is higher for hypofunctioning ("cold") nodules than for hyperfunctioning ("hot") nodules; hot nodules are almost always benign; (2) On ultrasonography a solid tumor is more likely to be malignant than a cystic tumor, although papillary carcinoma may present as a partially or predominantly cystic tumor.
- **Laboratory tests:** Most patients with thyroid cancer are euthyroid: (1) serum thyroglobulin levels are of limited value in the diagnosis of follicular epithelial tumors because they do not assist in the diagnosis of non-neoplastic versus neoplastic follicular lesions; (2) elevated serum calcitonin, seen in virtually all cases, is a key diagnostic feature in thyroid medullary carcinoma.

■ **Fine needle aspiration (FNA):**

- Represents an extremely useful initial approach in the diagnosis of a thyroid mass.
- Is quick and inexpensive and has minimal complications.
- Diagnostic sensitivity and specificity are reported to be high (on the order of >90%).
- Limitations in tumor diagnosis: (1) inability to differentiate a follicular adenoma from a follicular carcinoma on the basis of cytologic appearance. The hallmark of

follicular carcinoma is the presence of *capsular or vascular invasion,* but these diagnostic features do not appear in the FNA of *any* mass lesion. (2) On the other hand, FNA can be diagnostic for many other thyroid tumors such as papillary carcinoma, undifferentiated carcinoma, medullary carcinoma, lymphoma, metastatic tumors to the thyroid, and others. (3) FNA may produce changes that create diagnostic problems in the evaluation of tissue sections such as disruption of the tumor capsule, necrosis, pseudopapillae (particularly in oxyphilic tumors), and cytologic irregularities.

■ **Frozen section diagnosis:** The use of intraoperative frozen sections in the diagnosis of thyroid tumors has decreased with the increasing use of FNA.

■ **Treatment**

- **Surgery.** Treatment for the great majority of thyroid tumors is surgical excision. There are marked differences in opinion about what constitutes appropriate surgical management. The extent of surgery varies and includes:
  - **Lumpectomy:** Removal of a nodule or mass alone with minimal surrounding thyroid tissue. This procedure is generally not recommended for removal of thyroid tumors.
  - **Partial thyroidectomy:** Removal of a nodule or mass with a larger margin of surrounding thyroid tissue.
  - **Isthmusectomy:** Removal of a tumor within the isthmus, including a margin of surrounding thyroid tissue.
  - **Lobectomy:** Removal of one thyroid lobe.
  - **Hemithyroidectomy:** Removal of one thyroid lobe and the isthmus.
  - **Subtotal thyroidectomy:** Resection of more than half of each thyroid lobe plus the isthmus.
  - **Near-total thyroidectomy:** Removal of one entire lobe, the isthmus, and virtually the entire contralateral lobe except for about 10% of the posterior lateral portion of the contralateral lobe.
  - **Total thyroidectomy:** Removal of the entire thyroid gland. Advantages of total thyroidectomy include:
    - Higher survival rate for larger lesions (>1.5 cm).
    - Lowest recurrence rate, including tumor in the contralateral lobe.
    - Improved sensitivity of serum thyroglobulin as a marker for persistent or recurrent disease.
    - Allows use of radioactive iodine to treat persistent or recurrent disease.
    - Reduces the (unlikely) possibility that residual tumor in the contralateral lobe will transform to an anaplastic carcinoma.
- **Lymph node dissection:** This is advocated in the central neck ipsilateral to the thyroid tumor in all patients; lateral neck dissection is advocated when there are palpable nodes.
- **Radioactive iodine (^{131}I) therapy:** Thyroid ablation with ^{131}I is used in the treatment of differentiated thyroid carcinoma because (1) it destroys residual microscopic thyroid cancer; (2) it facilitates the identification of metastatic foci by radioactive iodine scanning; and (3) it has the best results in the treatment of distant metastasis in patients who are younger than 40 years of age at the time their metastasis is discovered and whose metastatic foci concentrate ^{131}I; poorer outcomes are seen in patients older than 40 years of age at the time of

discovery of their metastasis or who have extensive metastatic disease, moderately to poorly differentiated tumors, or tumors that do not concentrate ^{131}I.

- **External irradiation:** External radiation may be used postoperatively in patients with differentiated thyroid carcinomas with or without metastasis.
- **Chemotherapy:** Generally has a limited role in the treatment of thyroid cancers. It is most often used in conjunction with other modes of therapy (surgery and radiation) in the treatment of poorly differentiated or undifferentiated (anaplastic) carcinomas.
- **Thyroid hormone therapy:** Differentiated thyroid carcinomas contain functional thyroid-stimulating hormone (TSH) receptors, which are more abundant in follicular carcinomas than papillary carcinomas. TSH stimulates the growth of differentiated thyroid carcinomas. In theory, suppression of TSH receptors by thyroxine may result in tumor regression.

■ **Prognosis:** With the more common types of thyroid cancers prognosis is good; the best overall survival rates are associated with papillary carcinoma. Important prognostic factors include:
- The presence or absence of extrathyroidal spread.
- The presence or absence of metastatic disease.
- Age and gender of the patient.
- Pathologic features: histology, tumor size, presence or absence of encapsulation.

■ **Follow-up:** There is no standard protocol in the follow-up of patients with thyroid cancer. In general, scintiscans should be done within 3 months following the initial therapy with reexamination at one year. Disease-free patients then undergo whole body radioactive iodine scans at 3 and 5 years. Recurrent tumor is treated with radioactive iodine.

■ **Clinical staging of thyroid carcinoma,** as determined by physical examination, thyroid imaging, or endoscopic examination is as follows (Tables 8–2 and 8–3):

T—Primary tumor.
TX—Primary tumor cannot be assessed.
T0—No evidence of primary tumor.
T1—Tumor limited to the thyroid and measures 1 cm.
T2—Tumor limited to the thyroid and measures 1 cm but not more than 4 cm in greatest dimension.
T3—Tumor limited to the thyroid and measures more than 4 cm in greatest dimension.
T4—Tumor of any size extending beyond the thyroid capsule. This category may be further subdivided into a (solitary tumor) and b (multifocal tumor).

Table 8–2
CLINICAL STAGING: PAPILLARY OR FOLLICULAR CARCINOMA

For Patients <45 Years of Age		For Patients ≥45 Years of Age	
Stage	*Code*	*Stage*	*Code*
I	Any T, any N, M0	I	T1, N0, M0
II	Any T, any N, M1	II	T2 or T3, N0, M0
		III	T4, N0, M0 or any T, N1, M0
		IV	Any T, any N, M1

See text for abbreviations.

Table 8–3
CLINICAL STAGING: MEDULLARY CARCINOMA

Stage	Code
I	T1, N0, M0
II	T2, T3, or T4, N0, M0
III	Any T, N1, M0
IV	Any T, any N, M1

See text for abbreviations.

N—Regional lymph node metastasis.
NX—Regional lymph nodes cannot be assessed.
N0—No regional lymph node metastasis.
N1—Regional lymph node metastasis.
N1a—Ipsilateral lymph node metastasis.
N1b—Bilateral, midline, or contralateral cervical or mediastinal lymph node metastasis.
M—Distant metastasis.
MX—Presence of distant metastasis cannot be assessed.
M0—No distant metastasis.
M1—Distant metastasis; this category may be further specified according to the exact metastatic site(s) (e.g., pulmonary [PUL], osseous [OSS], liver [HEP], brain [BRA], and lymph nodes [LYM]).

■ **Pathologic staging (p):** Corresponds to the T (pT), N (pN), and M (pM) categories.

NOTE: A diagnosis of undifferentiated (anaplastic) carcinoma by definition is a Stage IV tumor.

C. BENIGN FOLLICULAR EPITHELIAL NEOPLASMS

1. Follicular Adenoma

Definition: Benign encapsulated tumor with evidence of follicular cell differentiation.

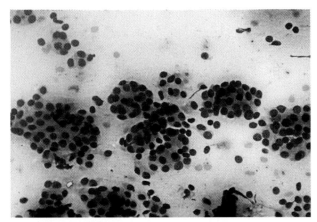

Figure 8–1. Fine needle aspiration, follicular adenoma. Fine needle aspirates of follicular neoplasms are typically much more cellular than adenomatoid nodules and have a preponderance of small follicular structures. Colloid is scanty or absent in more cellular follicular neoplasms. This lesion was found to be a follicular adenoma by histology. Diff-Quik stain.

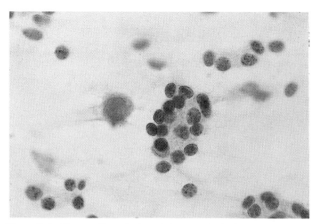

Figure 8–2. Fine needle aspiration of the same follicular adenoma shown in Figure 8–1. Note the syncytial grouping of the cells in this small follicle and the extruded fragment of dense colloid. The opaque chromatin pattern and round nuclear contours are typical of a follicular proliferation. Papanicolaou's stain.

Clinical

■ Affects women more often than men; occurs over a wide age range but is seen most commonly in the 5th to 6th decades.

■ Clinical presentation is usually that of a painless neck (thyroid) mass; duration of symptoms varies from months to years.

■ Adenomas are most often solitary and are limited to one part of the thyroid lobe but may involve the entire lobe.

■ No specific etiologic factors are associated with development of an adenoma.

■ Patients are usually euthyroid; serum thyroglobulin levels may be raised, but clinical evidence of hyperthyroidism is rarely seen.

Radiology

■ Thyroid imaging (with iodine 123 or technetium 99m) shows a poorly functional or "cold" nodule; adenomas are most often cold or hypofunctional nodules.

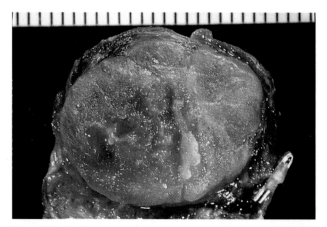

Figure 8–3. Follicular adenoma appearing as a solitary, encapsulated lesion.

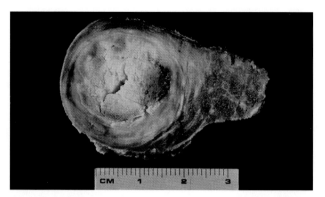

Figure 8–4. Follicular adenomas may have associated degenerative changes that include cyst formation, infarction, hemorrhage, and fibrosis.

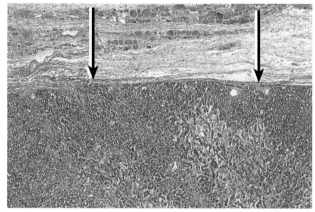

Figure 8–5. The hallmark of a follicular adenoma is encapsulation. The presence of a complete capsule encircling the tumor is a feature that separates an adenoma from an adenomatoid nodule. The absence of invasive growth differentiates a follicular adenoma from a follicular carcinoma. The thyroid tissue outside the tumor is compressed and atrophic and lacks proliferative features. The capsule in this example is very thin (arrows).

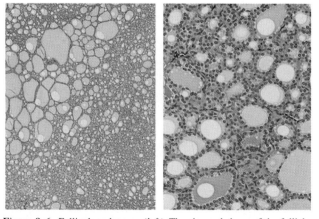

Figure 8–6. Follicular adenoma (left). The size and shape of the follicles and the cellularity of the tumor vary from case to case and even within a single case as is seen here (right). The nuclei in a follicular adenoma are round and regular with limited pleomorphism, have a coarse chromatin pattern, are not crowded or overlapped, and generally are aligned in a linear fashion along the basal aspect of the cells.

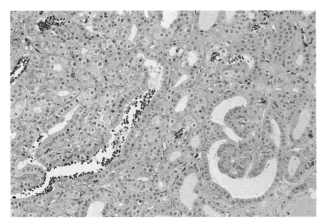

Figure 8–7. Follicular adenomas may have foci of papillary growth.

Pathology

Fine Needle Aspiration

- Features favoring a follicular neoplasm over a (cellular) adenomatoid nodule include:
  - Syncytial groups with or without distinct microfollicles; microfollicular or trabecular growth.
  - Cellular smears.
  - Increased cellularity; colloid is scanty, usually dense, and found in the follicular lumina.
  - Uniform cells with round nuclei, inconspicuous nucleoli, and ill-defined cell borders. Chromatin is opaque to coarsely granular and is usually evenly distributed.
  - Cytoplasmic features vary from scant to oxyphilic.

Gross

- Solitary encapsulated mass. The capsule varies in thickness but usually is thin. If a thick capsule is present, suspicion of a carcinoma should arise.
- Size varies, but adenomas generally measure 3 cm; larger tumors measuring more than 10 cm may be seen.
- Solid with a rubbery to firm consistency and a homogeneous appearance (except in the presence of secondary

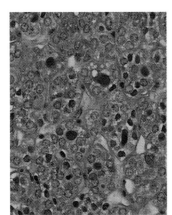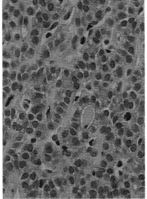

Figure 8–8. Follicular adenoma. *Left,* This cellular tumor was encapsulated with no evidence of invasive growth or features of papillary carcinoma. Colloid is present but may not be readily appreciated on hematoxylin and eosin stains. *Right,* Periodic acid–Schiff (PAS) stains assist in highlighting the colloid.

[degenerative] changes); pale tan to brown to orange (oxyphilic) in color.
- Secondary changes are uncommon and may include hemorrhage, fibrosis, cyst formation, calcification, and infarction may alter the appearance.

Histology

- Tumors are encapsulated with no evidence of capsular or vascular invasion. The capsule is composed of fibrous tissue within which small to medium-sized vascular spaces and smooth muscle bundles may be seen. The capsule is generally thin and clearly demarcated from the neoplasm on one side and the uninvolved thyroid tissue on the other side, which is usually compressed and may be atrophic. The capsule may vary in thickness from thin and regular to thick and irregular; a thickened capsule may indicate the possible presence of a carcinoma.
- The tumor is composed of relatively uniform colloid-filled follicles. Growth patterns may vary and include normofollicular (simple), macrofollicular (colloid), microfollicular (fetal), solid, trabecular, and organoid. In general, follicular adenomas usually have a single architectural pattern but may show an admixture of patterns; a neoplasm with a variety of growth patterns should raise suspicion for a papillary carcinoma.
- The cellularity and cytologic appearance of follicular adenomas vary from tumor to tumor and even within the same tumor; the neoplastic cells are generally uniform with defined cell borders.
- The nuclei are regularly shaped and aligned along the basal aspect of the cell. They are small to medium in size, hyperchromatic with absent to inconspicuous nucleoli and a variable amount of cytoplasm. The cytoplasm may be amphophilic, eosinophilic, oxyphilic (oncocyte), or clear. In the presence of oxyphilic cytoplasmic changes, the nuclei may be enlarged and pleomorphic, but they retain their uniformity in shape and their hyperchromatic appearance.
- Colloid-filled follicles are generally readily apparent but in some instances may be difficult to identify; periodic acid–Schiff (PAS) stains help in delineating the presence of colloid.
- Follicular adenomas are well vascularized, and the stromal component includes small to large vascular spaces. Neoplastic cells can be seen within the stromal vascular spaces, but any neoplastic foci in vascular spaces *within* the tumor itself does not qualify the tumor as a carcinoma.
- Rare mitotic figures can be seen. The presence of increased mitotic activity should be a matter of concern and should raise the suspicion of a carcinoma.
- Degenerative stromal changes that may be seen include edema, fibrosis, hemorrhage, cyst formation, calcification, ossification, mucinous stromal change, and squamous metaplasia; the last is unusual in adenomas but can occur following FNA. The presence of squamous metaplasia should at least raise concern about the possibility of a (papillary) carcinoma.
- Architectural and cytologic features of thyroid papillary carcinoma are absent.
- Capsular or vascular invasion is absent.

Table 8–4
FOLLICULAR ADENOMA VERSUS ADENOMATOID NODULE(S)

	Follicular Adenoma	Adenomatoid Nodules
Number	Solitary	Multiple
Capsule	Well-developed capsule	Poor encapsulation
Adjacent thyroid gland	Compression of surrounding gland	No compression of surrounding gland
Growth compared to remainder of thyroid	Different growth pattern in adjacent gland	Comparable growth pattern adjacent gland
Appearance compared to remainder of thyroid	Remainder of gland without histopathologic abnormalities	Dilated follicles and colloid nodules in gland are common
Degenerative changes	Uncommon	Frequently present

Differential Diagnosis

- Adenomatoid nodules (Table 8–4) (Chapter 7A).
- Follicular carcinoma (Chapter 8D, #1).
- Papillary carcinoma (Chapter 8D, #2).
- Medullary carcinoma (Chapter 8C, #3).

Treatment and Prognosis

- Conservative surgery (lobectomy) is the treatment of choice.
- No recurrences or metastases.

Histologic Types of Follicular Adenoma
(Table 8–5)

- Generally, the histologic variants of follicular adenoma are no different in clinical parameters or biologic behavior than the conventional type of follicular adenoma. The histologic subtypes of follicular adenoma, including the oxyphilic type, clear cell type, and signet ring cell type, are tumors in which one of these cell types is the dominant cell (defined roughly as 75% of the tumor).

2. Follicular Adenoma with Atypical Features

Definition: Any encapsulated follicular neoplasm that has histologic features suggestive of a more aggressive neoplasm (carcinoma) but does not demonstrate unequivocal evidence of either capsular or vascular space invasion.

Synonyms: Atypical follicular adenoma; follicular neoplasms of undetermined malignant potential.

- Histologic features that should suggest the possibility of a carcinoma include the following:
  - Thickened capsule.
  - Increased cellularity, particularly hypercellularity along the peripheral (tumor-capsule interface) aspects of the tumor.
  - Increased mitotic activity (especially with atypical forms).
  - Nuclear atypia with prominent nucleoli

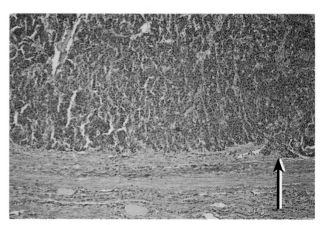

Figure 8–9. Atypical follicular adenoma characterized by its hypercellularity, especially along the tumor-capsule interface. The capsule is thickened but not excessively so; the tumor has an even contour along its periphery except toward the right *(arrow),* where there is an irregular growth. Multiple sections failed to show invasive growth.

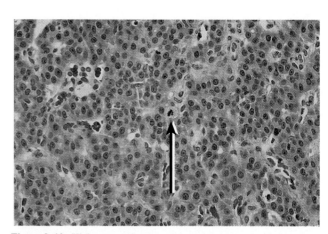

Figure 8–10. Higher magnification of the previous illustration showing a mitotic figure *(arrow).* The combination of increased cellularity, thickened capsule, irregular peripheral growth pattern, and mitotic activity resulted in a diagnosis of atypical follicular adenoma.

Table 8–5
HISTOLOGIC TYPES OF FOLLICULAR ADENOMA

Atypical
Hyalinizing trabecular adenoma (paraganglioma-like)
Oxyphil (Hürthle) cell
Signet ring cell
Clear cell

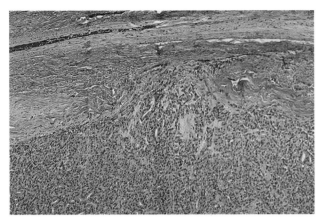

Figure 8–11. Atypical follicular adenoma characterized by increased cellularity along the tumor-capsule interface, a thickened capsule and, as seen here, an irregular peripheral growth. The neoplastic cells appear to be extending toward the capsule but are not within the capsule. Multiple sections failed to identify unequivocal evidence of invasive growth. Due to the hypercellularity and irregular growth, this follicular tumor was considered an atypical adenoma.

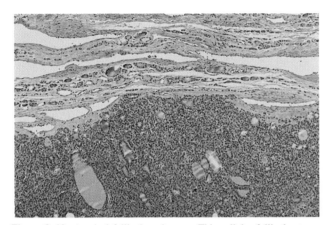

Figure 8–12. Atypical follicular adenoma. This cellular follicular tumor has a relatively thin capsule but shows an uneven contour along its periphery. The neoplastic cells are at the same level as capsular blood vessels seen on either side of the tumor. The presence of a hypercellular tumor with neoplastic cells at the same level as capsular blood vessels but without definitive invasive foci prompted the diagnosis of atypical follicular adenoma.

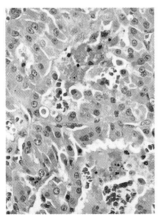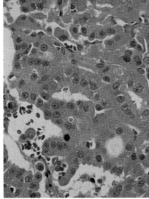

Figure 8–13. The classification of this oxyphilic follicular adenoma as atypical has no correlation with its oxyphilic cytoplasm. Rather, it is due to the presence of necrosis *(left)* and increased mitotic activity *(right)*. No definitive foci of invasive growth was seen after extensive sectioning; nevertheless, the presence of necrosis suggests a carcinoma.

- The presence of a thickened capsule with increased cellularity, even without mitosis, nuclear atypia, or prominent nucleoli, is a worrisome feature. Benign endocrine organ neoplasms generally are amitotic, and the presence of mitosis raises a concern about the possibility of a malignant tumor. However, as an isolated finding it is not indicative of malignancy. Nuclear pleomorphism, atypia, and prominent nucleoli are not diagnostic features of a malignant endocrine organ neoplasm. Benign tumors or even nonneoplastic lesions may have these nuclear changes. This is especially true of follicular neoplasms (i.e., adenoma and carcinoma) of the thyroid gland, in which the only criteria of malignancy are invasive growth or metastases. The nuclear features do not differentiate a follicular adenoma from a follicular carcinoma, which is the reason why these tumors cannot be differentiated on the basis of FNA cytology.

- In a follicular neoplasm with atypical features, the most critical issue is adequate and appropriate sectioning of the tumor to evaluate the tumor-capsule-thyroid parenchymal interface for evidence of invasive growth. This is equally true of any encapsulated thyroid neoplasm that has features suggestive of malignancy. Guidelines to the number of sections considered adequate to exclude the presence of invasion are as follows:
  - For a tumor measuring less than 6 cm, submit the entire tumor.
  - For a tumor measuring 6 cm, submit at least 10 blocks.
  - For a tumor measuring more than 6 cm, submit one additional block per centimeter of tumor.

Differential Diagnosis

- Minimally invasive follicular carcinoma (Chapter 8D, #1).
- Adenomatoid nodules (Chapter 7A).
- Papillary carcinoma (Chapter 8D, #2).
- Medullary carcinoma (Chapter 8E, #3).

Treatment and Prognosis

- Treatment for an atypical follicular adenoma is surgical removal (similar to treatment for the usual types of follicular adenomas).
- Generally, surgery is conservative in extent and is limited to the affected portions of the thyroid gland (lobectomy or subtotal thyroidectomy).
- Long-term prognosis is excellent.
- Close clinical follow-up is indicated.

3. Hyalinizing Trabecular Adenoma

Synonyms: Paraganglioma-like adenoma.

Clinical

- Affects women more than men; occurs over a wide age range from the 3rd to the 8th decades.
- Clinical presentation is that of an asymptomatic neck mass.
- May occur in any portion of the thyroid gland.

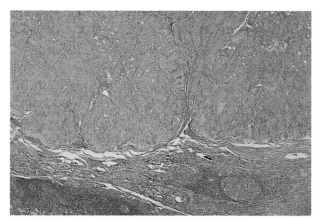

Figure 8–14. Hyalinizing trabecular adenoma. Well-demarcated tumor showing a lobulated or bosselated growth at its periphery.

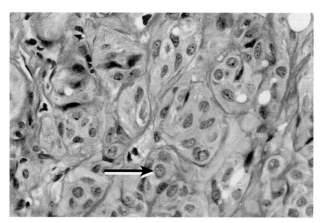

Figure 8–17. The nuclear features seen in the hyalinizing trabecular adenoma include enlarged round, oval, or elongated nuclei with irregularities in size and shape, nuclear grooves, and eosinophilic nuclear inclusions *(arrow)*. In addition, perinucleolar vacuoles or halos are present. The cytoplasm may be finely granular with acidophilic, amphophilic, or clear appearance.

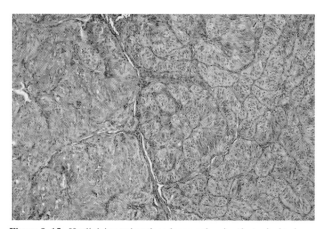

Figure 8–15. Hyalinizing trabecular adenoma showing the typical trabecular and organoid (paraganglioma-like) growth with areas of prominent hyalinization.

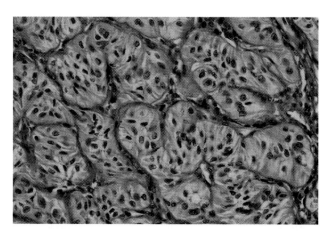

Figure 8–18. Hyalinizing trabecular adenoma. Cell nests composed of variably appearing oval to spindle-shaped nuclei showing irregularities in size and shape, and coarse to dispersed nuclear chromatin pattern.

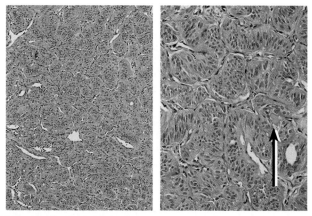

Figure 8–16. Hyalinizing trabecular adenoma. *Left,* Trabeculae and cell nests separated by a fibrovascular stroma. *Right,* The nuclei are round to elongated, often oriented perpendicular to the fibrovascular stroma. By and large, colloid is absent, but focally colloid-filled follicles can be seen *(arrow).*

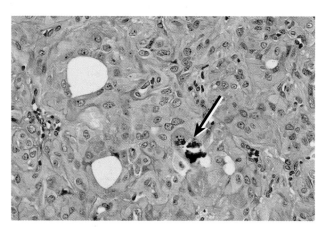

Figure 8–19. Hyalinizing trabecular adenoma. In addition to the nuclear cytomorphology, the presence of calcific concretions *(arrow)* may suggest a diagnosis of papillary carcinoma.

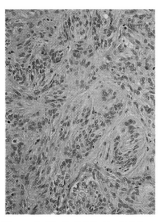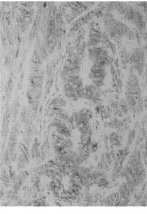

Figure 8–20. *Left,* The hyalinizing trabecular adenoma is a follicular epithelial cell-derived tumor that has minimal to absent follicle formation with little to no colloid. The differential diagnosis includes a medullary carcinoma. *Right,* The presence of thyroglobulin immunoreactivity, as seen here, would confirm a diagnosis of a follicular epithelial cell tumor excluding a C cell-derived neoplasm. This tumor is non-reactive with calcitonin, chromogranin, or synaptophysin.

Radiology

- Thyroid imaging (with iodine 123 or technetium 99m) shows a "cold" nodule, but the tumor may appear as a "hot" nodule.

Pathology

Gross

- Well-circumscribed tumor measuring 1 to 5 cm in diameter.

Histology

- Encapsulated or circumscribed tumor characterized by trabecular, organoid (cell nest) growth pattern with fibrovascular stroma.
- Lobulated growth can be seen at the periphery of the tumor.
- Prominent extracellular and intracellular hyalinization is present.
- Follicle formation is minimal or absent. The tumor has little colloid formation.
- Cells are elongated and sharply outlined with round, oval, or elongated nuclei demonstrating grooves, eosinophilic nuclear inclusions, and perinucleolar vacuoles. The cytoplasm is finely granular with an acidophilic, amphophilic, or clear appearance. Mitoses are infrequently seen.
- Nuclei are often oriented perpendicular to the fibrovascular stroma.
- Psammoma body-like formations can be seen.
- Chronic lymphocytic thyroiditis is often seen in the surrounding thyroid gland.
- *Immunohistochemistry:* Thyroglobulin, cytokeratin, and vimentin positive; chromogranin and calcitonin negative.

Differential Diagnosis

- Papillary carcinoma (Chapter 8D, #2).
- Medullary carcinoma (Chapter 8E, #3).

Treatment and Prognosis

- Conservative surgery (lobectomy or subtotal thyroidectomy).
- Excellent prognosis following surgical removal.

Additional Notes

- There is some reason for categorizing the hyalinizing trabecular adenoma as a variant of papillary carcinoma rather than as part of the spectrum of follicular adenoma; features that support this classification include:
  - Nuclear morphology with irregular shape, nuclear inclusions, and nuclear grooves.
  - Presence of psammoma body–like formations.
  - Purported reports of nodal metastasis, although we have not experienced this occurrence to date.
  - Occurrence of hyalinizing trabecular adenoma in patients with lymphocytic thyroiditis or in those with a history of radiation therapy; these two settings are more typically associated with papillary carcinoma.
- Hyalinizing trabecular neoplasms with minimally invasive growth have been identified and are termed **hyalinizing trabecular carcinoma.**
  - These tumors are considered the malignant counterparts of hyalinizing trabecular adenomas.
  - Tumors measure from 2.5 to 4 cm.
  - Histology is identical to that of hyalinizing follicular adenomas except that capsular or vascular space invasion is present.
  - These minimally invasive tumors are biologically low grade.
  - Conservative surgical removal with close follow-up is indicated.

4. Follicular Adenoma with Oxyphilia

Definition: The term oncocytic is derived from the Greek word meaning "swollen." Oncocytic and oxyphilic are synonymous terms. Oxyphilia results from an increase in the mitochondrial content of a cell. On light microscopy an oxyphilic cell is one that has a prominent granular eosinophilic-appearing cytoplasm.

Synonyms: Hürthle cell adenoma; oncocytic adenoma; oxyphilic cell adenoma.

Clinical

- A follicular adenoma with oxyphilia has the same demographic features, clinical presentation, treatment, and biologic behavior as "conventional" follicular adenomas.

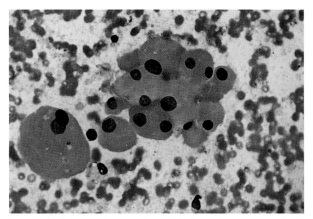

Figure 8–21. Fine needle aspiration, follicular neoplasm with oxyphilia. The cells of this oxyphilic follicular neoplasm are large and show abundant granular cytoplasm, which appears gray-blue on Diff-Quik stain. Note the low nuclear to cytoplasmic ratio. Very cellular oxyphilic neoplasms have little or no colloid; the cells tend to form small, loosely cohesive groups or shed singly. Diff-Quik stain.

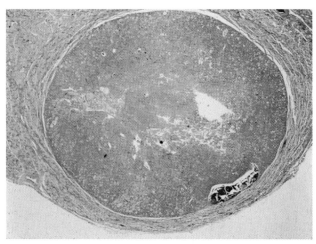

Figure 8–24. Like "conventional" follicular adenomas, follicular adenomas with oxyphilia are encapsulated tumors; the capsule may vary in thickness, and in this case there is a thin fibrous capsule encircling the tumor.

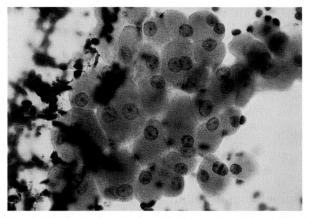

Figure 8–22. Fine needle aspiration, follicular neoplasm with oxyphilia. A Papanicolaou-stained smear of the neoplasm seen in the previous illustration shows cytoplasmic oxyphilia manifested as cytoplasmic granularity. The cytoplasm is usually more abundant than in nonoxyphilic follicular cells. The nuclei are enlarged, round, with readily apparent nucleoli.

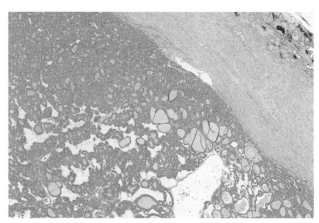

Figure 8–25. Another example of a follicular adenoma with oxyphilia shows the presence of colloid-filled follicles; in contrast with Figure 8–24, this tumor has a markedly thickened capsule. The presence of a thickened capsule should raise the possibility of invasive growth. Multiple sections in this tumor failed to show neoplastic transgression of the capsule or evidence of vascular invasion.

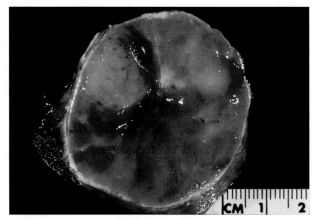

Figure 8–23. Follicular adenoma with oxyphilia. The tumor is completely encapsulated and is characterized by an orange coloration due to the presence of cytoplasmic oxyphilia.

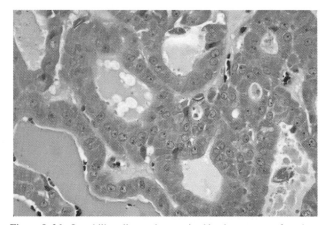

Figure 8–26. Oxyphilic cells are characterized by the presence of an abundant eosinophilic granular appearing cytoplasm. The cytoplasmic oxyphilia causes nuclear enlargement; however, despite the nuclear enlargement, the nuclei are round and uniform, and are basally located within the cell. In addition to the enlarged nuclei, central eosinophilic nucleoli often are seen in oxyphilic cells. Special stains can be used for mitochondria (see Fig. 8–91).

Pathology

Fine Needle Aspiration

- Smears or aspirates are dominated by enlarged oval to polygonal cells, often in sheets, that have an abundant granular-appearing cytoplasm.
- Because of the cytoplasmic oxyphilia, there is nuclear enlargement; the nuclei are round to oval and are eccentrically located. Binucleate cells can be seen.
- Prominent round, eosinophilic nucleoli are seen.
- Colloid is minimal to absent.

Gross

- The macroscopic appearance of a follicular adenoma with oxyphilia is similar to that of a conventional follicular adenoma except that the oxyphilia may impart a distinct orange color to the tumor.

Histology

- Histologic features are similar to those of conventional follicular adenomas. Follicular adenomas with oxyphilia are encapsulated tumors; the capsule may vary in thickness, but there is no transgression of the capsule nor evidence of vascular space invasion.
- Oxyphilic cells are characterized by the presence of an abundant eosinophilic, granular-appearing cytoplasm; the cytoplasmic margins are often distinctly visible.
- Cytoplasmic oxyphilia tends to cause nuclear enlargement and nuclear pleomorphism; however, despite nuclear enlargement, the nuclei are round and uniform, and hyperchromatic.
- In addition to the enlarged nuclei, prominent central eosinophilic nucleoli often are seen in oxyphilic cells.
- *Histochemistry:* Special stains for mitochondria include phosphotungstic acid hematoxylin (PTAH), in which the oxyphilic cell has a red appearance, and Novelli's stain, in which the mitochondria stain dark purple.
- *Immunohistochemistry:* Thyroid oxyphilic cells react positively to cytokeratin and thyroglobulin, although the thyroglobulin reactivity is less intense than in nonoxyphilic follicular cells, and negatively to chromogranin and calcitonin.
- *Electron microscopy:* Oxyphilic cells are packed with mitochondria; mitochondrial abnormalities can be seen, including quantitative and qualitative changes (in size, shape, and content).
- Oxyphilic cells, perhaps due to the oxygen-sensitive nature of mitochondria, may be easily traumatized, leading to marked degenerative changes following such events as FNA; degenerative changes of oxyphilic lesions may include infarction and pseudopapillary growth.
- Clear cell changes in follicular epithelial cells may be associated with the oxyphilic changes.

Additional Facts

- Hürthle originally described the cell that is now believed to represent the parafollicular cell or C cell of ultimobranchial derivation and not the oncocyte; the latter was originally described by Askanazy.
- The use of the designation Hürthle, oxyphilic, or oncocytic is purely descriptive and is indicative of a type of change in a cell; it is *not* indicative, in itself, of any speci-

Table 8–6
THYROID LESIONS WITH OXYPHILIC CELL CHANGES

Non-Neoplastic Lesions
Nodular goiter (adenomatoid nodules)
Chronic lymphocytic thyroiditis (Hashimoto's thyroiditis)
Graves' disease
Postradiation
Aging
Neoplasms
Follicular adenoma variants
Follicular carcinoma variants
Papillary carcinoma variants
Medullary carcinoma

fied biologic behavior in a thyroid tumor with oxyphilia. Too often the assumption is made that a diagnosis of Hürthle cell neoplasm is essentially synonymous with a follicular carcinoma and qualifies a tumor as malignant; this is erroneous because oxyphilic cell changes are seen in both non-neoplastic and neoplastic (benign and malignant) thyroid lesions (Table 8–6).
- A diagnosis of follicular carcinoma with oxyphilia can only be made in the presence of capsular or vascular invasion. In the absence of invasive growth, features found in an encapsulated follicular neoplasm (including the oxyphilic follicular adenoma) that may increase concern about malignancy include:
  • Increased cellularity.
  • Increased mitotic activity, including atypical mitoses.
  • Necrosis, either in individual cells or confluent foci.
- Cytoplasmic oxyphilia often causes nuclear enlargement and nuclear pleomorphism. This alteration in size and shape of the nucleus may lead to an erroneous diagnosis of carcinoma. Diagnostic confusion may be minimized by evaluating the tumor for other changes that may support a diagnosis of papillary carcinoma (e.g., architectural and cytomorphologic features).

5. Follicular Adenoma with Clear Cells

Clinical

- A follicular adenoma with clear cells has the same demographic features, clinical presentation, treatment, and biologic behavior as conventional follicular adenomas.

Pathology

Gross

- The macroscopic appearance of a follicular adenoma with clear cells is similar to that of a conventional follicular adenoma.

Histology

- Histologic features are similar to those of conventional follicular adenomas. Follicular adenomas with clear cells are encapsulated tumors; the capsule may vary in thickness, but there is no transgression of the capsule nor evidence of vascular space invasion.

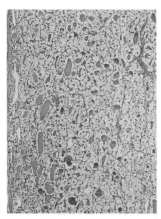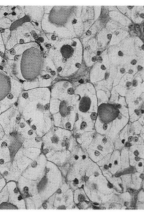

Figure 8–27. Follicular adenoma with clear cells. *Left,* This was a solitary encapsulated thyroid tumor with a nested growth and readily apparent colloid-filled follicles. *Right,* The characteristic feature of this tumor is the presence of a clear cytoplasm. Renal cell carcinomas may metastasize to the thyroid and simulate the appearance of a primary thyroid tumor. The presence of follicles filled with colloid and immunoreactivity for thyroglobulin (*not shown*) would confirm a tumor of thyroid follicular cell origin.

- The growth pattern is usually follicular but may include trabecular or solid growth.
- Cytologic appearance is that of a tumor predominantly or exclusively composed of cells with clear (empty) to finely granular-appearing cytoplasm. The nuclei are centrally situated, small, round, and regular, and are marked by hyperchromasia with or without sharp cell outlines.
- Colloid-containing follicles may be absent or only focally identified; PAS stain is helpful in identifying the presence of colloid.
- *Histochemistry:* Diastase-sensitive, PAS-positive intracytoplasmic material is present in the cells.
- *Immunohistochemistry:* Cells react positively with thyroglobulin, but the staining may be focal and of limited intensity; reactions to calcitonin and neuroendocrine cell markers (chromogranin and synaptophysin) are negative.

Differential Diagnosis

- Metastatic renal cell carcinoma (Table 8–7).
- Follicular carcinoma with clear cells (Chapter 8D, #1).
- Papillary carcinoma (Chapter 8D, #2).
- Parathyroid lesions (Chapters 9 and 10).
- Medullary carcinoma with clear cells (Chapter 8E, #3).

Additional Facts

- The clear cytoplasm may be due to:
  - Massively dilated mitochondria, appearing as intracytoplasmic vesicles on electron microscopy.
  - Intracytoplasmic glycogen accumulation.
  - Intracytoplasmic lipid accumulation.
  - Intracytoplasmic thyroglobulin deposition: the intracellular thyroglobulin accumulation may be related to the effects of TSH, which causes increased thyroglobulin deposition within the cell cytoplasm owing to the inability of the cell to release or excrete it.
- The clear cell change seen in follicular tumors may be closely linked to oxyphilic metaplasia and may represent the "end-stage" cytoplasmic changes of a tumor that once was predominantly oxyphilic.

6. Follicular Adenoma with Signet Ring Cells

Synonyms: Signet ring cell mucinous adenoma; mucin-producing microfollicular adenoma; mucin-producing adenoma.

Clinical

- Follicular adenomas with signet ring cells have the same demographics, clinical presentation, treatment, and biologic behavior as conventional follicular adenomas.

Pathology

Gross

- The macroscopic appearance of a follicular adenoma with signet ring cells is similar to that of a conventional follicular adenoma.

Histology

- Histologic features are similar to those of conventional follicular adenomas. Follicular adenomas with signet ring cells are encapsulated tumors; the capsule may vary in thickness, but there is no transgression of the capsule nor evidence of vascular space invasion.
- The growth pattern is microfollicular and nested; colloid is readily apparent.
- This tumor is characterized by cells that have large intracytoplasmic vacuoles that result in eccentric displace-

Table 8–7
FOLLICULAR TUMORS WITH CLEAR CELLS VERSUS METASTATIC RENAL CELL CARCINOMA

Features	Follicular Adenoma or Carcinoma with Clear Cells	Metastatic Renal Cell Carcinoma
Luminal secretion	Colloid; will be PAS positive	No colloid; find red blood cells; pseudofollicles
Nested growth with fibrovascular stroma	Present	Present
Cytoplasm	Foamy appearing	Clear
Nuclear	Round; dispersed or coarse chromatin	Small, round, hyperchromatic
Glycogen (intracytoplasmic diastase sensitive, PAS positive)	Yes, but will also be diastase resistant	Yes; intensely positive
Thyroglobulin immunoreactivity	Present but may be focal and of weak intensity	Absent

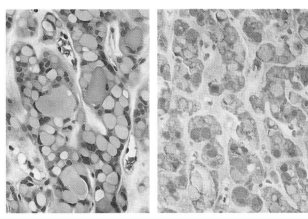

Figure 8–28. Follicular adenoma with signet ring cells, characterized by cells that have large intracytoplasmic vacuoles that result in eccentric displacement of the cell nucleus, creating a signet ring appearance. *Left,* Signet ring cells in which the cytoplasm is acidophilic and the nuclei are hyperchromatic with a flattened or semilunar appearance. *Right,* Strong thyroglobulin reactivity is present.

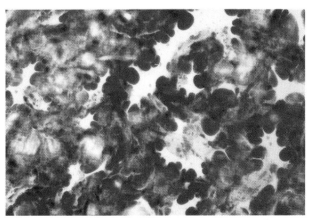

Figure 8–29. Lipid-rich cell adenoma. Oil red O stain for fat is positive. This tumor is characterized by cells that have small to medium sized intracytoplasmic vesicles that result in indentation of the centrally situated nucleus.

ment of the cell nucleus, creating a signet ring appearance.

- The cytoplasm appears clear to acidophilic to finely granular; the nuclei are hyperchromatic and are flattened or semilunar in appearance but may retain a rounder appearance.
- *Histochemistry:* Diastase-resistant, PAS-positive intracytoplasmic material is present; mucin stains are positive.
- *Immunohistochemistry:* Strong thyroglobulin reactivity is present; calcitonin and neuroendocrine cell markers (chromogranin and synaptophysin) are negative.

Differential Diagnosis

- Metastatic adenocarcinoma (lung and gastrointestinal tract).

Additional Facts

- The intense thyroglobulin immunoreactivity correlates with the intracytoplasmic thyroglobulin deposition, which in turn gives the cell its signet ring appearance. The intracellular thyroglobulin accumulation may be related to the effects of TSH, which causes increased thyroglobulin deposition within the cell cytoplasm due to the inability of the cell to release or excrete it.
- Thyroglobulin is a sialic acid–containing glycoprotein, and therefore thyroglobulin stains positively with PAS and acid mucin stains (e.g., Alcian blue at pH 2.5, sulfomucin). Mucicarmine, a stain for neutral mucins, is positive but usually weakly so; the mucicarminophilic seen in signet ring cells is attributed to the intracytoplasmic thyroglobulin accumulation.

7. Follicular Adenoma with Fat

Synonyms: Lipid-rich adenoma.

- Follicular adenoma with fat is extremely rare.
- Fat in follicular epithelial cells may occur as a result of aging.

- This tumor is characterized by cells that have small to medium-sized intracytoplasmic vesicles that result in indentation of the centrally situated nucleus.
- *Histochemistry:* Oil red O or other fat stains are positive.
- *Immunohistochemistry:* Thyroglobulin positive.

Differential Diagnosis

- Thyrolipoma.

D. MALIGNANT FOLLICULAR EPITHELIAL NEOPLASMS

1. Follicular Carcinoma (FC)

Definition: Follicular epithelial cell thyroid neoplasm, not belonging to papillary carcinoma, with evidence of capsular and/or vascular invasion.

Clinical

- Represents approximately 10% to 20% of all malignant thyroid tumors.
- More common in women than in men; occurs over a wide age range, including children and adolescents, but is most common in the 5th and 6th decades (patients are approximately 1 decade older than patients with papillary carcinoma).
- Usually presents as a solitary painless neck mass but pain may occur later in the disease course. Alternatively, the initial presentation may be a pulmonary metastasis or pathologic fracture secondary to osseous metastasis.
- Patients are usually euthyroid; uncommonly, they may present with clinical manifestations of hyperthyroidism.
- Incidence is greater in iodine-deficient regions of the world, and, partly for this reason, it occurs in glands that have been enlarged for long periods.

Radiology

- On thyroid scans (^{123}I) follicular carcinomas are most often cold or hypofunctioning nodules.

Pathology

Fine Needle Aspiration

NOTE: The contributions of FNA in the diagnosis of follicular carcinoma are limited. In a neoplasm in which the diagnosis of a carcinoma is based on the presence of invasive growth (capsular or vascular) rather than on cytomorphology, needle aspiration cannot supply the cytopathologist with that information. FNA is an excellent screening tool in the evaluation of a mass lesion of the thyroid, but when differentiating a follicular adenoma from a follicular carcinoma, often the FNA diagnosis is "follicular neoplasm, not further specified," which informs the treating physician that a neoplasm requiring additional therapy (i.e., surgical removal) is present.

■ Cellular with minimal to absent colloid.
■ Cells are often arranged in a microfollicular pattern, but a trabecular pattern may also be present. Small three-dimensional clusters with a syncytial configuration can be seen, and isolated cells are often found.
■ In general, the cells are monomorphic and larger than nonneoplastic follicular epithelial cells. They have uniform, round to oval nuclei with evenly distributed, finely granular (coarse) chromatin, small to inconspicuous nucleoli, and pale to clear cytoplasm with indistinct cell margins.
■ Nuclei may vary in appearance; anisokaryosis and anisochromatosis can be seen.

Histology

■ A diagnosis of follicular carcinoma is based on the presence of invasive growth (capsular or vascular invasion), extension into the adjacent thyroid parenchyma, or the presence of metastatic tumor.

Capsular Invasion

• The extent of capsular invasion is a source of contention. Some believe that any degree of invasion into the capsule qualifies the tumor as a minimally invasive follicular carcinoma; others think that the tumor must penetrate the entire thickness of the capsule to be regarded as unequivocal evidence of capsular invasion.
• Elastic stains may be helpful in determining whether capsular invasion has occurred.
• Problematic features relative to diagnostic interpretation include:
  • Irregularity of tumor contour.
  • Tangential sectioning.
  • Presence of a separate nodule lying immediately outside the capsule of the main tumor mass. In this situation, serial sections are needed to determine whether a connection is present. The presence of continuity between the main mass and the nodule outside the capsule is indicative of a carcinoma, but the absence of any connection does not exclude a diagnosis of carcinoma. The appearance of the entire gland must be considered in that the presence of other nodules may indicate multiple adenomatoid nodules.

Vascular Invasion

• Represents a more reliable feature of malignancy than capsular invasion.

• In low-grade or minimally invasive follicular carcinomas, vascular space invasion involves small to medium-sized blood vessels but not large vascular spaces.
• The "violated" vascular space must lie within the capsule or beyond the capsule.
• Tumor cells must be adherent to a vessel wall that is lined by identifiable endothelial cells. Tumor cells protruding into a vascular space in which an endothelial layer can be identified over the bulging tumor nests should be regarded as invasive.
• *Histochemistry:* Special stains such as elastic tissue stains or trichrome may be helpful, but because a continuous smooth muscle layer may not be present, these stains usually are of only limited help.
• *Immunohistochemistry:* Stains for endothelial markers (factor VIII–related antigen, *Ulex europaeus* agglutinin I, CD31, and CD34) may be of only limited assistance.

■ Two varieties of follicular carcinoma are recognized, differing in extent of invasive component, biologic behavior, and treatment. These variants are the **minimally invasive** and **widely invasive follicular carcinomas.**

a. Minimally Invasive or Low-Grade Follicular Carcinoma

Pathology

Gross

■ Appearance is essentially the same as that of follicular adenoma.

Histology

■ Many histologic features are similar to those of follicular adenoma; however, a larger proportion of these tumors has the atypical features previously described (see Chapter 8C, #2) but, by definition, capsular or vascular invasion must be present to qualify the tumor as a low-grade or minimally invasive follicular carcinoma.
■ Although an invasive component is present, the extent of invasion in these tumors is limited.

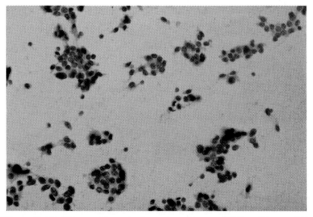

Figure 8–30. Fine needle aspiration of a solitary, solid thyroid mass. The aspirate is cellular with absent colloid. Small cell clusters with syncytial configuration are present, as are isolated cells. A microfollicular pattern is focally present.

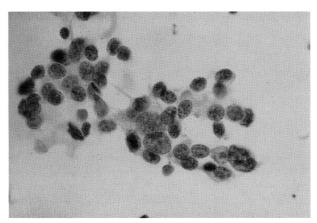

Figure 8–31. The cells are monomorphic, enlarged with uniform, round to oval nuclei with evenly distributed, finely granular (coarse) chromatin, small to inconspicuous nucleoli, and pale to clear cytoplasm with indistinct cell margins. Anisokaryosis and anisochromatosis can be seen.

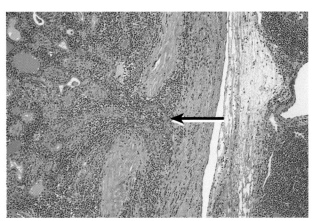

Figure 8–34. Higher magnification of the previous illustration shows the neoplastic follicular epithelial cells extending from the main mass into its capsule *(arrow)*. The capsule is bifurcated, appearing on either side of the invasive tumor. The presence of lymphocytic cell infiltrate somewhat obscures the neoplastic proliferation, but the presence of thyroid follicular epithelium within this focus confirms the diagnosis. The differential diagnosis may include FNA-related alterations (see Fig. 8–215).

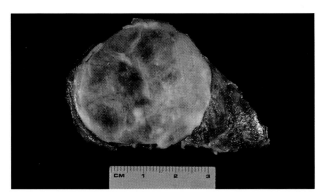

Figure 8–32. Follicular carcinoma. The gross appearance of this thyroid tumor, which showed minimal invasive growth on light microscopy, is similar to that of follicular adenoma.

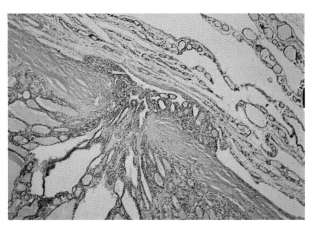

Figure 8–35. This follicular neoplasm had a growth pattern similar to that of adenomatoid nodule except that it was completely encapsulated and, as seen here, focally invaded through its capsule and into a small caliber vascular space, qualifying it as a minimally invasive follicular carcinoma.

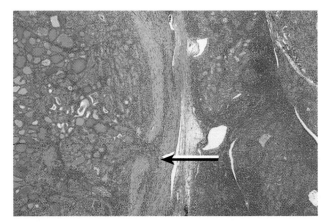

Figure 8–33. Follicular carcinoma, minimally invasive. This follicular tumor shows capsular invasion. The tumor penetrates its capsule but does not extend into adjacent thyroid tissue *(arrow)*. Lymphocytic thyroiditis is seen in the non-neoplastic thyroid (right side).

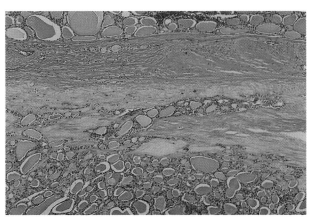

Figure 8–36. Follicular tumor with a thickened capsule. The tumor extends from the main mass and invades into its capsule. The extent of invasion is limited and this tumor qualifies as a minimally invasive follicular carcinoma.

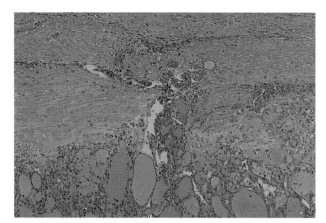

Figure 8–37. In addition to capsular invasion, the diagnosis of a follicular carcinoma can be based on the presence of vascular invasion. The vascular spaces must be outside the tumor mass to include capsular vessels or vascular spaces beyond the capsule and should have an endothelial lining. The invasive tumor should adhere to the vessel wall and not be "free-floating" in the space. In this example, there is direct penetration of a capsular vessel from the main tumor mass. In this example of a low-grade or minimally invasive follicular carcinoma, the vascular spaces are of small caliber.

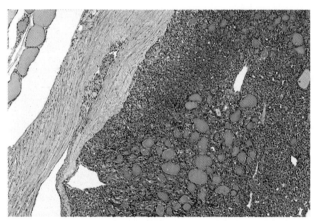

Figure 8–38. Minimally invasive follicular carcinoma. An endothelial-lined capsular vascular space is invaded by a follicular tumor. There is no direct continuity from the tumor to the vascular space in this example.

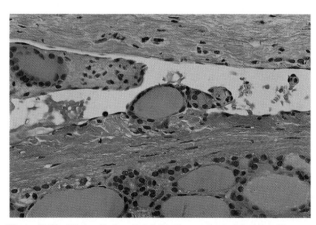

Figure 8–39. Minimally invasive follicular carcinoma. Small-caliber, endothelial-lined capsular blood vessel is invaded by follicular carcinoma. The tumor is adherent to the vascular wall, bulges into the vascular space, and is focally covered (luminal side) by flattened endothelial cells.

Differential Diagnosis

- Primarily but not exclusively follicular adenoma (Chapter 8C, #1).
- Papillary carcinoma (Chapter 8D, #2).
- Medullary carcinoma (Chapter 8E, #3).

Treatment and Prognosis

- Another contentious issue in regard to minimally invasive follicular carcinomas is the appropriate mode of therapy. Treatment options include conservative treatment and more radical approaches. Conservative therapy includes limited resection (lobectomy or subtotal thyroidectomy) without radioactive iodine therapy. Radical treatment includes total thyroidectomy followed by administration of radioactive iodine. The only caveat to the use of conservative modalities is the presence of limited invasion and the absence of metastatic tumor. In the presence of metastasis, treatment should include the use of radioactive iodine. The most common sites of metastasis in patients with follicular carcinoma are osseous sites and the lungs.
- The prognosis for minimally invasive or low-grade follicular carcinoma is excellent, with 70% to 100% 10-year survival rates reported (cure rates are reported to be >95%).
- Adverse prognostic findings include the presence of metastatic disease. In the presence of pulmonary or osseous metastasis, other adverse prognostic factors include:
  - Older age when metastasis is discovered.
  - Multiple sites of metastasis.
  - Absence of radioactive iodine uptake by the metastatic deposits.

b. Widely Invasive Follicular Carcinoma

- Widely invasive follicular carcinomas are much less common than their minimally invasive counterparts.

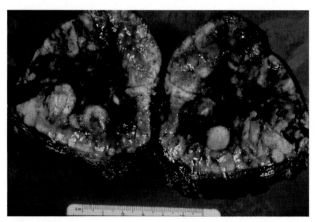

Figure 8–40. This fleshy, solid mass shows degenerative changes. Although on gross examination extensive invasive growth was not seen, microscopically this tumor was widely invasive.

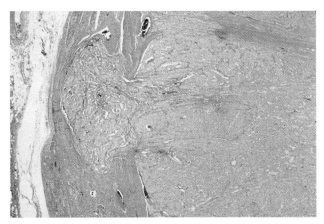

Figure 8–41. Follicular carcinoma, widely invasive, in which there is clear-cut invasion beyond the capsular delimitation of the tumor with extension into adjacent thyroid parenchyma. This type of invasion has a mushroom-like appearance.

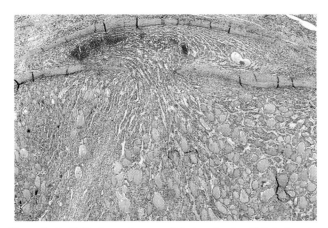

Figure 8–42. Follicular carcinoma, widely invasive, in which the invasive growth is obvious. This illustration shows a Movat stain that stains the elastic fibers of the capsule. This stain may help to delineate the capsule in less overt cases of follicular carcinoma, assisting in the determination of capsular invasion.

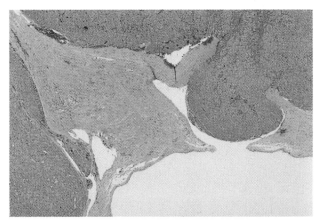

Figure 8–43. In addition to capsular invasion, a diagnosis of a widely invasive follicular carcinoma can be made on the basis of the presence of invasive growth into thick-walled, large-caliber blood vessels as seen here. In this example, the tumor invades directly from the main mass into the vascular space.

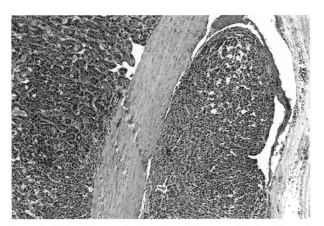

Figure 8–44. In this example, there is no direct extension from the main tumor mass *(left)* to an extracapsular large-sized, thick-walled vascular space *(right)*, which is invaded by the follicular carcinoma.

Pathology

Gross

- Fleshy, solid mass varying from 1 to 10 cm in diameter.
- Thick capsule.
- Extensive invasive growth.
- Yellow to red-pink, tan-brown, or orange.
- Central fibrosis may be seen, but irregular fibrosis and cyst formation are uncommon.
- Degenerative changes may be seen.

Histology

- Less of a diagnostic dilemma involving less subjectivity than minimally invasive follicular carcinoma.
- Clear-cut invasion beyond the capsular delimitation of the tumor with extension into adjacent thyroid parenchyma. Not infrequently, there is a mushroom-like protrusion of the tumor through and beyond its capsular delimitation.
- In addition, vascular space invasion, especially into the larger vascular spaces, is evident.
- These tumors also tend to have a greater percentage of solid or trabecular growth patterns, increased mitotic activity, nuclear hyperchromasia, and necrosis.

Differential Diagnosis

- Minimally invasive or low-grade follicular carcinoma (Chapter 8D, #1a).
- Papillary carcinoma (Chapter 8D, #2).
- Medullary carcinoma (Chapter 8E, #3).

Treatment and Prognosis

- Aggressive management is indicated, including total thyroidectomy and radioactive iodine therapy.
- Prognosis varies but is generally considered to be poor. These tumors tend to disseminate hematogenously, with metastasis occurring to osseous sites, lungs, and brain.
- Metastatic tumor is treated with radioactive iodine therapy, which may offer long-term palliation but not cure.
- Survival statistics rival those of poorly differentiated thyroid carcinomas, with 25% to 45% 10-year survival rates.

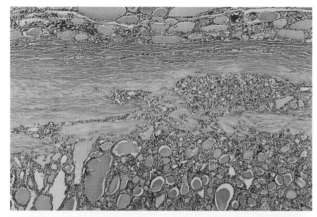

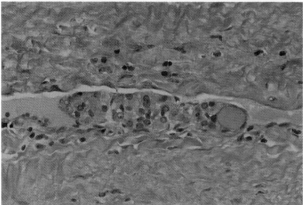

Figures 8–45 and 8–46. In this illustration, this follicular tumor shows capsular *(top)* and vascular *(bottom)* invasion. The extent of invasion was limited. The tumor is clearly invasive but did not invade beyond its capsule, and the vascular spaces involved were small. These features are those of a low-grade or minimally invasive follicular carcinoma.

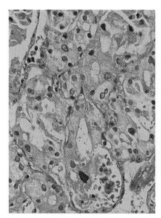

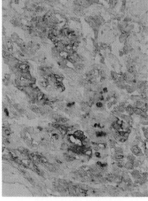

Figure 8–47. Several months following the diagnosis of the follicular carcinoma shown in Figures 8–45 and 8–46, the patient presented with bone pain. Radiographic studies showed multiple vertebral (osseous) lesions. Biopsy of one of these lesions is shown here. *Left,* Cellular tumor in which, focally, a microfollicular growth is seen. *Right,* The tumor is thyroglobulin positive, confirming metastasis from the "minimally invasive" or "low-grade" follicular carcinoma. This example is an exception to the rule because the great majority of low-grade follicular carcinomas have an excellent prognosis following surgical excision without recurrence or metastasis. However, this is an important example in that all follicular carcinomas, whether minimally or widely invasive, have the potential for aggressive behavior.

■ Adverse prognostic factors include:
  • Extensive intrathyroidal invasion.
  • Tumor size: Tumors greater than 6 cm have a worse prognosis.
  • Presence of distant metastasis.
  • Presence of local extraglandular spread.
  • Older age.

Additional Facts

■ Histologic variants of follicular carcinoma (both minimally and widely invasive) include:
  • Follicular carcinoma with oxyphilic (Hürthle) cells.
  • Follicular carcinoma with clear cells.
  • Hyalinizing trabecular carcinoma (Chapter 8C, #3).
■ Follicular carcinoma with oxyphilic cells (also known as Hürthle cell carcinoma) and clear cell carcinoma include tumors in which one of these cell types represents the dominant cell (defined roughly as 75% of the tumor).
■ These and all other variants of follicular carcinoma, except those that fulfill the criteria for poorly differentiated thyroid carcinomas, have the same diagnostic criteria, therapeutic interventions, and prognostic indicators as the more conventional types of follicular carcinoma.
■ The fact that these carcinomas have oncocytic (Hürthle) cells or clear cells does not alter any of the diagnostic, therapeutic, or prognostic parameters associated with follicular carcinoma. In other words, the cell type has little, if any, effect on treatment and prognosis; rather, the prognosis correlates with gender, age, extent of invasive growth, and presence or absence of metastasis.
■ The presence of oncocytic (Hürthle) cells does not in itself correlate with any one diagnosis, nor is it suggestive of a specific biologic behavior for that tumor; non-neoplastic and benign neoplasms of the thyroid may also have oncocytic (Hürthle) cells.
■ A follicular adenoma or carcinoma with clear cells must be differentiated from a metastatic renal cell carcinoma (see Table 8–7, page 94).

c. Follicular Carcinoma with Oxyphilic Cells

Synonym: Hürthle cell carcinoma.

■ More common in women than in men but less so than in follicular adenoma.
■ Tends to occur in patients approximately 10 years older than those with oxyphilic adenomas.
■ Clinical and radiographic features are similar to those typical of other follicular carcinomas.
■ Macroscopic appearance is similar to that of oxyphilic adenoma; however, in older patients these tumors tend to be larger.
■ Histologic features that may be different from oxyphilic adenomas include (1) thick capsule; (2) solid or trabecular growth; (3) increased nuclear-to-cytoplasmic ratio;

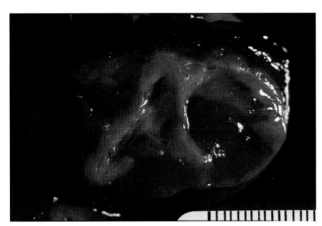

Figure 8–48. Follicular carcinoma with oxyphilic cells. This large thyroid tumor is characterized by an orange coloration due to the presence of cytoplasmic oxyphilia. Microscopically, there was invasive growth.

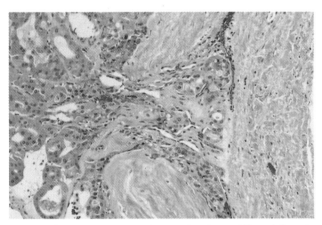

Figure 8–49. This thyroid tumor has cytoplasmic oxyphilia and shows invasion into its capsule. These combination of features are diagnostic for a follicular carcinoma with oxyphilia.

(4) characteristic uniformity of the nuclei with round nuclei and prominent central eosinophilic nucleoli; the cells in oxyphilic follicular adenoma may show pleomorphism and do not typically have prominent eosinophilic nucleoli; (5) presence of increased mitotic activity; and (6) presence of necrosis (individual cell or confluent areas). Regardless of the cytomorphologic features, the diagnosis of carcinoma is entirely predicated on the presence of invasive growth.
- As a general rule, the nuclei in follicular carcinomas are always smaller than those of papillary carcinomas.
- Differential diagnosis
  - Follicular adenoma with oxyphilia.
  - Oxyphilic medullary carcinoma.
  - Oncocytic tumor of parathyroid gland origin.
- Treatment, prognosis, and biologic course are the same as for conventional follicular carcinomas, although some authors believe that:
  - Total or near-total thyroidectomy should be performed for all oxyphilic follicular carcinomas regardless of whether they are minimally or widely invasive.

- Oxyphilic follicular carcinomas are more aggressive than follicular carcinomas without oxyphilia that are the same size and have the same extent of invasion.

2. Thyroid Papillary Carcinoma (TPC)
a. Usual or Conventional Type

Definition: Malignant epithelial tumor with evidence of follicular cell differentiation, typically with papillary or follicular structures (or both), and characteristic nuclear features. Numerous variations in the architectural patterns of papillary carcinoma can occur, but the nuclear changes (usually) remain constant.

Clinical

- TPC is the most common malignant thyroid neoplasm in countries with iodine-sufficient or iodine-excessive diets, comprising up to 80% of all thyroid malignant tumors.

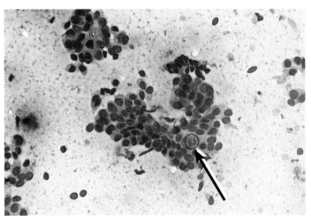

Figure 8–50. Fine needle aspiration, thyroid papillary carcinoma. An epithelial fragment in this fine needle aspirate of papillary carcinoma exhibits nuclear crowding and loss of polarity as well as an intranuclear cytoplasmic inclusion (arrow). Diff-Quik stain.

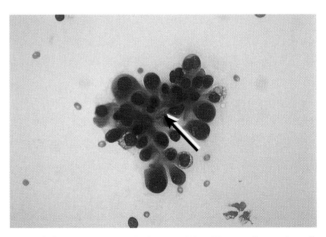

Figure 8–51. Fine needle aspiration, thyroid papillary carcinoma. A papillary fragment in this aspirate smear of papillary carcinoma contains a tiny vascular core (arrow). Nuclear enlargement is striking. Diff-Quik stain.

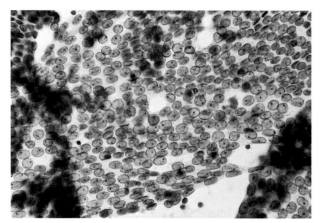

Figure 8–52. Fine needle aspiration, thyroid papillary carcinoma. The fine, evenly distributed chromatin with margination along the nuclear membrane gives the nuclei in this aspirate the clear, watery appearance that is the cytologic hallmark of papillary carcinoma. Papanicolaou's stain.

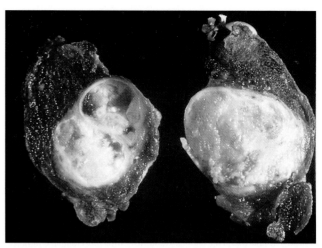

Figure 8–55. This thyroid papillary carcinoma is encapsulated, predominantly solid but focally cystic. In the cystic area, papillary growth can be seen. Prominent intratumoral fibrosis is present.

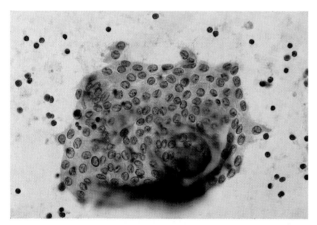

Figure 8–53. Fine needle aspiration, thyroid papillary carcinoma. A fragment of epithelium surrounds a refractile psammoma body in this aspirate smear of papillary carcinoma. The irregularities of nuclear contour ("grooves") are readily apparent. Papanicolaou's stain.

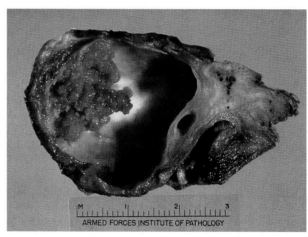

Figure 8–56. This thyroid papillary carcinoma is predominantly cystic with a portion showing papillary growth.

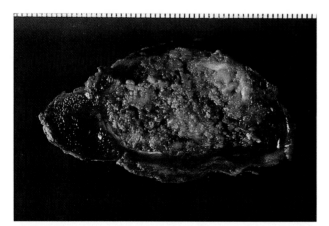

Figure 8–54. Thyroid papillary carcinomas demonstrate both macroscopic and microscopic diversity. This example of papillary carcinoma shows a predominantly solid tumor with obvious papillary growth. The tumor is only partially encapsulated, and toward its left upper outer area it loses its capsule and appears to be invasive.

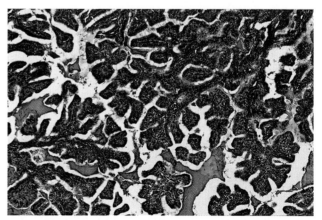

Figure 8–57. Papillary carcinoma showing the classic papillary growth pattern. The papillae are narrow with thin fibrovascular cores and show complexity in growth with arborization.

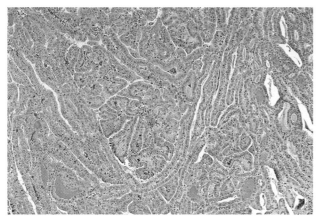

Figure 8–58. Another classic example of thyroid papillary carcinoma showing complexity in the papillary pattern, narrow and elongated follicles, and fibrovascular stroma.

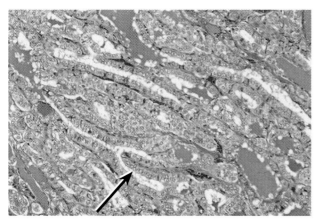

Figure 8–59. This example of papillary carcinoma shows elongated follicles, a feature that is not seen in follicular adenoma or carcinomas. An aborted papillary structure is seen toward the lower portion of the illustration *(arrow)*.

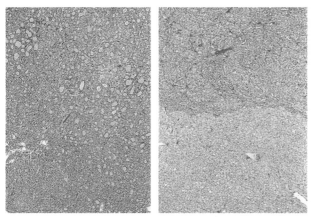

Figure 8–60. Although not diagnostic for papillary carcinoma, the presence of multiple different growth patterns in a single thyroid tumor should be highly suggestive of a diagnosis of papillary carcinoma. In this example of papillary carcinoma, a papillary growth was focally present *(not shown)*, but the dominant patterns included follicular *(left)* and solid and organoid patterns *(right)*.

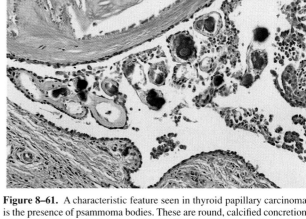

Figure 8–61. A characteristic feature seen in thyroid papillary carcinomas is the presence of psammoma bodies. These are round, calcified concretions with concentric lamination located in the tip of papillary stalk, in solid neoplastic component or in the stroma between neoplastic follicles. "Naked" psammoma bodies (unassociated with a cellular component) in the thyroid or in lymph nodes represent the presence of TPC.

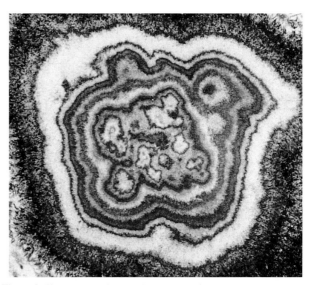

Figure 8–62. Electron microscopic depiction of a psammoma body shows the concentric layering of this calcified nidus of tumor.

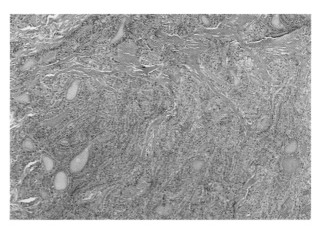

Figure 8–63. Inratumoral dense fibrosis arranged in an irregular pattern is a common feature of papillary carcinoma.

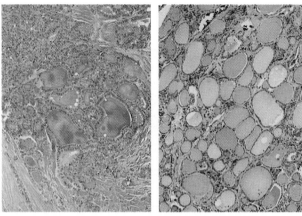

Figure 8–64. The colloid seen in papillary carcinoma *(left)* is thicker (more intensely eosinophilic) than the colloid seen in non-neoplastic thyroid follicles *(right)*. This is a weak criteria, but it may be helpful in the overall histologic picture in making a diagnosis of TPC.

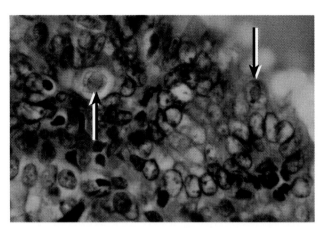

Figure 8–67. In addition to the optically clear-appearing nuclei, the presence of eosinophilic nuclear inclusions is another feature of papillary carcinoma *(arrows)*.

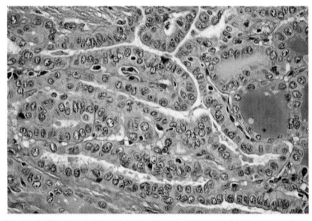

Figure 8–65. The architectural features are helpful in the diagnosis of papillary carcinoma, but the diagnosis ultimately hinges on the cytomorphology, specifically the nuclear details, including enlarged nuclei with irregularities in size and shape, dispersed to optically clear-appearing nuclear chromatin, nuclear crowding or overlapping with loss of the basal polarity of the nuclei, which appear randomly dispersed in all portions of the cell, and nuclear grooves.

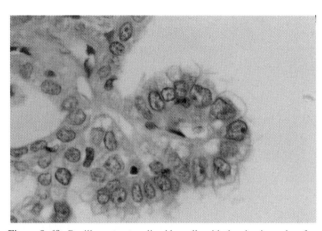

Figure 8–68. Papillary structure lined by cells with the classic nuclear features of papillary carcinoma, including enlarged, irregularly sized and shaped nuclei with optically clear nuclear chromatin and a distinct nuclear membrane. Prominent eosinophilic nucleoli are seen, some peripherally located touching the nuclear membrane and others more centrally located within the nucleus. Neither the nucleolar nor the cytoplasmic features are of much assistance in making a diagnosis of papillary carcinoma.

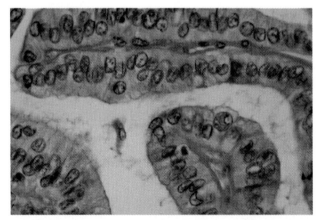

Figure 8–66. Classic nuclear features of papillary carcinoma including optically clear-appearing nuclei ("Orphan Annie" nuclei) with margination of the nuclear chromatin along the nuclear membrane. The latter appear distinct and sharply delineated. Convoluted, semilunar, and crenated-appearing nuclei are seen, as are nuclear grooves.

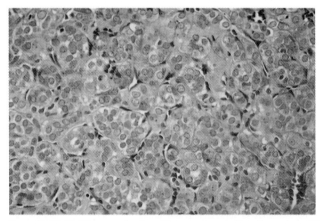

Figure 8–69. In this example of papillary carcinoma, there is an organoid growth and the nuclei appear more round and regular than in some of the previous examples. However, the nuclei are enlarged and show variations in size and shape, and the presence of a very fine and evenly dispersed nuclear chromatin ("powdery appearance") is diagnostic of papillary carcinoma.

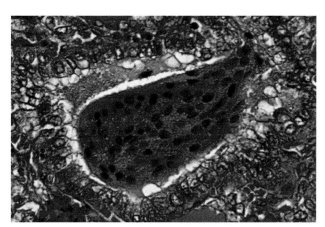

Figure 8–70. Thyroid papillary carcinoma in which there is an intrafollicular multinucleated giant cell.

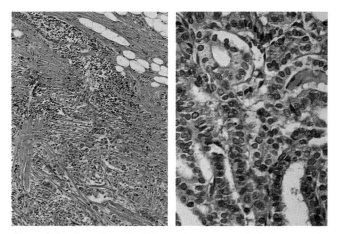

Figure 8–71. Regardless of cell type, adverse prognostic features associated with all types of papillary carcinoma include the presence of extrathyroidal invasion, as seen in this illustration. Note that the histology in this case is that of the usual or conventional type of papillary carcinoma, which, by virtue of its extrathyroidal invasion, will potentially have as adverse a prognosis as the so-called aggressive variants of TPC. In fact, encapsulated or minimally invasive "aggressive variants" of TPC, such as tall cell or columnar cell variants, probably share a relatively indolent biology with similar encapsulated or minimally invasive usual types of TPC.

- TPC tends to occur more frequently in women than in men; it occurs in all age groups, including children and adolescents but is most common in the 3rd to 5th decades. Papillary carcinoma is the most common thyroid malignant tumor in the prepubertal age group.
- Clinically apparent TPC presents as an asymptomatic, palpable thyroid mass or as enlargement of the regional lymph nodes.
- Any part of the thyroid gland can be affected.
- Etiology remains speculative and includes the following factors:

1. Iodine excess—in areas of endemic goiter, iodine added to the diet has been associated with an increase in the incidence of papillary carcinoma and a decrease in the incidence of follicular carcinoma.
2. External radiation—radiation exposure to the neck is a known etiologic factor for the development of thyroid cancer in general and papillary carcinoma in specific.

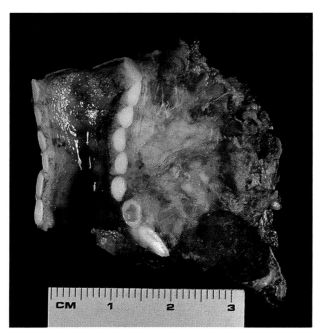

Figure 8–72. This usual or conventional type of papillary carcinoma invaded beyond the thyroid gland into the trachea, resulting in the death of the patient.

The cancer may arise in a relatively short period following the radiation exposure or decades later. Thyroid cancer risk following external radiation is highest when exposure occurs at a young age, decreases with increasing age at treatment, and increases with follow-up duration.

3. Genetic predisposition—papillary carcinoma may occur within families, suggesting the possibility that there may be a genetic susceptibility to the development of thyroid papillary carcinoma. Limited documentation has shown an association between papillary carcinoma and HLA-DR7 and between thyroid papillary carcinoma and colorectal diseases (including familial polyposis, Gardner's syndrome, and Cowden disease), as well as parathyroid disease (adenoma or hyperplasia), although this last "association" may occur in patients with external radiation exposure and not because of a genetic predisposition.
4. Pre-existing thyroid lesions—thyroid papillary carcinoma is more common in thyroid glands affected by chronic lymphocytic thyroiditis, although any direct correlation between these diseases has not been definitively proved. Similarly, thyroid papillary carcinoma may occur in patients with Graves' disease or in those with other thyroid lesions such as adenomatoid nodules, follicular adenoma, or follicular carcinoma. In the latter instances, the presence of thyroid papillary carcinoma is probably a chance occurrence rather than a representation of any specific association.

Radiology

- On thyroid scans (^{123}I), papillary carcinomas are most often "cold" or hypofunctioning nodules.

Pathology

Fine Needle Aspiration

NOTE: In contrast to follicular neoplasms (adenoma and carcinoma), the cytologic features of papillary carcinoma are diagnostic by FNA, making needle aspiration an excellent diagnostic tool for all variants of thyroid papillary carcinoma.

- Aspirates and smears are cellular; colloid is scant and may be absent.
- Cells may be arranged in papillary formations, monolayers, follicles, small or large cell clusters (syncytium-like formations), or are individually dispersed.
- The papillary formations may be sharply outlined with complex branching and a central vascular core.
- The component most diagnostic of papillary carcinoma is the nuclear features, which include:
  - Enlargement with irregularities in size and shape.
  - Powdery or dusty chromatin pattern (the nuclear clearing "Orphan Annie" patterns seen in histologic preparations are not found in cytologic preparations).
  - Intranuclear ("pseudo") inclusions (cytoplasmic invaginations).
  - Nuclear grooves.
  - Nuclear crowding or overlapping.
- The cytoplasm is usually abundant and includes a pale, vacuolated, or foamy appearance; the cytoplasmic features are not of much help in the diagnosis.
- Psammoma bodies can be seen and are helpful in the diagnosis of papillary carcinoma.
- Multinucleated cells are seen and sometimes are abundant.

Gross

- The majority of TPCs are solid with poor circumscription and/or apparent infiltration into the adjacent thyroid parenchyma, or they are extrathyroidal.
- TPCs may vary from solid to partly cystic or wholly cystic tumors. Cystic TPCs are usually encapsulated, filled with clear to yellow-brown fluid, and may demonstrate papillae. Fibrosis is a common finding in and around TPCs.
- TPCs may have a gritty consistency and may have extensive foci of calcification or ossification.

- TPCs can be divided by size into:
  - Small tumors: occult, minute, or microscopic, and less than 1.0 cm in diameter.
  - Intrathyroidal tumors: encapsulated, invasive, diffuse, cystic.
  - Extrathyroidal tumors: massive.

Histology

- The histologic diagnosis of TPC is based on both the architectural and cytomorphologic features (Table 8–8).

Architectural
Growth Patterns

- The classic example of a TPC includes papillary growth. The papillae are narrow with thin fibrovascular cores and show complexity in growth with arborization.
- TPCs may lack papillary growth and be entirely composed of a follicular growth pattern (see Chapter 8D, #2b for follicular variant of TPC).
- Other growth patterns in TPCs include solid, trabecular, follicular, macrofollicular, and cystic. These patterns may be seen singly or in combination in any given tumor.
- A diagnosis of TPC should be strongly considered in a single tumor that shows multiple growth patterns.
- Predominantly solid tumors are those in which solid elements make up nearly all of the neoplasm.
- The follicles in TPC are often elongated or twisted in appearance. This is an extremely valuable clue in papillary cancers that lack a papillary architecture. Elongated or twisted follicles are not seen in follicular adenomas or carcinomas.

Psammoma Bodies

- Psammoma bodies are round, calcified concretions with a concentric lamination; they are believed to be necrotic tumor cells that form the nidus for deposition of calcium salts.
- The name psammoma is derived from Greek and means "saltlike."
- Psammoma bodies are identified in up to 50% of TPCs.
- They are located in the tip of the papillary stalk but are also found in the solid neoplastic component or in the stroma between neoplastic follicles. **Psammoma bodies found in follicle lumina are not diagnostic and should be disregarded.**

Table 8–8
HISTOMORPHOLOGIC FEATURES OF PAPILLARY CARCINOMA

Architectural Features	Cytomorphologic Features
1. Growth patterns: papillary, follicular, solid, trabecular, organoid; multiple growth patterns can occur	1. Nuclear enlargement
2. Elongated or twisted follicles with little colloid	2. Nuclear irregularities in size and shape
3. Psammoma bodies	3. Dispersed to optically clear-appearing ("Orphan Annie") nuclear chromatin
4. Intratumoral irregular fibrosis	4. Margination of the chromatin along the nuclear membrane
5. Inspissated colloid (darker colloid compared to the surrounding thyroid)	5. Loss of nuclear basal polarity with haphazardly arrayed nuclei within the cell
6. Papillary protrusions into follicles	6. Crowded and overlapping nuclei
7. Squamous metaplasia	7. Eosinophilic nuclear (pseudo) inclusions
	8. Nuclear grooves
	9. When present, nucleoli tend to localize along the nuclear membrane
	10. Nondescript cytoplasmic changes

- "Naked" psammoma bodies indicate the presence of TPC, whether found in normal thyroid or in cervical lymph nodes.
- While not unequivocally diagnostic of papillary carcinoma, the presence of psammoma bodies is highly suspicious for the diagnosis of papillary carcinoma; rarely, calcific concretions are seen in association with benign thyroid diseases but, in contrast to true psammoma bodies, these concretions lack laminations and localize to follicle lumina.

Intratumoral Fibrosis
- Dense fibrosis is arranged in an irregular pattern and is a common feature of TPC.

Inspissated-Appearing Colloid
- The colloid seen in TPC is thicker (more intensely eosinophilic on hematoxylin and eosin stain than the colloid of adjacent non-neoplastic thyroid follicles. This is a weak criterion, but it may be helpful in the overall histologic picture in the diagnosis of TPC.

Cytomorphology (Nuclear Features)
- Cytomorphology is paramount in the diagnosis of TPC and remains constant regardless of the type of TPC found. Nuclear changes seen in TPC include the following:
  - Nuclear Enlargement:
    - As a general rule, the nuclei of papillary carcinomas are always larger than those of adenomatoid nodules and follicular tumors (adenomas, carcinomas).
    - Irregularities in size and shape are present; the nuclei may appear semilunar, crenated, or convoluted.

NOTE: The presence of cytoplasmic oxyphilia, as seen in numerous thyroid lesions, may induce nuclear enlargement, suggesting a diagnosis of TPC. However, other cytomorphologic features are required for the diagnosis of TPC.

  - Nuclear Chromatin:
    - Chromatin varies from very fine and evenly dispersed to optically clear (so-called "Orphan Annie eyes"). The nuclear chromatin typically marginates along the nuclear membrane, creating a fine but distinct nuclear membrane.
  - Nuclear Orientation:
    - Crowding or overlapping is present.
    - Basal polarity of the nuclei is lost; the nuclei appear randomly dispersed in all portions of the cell.
  - Nuclear Grooving:
    - Nuclear grooving is often used as an essential and diagnostic feature of TPC; however, although it is helpful in the diagnosis of TPC, **nuclear grooves are neither specific for nor diagnostic of TPC** but can be seen in non-neoplastic thyroid lesions and in other thyroid neoplasms as well, both benign and malignant.
  - Intranuclear Inclusions:
    - These appear as large, round eosinophilic inclusions and represent cytoplasmic invaginations into the nucleus.
    - Distortional changes in processing may result in intranuclear "bubbles" that simulate the appearance of the true intranuclear inclusions of TPC.

- Nucleoli:
  - When present, nucleoli are located along the nuclear membrane; however, this is a soft criterion and does not always hold true.
  - In comparison, the nucleoli (when present) in follicular adenomas and carcinomas tend to be centrally situated within the nucleus.
- Cytoplasmic Appearance:
  - There are no specific cytoplasmic changes that assist in diagnosing a papillary carcinoma.
  - Certain variants of papillary carcinoma are named according to their cytoplasmic appearance (e.g., oxyphilic cell TPC, clear cell TPC).
- Additional features associated with TPC include:
  - Lymphocytic infiltration.
  - Capsular or vascular invasion.
  - Multicentricity.
  - Pleomorphism, mitotic activity, and necrosis are generally not seen.

Differential Diagnosis

- Lesions that may have a papillary architecture, including adenomatoid nodules, Graves' disease, and dyshormonogenetic goiter (Chapters 7A, 6H, and 7B, respectively).

NOTE: Not all lesions with a papillary architecture are papillary carcinomas, and the absence of a papillary architecture does not exclude a diagnosis of TPC.

- Follicular adenoma, including the hyalinizing trabecular adenoma (Chapter 8C, #3).
- Follicular carcinoma (Chapter 8D, #1).
- Medullary carcinoma (Chapter 8E, #3).

NOTE: Differentiation from these tumors rests with the absence of the typical morphologic features associated with TPC or the absence of thyroglobulin immunoreactivity.

Treatment and Prognosis

- The standard treatment for TPC is surgery; however, the extent of surgery remains controversial and varies from lobectomy to subtotal thyroidectomy to total thyroidectomy. The standard approach in the past aimed toward aggressive management with total thyroidectomy and neck dissection. At present, there is no standard surgical method. Some surgeons advocate total thyroidectomy with postoperative radioactive iodine therapy; other surgical groups take a less radical approach by performing lobectomy with or without isthmusectomy or subtotal thyroidectomy followed by suppression of TSH secretion. This approach seems the most reasonable given the circumstances in which the tumor occurs—a low-risk patient population, localized to a single lobe, and not part of a histologic unfavorable category. Otherwise, more radical surgical intervention might be justified.
- In the absence of cervical lymph node enlargement, a (modified) neck dissection is not necessary. However, in the presence of apparent nodal involvement by tumor, a

modified lymph node dissection with preservation of the sternocleidomastoid muscle is performed.

■ Complications of thyroidectomy may include hypoparathyroidism and vocal cord paralysis.

■ TPCs tend to be biologically indolent and have an excellent prognosis (>90% survival at 20 years).

■ The rate of relapse after initial therapy is highest in the first decade and may be associated with increased mortality.

■ Metastatic spread occurs preferentially by way of lymphatic drainage and manifests as intrathyroidal or regional lymph node metastasis.

■ Distant (visceral) metastatic disease is unusual, occurring in 5% to 7% of cases; the lung is the most common visceral metastatic site (bone, liver, and brain metastasis may also occur).

■ Overall mortality rate for thyroid carcinoma is 0.2%.

■ **Adverse prognostic factors** include:

1. **Age and gender:** Mortality increases with age (patients <40 years generally do not die from TPC compared with patients >40 years); women fare better than men. *Low-risk group:* men 40 years of age or less; women 50 years of age or less. *High-risk group:* men over 40 years of age; women over 50 years of age.

2. **Tumor size:** Tumor recurrence and spread increase when the tumor is over 5 cm (best prognosis occurs with tumors 1.5 cm in diameter or less).

3. **Extrathyroidal extension:** The presence of extrathyroidal extension of tumor is one of the worst prognostic indicators in TPC of all histologic types.

4. **Histology** (type and differentiation): An adverse prognosis has been related to the cell type or growth pattern (e.g., columnar cell, tall cell, insular, and diffuse sclerosing variants), with some variants of TPC associated with a more aggressive clinical course and higher mortality rates. This association has not been definitively proven, but these histologic types of TPC may have an associated adverse prognostic feature (e.g., older age, male predilection, extrathyroidal extension) that better correlates with more aggressive behavior. The same cannot be said of poorly differentiated tumors (undifferentiated or anaplastic carcinoma), which, by virtue of their histologic features, are associated with a poor prognosis.

5. **Distant metastasis:** The site of the distant metastasis affects prognosis. Osseous metastasis is an ominous prognostic finding. However, pulmonary metastasis does not have as dire a prognosis as osseous or other distant metastatic disease but is associated with a moderately adverse outcome.

6. **Oncogene abnormalities:** The presence of point mutations such as an N-*ras* gene may be associated with a more aggressive TPC.

■ Factors associated with limited or questionable prognostic significance include:
• Vascular invasion.
• Tumor ploidy.
• Histologic patterns of growth, including solid or trabecular areas, number of papillae or psammoma bodies, and presence or absence of cervical lymph node metastasis.

Table 8–9
HISTOLOGIC TYPES OF THYROID PAPILLARY CARCINOMA

Occult, small, or microscopic
Encapsulated type
Follicular type
Macrofollicular type
Oncocytic or oxyphilic type
Clear cell type
Diffuse sclerosing type
Tall cell type
Columnar cell type
Poorly differentiated or anaplastic carcinoma

■ The effect of treatment (surgery, external radiation, radioactive iodine or chemotherapy) does not appear to be a significant predictor of survival in patients with TPC.

b. Types of "Conventional" Thyroid Papillary Carcinoma (Table 8–9)

NOTE: The demographic factors, including gender predilection and age range, and the clinical presentation (except for occult TPC), risk factors, treatment, prognosis, and prognostic factors are the same as those described for conventional TPC.

Occult, Small, or Microscopic
■ Defined as a papillary carcinoma measuring less than 1.0 cm in size.
■ Usually an incidental finding in a thyroid removed for other reasons; may present as an occult primary tumor with cervical lymph node metastasis.
■ Nonencapsulated or encapsulated; typical nuclear features of TPC are present, but increased sclerosis may be seen as well in and around the tumor.
■ May metastasize to regional lymph nodes.

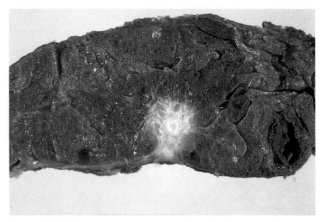

Figure 8–73. Gross appearance of an occult and sclerotic papillary carcinoma measuring less than 1.0 cm, discovered incidentally in a thyroid gland removed for other reasons.

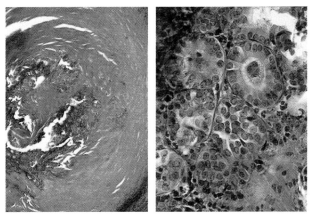

Figure 8–74. *Left,* Incidentally found (markedly) focus of encapsulated papillary carcinoma. *Right,* Details of the nuclear cytomorphology.

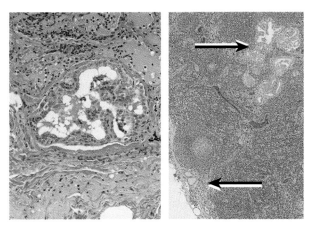

Figure 8–77. Microscopic thyroid papillary carcinoma *(left)* represented the primary focus for the metastatic carcinoma to cervical lymph nodes *(right)* seen in the subcapsular sinus and center of the lymph node *(arrows).*

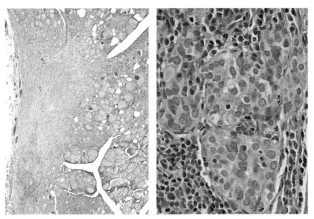

Figure 8–75. *Left,* Another incidentally found focus of papillary carcinoma with subcapsular localization; this is an example of a sclerotic, nonencapsulated microscopic papillary carcinoma. *Right,* Details of the nuclear cytomorphology.

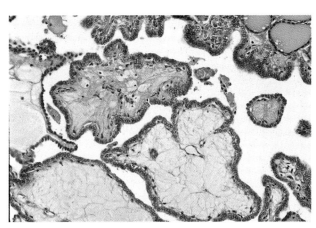

Figure 8–78. Papillary carcinoma with degenerative changes in which foamy macrophages appear within the papillae.

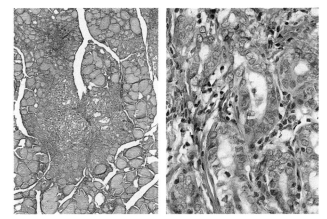

Figure 8–76. *Left,* Another incidentally found focus of microscopic papillary carcinoma with minimal sclerosis. *Right,* Details of the nuclear cytomorphology.

- Excellent prognosis; the presence of a microscopic focus of TPC is generally of limited, if any, biologic import.
- A diagnosis of microscopic TPC is not in itself an indication for additional surgical intervention.

Encapsulated Type
- Comprises approximately 10% of all TPCs.
- Well-defined capsule separates the neoplastic follicles from the adjacent thyroid parenchyma.
- Capsular invasion may be seen; despite this, these are still considered encapsulated tumors, and invasive growth does not alter the prognosis.
- Architecturally, this variant may be papillary, follicular, or cystic.
- Cytomorphologic features are typical of TPC.
- Treatment and prognosis are the same as those characteristic of conventional TPC.
- Cervical lymph node metastases may occur.
- Excellent prognosis.

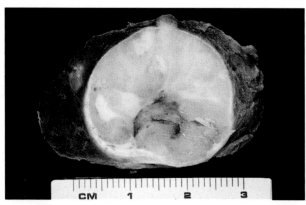

Figure 8–79. Encapsulated thyroid tumor that histologically showed features of papillary carcinoma (encapsulated papillary carcinoma). Toward the superior aspect of the film, the tumor invades into the capsule. The presence of capsular invasion in an encapsulated thyroid papillary carcinoma does not adversely alter the prognosis, nor should it warrant more aggressive forms of therapy.

Follicular Type
- Architectural features are predominantly composed of a follicular pattern of growth.
- Despite absence of papillary growth, other architectural features of TPC that can be seen include:
  - Elongated and/or twisted follicles.
  - Internal irregular fibrosis.
  - Presence of psammoma bodies in interfollicular stroma.
- If enough sections are taken, foci of papillary growth may be found.
- Diagnosis is primarily based on the cytomorphologic (nuclear) features, which are those of conventional TPC.
- Treatment and prognosis are those of conventional TPC.
- Biologic behavior is similar to that of conventional TPC.
  - May be completely encapsulated or invasive.
  - Cervical lymph node metastasis (often with papillary growth).
  - Treatment and long-term follow-up are similar to those of conventional TPC.

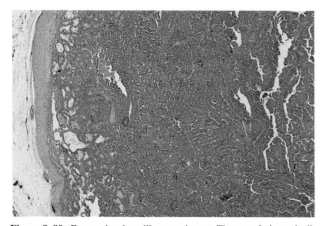

Figure 8–80. Encapsulated papillary carcinoma. The capsule is markedly thickened.

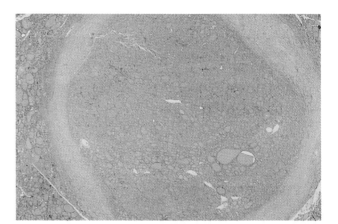

Figure 8–82. Thyroid papillary carcinoma. The tumor is encapsulated and is composed of a follicular growth pattern.

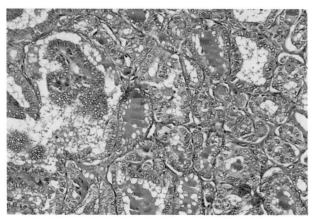

Figure 8–81. The architectural and cytomorphologic features of this encapsulated tumor are those of a papillary carcinoma, showing a predominantly follicular pattern and scattered papillae.

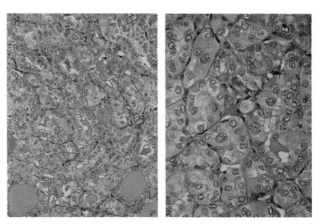

Figure 8–83. Thyroid papillary carcinoma. *Left,* The tumor is exclusively composed of a follicular growth, and some follicles have an elongated and twisted appearance. *Left and right,* The nuclei show characteristic features of papillary carcinoma.

Macrofollicular Type

- This variant is essentially the same as the follicular variant except that the neoplastic follicles are large (macrofollicles).
- This variant bears the most resemblance to adenomatoid or hyperplastic nodules, and, without evaluation of the cellular content, it may be misdiagnosed as such.
- A potential feature that may suggest the diagnosis is the presence of cellular foci in both central and peripheral locations.
- These cellular foci show the characteristic nuclear features of TPC (see Table 8–8).
- The presence of papillae is not required for a diagnosis, but abortive papillary structures can usually be found.
- Treatment and prognosis are the same as those of conventional TPC.

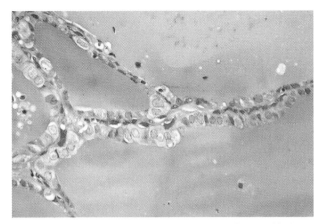

Figure 8–86. Portions of macrofollicles composed of cells with the nuclear features of papillary carcinoma.

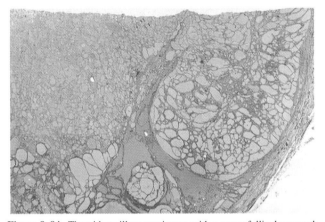

Figure 8–84. Thyroid papillary carcinoma with a macrofollicular growth pattern. At low magnification the tumor has the appearance of an adenomatoid nodule.

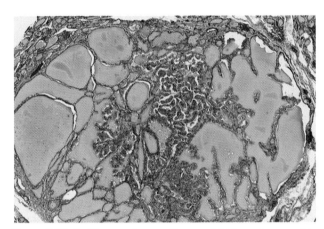

Figure 8–87. Papillary carcinoma with macrofollicles and areas of increased cellularity and papillary growth.

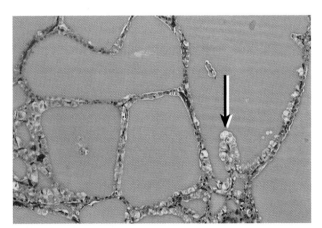

Figure 8–85. Macrofollicles lined by cells with the nuclear characteristics of papillary carcinoma. A papillary structure is seen toward the lower right of the illustration *(arrow)*. Some of the nuclei lining the follicles are flattened in appearance. These are the characteristic features for papillary carcinoma with a macrofollicular growth.

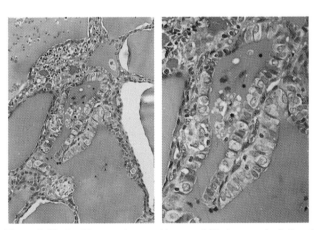

Figure 8–88. Papillary carcinoma with macrofollicular growth. *Left and right,* Areas of the tumor showing both architectural and cytomorphologic features diagnostic of papillary carcinoma.

Oxyphilic or Oncocytic Type

- Rare variant of papillary carcinoma.
- Tumors tend to be circumscribed or encapsulated, measuring from 0.5 to 6.0 cm in greatest dimension. Tumor consistency varies from soft to fleshy to firm, and color appears yellow to orange to brown; cystic changes can be seen.
- Architecturally, the tumors show a prominent papillary growth pattern with complex configurations and fibrovascular cores; focally, follicular, trabecular, and solid patterns of growth may also be seen. Psammoma bodies may be present.
- The characteristic cytomorphologic feature is the presence of cells with an abundant eosinophilic, finely to coarsely granular cytoplasm, representing increased cellular mitochondria. Focally, clear cytoplasmic changes may be seen.
- The nuclei are enlarged and irregular in size and shape. The nuclear chromatin is dispersed but not optically clear

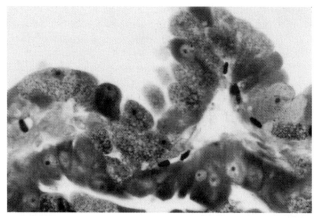

Figure 8–91. Novelli's stain for mitochondria shows the presence of dark purple granularity in the cytoplasm of the oxyphilic cells.

and is marginated along the nuclear membrane. Nuclear inclusions and grooves are present, and prominent eosinophilic nucleoli (one or two) may be seen.

- Although not seen in all cases, the nuclei have a tendency to localize at the apical portion ("tip") of the cell.
- The cells are enlarged but are not twice as tall as they are wide. A lymphocytic infiltrate may be focally present.
- *Histochemistry:* Stains for mitochondria are positive; Novelli's stain imparts a dark purple granularity to the cell.
- *Immunohistochemistry:* Cells react positively to thyroglobulin, cytokeratin, and vimentin.
- *Electron microscopy:* Increased mitochondrial content in the cells.
- Tumors may invade the adjacent thyroid parenchyma; extrathyroidal extension may occur but is uncommon.
- Treatment and prognosis are the same as those described for conventional TPC.

Clear Cell Variant

- See Chapter 8C, #5 (page 93) for a discussion of clear cell changes in thyroid lesions.
- Clear cell features may be associated with a number of thyroid tumors and are not limited to any one type.
- Clear cell features may be seen in limited areas of TPC or may comprise most or all of the neoplasm.

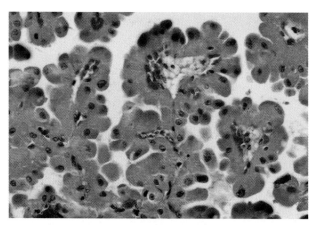

Figure 8–89. Papillary carcinoma with oxyphilia. Architecturally, these tumors tend to have a prominent papillary growth with complex configurations and fibrovascular cores. The characteristic cytomorphologic feature is the presence of cells with an abundant eosinophilic, finely to coarsely granular cytoplasm representing increased cellular mitochondria. The nuclei are enlarged and irregular in size and shape and have a tendency to localize at the apical ("tips") portion of the cell.

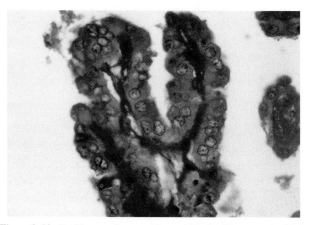

Figure 8–90. Papillary carcinoma with oxyphilia. Papillary growth with fibrovascular stroma, characteristic eosinophilic, granular cytoplasm and nuclei diagnostic of papillary carcinoma, including the tendency to localize at the apical ("tips") portion of the cell.

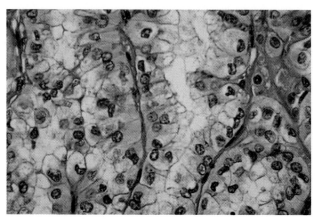

Figure 8–92. Papillary carcinoma with clear cells.

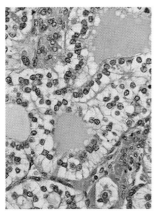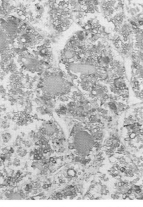

Figure 8–93. Papillary carcinoma with clear cells showing colloid-filled follicles *(left)* and thyroglobulin immunoreactivity *(right)*.

- Other than the distinct clear cell features, both architecture and nuclear morphology are the same as those of conventional TPCs.
- This variant may require immunohistochemical examination to prove that the tumors are of follicular cell origin (thyroglobulin positive) rather than thyroid C-cell origin (medullary carcinoma) and that they do not represent metastatic disease to the thyroid, particularly a renal cell carcinoma.
- Rarely, a metastatic TPC may occur to the kidney that simulates a primary renal cell carcinoma.
- Treatment and prognosis are the same as those described for conventional TPC.

Purported Biologically Aggressive Types of TPC
General Considerations
- Have a tendency to occur in older patients (except the diffuse sclerosing variant).
- Generally are large, measuring more than 5 cm.
- Often present with extrathyroidal extension.
- Tend to disseminate early in the disease course, leading to regional lymph node metastasis as well as distant metastasis, particularly to the lung.
- Are treated more aggressively than conventional types of TPC or less aggressive variants of TPC.
- Some of the tumors included within the category of aggressive types of TPC have been designated by a particular cell type (e.g., tall cell, columnar cell), whereas others have been designated by a growth pattern (e.g., insular). However, these tumors should not be included within the group of aggressive variants and treated accordingly simply on the basis of a particular cell type or growth pattern; rather, each tumor should be evaluated like any other papillary carcinoma, noting particularly the presence or absence of extrathyroidal extension. Given the tendency of these tumors as a group to be large, they may also show a tendency toward extrathyroidal extension. This finding, perhaps combined with some additional features of these tumors (e.g., older age at presentation), probably is much more significant than the individual cell type or growth pattern in predicting the aggressiveness of the tumor. The exception to this would be the poorly differentiated or

anaplastic thyroid carcinoma, which by definition is a high-grade, aggressive tumor.

Diffuse Sclerosing Type
Clinical

- Occurs more commonly in women than in men; tends to occur in younger age groups (childhood to mid-thirties).
- Clinical presentation is most often that of a bilateral goiter or diffuse enlargement of the thyroid gland rather than a single mass; however, some patients may present with a "dominant" nodule.
- Delay in diagnosis may be due to the similarity of the clinical presentation with that of chronic thyroiditis.
- Etiologic factors are unknown, although these tumors are associated with chronic lymphocytic thyroiditis.
- Serum antithyroid antibodies may be present.

Pathology

Gross
- Bilateral diffusely enlarged thyroid gland or a discrete dominant mass or nodule may be present.

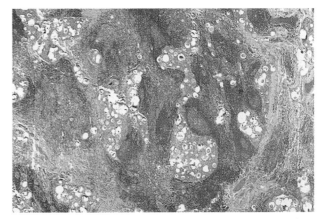

Figure 8–94. Diffuse sclerosing thyroid papillary carcinoma showing a diffuse growth pattern with associated lymphocytic thyroiditis. This tumor type has associated fibrosis and innumerable psammoma bodies.

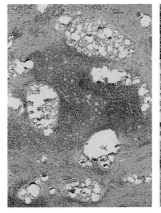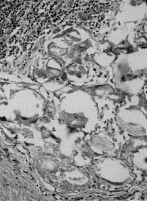

Figure 8–95. Diffuse sclerosing thyroid papillary carcinoma. *Left,* Characteristic diffuse growth pattern with lymphocytic thyroiditis, fibrosis, and psammoma bodies is seen. *Right,* The neoplastic cells have the typical nuclear features of conventional papillary carcinoma and are associated with classic psammoma bodies.

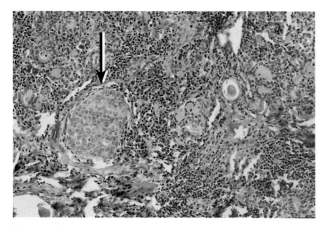

Figure 8–96. In this type of papillary carcinoma there is often extensive associated squamous metaplasia that may include squamous morules *(arrow)*.

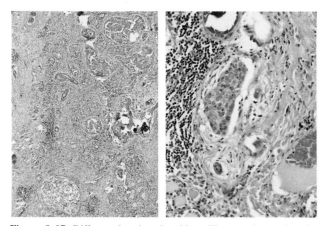

Figure 8–97. Diffuse sclerosing thyroid papillary carcinoma has the propensity to invade the intrathyroidal lymphatic spaces as seen here. Although not illustrated, this variant of papillary carcinoma tends to have extrathyroidal invasion.

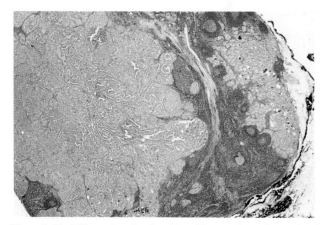

Figure 8–98. Diffuse sclerosing thyroid papillary carcinoma is associated with a high incidence of cervical lymph node metastasis as seen here.

- Regardless of the extent of involvement, the mass is firm, tan-white to gray in appearance, with ill-defined borders and marked fibrotic changes. An identifiable mass may measure up to 1 cm in greatest dimension.
- Due to the presence of innumerable psammoma bodies (see the following section on Histology), these tumors characteristically have a gritty consistency on cut section.

Histology

- This type of papillary carcinoma has a diffuse growth pattern with involvement of one lobe or the entire gland.
- The tumor may demonstrate a prominent papillary growth with solid areas; often, there is extensive associated squamous metaplasia, including squamous morules.
- The neoplastic cells have the typical nuclear features of conventional papillary carcinoma.
- There is pronounced fibrosis throughout the gland as well as innumerable psammoma bodies; the latter give the gland a gritty consistency on cut sections and create difficulties (artifactual distortions) in the processing of the tissue.
- The tumor has a propensity to invade the intrathyroidal lymphatic spaces as well as to show extrathyroidal invasion.
- A prominent lymphocytic infiltrate that may include germinal centers is associated with the tumor.
- *Immunohistochemistry:* The presence of S-100 protein-positive dendritic cells has been noted to have a possible correlation with a better prognosis.

Differential Diagnosis

- Chronic lymphocytic thyroiditis (Chapter 6A).
- Squamous metaplasia (Chapter 3B, #8a).

Treatment and Prognosis

- Total thyroidectomy or near-total thyroidectomy is the treatment of choice, often supplemented by radioactive iodine therapy.
- This variant of papillary carcinoma is associated with:
  - A high incidence of cervical lymph node metastasis.
  - A greater incidence of distant metastasis, in particular to the lung.
  - Shorter periods of disease-free survival.
- Despite the greater incidence of pulmonary metastases, the mortality rate for this tumor is low (possibly due to the ameliorating effects of younger age).

Tall Cell Type

Definition: A tall cell is defined as a cell that is twice as tall as it is wide. This is a vague definition; cells qualifying as "tall cells" can be seen in more conventional forms of papillary carcinoma. Although the tall cell type of papillary carcinoma has been described as a distinct tumor type, this remains a controversial issue. We are not sure it truly exists as a distinct clinicopathologic entity. The clinical and pathologic features ascribed to this tumor type are detailed in the following sections.

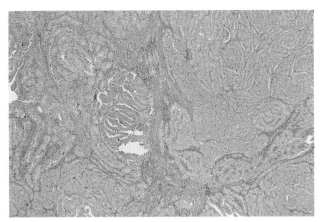

Figure 8–99. The tall cell type of papillary carcinoma represents a loosely defined entity. Among the features ascribed to this tumor is the presence of prominent papillarity, as well as a follicular growth pattern with elongated follicles; fibrosis is present and an associated lymphocytic cell infiltrate may or may not be present.

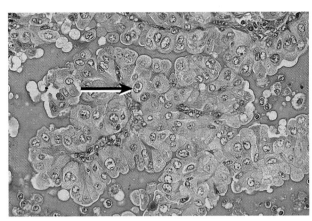

Figure 8–102. Tall cell type of papillary carcinoma with elongated and colloid-filled follicles. The cytologic features are those of the tall cell as detailed in the previous illustration, including the presence of eosinophilic intranuclear inclusions *(arrow)*.

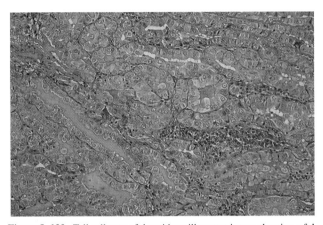

Figure 8–100. Tall cell type of thyroid papillary carcinoma showing a follicular growth with elongated follicles containing colloid, associated fibrosis, and a lymphocytic cell infiltrate.

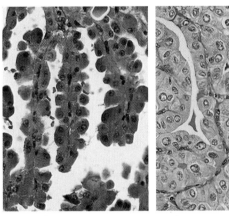

Figure 8–103. In comparing a papillary carcinoma with oxyphilia *(left)* with the so-called tall cell type of papillary carcinoma *(right)*, the cytoplasm in the oxyphilic papillary carcinoma is seen to be more intensely eosinophilic, the cells are enlarged but are not twice as tall as they are wide, and the cytoplasmic borders are not sharply demarcated.

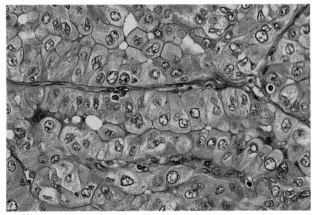

Figure 8–101. A "tall" cell is defined as being twice as tall as it is wide. In this example, there are follicles, but scanty colloid is present. The cell lining follicles are twice as tall as they are wide, but, depending on the section, some cells appear wider than they are tall. Other features seen in the so-called tall cell include nuclei situated in the center or basal portion of the cell, dispersed to optically clear-appearing nuclear chromatin, and a finely granular eosinophilic cytoplasm with sharp demarcation of the cytoplasmic borders.

Clinical

- Uncommon tumor.
- More common in women than men; generally occurs in older age groups (6th decade or later).
- The most common clinical presentation is that of an asymptomatic neck mass; other complaints include an enlarging neck mass.
- All portions of the thyroid gland may be involved.
- The tumors appear as "cold" nodules on thyroid scanning.
- The etiology is unknown; there is no known association with a pre-existing thyroid pathologic process.

Pathology

Fine Needle Aspiration

- Cytomorphologic features may include the presence of papillary fronds, oxyphilic cells with prominent nuclear grooves, and intranuclear cytoplasmic inclusions.

Gross

- These tumors tend to be large, measuring more than 5 cm in greatest dimension, and have extrathyroidal extension.

Histology

- A prominent papillary growth pattern is present; other growth patterns include follicular, cribriform, and solid patterns. Colloid-filled follicles are readily identifiable, and marked fibrosis is seen.
- Another pattern of growth includes markedly elongated follicles arranged in parallel lines ("railroad tracks") with minimal colloid content.
- The cells lining the follicles or papillae are twice as tall as they are wide (tall cells); in our experience, depending on the plane of sectioning, the cells may appear more wide than tall.
- The nuclei are situated in the center or, occasionally, basal portion of the cell and are normochromic or hyperchromatic with nuclear grooves and prominent eosinophilic intranuclear cytoplasmic pseudoinclusions (invaginations).
- The cells are also characterized by the presence of light to dark eosinophilic, finely granular cytoplasm. The cytoplasmic margins or borders are often readily seen sharply demarcating the cells.
- Mitotic figures may be present; psammoma bodies are usually not present.
- An associated lymphocytic infiltrate is often seen in and around the tumor as well as within the papillary cores.
- Extrathyroidal extension and vascular space invasion are seen.

Differential Diagnosis

- Columnar cell type of TPC (Chapter 8D, #2b).
- Oxyphilic type of TPC (Chapter 8D, #2b).

Treatment and Prognosis

- Total thyroidectomy or near-total thyroidectomy is the treatment of choice, often supplemented by radioactive iodine therapy.
- This type of papillary carcinoma is associated with the following:
  - High incidence of cervical lymph node metastasis.
  - High incidence of distant metastasis (lung and bone).
  - Tendency toward local recurrence in the neck, often with invasion into the trachea.
  - High mortality rate.

Additional Facts

- The tall cell variant of papillary carcinoma may behave aggressively. However, the aggressive behavior may correlate less with morphologic cell type (i.e., the tall cell) than with other factors. These other factors are those considered to be adverse prognostic features and include:
  - The tendency of these tumors to occur in older patients.
  - The tendency of these tumors to be large (>5 cm).
  - The tendency of these tumors to have extrathyroidal extension.

- Cells that may be twice as tall as they are wide can be identified in other types of papillary carcinomas (e.g., more conventional types, as well as the columnar cell type) without being classified as the tall cell type. The histologic features of the tall cell in this type of papillary carcinoma are detailed above. The cells in the columnar cell carcinoma are twice as tall as they are wide, but they have features that are not present in the tall cell type, and they do not have the other histologic features seen in the tall cell type of papillary carcinoma.
- There are no specific quantitative requirements for classifying a tumor as the tall cell type, but the majority of the tumor (>50%) should be composed of tall cells.
- Microscopic types of the tall cell papillary carcinoma exist that would have the biologic behavior of a conventional microscopic TPC; the existence of the microscopic type of tall cell TPC would refute the notion that the tall cell TPC is invariably an aggressive tumor.

Columnar Cell Type

Definition: Purported aggressive type of TPC characterized by cells having nuclear stratification.

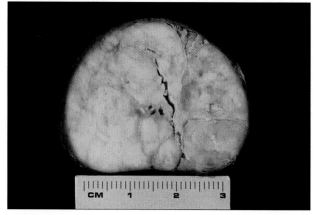

Figure 8–104. Columnar cell type of papillary carcinoma appearing as a large, solid, and encapsulated tumor.

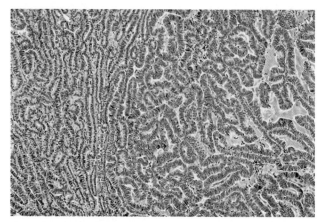

Figure 8–105. Columnar cell carcinoma is characterized by prominent papillary growth, markedly elongated follicles arranged in parallel ("railroad tracks") and minimal colloid content.

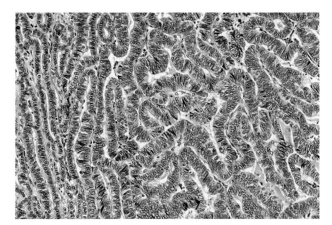

Figure 8–106. Columnar cell type of papillary carcinoma. The histologic hallmark is the columnar-appearing cells that have prominent nuclear stratification. Intensely hyperchromatic appearing cells, representing pyknotic nuclei, can be seen intermixed throughout the proliferation.

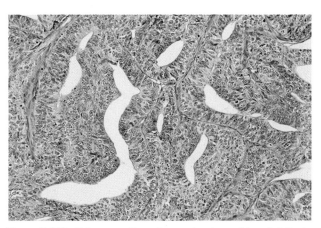

Figure 8–109. Columnar cell carcinoma showing solid and follicular growth patterns.

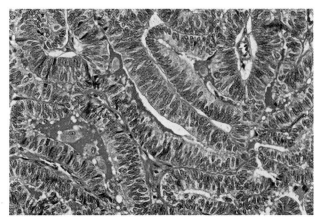

Figure 8–107. The nuclei in the columnar cell carcinoma tend to be elongated with coarse chromatin and are not particularly reminiscent of the nuclear features in conventional types of papillary carcinoma.

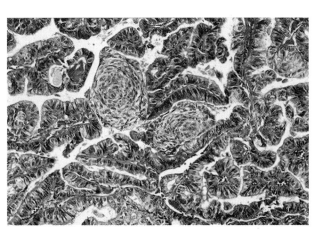

Figure 8–110. The columnar cell carcinoma may have associated squamoid foci as illustrated here.

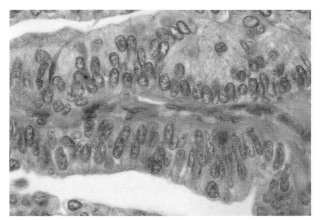

Figure 8–108. As seen here, in areas of any given columnar cell carcinoma, the nuclei may show features of a usual papillary carcinoma. When present, these nuclear features are limited in extent.

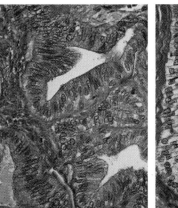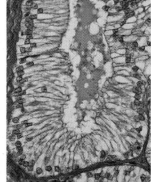

Figure 8–111. The cytoplasmic changes in the columnar cell carcinoma vary from a nondescript eosinophilic appearance *(left)* to a clear or vacuolated appearance with subnuclear vacuolization similar to that seen in secretory-type endometrium *(right)*.

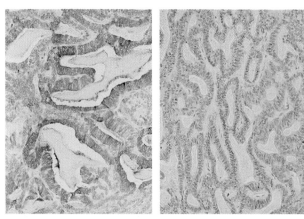

Figure 8–112. Thyroglobulin immunoreactivity in columnar cell carcinoma is quite variable from case to case and even within the same case. These illustrations are taken from the same tumor. *Left,* Portions of the tumor are thyroglobulin positive, whereas other portions of the tumor do not show any thyroglobulin reactivity.

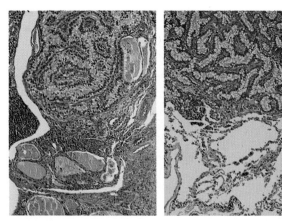

Figure 8–114. *Left,* Columnar cell carcinoma of the thyroid showing tumor cells with clear-appearing cytoplasm. The majority of this tumor showed typical features of columnar cell carcinoma, including nuclear stratification (not shown). In addition, at presentation, this tumor had extrathyroidal invasion (not shown). *Right,* The tumor metastasized to the lung 2 years following the resection of the thyroid tumor. The metastatic foci had the similar clear cytoplasmic changes as the primary tumor. The presence of extrathyroidal invasion, not the cell type, was the key prognostic factor in this case.

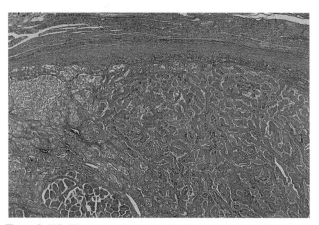

Figure 8–113. The prognosis associated with the columnar cell carcinoma correlates with the extent of invasion and not to the cell type. Those columnar cell carcinomas that are encapsulated (as shown here), are minimally invasive or whose invasive component is limited to the thyroid gland have a favorable prognosis correlating to similar staged conventional types of thyroid papillary carcinoma.

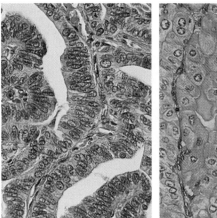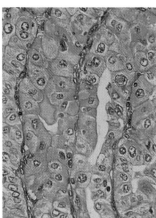

Figure 8–115. Both the columnar cell variant *(left)* and the tall cell variant *(right)* of papillary carcinoma have cells that are twice as tall as they are wide. However, this is the only similarity that these tumors "share." The cytomorphology of the two tumors is quite different and distinctive, as seen in this illustration.

Clinical

- Rare with only a limited number of published cases in the literature.
- Considered more common in men than in women; however, recent findings may suggest that this tumor follows the same gender predilection patterns as conventional TPC (i.e., female predominance). Occurs over a wide age range.
- The most common clinical presentation is that of an asymptomatic neck mass; other complaints include an enlarging neck mass.
- All portions of the thyroid gland may be involved.
- The tumors appear as cold nodules on thyroid scanning.
- The etiology is unknown; there is no known association with a pre-existing thyroid pathologic process.

Pathology

Gross

- These tumors may be large, measuring more than 5 cm, and may show invasive growth (intrathyroidal and extrathyroidal); however, they may also be small (<5 cm), encapsulated, and even microscopic.

Histology

- There is a prominent papillary growth pattern, but other growth patterns may be seen including follicular, cribriform, and solid. Colloid may be seen only focally and can be absent.
- Another pattern of growth includes markedly elongated follicles arranged in parallel lines (railroad tracks) with minimal colloid content.

■ The cells are twice as tall as they are wide (tall cells) but are columnar shaped and have prominent **nuclear stratification.**

■ The nuclei tend to be elongated and hyperchromatic; in focal areas of any given tumor, the nuclei may show the classic features of TPC.

■ The cytoplasmic changes may vary from a nondescript eosinophilic appearance to a clear or vacuolated appearance with subnuclear vacuolization similar to that seen in secretory-type endometrium.

■ Squamoid foci may be present.

■ Increased mitotic activity may be present; necrosis is generally not found.

■ These tumors may be completely encapsulated, show limited invasive growth (capsular or vascular), or have associated extrathyroidal invasion.

■ *Immunohistochemistry:* All tumors are thyroglobulin positive, but there is marked variability in thyroglobulin reactivity in any one case. Portions of the tumor may be intensely thyroglobulin reactive, whereas other areas, including those immediately next to the intensely positive foci, may be completely negative. Other stains that elicit positive reactions include cytokeratin and vimentin. There is no immunoreactivity with calcitonin or chromogranin.

Differential Diagnosis

■ Tall cell type of papillary carcinoma (see preceeding section).

■ Hyalinizing trabecular adenoma (Chapter 8C, #3).

■ Medullary carcinoma (Chapter 8E, #3).

Treatment and Prognosis

■ Treatment should include complete excision of the tumor. Depending on certain factors, excision can be conservative (lobectomy or subtotal thyroidectomy) or more aggressive (total thyroidectomy with postoperative radioiodine therapy).
  • For conservative management, the tumor should be confined to the thyroid with no evidence of extrathyroidal extension.
  • More aggressive management is indicated for tumors with extrathyroidal extension.

■ These tumors may metastasize to cervical lymph nodes. Distant metastasis, including metastasis to the lung and bone, may occur, particularly in cases with extrathyroidal extension.

■ The columnar cell type has been associated with high mortality rates, with death occurring within 4 years from the time of diagnosis. However, such cases involved large tumors with extrathyroidal extension. Tumors confined to the thyroid with no extrathyroidal invasion have a prognosis similar to that typical of more conventional TPC even in the presence of nodal metastatic disease.

Additional Facts

■ The histologic appearance of the metastatic foci may include columnar cells (tall cells with nuclear stratification), cells with the clear-appearing (secretory endometrium-like) cytoplasm, or cells with the classic features of TPC.

■ The aggressive behavior of the columnar cell type of papillary carcinoma (and, for that matter, the tall cell variant) may correlate less with the morphologic cell type (i.e., columnar or tall cell) and more closely with other factors. These other factors are those considered adverse prognostic features and include:
  • The tendency of these tumors to occur in older patients.
  • The tendency of these tumors to be large (>5 cm).
  • The tendency of these tumors to have extrathyroidal extension.

■ There are no specific quantitative requirements for classifying a tumor as the columnar cell type, but the majority of the tumor (>50%) should be composed of columnar cells.

Undifferentiated (Anaplastic) Carcinoma

Definition: Highly aggressive, poorly differentiated thyroid neoplasm with evidence (keratin immunoreactivity) of epithelial differentiation.

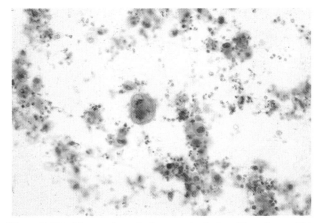

Figure 8–116. Fine needle aspiration, anaplastic thyroid carcinoma. This anaplastic thyroid carcinoma is characterized by pleomorphic cells with highly atypical nuclear features. The presence of necrotic debris in the background is a common finding. The chief differential diagnostic consideration is metastatic carcinoma. Papanicolaou's stain.

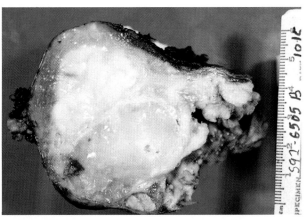

Figure 8–117. Anaplastic thyroid carcinoma appearing as a large, tan-white, firm tumor replaces most of the involved thyroid and shows invasive growth. The tumor presented as a rapidly enlarging neck mass.

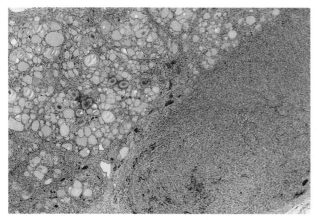

Figure 8–118. Anaplastic carcinoma. The tumor is unencapsulated, replacing the thyroid tissue. The tumor is solid, has a fascicular and storiform growth pattern, and is poorly differentiated without evidence of colloid formation.

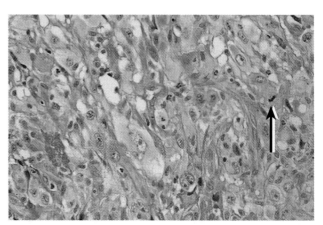

Figure 8–121. Anaplastic carcinoma. The tumor is predominantly composed of epithelioid cells consisting of large, round to oval nuclei with a vesicular chromatin pattern and prominent eosinophilic nucleoli. A mitotic figure is present *(arrow)*.

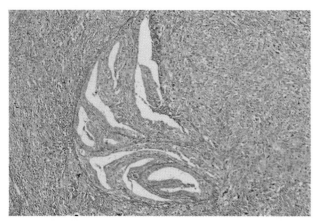

Figure 8–119. Anaplastic carcinoma. In this example, a remnant of a differentiated thyroid lesion (papillary carcinoma) is seen within the anaplastic neoplastic infiltrate. The latter is poorly differentiated and is composed of epithelioid and spindle-shaped cells without evidence of colloid formation.

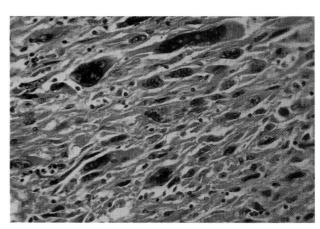

Figure 8–122. Anaplastic carcinoma. Scattered giant cells characterized by the presence of multiple nuclei with atypical cytologic features are seen.

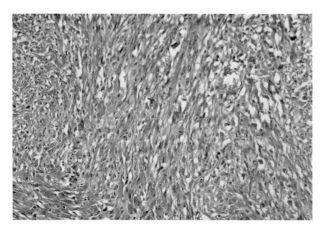

Figure 8–120. Anaplastic carcinoma. The tumor consists an undifferentiated malignant cellular infiltrate predominantly composed of spindle-shaped (sarcoma-like) cells with elongated, pleomorphic, and hyperchromatic nuclei.

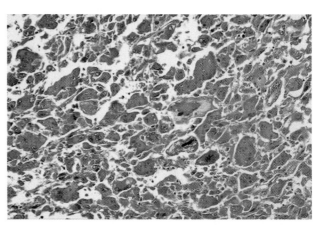

Figure 8–123. Anaplastic carcinoma. In this example, the giant cell proliferation represents the predominant neoplastic cellular component.

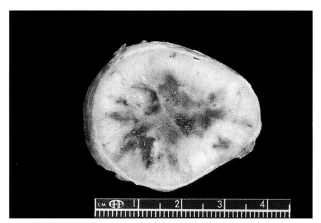

Figure 8–124. In rare examples, anaplastic carcinomas may present as an encapsulated tumor, as seen in this illustration. The central aspects of this solid mass show secondary degenerative changes, including hemorrhage, cyst formation, fibrosis, and necrosis.

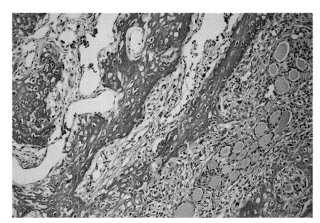

Figure 8–127. Anaplastic carcinoma. Heterologous bone is seen in association with sarcomatous foci. Residual non-neoplastic thyroid follicles are present.

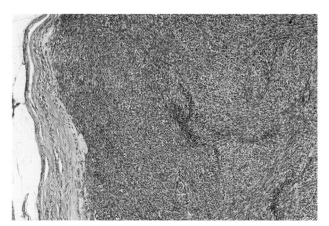

Figure 8–125. Anaplastic carcinoma. Microscopic depiction of the gross specimen shown in the previous illustration. The tumor is encapsulated and consists of a malignant spindle cell infiltrate with a fascicular and storiform growth. The encapsulation of an anaplastic carcinoma is uncommon. More typically, anaplastic carcinomas are widely invasive into and beyond the thyroid gland with extensive infiltration into the perithyroidal soft tissues (muscle, vessels, nerves), invasion into the larynx, trachea, and esophagus, and vascular space invasion with the development of tumor thrombi.

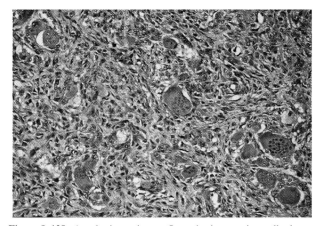

Figure 8–128. Anaplastic carcinoma. Osteoclastic-type giant cells characterized by numerous nuclei with limited atypical cytologic features and abundant eosinophilic to granular-appearing cytoplasm are seen admixed with a predominantly malignant spindle-shaped cellular infiltrate.

Synonyms: Sarcomatoid carcinoma; pleomorphic carcinoma; metaplastic carcinoma; spindle cell carcinoma; giant cell carcinoma.

Clinical

■ Uncommon thyroid malignant tumor.
■ More common in women than in men. Typically occurs in older patients (7th decade or older); rarely occurs in patients younger than 50 years of age.
■ Clinical presentation is that of a neck or thyroid mass that rapidly enlarges over a short period (weeks to months). The rapid thyroid enlargement may be seen in patients with a long-standing goiter or low-grade carcinoma (papillary or follicular). Rarely, anaplastic carcinomas may present with metastatic disease in the absence of an overt thyroid or neck mass. Often, the neck enlargement is associated with dyspnea, dysphagia, and hoarseness.

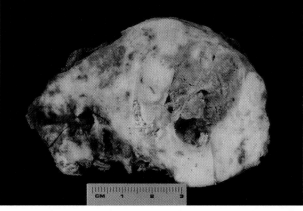

Figure 8–126. Anaplastic carcinoma. The tumor is large and solid and shows necrosis and cystic degenerative changes. Focally, there are tan-yellow, hard areas representing the presence of heterologous bone in this neoplasm.

■ These tumors are large, bulky masses that distort the appearance of the neck and may cause reddening of the overlying skin. The tumors are firm to hard and are fixed to the adjacent structures, including the skin. Cutaneous ulceration and necrosis may be seen, and the tumor may grow through the skin. Because of the tendency for these tumors to grow very large, cervical adenopathy may be difficult to appreciate.

■ Most patients are euthyroid, although uncommonly both thyroid hypofunction and hyperfunction may occur. Thyroid hyperfunction associated with an anaplastic carcinoma is believed to be due to destruction of the thyroid follicular epithelium with release of colloid and thyroid hormone into the circulation.

■ In a high percentage of cases, an anaplastic carcinoma develops in patients with a preexisting thyroid lesion. The majority of these lesions are follicular-derived tumors (follicular adenoma or carcinoma, papillary carcinoma), but patients may have a history of a long-standing goitrous thyroid. Despite the fact that anaplastic thyroid carcinoma occurs in the setting of antecedent thyroid disease, the probability of anaplastic transformation is considered low.

■ Anaplastic carcinomas are more frequent in areas of endemic goiter, but the prophylactic administration of iodine decreases the incidence.

■ Radiotherapy (external and radioactive iodine) has been implicated as a potential causative factor in the development of anaplastic carcinoma of the thyroid; however, the probability of this is so low that it should play no role in considering whether to use these modalities in treatment.

Radiology

■ Radioactive iodine scans show a hypofunctioning (cold) lesion; uptake in either the primary tumor or metastatic foci may represent remnants of the better differentiated component.

■ Computed tomography (CT) scans show a large irregular mass of low attenuation that may have cystic and necrotic areas.

■ Invasion into adjacent vital structures can be seen.

Pathology

Fine Needle Aspiration

■ Cellular aspirates with sheets, cell clusters, or isolated cells are present.

■ Large pleomorphic cells with bizarre hyperchromatic nuclei, prominent single or multiple nucleoli, and a variable amount of nondescript cytoplasm.

■ Spindle-shaped cells are commonly seen.

■ Mitoses and necrotic background are present.

Gross

■ These large and widely invasive tumors vary in appearance. They often are tan-white and firm to hard but may appear mottled and soft to rubbery owing to extensive hemorrhage and necrosis.

■ Rarely, the anaplastic foci may appear as small, firm to hard, solid areas in a nodule or differentiated neoplasm.

■ The remnant of the non-neoplastic thyroid gland may be limited in extent or absent owing to replacement by the anaplastic carcinoma.

■ Extrathyroidal invasion is commonly present.

Histology

■ The histology of these tumors varies considerably. Growth patterns include solid, fascicular, and storiform patterns. Admixtures of different growth patterns may be seen in any one case.

■ Cell types also vary and include the following types:
  • **Epithelioid:** Resembles the undifferentiated cell type of other sites (lung, nasopharynx) and is composed of large, round to oval nuclei with a vesicular chromatin pattern and prominent eosinophilic nucleoli. Squamous differentiation that includes keratin pearls may be focally present but does not make up the majority of the tumor. Epithelioid cell foci generally are devoid of giant cells but may be admixed with spindle-shaped (sarcomatous) foci. If present, areas of nested or cohesive growth pattern are most suggestive of an epithelial neoplasm.
  • **Spindle-shaped** (sarcoma-like): Elongated, pleomorphic, and hyperchromatic nuclei are characteristic.
  • **Giant cells:** Pleomorphic, round to oval cells characterized by bizarre-looking, often multiple nuclei and abundant eosinophilic to granular-appearing cytoplasm. The giant cell proliferation may represent the only neoplastic cellular component, or the giant cells may be admixed with spindle-shaped (sarcomatous) foci. **Osteoclastic-type giant cells** characterized by numerous nuclei with limited atypical cytologic features may be present in a small percentage of cases. Typically the osteoclastic-type giant cells are seen in or near hemorrhagic areas.

■ As noted previously, in any given tumor both mixed growth patterns and mixed cell types can be seen.

■ Regardless of the cell type, the neoplastic cellular infiltrate:
  • Is poorly differentiated and shows no evidence of colloid formation.
  • Is markedly pleomorphic and shows an increased nuclear:cytoplasmic ratio; prominent eosinophilic nucleoli may be present.
  • Has a high mitotic rate with numerous atypical forms.
  • Has associated foci of confluent necrosis and individual cell necrosis.

■ The stroma may show myxoid change or prominent collagen deposition; an associated inflammatory cell infiltrate including many neutrophils may be present.

■ Prominent vascularity is present that may have a pericytic ("staghorn") growth pattern or may resemble the appearance of an angiosarcoma (interconnecting vascular channels lined by neoplastic cells).

■ Heterologous elements, including bone and cartilage may be present. When present, these elements are usually associated with sarcomatous foci but may also be admixed with epithelial and giant cell infiltrates.

■ Invasive growth is present, including extensive intrathyroidal invasion as well as extrathyroidal infiltration; the latter includes extensive infiltration into the perithyroidal

soft tissues (muscle, vessels, nerves) and invasion into the larynx, trachea, and esophagus.
- Vascular space invasion (veins, arteries, and lymphatics) with replacement of endothelial cells and development of tumor thrombi is often present.
- Remnants of a preexisting thyroid follicular-derived lesion (adenomatoid nodule, follicular adenoma, follicular carcinoma, or papillary carcinoma) may or may not be present. The identification of this component may be a function of sampling.
- *Immunohistochemistry:*
  • Reactivity with epithelial markers, including cytokeratin (both high- and low-molecular-weight or mixtures of these keratins) and epithelial membrane antigen (EMA) is seen in all cellular components (epithelial, spindle-shaped, and giant cells); reactivity is variable and usually is limited to focal areas or scattered cells.
  • Vimentin reactivity is usually present in all cellular components but is most pronounced with spindle-shaped cells.
  • Thyroglobulin reactivity is extremely variable, usually absent, and generally is not helpful in the diagnosis of undifferentiated carcinoma.
  • Reactivity with chromogranin and calcitonin is negative.
- *Electron microscopy:* Evidence of epithelial (follicular cell) differentiation, including specialized cell junctions (desmosomes) or microvilli, may be present, but owing to the poorly differentiated nature of these tumors, these findings may not be identified.

Differential Diagnosis

- Malignant lymphoma (diffuse, predominantly large cell type) (Chapter 8F, #2).
- Angiosarcoma (malignant hemangioendothelioma) (Chapter 8G, #2c).
- Other sarcomas (primary and secondary involvement from a neck soft tissue tumor), including malignant fibrous histiocytoma, fibrosarcoma, high-grade malignant peripheral nerve sheath tumor, leiomyosarcoma.
- Medullary carcinoma (Chapter 8E, #3).

Treatment and Prognosis

- If possible, complete surgical excision is indicated. Unfortunately, these tumors tend to be so large and invasive that complete surgical excision is not possible, and debulking of the tumor is all that can be done. In a small number of patients, the tumor is confined to the thyroid or shows only limited invasion, and complete surgical excision can be performed.
- Postoperative external irradiation and chemotherapy are administered, but their efficacy is questionable at best.
- Radioactive iodine therapy has no role in the management of undifferentiated carcinoma.
- The combination of surgery, external irradiation, and chemotherapy offers the best chance of survival, but, even with this multimodal therapy, most patients die within a short period (6 months). Long-term survival may occur in patients in whom the tumor is confined to the thyroid or

shows limited invasive growth and who have undergone complete resection of the tumor with supplemental radiotherapy and chemotherapy.
- Metastatic disease occurs early (at presentation or soon thereafter); both lymphatic (regional and distant) and hematogenous spread occur. Common metastatic sites include the adrenal glands, lung, and gastrointestinal tract. The histology of the metastatic tumor resembles that of the primary neoplasm, and all of the cellular components of the primary tumor may appear in the metastatic foci (except for heterologous elements [bone and cartilage]).
- Extensive local and regional disease is commonly seen at or soon after presentation with extensive infiltration into the perithyroidal soft tissues (muscle, vessels, nerves) and invasion into the larynx, trachea, esophagus, and major blood vessels.

Additional Facts

- The nature of the osteoclastic giant cells remains uncertain. These may represent reactive cells of macrophage-histiocyte origin as evidenced by their ability to phagocytize inflammatory cells, their positive immunoreaction with macrophage (CD68 [KP1]) markers, their ultrastructural features, and the presence of high levels of acid phosphatase activity. More likely, these giant cells are neoplastic epithelial cells, an interpretation supported by the fact that they have been found in vascular spaces in and around the tumor as well as in metastatic foci.
- **Undifferentiated small cell carcinoma** has been considered a type of undifferentiated carcinoma. However, the existence of a true small cell carcinoma in the thyroid is questionable. These tumors may more likely represent a lymphoma or a variant of medullary carcinoma.
- **Insular carcinoma**
  • This tumor has been classified in the spectrum of high-grade, poorly differentiated thyroid carcinomas. However, insular growth patterns may be seen in non-neoplastic thyroid lesions (e.g., dyshormonogenetic goiter) and in differentiated thyroid tumors (usually

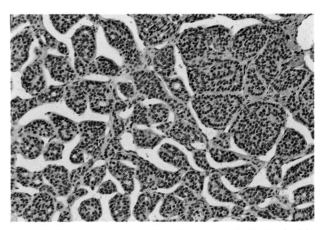

Figure 8–129. Thyroid tumor with an insular growth characterized by solid growth with microfollicles arranged in round to oval cell nests or islands (insulae). The presence of an insular growth is not indicative of malignancy. This follicular tumor was invasive (not shown), the feature that determines malignancy in this neoplasm.

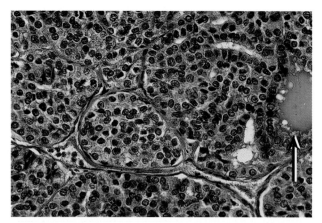

Figure 8–130. Thyroid tumor with an insular growth pattern. Higher magnification of Figure 8–129 showing the tumor composed of a monotonous population of small cells with round nuclei and indistinct cytoplasm. Colloid production is evident in a neoplastic follicle *(arrow)*.

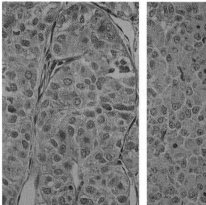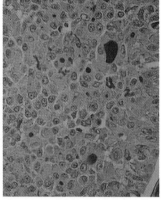

Figure 8–131. Follicular neoplasm with insular growth pattern. This was an invasive tumor and based on invasion, rather than its growth pattern (i.e., insular), represents a follicular carcinoma. *Left,* Follicle lumina containing colloid may be readily overlooked, appearing as eosinophilic material by conventional light microscopic stains. *Right,* Periodic acid–Schiff (PAS) stain enhances the appearance of the colloid. A thyroid tumor that produces colloid should not be considered as a poorly differentiated neoplasm.

papillary carcinoma but occasionally follicular carcinoma) that are entirely confined to the thyroid and completely amenable to conservative surgical resection. The presence of insular growth does not unequivocally qualify a given tumor as a poorly differentiated carcinoma.

- *Gross:* These are solid tumors often with associated necrosis. Most measure more than 5 cm in diameter.
- *Histology:*
  - Solid growth with microfollicles containing dense colloid arranged in round to oval cell nests or islands (insulae).
  - Monotonous population of small cells with round nuclei and indistinct cytoplasm.
  - Invasive growth, including infiltration (intrathyroidal and extrathyroidal); vascular spaces may or may not be present.
  - Necrosis and increased mitotic activity may occur but generally are not prominent.

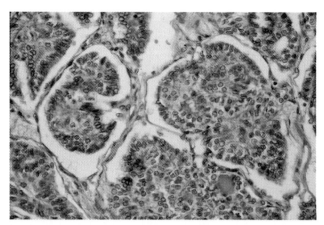

Figure 8–132. This thyroid papillary carcinoma shows areas of insular growth. The presence of an insular growth pattern in itself does not necessarily confer a higher grade or a more aggressive behavior on any given thyroid tumor. This thyroid papillary carcinoma with an insular growth pattern behaves no differently than a papillary carcinoma without insular growth. Prognostic features do not unequivocally correlate with patterns of growth (i.e., insular) or cell type (e.g., tall or columnar cell) but do correlate with features such as extrathyroidal extension of the tumor.

- *Immunohistochemistry:* Cells react positively with keratin and thyroglobulin and negatively with chromogranin and calcitonin.
- Treatment and prognosis depend on the usual parameters for thyroid carcinoma; aggressive management is not necessarily indicated simply because of the insular growth pattern.

3. Unusual Epithelial Tumors of the Thyroid Gland

a. Primary Thyroid Mucoepidermoid Carcinoma

Definition: Low-grade malignant thyroid tumor originating from follicular epithelial cells. The histologic appearance is similar to that of its low-grade salivary gland counterpart, including the presence of squamous or epidermoid cells and mucous cell differentiation.

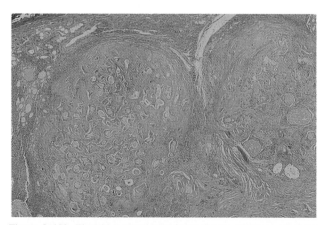

Figure 8–133. Thyroid mucoepidermoid carcinoma. The tumor is delineated but unencapsulated and is composed of solid and cystic foci with intratumoral fibrosis. Chronic lymphocytic thyroiditis is seen in the non-neoplastic thyroid tissue.

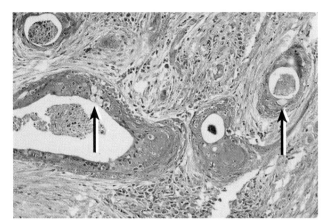

Figure 8–134. Thyroid mucoepidermoid carcinoma. The neoplastic proliferation includes squamous or epidermoid cells, within which are scattered mucocytes. The squamous or epidermoid cells show keratinization and intercellular bridges. Mucous cells (mucocytes) include cells with abundant clear to foamy appearing cytoplasm and peripherally located hyperchromatic nuclei *(arrows)*.

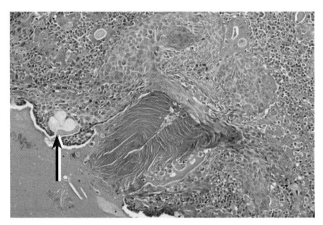

Figure 8–135. Thyroid mucoepidermoid carcinoma. In this example, the squamous or epidermoid component includes horny pearl formation as well as individual cell keratinization. Scattered mucocytes are seen intimately admixed with the epidermoid component *(arrow)*.

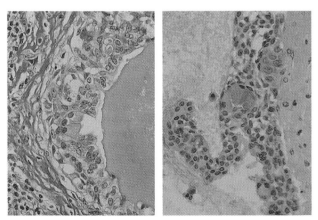

Figure 8–136. Thyroid mucoepidermoid carcinoma. *Left,* Typical hematoxylin and eosin stained sections. *Right,* Mucicarmine stains showing the intracytoplasmic and intraluminal mucin-positive (red) material.

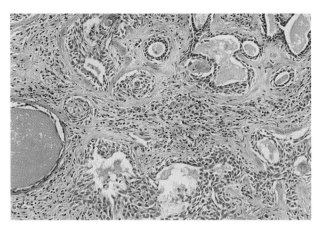

Figure 8–137. Thyroid sclerotic mucoepidermoid carcinoma with eosinophilia. Intratumoral sclerosis and eosinophils are seen intimately associated with the neoplastic cellular infiltrate.

Synonym: Sclerosing mucoepidermoid carcinoma with eosinophilia.

Clinical

- Uncommon thyroid malignant tumor.
- Affects women more than men; occurs over a wide age range (2nd to 8th decades) but appears most frequently in patients in the 5th to 7th decades.
- Most common presenting complaint is a painless neck mass; less commonly, pain, hoarseness, and vocal cord paralysis may occur.
- Any portion of the thyroid gland, including the isthmus may be affected.
- No known etiologic factors.

Radiology

- Hypoactive "cold" nodule on thyroid imaging.

Pathology

Gross

- Solitary mass measuring up to 3.5 cm in greatest dimension.
- Cut section shows a solid, nodular-looking tissue that varies from tan-brown to yellow-orange in color and has a rubbery to firm consistency. Cystic changes can be seen.

Histology

- Circumscribed but unencapsulated, predominantly solid mass; prominent cystic foci may be present.
- The neoplastic proliferation includes squamous or epidermoid cells admixed with mucocytes.
  - **Squamous or epidermoid cells:**
    - Round to oval cells with round nuclei, prominent centrally located nucleoli, and eosinophilic cytoplasm.
    - Horny pearl formation, individual cell keratinization, and intercellular bridges.
    - Mild nuclear pleomorphism, slight increase in the nucleus-to-cytoplasm ratio, and scattered mitotic figures.

- **Mucous cells:**
  - Cells with abundant clear to foamy appearing cytoplasm and peripherally located hyperchromatic nuclei.
  - Mucocytes intimately admixed with squamous or epidermoid cells.
- A mixed inflammatory cell infiltrate including mature lymphocytes and plasma cells is seen within the neoplastic proliferation. Eosinophils may predominate in any given tumor.
- Intratumoral sclerosis composed of thick, acellular hyalinized bands of tissue can be seen; it is not necessarily limited to cases with abundant eosinophils.
- Tumors are generally confined to the thyroid gland, but extrathyroidal extension may occur.
- Chronic lymphocytic thyroiditis is commonly present in the surrounding non-neoplastic thyroid gland and may include foci of squamous metaplasia.
- Separate foci of papillary carcinoma and adenomatoid nodules may be seen.
- *Histochemistry:* Intracytoplasmic and intraluminal mucin-positive material is seen with mucin stains (mucicarmine and PAS stain with diastase). The cystic spaces also show mucicarminophilic material.
- *Immunohistochemistry:* Cells react positively with cytokeratin, CAM 5.2, and thyroglobulin and negatively with calcitonin, chromogranin, and (monoclonal) carcinoembryonic antigen.

Differential Diagnosis

- Metastatic mucoepidermoid carcinoma of salivary gland origin.
- Primary thyroid squamous cell carcinoma (Chapter 8D, #3c).
- Papillary carcinoma with squamous metaplasia (Chapter 8D, #2a).
- Adenosquamous carcinoma—primary thyroid origin or (direct) invasion from a minor salivary gland mucoepidermoid carcinoma from the larynx or trachea (Chapter 8D, #3b).
- Lymphocytic thyroiditis with epithelial lined cysts (Chapter 6B).
- Medullary carcinoma with squamous differentiation (Chapter 8E, #3).
- Branchial cleft–derived cysts.

Treatment and Prognosis

- Surgery is the treatment of choice; conservative therapy (lobectomy or subtotal thyroidectomy) can be performed.
- Metastatic tumor to cervical lymph nodes and to the lung may occur.
- Extrathyroidal extension and metastatic disease, considered adverse biologic factors in other follicular epithelial-derived tumors, do not adversely affect the prognosis of thyroid mucoepidermoid carcinoma.
- This is an indolent tumor with an excellent prognosis.

Additional Facts

- Solid cell nests have been considered the progenitor of thyroid mucoepidermoid carcinomas, and there are some his-

tologic and histochemical features that suggest this possibility. However, the presence of keratinization, intercellular bridges, and thyroglobulin reactivity with absent calcitonin and chromogranin are more supportive of a follicular epithelial cell origin than of origin from solid cell nests.
- One likely origin of thyroid mucoepidermoid carcinoma is squamous metaplasia of follicular epithelial cells. Supporting this idea is the occurrence of thyroid mucoepidermoid carcinomas in patients with lymphocytic thyroiditis, which is also a common setting for squamous metaplasia.
- Rarely, other salivary gland-type tumors may occur in the thyroid gland such as benign mixed tumors.

b. Adenosquamous Carcinoma of the Thyroid

- Extraordinarily rare tumor of the thyroid gland.
- There are too few cases in the literature to suggest any correlation with low-grade mucoepidermoid carcinomas. Therefore, the spectrum of histologic types seen in the salivary glands (low-grade, intermediate-grade, and high-grade) is not seen in the thyroid.
- Histologically, these tumors include a squamous cell carcinoma with foci of mucin production. The neoplastic infiltrate is characterized by cells with obvious squamous differentiation (keratinization, intercellular bridges), pleomorphism, increased mitotic activity, and invasive growth. Because foci of undifferentiated carcinoma can occur, this tumor has been considered an anaplastic or undifferentiated carcinoma.
- Regardless of which category this tumor is assigned to, it behaves like a high-grade tumor and its behavior is similar to that of the thyroid anaplastic carcinoma. In this regard, this thyroid tumor is similar to adenosquamous carcinomas of the upper aerodigestive tract, which are high-grade malignant tumors originating from the surface epithelium.
- Treatment should be similar to that of anaplastic or undifferentiated thyroid carcinomas.
- In the presence of an adenosquamous carcinoma in the thyroid, a primary tumor originating in an adjacent organ (larynx or trachea) should be excluded.

c. Squamous Cell Carcinoma

- Extraordinarily rare primary thyroid follicular cell–derived tumor entirely composed of cells with squamous differentiation.
- No gender predilection; occurs in older people.
- The spectrum of histologic changes includes well, moderately, and poorly differentiated squamous cell carcinomas. In contrast with squamous metaplasia, squamous cell carcinomas show pleomorphism, an increased nuclear-to-cytoplasmic ratio, hyperchromatic nuclei, increased mitotic activity, and invasive growth.
- These tumors tend to arise in patients with long-standing thyroid disease, including goitrous thyroids and chronic lymphocytic thyroiditis.
- Squamous cell carcinomas of the thyroid probably originate from squamous metaplastic foci of follicular epithelial cells.

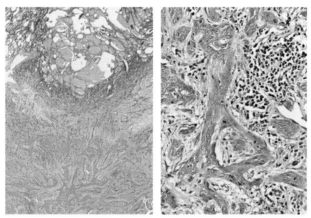

Figure 8–138. *Left,* Primary thyroid squamous cell carcinoma occurring in the setting of an adenomatoid nodule. The neoplasm is solid and invasive. *Right,* Well-differentiated squamous cell carcinoma with cellular pleomorphism and mitotic figures.

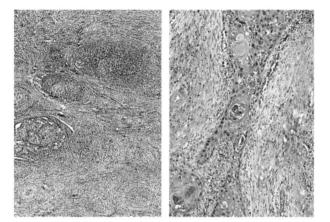

Figure 8–139. *Left,* Primary thyroid squamous cell carcinoma occurring in the setting of an chronic lymphocytic thyroiditis. *Right,* Well-differentiated keratinizing squamous cell carcinoma.

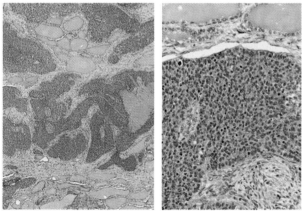

Figure 8–140. Primary thyroid squamous cell carcinoma. *Left,* The tumor is invasive and is composed of solid interconnecting cords; it is nonkeratinizing with areas of central necrosis. *Right,* Poorly differentiated nonkeratinizing squamous cell carcinoma. Numerous mitotic figures are seen. The tumor is reminiscent of transitional carcinomas occurring in other sites (e.g., urinary bladder, nasopharynx). In this example, the patient did not have a primary tumor in any other site.

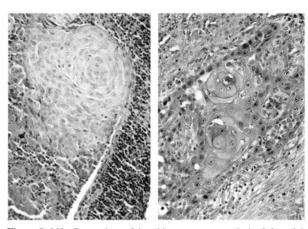

Figure 8–141. Comparison of thyroid squamous metaplasia *(left)* and thyroid well-differentiated squamous cell carcinoma *(right)* shows that the former is bland in appearance and is composed of rounded nests without invasive growth; it lacks significant cellular pleomorphism and/or mitotic activity. Foci of thyroid squamous carcinoma are invasive and are composed of a pleomorphic cell infiltrate with associated increased mitotic activity.

- These tumors have been classified with anaplastic thyroid carcinomas. However, the histology of these tumors is so readily recognizable that the tumor merits its own classification separate from the anaplastic carcinomas.
- Regardless of how this tumor is categorized, it behaves like a high-grade tumor, and its behavior is similar to that of thyroid anaplastic carcinomas. Treatment should be similar to that of anaplastic or undifferentiated thyroid carcinomas.
- In the presence of a squamous cell carcinoma of the thyroid, a primary tumor originating elsewhere should be excluded. Squamous carcinomas from a mucosal site may invade the thyroid directly or may metastasize to the thyroid.

E. C-CELL–RELATED LESIONS

1. Thyroid C Cells

Synonym: Parafollicular cell.

- Thyroid C cells originate from the neural crest via migration through the ultimobranchial apparatus.
- The ultimobranchial apparatus (or body) is so named because of its location in the terminal (ultimate) portions of branchial cleft (branchial cleft 5 or 6).
- The cellular derivatives of the ultimobranchial apparatus descend to the lateral lobes (middle and upper thirds) of the thyroid but do not migrate to more central (isthmic) aspects; therefore, C cells and lesions derived from C cells are not found in the central portion (isthmus) of the thyroid gland and usually not in the *extreme* upper or lower aspects of the lateral lobes.
- The main secretory product of C cells is the 32–amino acid peptide calcitonin; another C-cell peptide product is the 37–amino acid peptide calcitonin gene-related peptide (CGRP).
  - Calcitonin mRNA predominates in thyroid C cells.
  - CGRP mRNA predominates in extrathyroidal sites, including the brain, other neural tissues, gastrointestinal tract, lungs, urinary bladder, and thymus.

- Both calcitonin and CGRP are found in the serum of patients with thyroid medullary carcinoma in high quantities, but the levels of CGRP are much more variable and usually lower than the calcitonin levels.
- Calcitonin levels increase rapidly in response to pentagastrin stimulation, whereas CGRP response is more variable.
■ Calcitonin is the most potent endogenous inhibitor of osteoclastic bone resorption and acts on the kidneys to enhance the secretion of calcium. Calcitonin secretion is stimulated by elevated serum calcium and gastrin levels. The physiologic role of calcitonin in humans is unclear, and there is no evidence that decreased levels of calcitonin after thyroidectomy are detrimental.
■ CGRP is a potent peripheral vasodilator and may play a role in the cutaneous flushing seen in some patients with thyroid medullary carcinoma.
■ On light microscopy, C cells can be difficult to identify or distinguish from follicular epithelial cells. C cells are larger than follicular cells and have a polygonal to spindle shape with central, round to oval nuclei and pale granular to clear-appearing cytoplasm.
■ C cells are located adjacent to or within follicles (parafollicular); ultrastructurally, they lie between the follicular epithelial cell basement membrane and the follicular surface epithelium.
■ C cells are readily identifiable by immunohistochemistry and show intense reactivity with calcitonin and neuroendocrine markers such as chromogranin and synaptophysin. Cytokeratin (low-molecular-weight), neuron-specific enolase (NSE), and polyclonal carcinoembryonic antigen (CEA) are also reactive with C cells.
■ Intracytoplasmic membrane-bound neurosecretory granules are seen by electron microscopy.
■ Solid cell nests are remnants of the ultimobranchial apparatus that give rise to C cells and are incidentally found in thyroid glands removed for other reasons.
■ C-cell–derived thyroid lesions include C-cell hyperplasia and medullary carcinoma.

2. C-Cell Hyperplasia

Definition: Multifocal quantitative increase in thyroid C cells with replacement of thyroid follicles and follicular epithelial cells. C-cell hyperplasia may be more accurately considered a premalignant proliferation or the earliest phase in the evolution of thyroid medullary carcinoma rather than a non-neoplastic hyperplastic process.

Clinical

■ Uncommon lesion seen most often in association with other diseases, including:
- MEN syndromes.
- Hypercalcemia due to hyperparathyroidism.
- Hypercalcemia due to nonparathyroid causes.
- Hypergastrinemia (Zollinger-Ellison syndrome).
- Adjacent to nonmedullary thyroid neoplasms (follicular adenoma, follicular carcinoma, papillary carcinoma).
■ No specific demographic data are associated with C-cell hyperplasia except as it relates to thyroid medullary carci-

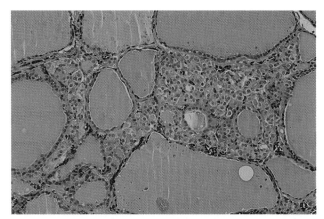

Figure 8–142. C-cell hyperplasia. A nodular interfollicular focus of C-cell hyperplasia is seen. Darker staining colloid-filled follicles are at the periphery *(left and right)* and bottom of the C-cell focus.

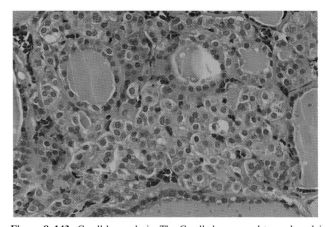

Figure 8–143. C-cell hyperplasia. The C cells have round to oval nuclei with stippled chromatin; mild nuclear pleomorphism with variability in nuclear size is seen. The C-cell proliferation is occurring adjacent to colloid-filled thyroid follicles (parafollicular).

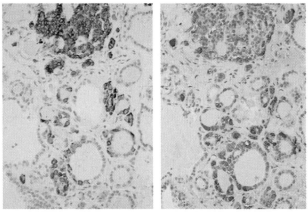

Figure 8–144. C-cell hyperplasia. Calcitonin *(left)* and chromogranin *(right)* reactivity is seen within the more solid area *(top)* as well as in individual C cells. The latter are seen intimately associated with the nonreactive follicular epithelial cells.

noma occurring sporadically or in association with the MEN syndrome.

- The presence of C-cell hyperplasia may or may not be associated with elevated serum calcium or calcitonin levels. In fact, most patients with C-cell hyperplasia do not have elevated basal levels of serum calcitonin but do have an abnormal increase in serum calcitonin following provocative testing with the secretagogues for calcitonin, calcium, and pentagastrin.
- Patients with elevated basal calcitonin levels whose values do not rise further following provocative testing should be retested after 3 months.
- C-cell hyperplastic foci may occur adjacent to some thyroid follicular neoplasms.

Pathology

Gross

- Generally, the lesion is nondescript with no demonstrable mass lesion or lesions.

Histology

NOTE: A fine line exists between C-cell hyperplastic lesions and small foci of medullary carcinoma; the former may be a preneoplastic process.

- The foci of C-cell hyperplasia may be nodular or diffuse.
- A focus should consist of at least 50 or more C cells within a single low-power field. However, recent evidence indicates that the number of C cells is of no importance for the diagnosis of C-cell hyperplasia; rather, the presence of mildly to moderately atypical C cells *that can be identified by light microscopy* is diagnostic of C-cell hyperplasia.
- The C cells are present in intrafollicular locations surrounding an identifiable follicle or completely replacing it.
- The C cells have round to oval nuclei with stippled chromatin; nuclear pleomorphism with variable nuclear size can be seen.
- *Immunohistochemistry:* Cells react positively with calcitonin and chromogranin; cytokeratin and CEA may be present. Reaction with thyroglobulin is negative (except when the C-cell hyperplasia has not completely obliterated the follicular epithelial cells, and thyroglobulin is seen within remnants of the follicular epithelium).

Differential Diagnosis

- Medullary carcinoma (see later).
- Solid cell nests (Chapter 3C, #3).
- Squamous metaplasia (Chapter 3A, #8).
- Intrathyroidal parathyroid tissue (Chapter 3C, #1).
- Intrathyroidal thymic tissue (Chapter 3C, #1).
- Palpation thyroiditis (Chapter 5B, #5).

Treatment and Prognosis

- A diagnosis of C-cell hyperplasia generally necessitates total thyroidectomy.
- The prognosis for patients with C-cell hyperplasia is excellent. Increased morbidity and mortality occur in pa-

tients with MEN syndromes due to nonthyroid neoplasms or medullary carcinoma but not as a result of C-cell hyperplasia.

Additional Facts

- Identification of C-cell hyperplasia in a thyroid that has been removed for other reasons should initiate serologic analysis for calcitonin abnormalities by provocative (calcium or pentagastrin) testing. The presence of calcitonin abnormalities following provocative testing indicates more widespread (multifocal and bilateral) involvement of the thyroid gland, prompting removal of the entire gland.
- Normal thyroid glands may contain foci of up to 50 C cells in a single low-power field, and nodules of C cells may be seen in the thyroids of older patients.

3. Thyroid Medullary Carcinoma (TMC)

Definition: Malignant neuroendocrine tumor of the thyroid gland showing C-cell differentiation.

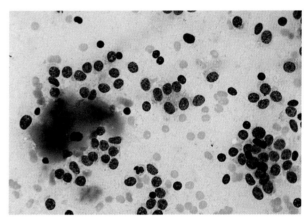

Figure 8–145. Fine needle aspiration, thyroid medullary carcinoma. A fragment of amyloid is found amid the tumor cells in this aspirate of medullary thyroid carcinoma. The cells have coarse chromatin and form loose groups rather than follicular or papillary structures. Diff-Quik stain.

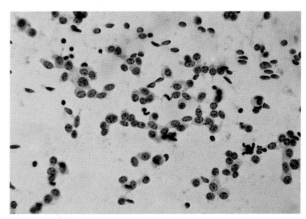

Figure 8–146. Fine needle aspiration, thyroid medullary carcinoma. The coarse "salt and pepper" chromatin typical of a neuroendocrine neoplasm is best seen in the Papanicolaou-stained smear of this medullary thyroid carcinoma.

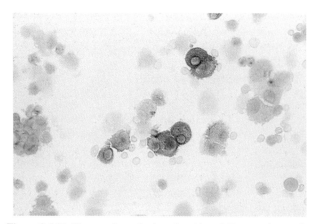

Figure 8–147. Fine needle aspiration, thyroid medullary carcinoma. Immunohistochemical staining for calcitonin confirms the diagnosis of medullary carcinoma in this fine needle aspirate of a thyroid nodule.

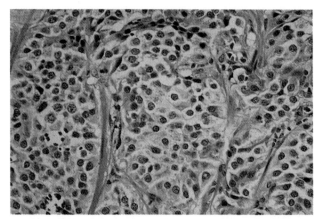

Figure 8–150. Thyroid medullary carcinoma. Classic appearance of the neoplastic infiltrate seen within the cell nest. These cytologic features include round to oval cells with round to oval and slightly pleomorphic nuclei that have a coarse or stippled chromatin pattern, and an ill-defined eosinophilic or amphophilic granular cytoplasm. Intranuclear pseudoinclusions can be seen.

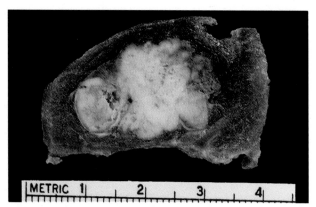

Figure 8–148. Thyroid medullary carcinoma. This tumor is solitary, well-delineated or circumscribed but not encapsulated; it has a tan-white and focally nodular appearance.

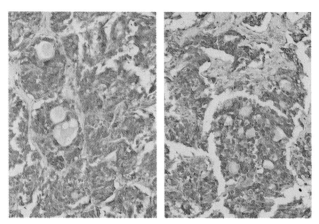

Figure 8–151. Thyroid medullary carcinoma. The neoplastic cells are calcitonin *(left)* and chromogranin *(right)* positive.

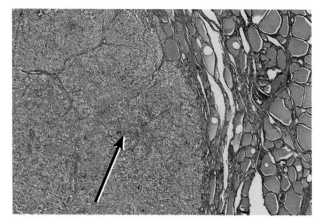

Figure 8–149. Thyroid medullary carcinoma. The tumor is circumscribed but unencapsulated, predominantly solid with small cell nests separated by a fibrovascular stroma; it is without evidence of colloid-filled follicles. Associated with the tumor is an irregular appearing amorphous and acellular homogeneous, eosinophilic deposition corresponding to amyloid *(arrow)*.

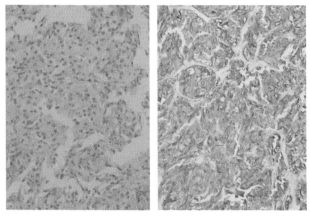

Figure 8–152. Thyroid medullary carcinoma. The neoplastic cells are thyroglobulin *(left)* negative and carcinoembryonic antigen (CEA) positive *(right)*. The presence of increased CEA reactivity and decreased calcitonin reactivity has been associated with more aggressive behavior.

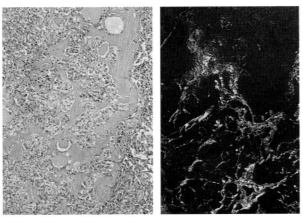

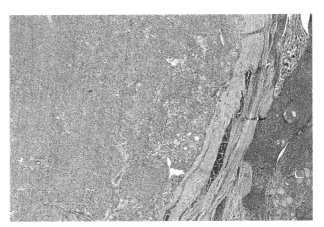

Figure 8–153. Thyroid medullar carcinoma with associated amyloid deposition appearing on hematoxylin and eosin–stained sections *(left)* as acellular, eosinophilic appearing material. *Right,* Special stains are helpful in determining the presence of amyloid, as seen in this Congo red–stained specimen, demonstrating the classic apple-green birefringence of the amyloid as seen under polarization.

Figure 8–156. Thyroid medullary carcinoma appearing as an encapsulated tumor predominantly composed of a spindle-shaped cellular proliferation.

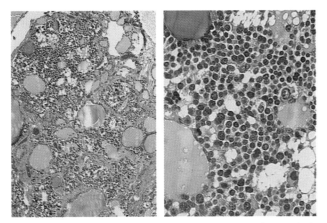

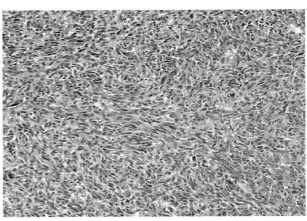

Figure 8–154. Thyroid medullary carcinoma. Incidental microscopic focus of medullary carcinoma was found in this thyroid gland removed for multiple adenomatoid nodules.

Figure 8–157. Thyroid medullary carcinoma. Portions of the previous illustration are shown here, showing a spindle-shaped cellular infiltrate with a fascicular to storiform growth and scattered mitotic figures. These features could be those of an anaplastic thyroid carcinoma or even a mesenchymal malignancy.

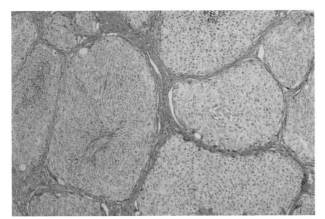

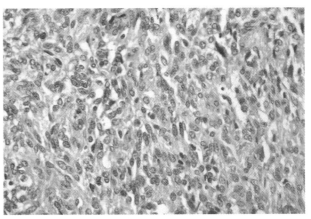

Figure 8–155. Thyroid medullary carcinoma may show histologic variability from case to case and even within the same case. In this example, the tumor is composed of large cell nests separated by fibrovascular stroma. Some of the nests have round to oval pleomorphic cells while others are dominated by spindle-shaped cells.

Figure 8–158. Higher magnification of the tumor shown in the previous two illustrations shows that the spindle-shaped and pleomorphic nuclei have a stippled chromatin, suggesting a C-cell–derived tumor.

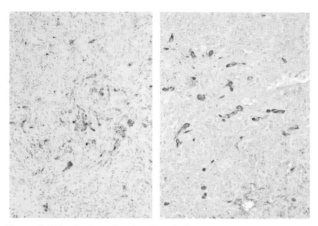

Figure 8–159. Confirmation that the spindle-shaped and pleomorphic tumor seen in the previous three illustrations is of C-cell derivation is done by immunohistochemical examination, showing the presence of chromogranin *(left)* and calcitonin *(right)* reactivity. In addition, cytokeratin and CEA were positive but thyroglobulin and mesenchymal markers were negative.

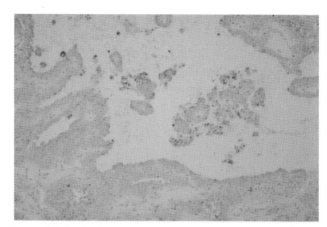

Figure 8–162. Confirmation that this thyroid tumor with a papillary growth is of C-cell derivation is made by immunohistochemistry. In this illustration, the tumor cells are calcitonin positive.

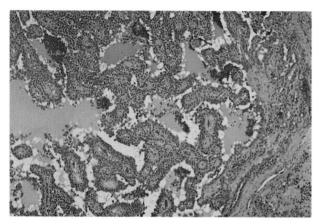

Figure 8–160. Thyroid medullary carcinoma with a papillary growth pattern.

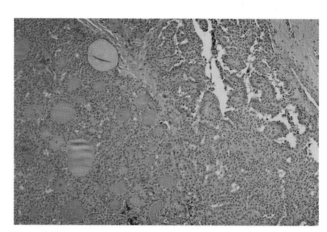

Figure 8–163. Thyroid medullary carcinoma with a focal papillary appearance *(upper right)* and a follicular or glandular growth pattern *(left).*

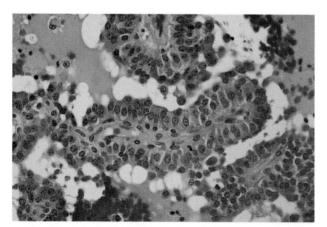

Figure 8–161. Higher magnification of the previous illustration showing a papillary frond with a fibrovascular core but lined by cells with the nuclear characteristics of medullary carcinoma.

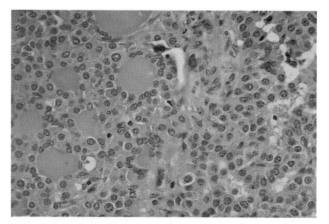

Figure 8–164. Higher magnification of the previous illustration shows the neoplastic cells to have characteristic features of medullary carcinoma despite the apparent follicular growth and colloid formation. Immunohistochemistry showed calcitonin and chromogranin reactivity *(not shown),* confirming C cell derivation. The colloid-looking material and surrounding cells were thyroglobulin negative. The colloid-looking material represents secretion by the C cells and will be calcitonin and chromogranin positive.

Synonyms: C-cell carcinoma; solid amyloidotic carcinoma.

Clinical

- TMC represents 5% to 10% of all thyroid neoplasms.
- TMC occurs in two forms (Table 8–10):
  - Sporadic or nonfamilial—unassociated with MEN syndrome.
  - Inherited or familial—associated with one of three clinical syndromes.
- Eighty percent of TMCs are sporadic; 20% are inherited.
- The genetic form of the disease should be suspected in all patients with a diagnosis of TMC until proved otherwise.
- **Sporadic TMC**
  - Is slightly more common in women than in men; occurs primarily in older individuals (compared with the familial form) who have a mean age at diagnosis in the 5th to 6th decades.
  - Presents clinically as a unilateral palpable thyroid mass; the incidence of cervical lymphadenopathy at presentation is high, but distant metastasis (lung, liver, bone) is uncommon.
  - Almost always produces elevated basal serum levels of calcitonin in patients with clinically evident disease.
- **Familial TMC**
  - The clinical presentation may correlate with the pathologic features in the other organs involved by the MEN syndrome (adrenal gland, parathyroid, pituitary gland, gastrointestinal tract, and pancreas).
  - In patients with MEN 2A (the most common of the familial TMC syndromes):
    - Is slightly more common in women than in men; mean age at diagnosis is in the 3rd decade.
    - Presents clinically as a slow growing, painless thyroid mass that may be multicentric and involves both thyroid lobes.
  - In patients with MEN 2B:
    - Is slightly more common in women than in men; mean age at diagnosis is in the 2nd decade. It is even seen in the neonatal period.
    - Presents clinically as a painless thyroid mass. In addition, these patients have mucosal neuromas (affecting the oral mucosa, lips, tongue, and eyelids), ganglioneuromatosis of the gastrointestinal tract, and skeletal deformities, including a Marfan's-like habitus, pes cavus). Because of the gastrointestinal ganglioneuromatosis, children with MEN 2B may present with a clinical picture that is identical to that of Hirschsprung's disease—rectal biopsy reveals proliferation rather than absence of ganglia.
  - Familial non-MEN TMC or TMC alone:
    - Is slightly more common in women than in men; mean age at diagnosis is in the 5th decade.
    - Presents clinically with a painless thyroid mass.
- Additional signs and symptoms seen in all patients with TMC may include severe watery diarrhea, flushing, renal stones, hypertension, Cushing's disease, or carcinoid syndrome. Many if not all of these associated signs and symptoms correlate with the other organ system lesions associated with MEN or with the elaboration of hormone secretion (other than calcitonin) by the TMC (e.g., adrenocorticotropic hormone [ACTH]).

Radiology

- Radionuclide imaging: hypofunctioning ("cold") nodule.
- *Ultrasonography:* solid mass.
- Imaging with iodine 131 metaiodobenzylguanidine (MIBG) is a useful tool in the diagnosis of thyroid medullary carcinoma.
  - MIBG ^{131}I is a guanethidine analog used in the detection of neoplasms of neural crest origin. Many neural crest–derived tumors (including TMC and pheochromocytoma) belong to the **dispersed neuroendocrine system (DNES),** formerly known as the **a**mine **p**recursor **u**ptake and **d**ecarboxylase (**APUD**) system, and sequester norepinephrine in intracellular granules.
  - MIBG is structurally similar to norepinephrine and competes with norepinephrine for uptake and storage in chromaffin granules in adrenergic cells.
  - The uptake of MIBG does not depend on the ability of a tumor to actively synthesize and secrete catecholamines.
- Plain films of the neck may reveal dense calcification, which is considered a feature of this tumor.

Table 8–10
THYROID MEDULLARY CARCINOMA

Features	Sporadic (Nonfamilial)	Familial (Inherited)
Percentage of cases	80%	20%
Inheritance	Noninherited	Autosomal dominant
Associated lesions	None	MEN 2A MEN 2B Familial non-MEN (TMC alone)
Genetic	No genetic abnormalities	The gene for MEN 2A (and the other forms of MEN) has been mapped to a locus near the centromere of chromosome 10
Gender, age (mean age at diagnosis)	Women more than men; fifth to sixth decades	MEN 2A: women > men; third decade and younger MEN 2B: women > men; second decade and younger Non-MEN: women > men; fifth decade
Treatment	Total thyroidectomy	Total thyroidectomy
Prognosis	Indolent course 5-year survival rates of 60% to 80% 10-year survival rates of 40% to 60%	In decreasing order of survival: non-MEN, MEN 2A, MEN 2B

Pathology

Fine Needle Aspiration

- Cytologic variability occurs from case to case, reflecting the histologic variability of TMC.
- There is increased cellularity with single cells or small cell clusters; follicular patterns, papillary structures, and colloid are not seen.
- The tumor cells vary and include round to oval, spindle-shaped, and polygonal cells with round to oval, pleomorphic nuclei, a stippled or coarse chromatin pattern, and an abundant eosinophilic cytoplasm. The nuclei may have intranuclear inclusions and may be eccentrically located, giving a plasmacytoid appearance to the cell.
- In air-dried smears, distinct metachromatic red cytoplasmic granules corresponding to neurosecretory granules can be seen. These granules are not seen in all cases or in all cells.
- Binucleate and multinucleate cells are seen.
- Extracellular homogeneous eosinophilic to pale orange, amorphous clumps, spheres, or rods are seen, corresponding to the presence of amyloid; Congo red staining can confirm the presence of amyloid.

Gross

- Sporadically occurring tumors are typically unilateral, solitary lesions; familial tumors are usually multifocal and bilateral.
- Size is variable. Some TMCs are barely visible, whereas others are large tumors occupying part or all of the affected lobe.
- The tumors may be encapsulated. Larger tumors are well delineated or circumscribed but not encapsulated. Some tumors have an infiltrative growth pattern.
- On sectioning, the tumors may be tan-white, yellow, gray, or pink in color and vary in consistency from soft to rubbery to firm. Hemorrhage and necrosis are not usually present, but calcifications may be seen.

Histology

NOTE: The histologic features of TMC vary considerably from case to case; however, regardless of the clinical setting in which it occurs, the histology of TMC is the same. Of note is the fact that in the familial forms of the disease, foci of C-cell hyperplasia are typically present either adjacent to the lesion or at a distance from it.

- The histologic variants of TMC are listed in Table 8–11.
- The tumors vary from encapsulated to circumscribed but unencapsulated to infiltrative. Extension of the tumor into adjacent thyroid parenchyma is often present. Colloid-filled follicles can be seen within the tumor but do not indicate dual C-cell and follicular differentiation; rather, they represent remnants of the follicular epithelium that are entrapped in the medullary carcinoma.
- The growth patterns of TMC include organoid, lobular, trabecular, solid, and insular or sheetlike; less often, TMC may exhibit papillary, follicular, or glandular growth patterns. Cell nests are separated by a fibrovascular stroma.
- Cytomorphologic variability includes round to oval to spindle-shaped to plasmacytoid cells with round to oval

Table 8–11

HISTOLOGIC VARIANTS OF THYROID MEDULLARY CARCINOMA

Classic or conventional type (organoid)
Spindle-shaped
Microscopic
Tubular (follicular)
Papillary
Small cell
Squamous
Oxyphilic (oncocytic)
Clear cell
Giant cell
Pigmented or melanotic
Encapsulated

nuclei and ill-defined eosinophilic or amphophilic granular cytoplasm.

- The nuclei may be pleomorphic and have a coarse or stippled chromatin pattern. Binucleate and multinucleate cells can be seen. The nucleus may be eccentrically situated, giving a plasmacytoid appearance to the cell, but a paranuclear clear zone or "hof" typical of plasma cells is not present. Intranuclear pseudoinclusions may be seen. Mitotic figures are seen but, in general, the mitotic rate is low.
- The cytoplasm is ill defined and most often eosinophilic to amphophilic and granular. Clear cell changes may be seen focally or may predominate in any given tumor.
- Invasive growth may be present, including extension into the adjacent thyroid parenchyma as well as vascular space invasion. Invasion into the perithyroidal soft tissue or into adjacent organs (larynx, trachea, esophagus) may occur, particularly with large tumors.
- Necrosis and hemorrhage are not characteristically present.
- Stromal amyloid can be seen in 25% or more of patients.
  - Amyloid appears as homogeneous, acellular eosinophilic bands or nodules.
  - Amyloid may be present focally, or it may be so diffuse that it almost completely replaces the tumor. In some cases there is no associated amyloid deposition.
  - Multinucleated giant cells may be associated with the amyloid, and amyloid can be seen within the cytoplasm of the multinucleated giant cells.
  - Special histochemical stains for amyloid include Congo red, which imparts an apple-green birefringence in polarized light, and crystal violet, which imparts a metachromatic appearance.
- *Immunohistochemistry:* Positive reactivity with amyloid a (AA) antibody.
- *Histochemistry:* Tumor cells are argyrophilic (Grimelius' stain) but less often are argentaffinic (Fontana-Masson stain). Intracellular and extracellular PAS, Alcian blue, and mucicarmine positive staining can be seen. Rarely, melanin pigment may be found by argentaffin (Fontana-Masson) stains.
- *Immunohistochemistry:* Calcitonin, CGRP, chromogranin, synaptophysin, NSE, cytokeratin, and CEA staining is present, but thyroglobulin staining is negative. Additional peptides that can be seen in TMC include somatostatin, ACTH, bombesin, leu-enkephalin, sero-

tonin, glucagon, gastrin, vasoactive intestinal peptide (VIP), substance P, human chorionic gonadotropin, and others, including reports of insulin reactivity.

■ *Electron microscopy:* Membrane-bound neurosecretory granules are a characteristic ultrastructural feature of TMC and have been shown to contain calcitonin. These granules have been divided into larger (type I) and smaller (type II) granules, measuring on average 280 nm and 130 nm in diameter, respectively.

Differential Diagnosis

■ Hyalinizing trabecular adenoma or carcinoma (Chapter 8C, #3).
■ Follicular carcinoma (Chapter 8D, #1).
■ Papillary carcinoma (Chapter 8D, #2).
■ Paraganglioma (Chapter 8G, #1).
■ Amyloid goiter (Chapter 7C).
■ Malignant lymphoma (Chapter 8F, #2).

Treatment and Prognosis

■ Surgery, including total thyroidectomy, is the treatment of choice for all forms of TMC.
■ Metastases to the regional lymph nodes from TMC occurs early in the course of the disease, and prophylactic central lymph node dissection is indicated as part of the initial therapeutic management. Central lymph node dissection includes nodes from the hyoid bone to the innominate vein.
■ Patients with palpable thyroid tumors often have metastases to the lateral cervical lymph nodes; however, modified or radical neck dissection is reserved for patients with jugular node metastasis (sampled intraoperatively) or disease that invades the jugular veins or sternocleidomastoid muscles.
■ During surgery, the parathyroid glands should be identified and, if enlarged, excised.
■ Metastatic tumors occur to the regional lymph nodes; less frequently, distant metastasis occurs to the liver, lungs, bone, or adrenal glands.
■ Postoperative management includes monitoring of serum calcitonin and CEA levels.
   • Stable CEA levels with or without changes in calcitonin levels suggest stable or slowly progressive disease.
   • Rapidly rising CEA levels with stable or falling calcitonin levels suggest the emergence of a more aggressive tumor.
   • Rapidly rising CEA and calcitonin levels suggest the emergence of a more aggressive tumor.
■ *Prognosis:* The most important prognostic factor is the clinical stage.
   • Tumors confined to the thyroid without evidence of metastatic disease have an excellent prognosis, with an almost 100% cure rate following surgery.
   • Patients whose thyroid lesion or tumor is discovered in the screening process for familial disease usually have C-cell hyperplasia or small neoplastic foci and have an excellent prognosis following surgery.
   • Patients whose tumors have not been totally excised, who have distant metastasis, or who have elevated postoperative calcitonin or CEA levels have a less favorable

prognosis, but even in this group there is variability in outcome. Some patients survive for long periods, whereas others succumb to the disease in a relatively short period.
   • Survival rates: 5 years, 60% to 80%; 10 years, 40% to 60%.
   • Other factors affecting prognosis:
      • The survival patterns of TMC are (in decreasing order of survival [best to worst]): (1) familial non-MEN related; (2) sporadically occurring or associated with MEN 2A; and (3) associated with MEN 2B (MEN 2B–associated TMCs are aggressive tumors marked by early dissemination).
      • The earlier the detection (smaller tumor, lower stage), the better the survival.
      • Patients who are younger than 40 years of age have a better prognosis.
      • Women have a better prognosis than men.
      • Calcitonin-rich tumors (>75% of cells) have a better prognosis than calcitonin-poor tumors (<25% of cells), with 5-year survival rates of 100% and 50%, respectively. However, these survival statistics do not necessarily apply for longer periods (beyond the 5-year range).
      • More aggressive behavior may be associated with persistently elevated CEA levels associated with decreasing calcitonin levels both in serum and tissue.
      • Pathologic factors other than calcitonin and CEA immunoreactivity that may correlate with prognosis include the following:

      1. Tumor size—the smaller the tumor the better the prognosis.
      2. Encapsulation—encapsulated tumors have a more favorable prognosis.
      3. Invasion beyond the thyroid gland—the higher the stage, the worse the prognosis.
      4. Amyloid content—the higher the amyloid content, the better the prognosis, a fact that is further enhanced by the presence of calcification.
      5. Pleomorphism, mitotic activity, and necrosis—the greater these features, the worse the prognosis.
      6. CD15 (Leu M1) immunoreactivity—little or absent Leu M1 reactivity (defined as <15% positive tumor cells) may be associated with a better prognosis than more diffuse reactivity (defined as >15% positive tumor cells).

■ Radioactive iodine therapy plays no role in the management of TMC. The neoplastic cells do not take up iodine, and, therefore, ablative therapy does not work.
■ TMC is not radiosensitive, but radiotherapy can be used for patients who have inoperable disease and whose tumor may be compressing and compromising some vital structures (trachea, esophagus, large vessels). There is no effective chemotherapeutic regimen for TMC.
■ There is no reliable or effective medical management for the diarrhea and flushing that may occur with TMC.

Additional Facts

■ The genetic form of TMC is discovered in approximately 10% to 15% of cases when evaluating the relatives of patients with an apparent sporadically occurring form of TMC, making it a valuable and worthwhile screening tool. A negative screening test result reduces the probability that familial disease exists.

■ Once MEN syndrome has been diagnosed in a family member, all other at-risk family members should be screened; testing should be performed annually until the age of 30, at which time more than 90% of all MEN gene carriers are detected by screening methods.

■ Screening method, according to Wells and associates, includes the following steps:

1. A 50-second infusion of calcium gluconate followed by a 10-second bolus of pentagastrin.
2. Calcitonin levels are then measured at 0, 2, 3.5, and 5 minutes later; peak levels occur at the 2- and 3.5-minute points.

■ Amyloid-free TMC may behave more aggressively than amyloid-associated TMC.

■ Tumors that metastasize to the cervical lymph nodes in patients without a known primary tumor that have the histologic and immunohistochemical features of TMC, including calcitonin, chromogranin, cytokeratin, and CEA reactivity, are not necessarily diagnostic of a primary thyroid tumor. Certainly, in this setting, TMC is the leading diagnosis; however, neuroendocrine tumors from mucosal sites of the head and neck (e.g., larynx) may demonstrate an identical histologic and immunohistochemical staining pattern of TMC. In this situation, the most important diagnostic test is the presence or absence of elevated serum calcitonin levels.

• TMC is almost invariably associated with elevated serum calcitonin levels.

• Upper aerodigestive tract mucosal neuroendocrine tumors are not associated with elevated serum calcitonin levels.

F. LYMPHOPROLIFERATIVE DISEASES OF THE THYROID GLAND

1. Benign Lymphoproliferative Disorders

a. Langerhans Cell Histiocytosis (LCH)

Definition: Rare systemic disease characterized by the proliferation of Langerhans' cell histiocytes. A number of criteria for the diagnosis of LCH have been established, which include the following:

1. A **"presumptive"** diagnosis is warranted when conventional light microscopic features are "consistent" with the presence of Langerhans' cell histiocytes.
2. A higher level of diagnostic confidence (designated **"diagnosis"**) is justified when the histologic findings are supplemented by the presence of two or more of the following features: positive staining with ATPase, S-100 protein, or α-D-mannosidase, or characteristic binding of peanut lectin.
3. A **"definitive"** diagnosis requires the finding of Birbeck's granules in lesional cells by electron microscopy

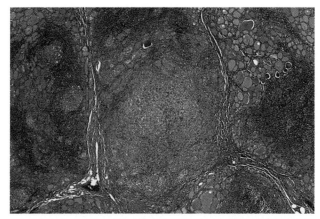

Figure 8–165. Eosinophilic granuloma of the thyroid. This focal lesion was an incidental finding in a thyroid removed for other reasons. The cellular infiltrate includes histiocytic cells with associated eosinophils. It is seen in and around a germinal center that was part of a chronic lymphocytic thyroiditis.

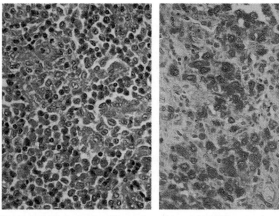

Figure 8–166. *Left,* The diagnostic cell in eosinophilic granuloma is the Langerhans histiocyte, which is characterized by enlarged cells with vesicular nuclei having an indented, notched, grooved, vesicular, or "coffee-bean" shape, one or two nucleoli, and pale to eosinophilic finely vacuolated cytoplasm. *Right,* Langerhans' histiocytes are positive with S-100 protein.

or a demonstration of T6 antigenic determinants on the surface of the cells in the appropriate histologic setting.

Synonyms: Eosinophilic granuloma; histiocytosis X.

Clinicopathology (limited to thyroid involvement)

■ Thyroid involvement by LCH is rare.

■ No gender predilection; occurs over a wide age range from 2 months to 55 years. The median age at occurrence is 37 years.

■ Thyroid involvement by LCH may occur as part of a systemic disease, with thyroid involvement found at autopsy. Alternatively, patients may present with thyroid enlargement, but the foci of LCH are not grossly appreciated, and microscopic foci of LCH are found only on histologic examination. The thyroid enlargement is due to another (coexisting) pathologic process such as adenomatoid nodules, lymphocytic thyroiditis, or papillary carcinoma, and the foci of LCH are identified incidentally.

- Histologically, thyroid involvement by LCH may be diffuse or focal. The Langerhans histiocytes are characterized by the presence of enlarged cells, containing vesicular nuclei with an indented, notched, grooved, vesicular, or "coffee bean"–shaped appearance, one or two nucleoli, and pale to eosinophilic finely vacuolated cytoplasm. Intracytoplasmic phagocytosed cellular debris may be found.
- A variable amount of eosinophils are seen intermingled with the Langerhans cell histiocytes and tend to be more concentrated near areas of necrosis.
- The histiocytic foci may infiltrate the thyroid parenchyma, causing effacement of the follicular architecture with destruction of the thyroid follicles. In addition, reactive changes of the follicular epithelium, including enlarged cell size, can be seen.
- Lymphocytic thyroiditis is commonly found in the thyroid tissue not involved by LCH.
- The histiocytic cell proliferation often extends beyond the confines of the capsule, causing adherence of the thyroid gland to the surrounding soft tissue or muscle.
- *Immunohistochemistry:* Langerhans cells react positively with S-100 protein, lysozyme, CD1a, and CD68 (KP1); no reactivity is seen with cytokeratin.
- *Electron microscopy:* Intracytoplasmic rod-shaped granules (Birbeck's granules) are identified.
- Localized disease is treated by surgical resection. For patients with isolated disease to the thyroid, the prognosis is favorable; these patients do not subsequently experience systemic involvement.
- Systemic disease is treated by combination chemotherapy. In patients with thyroid involvement associated with systemic disease the clinical course is aggressive and the prognosis is poor; death due to disease-related complications generally occurs in a short period (within 1 year).
- Given the disparity in clinical outcome between localized (isolated) disease to the thyroid and systemic involvement, it is imperative to exclude systemic disease in patients who may initially present with thyroid involvement.

b. Sinus Histiocytosis with Massive Lymphadenopathy (SHML)

Definition: Idiopathic, predominantly node-based histiocytic proliferative disorder associated with an indolent biologic course and spontaneous resolution. Extranodal involvement may occur as part of a generalized process involving the lymph nodes, or extranodal sites may be involved independent of the lymph node status.

Synonym: Rosai-Dorfman disease.

Clinicopathology (limited to thyroid involvement)

- Thyroid involvement by SHML is rare. It may represent secondary extension from the perithyroidal lymph nodes, or it may occur independent of nodal involvement.
- Clinically, SHML involving the thyroid may simulate the presentation of subacute thyroiditis, presenting with subclinical hypothyroidism and a painful goitrous thyroid.
- The histiocytic cells (so-called SHML cells) are characterized by round to oval, vesicular to hyperchromatic nuclei

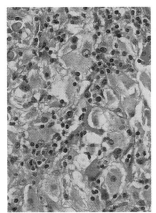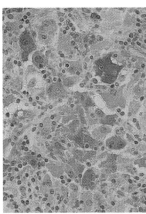

Figure 8–167. Extranodal (nonthyroidal) sinus histiocytosis with massive lymphadenopathy (Rosai-Dorfman disease). *Left,* The histiocytes have abundant, eosinophilic foamy, and granular-appearing cytoplasm with ill-defined cell borders; several of the histiocytes have lymphocytes within their cytoplasm (emperipolesis). *Right,* The histiocytes are typically S-100 protein positive.

and an abundant amphophilic to eosinophilic, granular to foamy to clear-appearing cytoplasm. The nucleoli may be prominent and eosinophilic or may be inconspicuous.
- Characteristically, SHML cells demonstrate emperipolesis. The phagocytized cells are most often lymphocytes, but plasma cells, erythrocytes, and polymorphonuclear leukocytes are also seen engulfed within the histiocytic cell cytoplasm. Emperipolesis is readily identifiable in nodal-based disease, but in extranodal disease it may be more difficult to identify, although it can usually be found.
- *Immunohistochemistry:* The most striking feature of SHML cells is the presence of diffuse S-100 protein reactivity. SHML cells also demonstrate consistent immunoreactivity with α_1-antichymotrypsin (ACT), CD68 (KP1), lysozyme, and MAC-387; less frequently, they may show immunoreactivity with Ki-1 and α_1-antitrypsin (AAT). SHML cells do not demonstrate immunoreactivity with Leu-M1.
- *Electron microscopy:* No Birbeck's granules are found.
- Too few cases of thyroid involvement have been reported to make any definitive comments on therapy and prognosis. In all likelihood, the treatment and prognosis are similar to those seen in the great majority of patients with SHML, who have an excellent prognosis, often with spontaneous resolution of disease, without any specific therapy.
- The etiology of SHML remains obscure. An infectious etiology has been considered, but an infectious agent has never been isolated. Other possible etiologic considerations include immunodeficiency, autoimmune disease, and a neoplastic process, but none of these have been substantiated.

2. Malignant Lymphoproliferative Disorders

a. Non-Hodgkin's Malignant Lymphoma

Definition: Primary thyroid involvement by a malignant tumor composed of lymphoid cells.

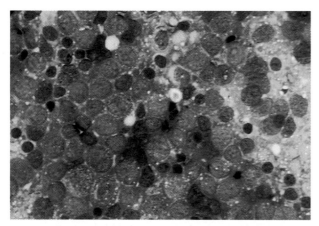

Figure 8–168. FNA, thyroid malignant lymphoma. Large cell lymphoma developing in the setting of lymphocytic thyroiditis is relatively easy to identify in FNA smears, which show a monotonous population of large lymphoid cells. Small cell and mixed lymphomas may be difficult to recognize. Diff-Quik stain.

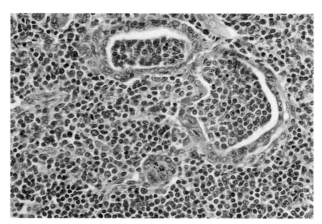

Figure 8–171. Thyroid malignant lymphoma showing a dyscohesive, monotonous cellular infiltrate with "colonization" of thyroid follicles (lymphoepithelial lesions).

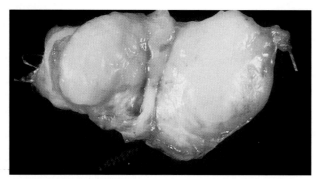

Figure 8–169. Primary thyroid malignant lymphoma appearing as large solid and nodular lesions with a homogeneous "fish flesh" appearance on cut section. The tumors have poor demarcation from the surrounding thyroid parenchyma and completely replace the involved thyroid tissue.

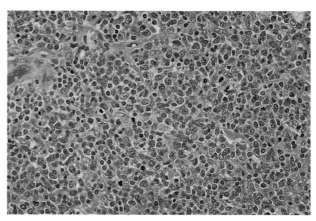

Figure 8–172. Thyroid malignant lymphoma with complete effacement of thyroid tissue. The neoplastic cells have a dyscohesive growth and are predominantly large cells.

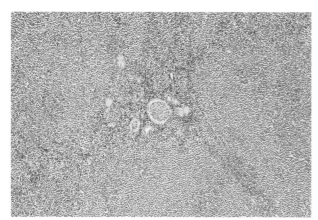

Figure 8–170. Thyroid malignant lymphoma. The tumor has a diffuse growth pattern composed of a monotonous-appearing cellular infiltrate. There is effacement of the thyroid parenchyma and, in the center of the field, the neoplastic cells are "packed" or "stuffed" within thyroid follicles (lymphoepithelial lesions).

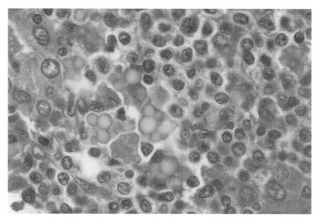

Figure 8–173. Thyroid malignant lymphoma. High magnification shows that the neoplastic infiltrate is composed of small and large cells. Extracellular eosinophilic globules corresponding to immunoglobulin are seen.

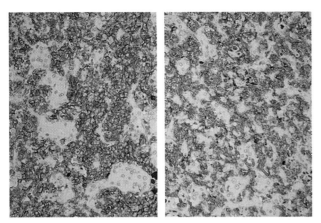

Figure 8–174. Immunohistochemical confirmation of a lymphoid malignancy of B-cell lineage is seen by the presence of *(left)* leukocyte common antigen (LCA) and *(right)* L26 reactivity, respectively. Note that the follicular epithelium in both illustrations does not react with these markers.

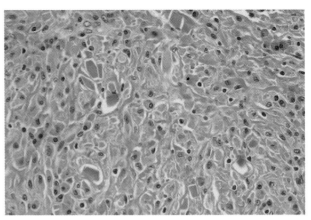

Figure 8–177. Thyroid malignant lymphoma with plasmacytoid features, including the presence of crystalloid immunoglobulin deposits.

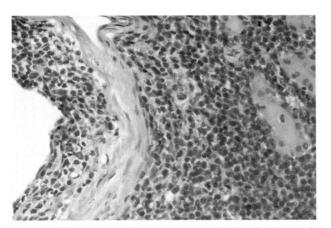

Figure 8–175. Thyroid malignant lymphoma showing lymph-vascular space infiltration.

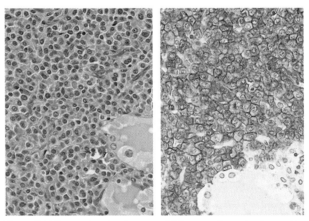

Figure 8–178. Despite the plasmacytoid features shown in the previous two illustrations and on the left side of this illustration, the neoplastic cells react with LCA (CD45), *right.* True plasma cell tumors generally do not show LCA reactivity.

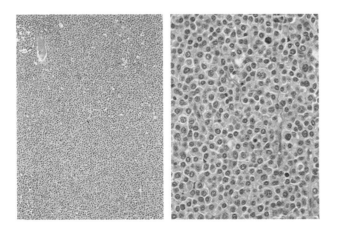

Figure 8–176. Thyroid malignant lymphoma. *Left,* diffuse growth with effacement of the thyroid tissue. *Right,* The neoplastic infiltrate has a plasmacytoid appearance suggesting the possibility of a plasma cell neoplasm. The neoplastic cells do not have a paranuclear clear zone ("hof").

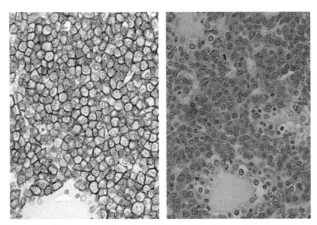

Figure 8–179. As a continuation of the previous illustration, this plasmacytoid malignant lymphoma shows B-cell lineage reactivity with the marker L26 (CD20) *(left)* and has kappa light chain restriction *(right).* This pattern of immunoreactivity can be seen in true plasma cell neoplasms.

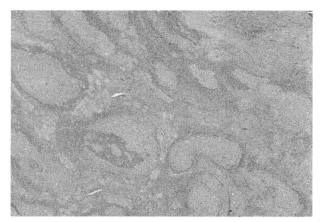

Figure 8–180. Thyroid malignant lymphoma. Unlike the previous illustrations, this lymphoma has a follicular growth pattern. The follicles are enlarged with convoluted shapes.

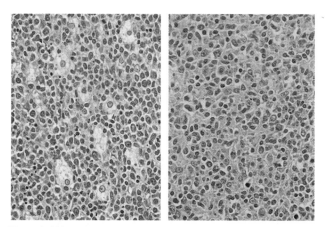

Figure 8–183. *Left,* Benign lymphoid follicle in chronic lymphocytic thyroiditis contains numerous tingible body macrophages. *Right,* Malignant follicle in a lymphoma does not have tingible body macrophages but includes malignant cells.

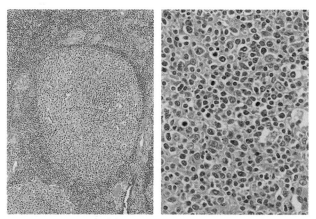

Figure 8–181. Thyroid malignant lymphoma, follicular. *Left,* The lymphomatous follicle is enlarged without tingible body macrophages. *Right,* Mixed neoplastic cellular infiltrate, including small and large cells.

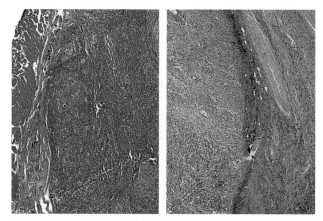

Figure 8–184. *Left,* The lymphoid infiltrate in chronic lymphocytic thyroiditis does not extend beyond the thyroid capsule into perithyroidal tissues. *Right,* The neoplastic cells of a thyroid malignant lymphoma will invade beyond the thyroid capsule into perithyroidal tissues.

Clinical

- Primary non-Hodgkin's malignant lymphomas comprise less than 1% to 8% of all thyroid malignant neoplasms.
- They are much more common in women than in men; this is predominantly but not exclusively a disease of older individuals (in the 7th decade or later).
- The clinical presentation is usually that of a rapidly enlarging, firm, nontender thyroid gland. The enlargement usually occurs over a short period (weeks to months). In addition to the rapidly enlarging mass, other complaints include hoarseness, dysphonia, vocal cord paralysis, dysphagia, dyspnea, and stridor; more uncommonly, superior vena cava obstruction may occur.

NOTE: In general, the only other thyroid neoplasm that presents as a rapidly enlarging thyroid mass is an anaplastic carcinoma, which also tends to occur in the same age population as thyroid malignant lymphoma.

- On palpation, the thyroid gland is usually found to be an asymmetrically hard, bulky mass that is often multinodu-

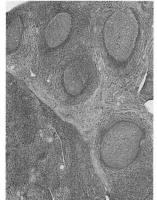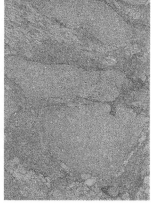

Figure 8–182. Lymphoid follicles are seen in both chronic lymphocytic thyroiditis *(left)* and malignant lymphoma with a follicular growth *(right).* However, in the former, the lymphoid follicles are small, round, and widely separated one from another, whereas in the latter, the lymphoid follicles are enlarged with odd shapes and encroach on one another.

lar but may be uninodular. Cervical adenopathy (unilateral or bilateral) may be present, including varying degrees of nodal fixation.

■ Most patients are euthyroid, but a minority of patients may be hypothyroid, probably owing to a preexisting chronic lymphocytic thyroiditis rather than to the lymphomatous infiltrate. In patients with chronic lymphocytic thyroiditis, antithyroid (antithyroglobulin and antimicrosomal) antibodies may be present on laboratory analysis. Rarely, hyperthyroidism may occur, perhaps owing to rapid destruction of thyroid follicular epithelium with release of colloid and thyroid hormone into the circulation.

■ Non-Hodgkin's malignant lymphoma of the thyroid is almost always associated with chronic lymphocytic thyroiditis (Hashimoto's thyroiditis), and patients with this disease have a 67 times greater risk than normal people of developing malignant lymphoma.
  • Chronic lymphocytic thyroiditis is an immunologically mediated (autoimmune) disease that may lead to the development of a malignant clone following persistent chronic antigenic stimulation of lymphocytes, thereby increasing their susceptibility to neoplastic transformation.
  • Areas that are transitional between reactive lymphoid hyperplasia and areas of unequivocal lymphoma can be seen.
  • A morphologic continuum exists between Hashimoto's thyroiditis, low-grade B-cell lymphoma, and high-grade lymphomas of the thyroid.
  • Clonal rearrangements of immunoglobulin genes may be present on rare occasions in patients with chronic lymphocytic thyroiditis.

■ Prior irradiation to the head and neck region is another possible etiologic factor in the development of thyroid malignant lymphoma.

■ Thyroid lymphomas share many features with lymphomas of salivary gland origin.
  • Both are associated with an immunologically mediated, extranodal lymphoid infiltrate (chronic lymphocytic thyroiditis for the thyroid and myoepithelial sialadenitis [MESA] for salivary glands).
  • Both involve the presence of lymphoepithelial lesions.
  • Patients with both diseases may present with the lymphoma limited to that particular site without concomitant or subsequent involvement of other sites. However, concomitant or metachronous involvement of other sites such as the gastrointestinal tract occurs in patients with both thyroid and salivary gland lymphomas.
  • For these reasons, both lesions are believed to be mucosa-associated lymphoid tissue (MALT) lymphomas.

Radiology

■ Thyroid lymphomas appear as hypofunctioning "cold" nodules on thyroid scans because lymphomatous infiltrates do not concentrate radioiodine.

■ CT scans may show nodularity, extension, or invasion within the gland or into the perithyroidal soft tissue, as well as necrosis and calcification.

■ On ultrasonographic examination, thyroid lymphomas appear as extremely hypoechoic masses; often this occurs in glands that have decreased echogenicity owing to the presence of chronic lymphocytic thyroiditis.

■ Magnetic resonance imaging shows an intensity similar to that of chronic lymphocytic thyroiditis; T2-weighted images show homogeneous areas of high intensity.

Pathology

Fine Needle Aspiration

NOTE: The cytologic diagnosis of a large cell malignant lymphoma is not as problematic as the diagnosis of a small cell malignant lymphoma; small cell and mixed small and large cell lymphomas may be impossible to distinguish from Hashimoto's thyroiditis. All cell types of malignant lymphoma may coexist with Hashimoto's thyroiditis.

Large Cell Lymphoma
■ Monotonous, dyscohesive atypical cells with large round to oval, vesicular nuclei and prominent nucleoli are found.
■ Necrotic debris is seen in the background.

Small Cell Lymphoma and Mixed Small and Large Cell Lymphomas
■ Features helpful in the diagnosis include a single cell or biphasic cell population lacking plasma cells or the cellular spectrum of differentiation seen in a normal germinal center.

Gross

■ In most cases, thyroid lymphomas appear as large solid tumors with a homogeneous "fish flesh" appearance on cut sections and poor demarcation from the surrounding thyroid parenchyma. Complete replacement of the thyroid gland may occur.

■ Extension beyond the thyroid capsule often occurs into the adjacent soft tissues, and the thyroid may be adherent to the surrounding structures. Hemorrhage and necrosis are usually not present.

■ The non-neoplastic thyroid may be nodular or lobular in appearance with associated fibrosis. These changes suggest the presence of lymphocytic thyroiditis.

Histology—General Features

■ Virtually every type of non-Hodgkin's malignant lymphoma occurs in the thyroid gland.

■ Most thyroid malignant lymphomas are of a B-cell immunophenotype; although uncommon, lymphomas with a T-cell immunophenotype may also occur in the thyroid gland.

■ The most common type of thyroid malignant lymphoma is a diffuse large cell lymphoma (the large noncleaved type is more common than the immunoblastic type).

■ Plasmacytic differentiation may be seen and may predominate in any given tumor simulating a plasmacytoma. In this situation immunohistochemical stains are helpful in differentiating malignant lymphoma with plasmacytic differentiation (leukocyte common antigen [LCA] and L26 positive) from a plasmacytoma (LCA negative, L26 positive).

■ The following morphologic features are characteristically seen in thyroid lymphomas:
  • Effacement of the thyroid architecture.
  • Neoplastic cellular infiltrate permeating between the non-neoplastic follicles.

- Presence of **"lymphoepithelial" lesions** when the neoplastic cells "pack" or "stuff" the thyroid follicles.
- Absence of germinal centers within the neoplastic cell infiltrate.
- Follicles composed of the neoplastic cellular infiltrate in a lymphoma with a follicular growth pattern. They do not demonstrate the spectrum of differentiation seen in a normal germinal center including tingible body macrophages.
- Lymph-vascular space invasion.
- Extension of neoplastic infiltrate beyond the thyroid capsule into the perithyroidal soft tissues. The thyroid may be adherent to the surrounding structures.
■ *Immunohistochemistry:*
- **B-cell phenotype:** Cells react positively with LCA (CD45) and B-cell markers (CD20 [L26]). Immunoglobulin light chain restriction (kappa or lambda light chains) can be seen. No reactivity is seen with T-cell markers (CD45RO [UCHL-1] or CD3), cytokeratin, thyroglobulin, calcitonin, or chromogranin).

NOTE: The absence of staining for cytoplasmic immunoglobulins does not exclude the diagnosis.

- **T-cell phenotype:** Cells react positively with LCA (CD45) and T-cell markers (CD45RO [UCHL-1] or CD3). No reactivity is seen with B-cell markers (CD20 [L26]), cytokeratin, thyroglobulin, calcitonin, or chromogranin.
■ *Molecular biology:* Immunoglobulin and T-cell gene rearrangements can be seen (these features are absent in Hashimoto's thyroiditis).

Differential Diagnosis

■ Chronic lymphocytic thyroiditis (Hashimoto's thyroiditis) (Table 8–12) (Chapter 6B).
■ Anaplastic carcinoma (Chapter 8D, #2b).

■ Thyroid carcinomas with an insular growth pattern (Chapter 8D, #2b).
■ Medullary carcinoma (Chapter 8E, #3).

Treatment and Prognosis

■ Prior to the initiation of any therapy, clinical staging is essential for the planning of treatment.
■ Clinical staging includes radiologic assessment of the neck, mediastinum, retroperitoneum, abdomen, and pelvis, complete blood count, and bone marrow biopsy. Staging is done to exclude more widespread disease.
■ For patients with low-stage disease (Stages I to II) with tumor localized to the thyroid and cervical lymph nodes, treatment includes high-dose radiotherapy to the thyroid and cervical lymph nodes with or without chemotherapy.
■ For patients with high-stage disease (Stages III and IV) with more widespread disease, treatment includes high-dose radiotherapy with chemotherapy.
■ The need for thyroidectomy remains controversial.
- Some surgeons advocate surgical resection of the gland in patients with low-stage disease because it allows removal of the entire tumor.
- Some surgeons advocate surgical excision of a sufficient amount of tissue for diagnostic purposes only, followed by initiation of radiotherapy or chemotherapy.
- Surgical intervention is justified for debulking large tumors or decompressing tumors that compromise vital structures.
■ The prognosis for patients with *low-stage (localized) disease* is considered very good: 5-year survival rates vary from 50% to 100%, and 10-year survival rates reach 50%.
■ The prognosis for *high-stage (widespread) disease* does not approach that of low-stage disease.
■ Factors that affect prognosis include the following:
- **Stage:** the lower the stage, the better the prognosis.
- **Age:** patients over 65 years old at the time of diagnosis have a worse prognosis.
- **Tumor recurrence:** portends an adverse prognosis.

Table 8–12
MALIGNANT LYMPHOMAS VERSUS CHRONIC LYMPHOCYTIC THYROIDITIS

Features	Malignant Lymphoma	Chronic Lymphocytic Thyroiditis
Thyroid architecture and follicular epithelium	Effaced; destruction of follicular epithelium; lymphoepithelial lesions—"packing" or "stuffing" of the follicles with the neoplastic cells	Preserved; no destruction of follicular epithelium; cytoplasmic oxyphilia and nuclear enlargement; "packing" or "stuffing" of the follicles by mature lymphocytes; multinucleated giant cells
Germinal centers	Absent in lymphomatous areas; follicles may be present but are composed of malignant cells without tingible body macrophages	Present; heterogeneous cell population; tingible body macrophages in lymphoid follicles
Cellular components	Monomorphic malignant cellular infiltrate or admixture of different malignant cell types (i.e., small cleaved and large noncleaved cells)	Polymorphous; composed of mature lymphocytes, histiocytes, and plasma cells
Extrathyroidal extension	Malignant cellular infiltrate often "spills out" into the perithyroidal soft tissues, thyroid may be adherent to surrounding structures	Sharp outline between benign lymphocytic cell infiltrate and perithyroidal soft tissue; thyroid not adherent to surrounding structures
Immunohistochemistry	Most lymphomas show B-cell lineage specificity and kappa or lambda light chain restriction; occasionally, a T-cell lineage-specific lymphoma may occur	No lineage specificity nor light chain restriction; both B cells and T cells are present in the benign cellular infiltrate; light chain restriction is not present
Associated parenchymal changes	Lymphocytic thyroiditis	Squamous metaplasia; fibrosis; lymphoepithelial cysts

- **Histology:** (1) tumors with plasmacytic differentiation have a better prognosis; (2) immunoblastic lymphomas behave worse than large cell lymphomas; and (3) the presence of necrosis may be associated with a worse prognosis.
- **Extrathyroidal extension** may not be as significant for prognosis as previously believed and certainly is not as poor a prognostic sign as when it occurs in epithelial malignancies of the thyroid.

b. Plasmacytoma

Definition: Malignant tumor of plasma cells (terminally differentiated B lymphocytes).

Clinicopathology

- Thyroid involvement by a malignant proliferation of plasma cells may be part of multiorgan systemic involvement (multiple myeloma) or may occur as an isolated phenomenon (extramedullary plasmacytoma).
- Gender, age, clinical presentation, and macroscopic features are essentially similar to those characteristic of non-Hodgkin's malignant lymphomas.
- Serum immunoelectrophoresis may show abnormalities (monoclonal spike) in both the systemic and localized forms of the disease.
- Histologically, plasma cell malignant tumors are composed of plasma cells in varying degrees of maturation and atypicality. Plasma cells are characterized by a round to oval shape with an eccentrically situated round nucleus. The nucleus has a characteristic "clock face" chromatin pattern, but dispersed nuclear chromatin can be seen. A characteristic paranuclear clear zone ("hof"), which represents the Golgi apparatus where immunoglobulin is processed and glycosylated for secretion, is seen. The cytoplasm is nondescript and is abundant and basophilic.
- The neoplastic cells may extend outside the thyroid capsule and may invade the perithyroidal soft tissues.

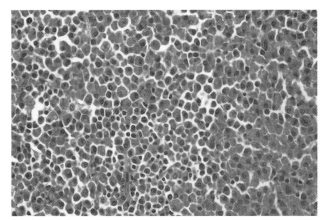

Figure 8–185. Extramedullary plasmacytoma of the thyroid showing true plasma cells characterized by round to oval cells with an eccentrically situated round nucleus; the nucleus has a characteristic "clock face" dispersed chromatin pattern. A characteristic paranuclear clear zone ("hof") representing the Golgi apparatus where immunoglobulin is processed and glycosylated for secretion is seen. Intracytoplasmic (immune) globules can be seen.

- An associated lymphocytic thyroiditis is present in the non-neoplastic thyroid gland in the majority of cases.
- Amyloid deposits, as shown by the presence of acellular hyalinized material, may be associated with the plasma cell malignant infiltrate. Histochemical stains (Congo red or crystal violet) and/or immunohistochemical examination (AA protein) assist in confirming the presence of amyloid.
- *Histochemistry:* Cytoplasmic pyroninophilia (methyl green pyronin [MGP]), appearing red on staining.
- *Immunohistochemistry:* B-cell markers (CD20 or L26) are positive. Immunoglobulin light chain restriction (kappa or lambda) can be demonstrated. Plasma cell malignancies generally are LCA (CD45) negative.

Differential Diagnosis

- Non-Hodgkin's malignant lymphoma with plasmacytoid features (Chapter 8F, #2).
- Plasma cell granuloma (see Additional Facts below).
- Medullary carcinoma (Chapter 8E, #3).

Treatment and Prognosis

- Like non-Hodgkin's malignant lymphoma, staging is required before therapy is initiated and may necessitate a bone marrow biopsy.
- Treatment depends on the clinical setting in which the plasma cell neoplasm occurs.
  - Localized disease: surgery with or without radiotherapy.
  - Systemic disease: combination surgery, radiotherapy, and chemotherapy.
- Prognosis for localized disease is considered good; survival rates are better than those reported for low-stage thyroid malignant lymphomas.
- Prognosis for systemic disease (multiple myeloma) is poor with extremely high mortality rates within 3 years of diagnosis; the 10-year survival rate is approximately 10%.
- The diagnosis of plasmacytoma of the thyroid does not necessarily portend the development of multiple myeloma.

Additional Facts

Plasma Cell Granuloma (Inflammatory Pseudotumor)

- Rare benign (polyclonal) plasma cell proliferation of the thyroid.
- Seen exclusively in women.
- Characterized by nodular lesions composed of mature plasma cells with identifiable Russell bodies (intracytoplasmic or extracellular cherry-red round bodies or globules representing immunoglobulin). Other benign inflammatory cells can also be seen including mature lymphocytes and histiocytes.
- The presence of Russell bodies is often an indication of a benign condition.
- Immunohistochemical evaluation shows light chain polyclonality (both kappa and lambda).

c. Hodgkin's Disease

- Involvement of the thyroid by Hodgkin's disease is rare.
- When Hodgkin's disease involves the thyroid it usually occurs secondary to cervical or mediastinal nodal disease.
- Rarely, primary Hodgkin's disease of the thyroid may occur.
- Histologically, the most common type of Hodgkin's disease involving the thyroid is the nodular sclerosing type.

d. Other Malignant Lymphoproliferative Lesions

- Thyroid involvement by other malignant lymphoproliferative tumors can occur but generally is uncommon. These tumors include chronic lymphocytic leukemia, mycosis fungoides, and chloroma.

G. NONEPITHELIAL NEOPLASMS OF THE THYROID, EXCLUDING LYMPHOPROLIFERATIVE DISEASES

1. Thyroid Paraganglioma

Definition: Benign tumor originating from the neural crest–derived paraganglia of the autonomic nervous system. Paraganglia are identified throughout the body in both adrenal and extra-adrenal sites.

Clinical (limited to the thyroid gland)

- Rare primary thyroid neoplasm.
- More common in women than in men; this is a tumor of adults.
- Patients present with an asymptomatic thyroid mass; systemic symptoms are not present.

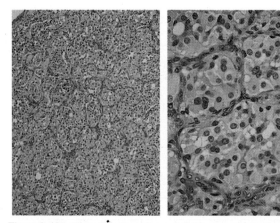

Figure 8–186. Thyroid paraganglioma. *Left,* The tumor has a characteristic cell nest or organoid growth (zellballen) with a fibrovascular stroma that surrounds and separates the tumor nests. *Right,* The neoplasm is composed predominantly of chief cells, which are round or oval with uniform nuclei, have a dispersed chromatin pattern, and abundant eosinophilic, granular or vacuolated cytoplasm. Sustentacular cells represent the other cellular component of the tumor, which are difficult to appreciate by light microscopy.

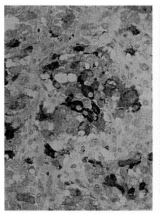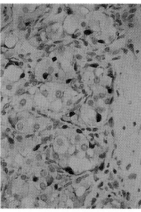

Figure 8–187. Thyroid paraganglioma immunoreactivity includes *(left)* chromogranin positive reactions in the chief cells and *(right)* S-100 protein positive reactions in the sustentacular cells. The sustentacular cells are modified Schwann's cells and are seen at the periphery of the cell nests as spindle-shaped cells.

- Patients are euthyroid.
- Radioisotopic scan shows the presence of a hypofunctioning ("cold") solitary mass.
- The presence of intrathyroidal paraganglia has not been definitively identified; however, paraganglia, derived from the inferior laryngeal paraganglial tissue, are found in the thyroid capsule and perhaps migrate to this site during embryogenesis.

Pathology

Gross

- Encapsulated, firm lesions have a nodular appearance, are tan-brown in color, and measure up to 3.5 cm in greatest dimension.

Histology

- Histologic features include the presence of a cell nest or organoid growth (zellballen) with a fibrovascular stroma that surrounds and separates the tumor nests.
- The neoplasm is composed predominantly of chief cells, which are round or oval, have uniform nuclei, a dispersed chromatin pattern, and abundant eosinophilic, granular, or vacuolated cytoplasm.
- Sustentacular cells, representing the other cellular component of the tumor, are difficult to appreciate by light microscopy. These cells are modified Schwann's cells and are seen at the periphery of the cell nests as spindle-shaped, basophilic-appearing cells.
- There is no evidence of follicular differentiation or colloid formation within the neoplasm.
- Cellular pleomorphism may be seen; mitoses and necrosis are infrequently identified.
- Spindling of the chief cells may be present; an amyloid stroma is not seen.
- *Histochemistry:* Tumor cells are argyrophilic (Churukian-Schenk's stain). Reticulin staining delineates the cell nests. Argentaffin (Fontana-Masson), mucin, and PAS stains are negative.

- *Immunohistochemistry:*
  - Chief cells react positively to chromogranin, synaptophysin, and NSE; focal S-100 protein reactivity can be seen.
  - Sustentacular cells show characteristic S-100 protein staining along the peripheral aspects of the cell nests.
  - There is no reactivity with cytokeratin, thyroglobulin, calcitonin, or CEA.
- *Electron microscopy:* Membrane-bound neurosecretory granules of varying sizes are seen.

Differential Diagnosis

- Hyalinizing trabecular adenoma (Chapter 8C, #3).
- Medullary carcinoma (Chapter 8E, #3).
- Carotid body paraganglioma arising adjacent to the thyroid; differentiation is based on clinical and/or operative findings.
- Thyroid papillary carcinoma (Chapter 8D, #2).

Treatment and Prognosis

- Conservative surgical excision (lobectomy) is curative.
- These tumors are benign; malignant behavior, as shown by local or regional invasion, is extraordinarily uncommon.
- Concomitantly occurring carotid body tumors may be present.

2. Mesenchymal Tumors of the Thyroid Gland

a. Benign Mesenchymal Tumors

- Rare group of tumors that may occur in the thyroid.
- May present as a solitary thyroid nodule or mass; may also be identified in a thyroid gland removed for another lesion such as an adenomatoid nodule or a neoplasm (e.g., follicular adenoma).
- Four types of lesions:
  - Vascular tumors: hemangioma, lymphangioma.

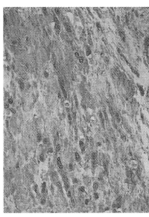
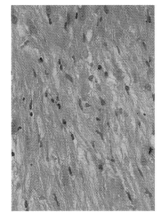

Figure 8–189. *Left,* Benign Schwannoma composed of bland-appearing spindle cells with wavy nuclei. *Right,* Neural-derived tumors are S-100 protein positive.

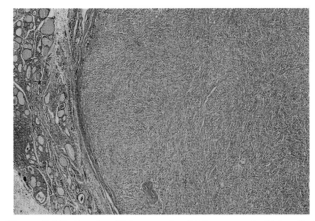

Figure 8–190. Intrathyroidal encapsulated leiomyoma. A thick-walled vascular structure is seen toward the lower center portion of the illustration. The development of primary thyroid smooth muscle tumors could be of vascular smooth muscle origin.

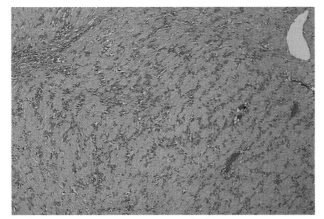

Figure 8–188. Intrathyroidal benign peripheral nerve sheath tumor (benign Schwannoma) showing elongated or spindle-shaped cells with nuclear palisading (Verocay bodies).

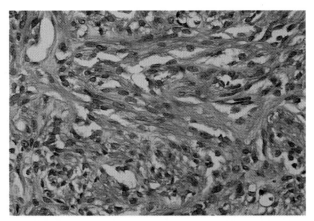

Figure 8–191. Higher magnification shows bland cells with elongated cigar-shaped nuclei. Immunoreactivity was present with muscle markers *(not shown)*.

- Neural tumors: benign peripheral nerve sheath tumor (benign Schwannoma).
- Muscle tumors: leiomyoma.
- Adipose tissue tumors: lipoma.
■ Diagnosis is often established by light microscopic evaluation; immunohistochemistry may be helpful in the diagnosis and differential diagnosis.
■ Surgical excision is curative.

b. Malignant Mesenchymal Tumors

Definition: Thyroid malignant tumors with mesenchymal differentiation as confirmed by light microscopy, immunohistochemistry, and electron microscopy with no evidence of epithelial differentiation by the same diagnostic modalities.

■ Primary sarcomas of the thyroid gland are rare. Involvement of the thyroid secondary to a primary cervical neck or mediastinal sarcoma should be excluded.
■ Immunohistochemistry plays an important role in the diagnosis of sarcomas; sarcomatous lesions described prior to the development of immunohistochemical techniques

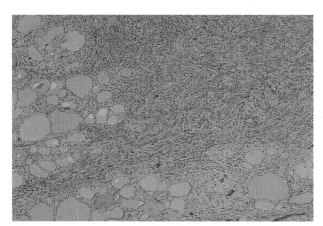

Figure 8–192. Thyroid leiomyosarcoma. In contrast to the leiomyoma, this thyroid tumor is unencapsulated and infiltrative. The neoplastic cells are spindle-shaped and have a fascicular growth.

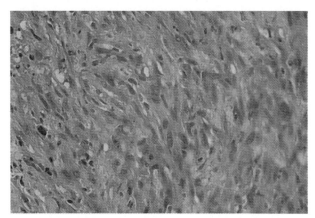

Figure 8–193. Higher magnification from the previous illustration shows a malignant pleomorphic and spindle cell infiltrate. Immunohistochemistry *(not shown)* demonstrated reactivity limited to myogenic markers.

may represent anaplastic carcinomas rather than true mesenchymal malignancies.
■ Sarcomas occurring in the thyroid include six types:
- Vascular tumors: angiosarcoma (see next section, Chapter 8F, #2c);
- Neural tumors: malignant peripheral nerve sheath tumor (malignant Schwannoma).
- Muscle tumors: leiomyosarcoma.
- Adipose tissue tumors: liposarcoma.
- Fibroblast tumors: fibrosarcoma.
- Matrix-forming tumors: osteosarcoma and chondrosarcoma.
■ The fact that these tumors are malignant is not in dispute, but whether they are true mesenchymal malignancies rather than carcinomas with sarcomatoid features remains a controversial issue. However, this is an academic argument because the treatment and prognosis generally follow those described for anaplastic carcinoma.
■ The one exception in the group of mesenchymal tumors is the angiosarcoma.

c. Angiosarcoma of the Thyroid Gland

Definition: Malignant neoplasm with endothelial differentiation.

Synonyms: Epithelioid angiosarcoma; malignant hemangioendothelioma.

Clinical

■ Extremely rare.
■ Demographic data are similar to those described for anaplastic carcinoma.
■ Typical clinical presentation is sudden enlargement of a long-standing goitrous thyroid with or without pain. Chest pain and massive hemothorax may be present owing to early metastatic tumor to the lung and pleura.
■ Has a predilection for (but is not found exclusively in) the mountainous or high-altitude regions of Europe. These areas are often iodine deficient, resulting in goitrous thy-

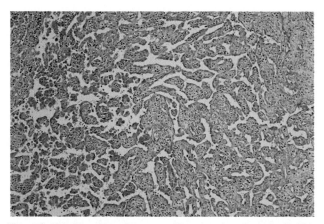

Figure 8–194. Thyroid angiosarcoma. The tumor is composed of widely dilated, ramifying, and intercommunicating vascular spaces with vascular tufts. The cells associated with these spaces and tufts have elongated to epithelioid-appearing nuclei with prominent eosinophilic nucleoli.

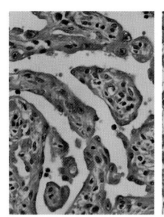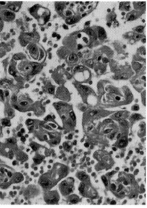

Figure 8–195. Thyroid angiosarcoma. The neoplastic infiltrate, whether lining the vascular spaces *(left)* or in intraluminal vascular tufts and *(right)* associated with more solid aspects of the tumor, is malignant and shares similar features including enlarged pleomorphic spindle-shaped or rounded nuclei with prominent eosinophilic nucleoli. Epithelioid cells are seen in both panels. *Right,* Intracytoplasmic vacuoles containing erythrocytes are seen. These vacuoles represent early attempts at lumen formation. Scattered red blood cells are seen within the spaces.

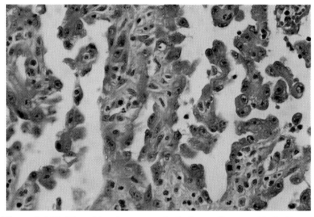

Figure 8–196. Thyroid angiosarcoma, including malignant epithelioid cells and mitotic figures.

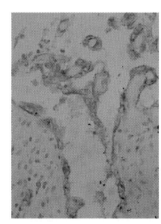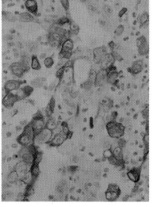

Figure 8–197. Thyroid epithelioid angiosarcoma showing *(left)* cytokeratin and *(right)* factor VIII-related antigen reactivity.

roids (endemic goiters). Angiosarcomas often develop in people with long-standing goiters.

Pathology

Gross

- These tumors are typically large and invasive and have associated necrosis and hemorrhage.
- Less commonly, they may appear as delineated or circumscribed nodular lesions.

Histology

- This tumor is characterized by the presence of dilated vascular spaces showing prominent anastomoses and lined by atypical to overtly malignant endothelial cells. Vascular tufting is seen.
- Anastomosing vascular channels may be present only focally, or they may be obscured by a dominant solid, cellular malignant infiltrate composed of spindle-shaped and epithelioid cells with large, pleomorphic, and vesicular nuclei, prominent nucleoli, and an eosinophilic cytoplasm.
- Multinucleated giant cells and bizarre-looking cells can be seen. Mitotic activity, including atypical forms, hemorrhage, and necrosis is consistently seen.
- The malignant infiltrate is invasive, destroying the thyroid follicular epithelium as well as invading outside the thyroid capsule.
- Intracytoplasmic vacuoles, representing early attempts at lumen formation, are seen; erythrocytes may or may not be present within these vacuoles.
- *Immunohistochemistry:* Reactions with vimentin, endothelial markers, including factor VIII-related protein, CD34 (QBEND—hematopoietic progenitor cell antigen), CD31 (vascular cell adhesion molecule), and *Ulex europaeus I* may be positive. Cytokeratin reactivity may also be present. Positive reactions to thyroglobulin are absent.

NOTE: The above immunohistochemical staining pattern is not specific for an endothelial neoplasm and can be seen in other malignant mesenchymal tumors as well as in malignant epithelial neoplasms; the latter includes anaplastic carcinomas with sarcomatoid features (angiomatoid carcinoma) of the thyroid gland.

- *Electron microscopy:* Weibel-Palade bodies appearing as intracytoplasmic rod-shaped, membrane-bound structures are specific for endothelial cells and represent the storage site for factor VIII–related protein. However, these are best identified in well-differentiated malignant vascular tumors and are difficult to identify in poorly differentiated vascular tumors. Other ultrastructural features that may be seen in endothelial neoplasms but are not specific for them include pinocytic vesicles, basal lamina, cytoplasmic filaments, and intracytoplasmic vacuoles.

Differential Diagnosis

- Anaplastic carcinoma (with angiomatoid features) (Chapter 8D, #2b).

■ Post-FNA–induced changes in the central portions of an adenomatoid nodule that may include the following:
  • Dilated vascular channels with thrombosis and organization, including interanastomosing channels (Chapter 8I).
  • Papillary endothelial hyperplasia-like changes (Chapter 8I).

Treatment and Prognosis

■ Treatment includes a combination of surgery, radiotherapy, and chemotherapy.
■ Prognosis is dismal; these tumors are highly aggressive with widespread local invasive growth and early dissemination to lung and lymph nodes.

Additional Facts

■ The diagnosis of angiosarcoma of the thyroid is the subject of controversy. Those who do not believe in its existence believe that these tumors are anaplastic carcinomas with angiosarcomatous features (angiomatoid carcinomas).
■ The specific designation as an angiosarcoma or an angiomatoid carcinoma appears moot because these are high-grade malignant neoplasms that are treated similarly, and they share the same poor prognosis and outcome.
■ **Carcinosarcoma or true malignant mixed tumors** of the thyroid gland probably represent anaplastic carcinomas with sarcomatoid differentiation rather than differentiation of a malignant tumor along both epithelial and mesenchymal cell lines.

d. Teratomas

Definition: A teratoma is a true neoplasm composed of a variety of tissue types representing all three germ layers (ectoderm, endoderm, and mesoderm); it occurs in areas in which these tissues are not natively identified.

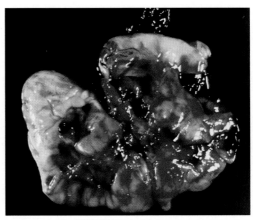

Figure 8–199. Large solid and cystic cervical teratomas with associated hemorrhage.

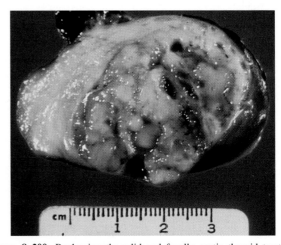

Figure 8–200. Predominantly solid and focally cystic thyroid teratoma with a homogenous white appearance.

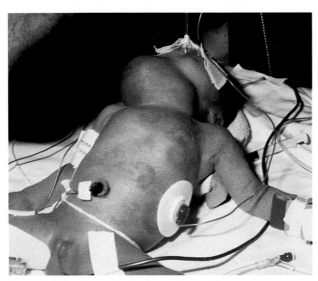

Figure 8–198. Infant with a massive midline and lateral teratoma that involved the thyroid gland.

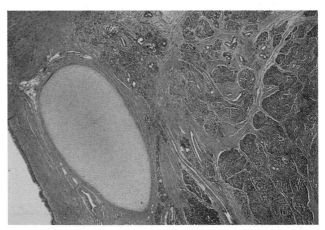

Figure 8–201. Intrathyroidal teratoma consisting of a respiratory epithelium *(lower left)*, pancreatic tissue *(right)*, and mature cartilage *(left of center)*.

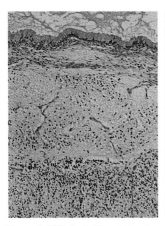
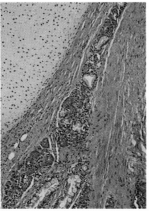

Figure 8–202. *Left,* Thyroid teratoma with intestinal-type mucin producing epithelium subjacent to which is neuroectodermal tissue. *Right,* Mature cartilage and mucoserous glandular tissue.

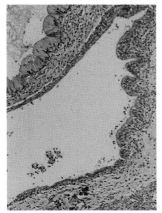
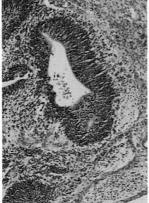

Figure 8–203. Another thyroid teratoma with *(left)* ciliated respiratory and mucin-producing epithelium and *(right)* primitive neuroectodermal tissue.

Adult Thyroid Teratomas
- Thyroid teratomas not related to secondary thyroid involvement from a cervical neck teratoma are uncommon.
- They are more common in women than in men and occur over a wide age range.
- Adult thyroid teratomas are often malignant and behave somewhat like the immature teratomas of gonads; the degree of immaturity of the tissue determines its malignant potential.
- These tumors behave aggressively and usually are fatal regardless of all attempts to control the disease (using total thyroidectomy, radiation, and chemotherapy).

Pediatric Thyroid Teratomas
- Thyroid involvement occurs secondary to extension from a cervical neck teratoma.
- Most cervical teratomas occur in stillborns, neonates, or infants younger than 1 year of age and present as a large midline or lateral neck mass with or without airway compression and compromise.
- Cervical teratomas are large, often measuring more than 10 cm in greatest dimension; on cut sections they are solid to cystic in appearance.

- Histologically, an admixture of all three germ layers is found. These components most commonly are mature.
- Surgical resection is the treatment of choice. These tumors are benign and have an excellent prognosis.

Additional Facts

- **Hamartomas** are defined as benign, tumor-like proliferations or overgrowths of tissue indigenous to a specific site. Hamartomatous lesions of the thyroid are extraordinarily rare and may in fact represent teratomas.
- Little clinical importance is ascribed to thyroid involvement by cervical teratomas in both adults and children. Similarly, little clinical importance is attached to the histogenesis (thyroid versus nonthyroid) in cervical teratomas that have an anatomic relationship with the thyroid gland.

H. SECONDARY OR METASTATIC TUMORS TO THE THYROID

- The thyroid gland may be secondarily involved by malignant tumors originating in other sites. This involvement may take the form of direct invasion by a malignant neoplasm in a nearby site or hematogenous spread from a distant primary malignant tumor.
- Among the tumors that invade directly into the thyroid from an adjacent organ are mucosal tumors of the larynx, pharynx, trachea, and esophagus. Squamous cell carcinoma (or one of its histologic variants) is by far the most common malignant tumor that invades directly into the thyroid gland.
- Tumors metastasizing to the thyroid from a distant primary site can originate from virtually every organ system (Table 8–13); those that metastasize most frequently to the thyroid gland include renal cell carcinoma, breast carcinoma, lung carcinoma, and malignant melanoma.
- Metastatic tumors to the thyroid may originate from an occult primary source and can simulate the appearance of a primary thyroid tumor. Similarly, metastatic thyroid tumors may metastasize to other sites, simulating primary tumors in those organs.
- A clinically detectable thyroid mass due to metastatic disease is found in a minority of patients; thyroid involvement by metastatic deposits from distant sites is more often seen in autopsy material.

Table 8–13
SECONDARY OR METASTATIC TUMORS
TO THE THYROID GLAND

Epithelial

Kidney, breast, lung, gastrointestinal, hepatobiliary and pancreas, genitourinary tract

Neuroectodermal

Malignant melanoma, neuroendocrine carcinoma (small cell carcinoma)

Lymphoproliferative

Non-Hodgkin's malignant lymphoma, Hodgkin's disease, leukemia

Mesenchymal

Kaposi's sarcoma

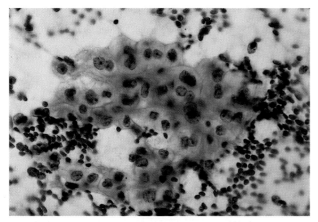

Figure 8–204. Fine needle aspiration, metastatic renal cell carcinoma. This renal cell carcinoma metastatic to the thyroid has clear cells with distinct cell borders and vesicular nuclei with prominent nucleoli, a pattern that would be unusual for a primary thyroid neoplasm. Inquiry about the clinical history can be invaluable in establishing a correct diagnosis. Papanicolaou's stain.

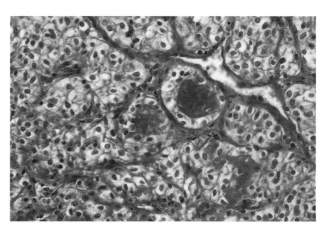

Figure 8–207. Instead of colloid, often the pseudofollicles of a metastatic renal cell carcinoma contains red blood cells. This is a helpful but not diagnostic feature seen in renal cell carcinomas and generally not in primary thyroid tumors.

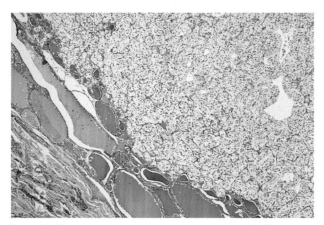

Figure 8–205. Metastatic renal cell carcinoma to the thyroid. The metastasis has localized within an adenomatoid nodule. The metastasis is composed of clear cells with focal follicle-like structures but without colloid. The tumor has a nested growth with fibrovascular stroma.

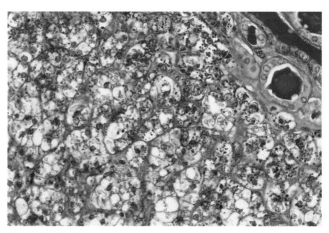

Figure 8–208. Renal cell carcinomas contain glycogen as seen by the presence of periodic acid–Schiff (PAS)-positive cytoplasmic material. If the cytoplasmic material is glycogen, predigestion with diastase *(not shown)* will wash away this material. Note that colloid is PAS positive.

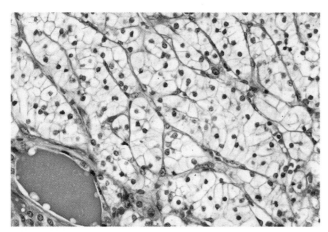

Figure 8–206. Higher magnification shows that the neoplastic infiltrate is composed of nests of clear cells separated by a fine fibrovascular stroma. The tumor cells have a single round hyperchromatic nucleus and sharply delineated cell borders. A remnant of a colloid-filled thyroid follicle is seen in the lower left.

- In patients with a clinically detectable mass, the metastatic tumor presents as a rapidly growing thyroid mass of recent onset. Patients are generally euthyroid, although some may present with disturbances in thyroid function (hyperthyroidism).
- A metastatic tumor may appear as a single hypofunctioning ("cold") mass on thyroid scan and as a solid or cystic lesion on ultrasonography. Radiologically, metastatic deposits may simulate the appearance of a primary thyroid lesion; multiple lesions may be more indicative of a metastatic tumor.
- Metastatic tumor to the thyroid may localize within a primary thyroid lesion such as an adenomatoid nodule or a thyroid neoplasm, including follicular adenomas, follicular carcinomas, and papillary carcinomas.
- Histologically, renal cell carcinoma may be the metastatic tumor that is most difficult to differentiate from a primary clear cell neoplasm of the thyroid (Table 8–14). Metastatic renal cell carcinoma to the thyroid is characteristically

Table 8–14
FOLLICULAR TUMORS WITH CLEAR CELLS VERSUS METASTATIC RENAL CELL CARCINOMA

Features	Follicular Tumors with Clear Cells	Metastatic Renal Cell Carcinoma
Luminal secretion	Colloid is present, is PAS positive	No colloid; find red blood cells; pseudofollicles
Nested growth with fibrovascular stroma	Present	Present
Cytoplasm	Foamy appearing	Clear
Nuclear	Round; dispersed or coarse chromatin	Small, round, hyperchromatic
Glycogen (intracytoplasmic, diastase sensitive, PAS positive)	Yes, but will also be diastase resistant	Yes; strongly positive
Thyroglobulin immunoreactivity	Present, but may be focal and of weak intensity; colloid is intensely positive	Absent

circumscribed or even encapsulated, mimicking a follicular neoplasm (adenoma or carcinoma). Further diagnostic confusion may occur because renal cell carcinomas may metastasize to a pre-existing thyroid lesion (nodule or tumor), partially replacing these lesions.

- In metastatic tumors that may simulate the appearance of a follicular cell–derived tumor (e.g., renal cell carcinoma), the presence or absence of thyroglobulin immunoreactivity is the single most helpful parameter in determining whether a tumor is a primary follicular cell–derived neoplasm or a metastatic tumor. However, the absence of thyroglobulin reactivity does not necessarily exclude the possibility of a primary follicular epithelial cell–derived tumor, and it certainly does not exclude a C-cell–derived tumor. Anaplastic carcinomas may be thyroglobulin negative; C-cell tumors are thyroglobulin negative but are calcitonin and neuroendocrine marker (chromogranin and synaptophysin) positive.
- Some metastatic tumors have a specific immunohistochemical antigenic profile.
  - Malignant melanoma: S-100 protein and HMB-45 positive.
  - Prostate carcinoma: Prostatic-specific antigen (PSA) and prostatic acid phosphatase (PAP) positive.
  - Gastrointestinal, hepatobiliary, and pancreatic adenocarcinoma: CA 19-9 and DUPAN-2 positive.

NOTE: There are no specific immunohistochemical markers for renal cell carcinoma.

- Surgical resection of a metastatic tumor may inadvertently occur if the metastatic tumor presents as a metastasis from an occult primary neoplasm. Surgical resection is an acceptable treatment modality even for some tumors that are known to be metastatic to the thyroid (i.e., renal cell carcinoma).
- Prolonged survival following surgical resection (lobectomy or total thyroidectomy) may occur in patients with some metastatic tumors (e.g., renal cell carcinoma) in which the metastatic disease is limited to the thyroid.
- In general, external irradiation and chemotherapy are used in the treatment of metastatic tumors to the thyroid.
- Despite all attempts to control disease, the prognosis in patients with metastatic tumor to the thyroid is generally poor, with death occurring within 2 years after identification of metastasis to the thyroid.

I. FINE NEEDLE ASPIRATION–RELATED HISTOLOGIC CHANGES TO THE THYROID GLAND

- FNA has tremendous importance as the first interventive procedure in the diagnosis of a thyroid mass.
- The diagnostic sensitivity and specificity of FNA of a thyroid mass are high.

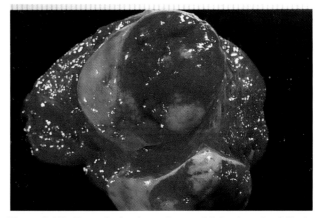

Figure 8–209. Postaspiration hemorrhage and infarction of a follicular adenoma with oxyphilia.

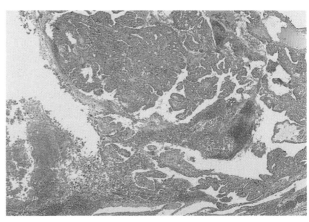

Figure 8–210. The postaspiration changes in this follicular adenoma with oxyphilia include hemorrhage, cystic degeneration, and papillary formation.

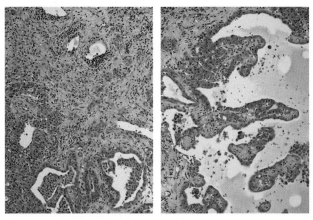

Figure 8–211. Separate areas in this oxyphilic follicular adenoma include hemorrhage with hemosiderin-laden macrophages, granulation tissue, and papillae.

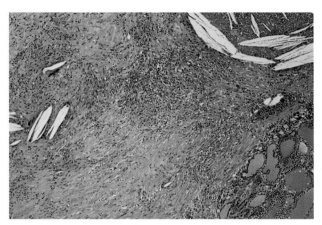

Figure 8–214. Cholesterol granulomas are seen in this adenomatoid nodule that was aspirated.

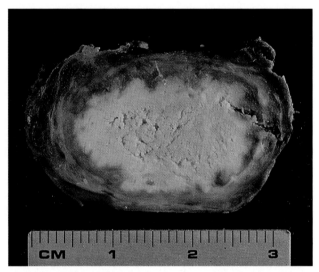

Figure 8–212. Postaspiration infarction of a papillary carcinoma.

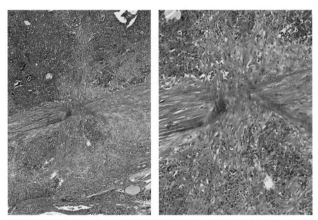

Figure 8–215. Capsular alterations may include foci of pseudoinvasive growth. *Left,* The needle tract is apparent. *Right,* The area in question shows fibrosis and an inflammatory cell infiltrate, but follicular epithelium is not present (compare with Fig. 8–34).

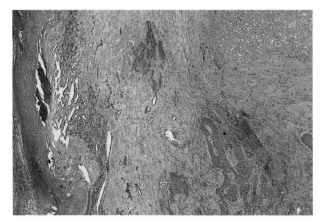

Figure 8–213. Postaspiration changes in an adenomatoid nodule include infarction *(upper right),* fibrosis, chronic inflammation, squamous metaplasia, and calcifications.

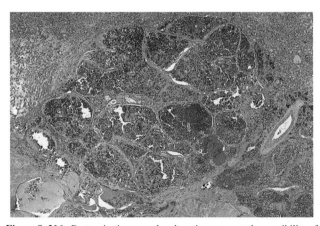

Figure 8–216. Postaspiration vascular alterations suggest the possibility of a vascular neoplasm such as a hemangioma.

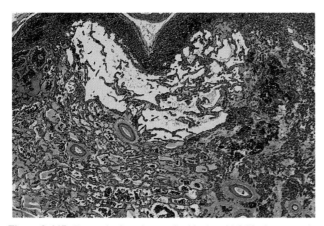

Figure 8–217. Postaspiration changes in this thyroid follicular tumor include dilated, ramifying, and interconnecting channels with papillary tufting, suggesting the possibility of a vascular neoplasm.

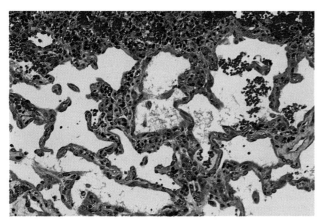

Figure 8–218. Higher magnification of Figure 8–217 shows that the postaspiration alterations involve the follicular epithelial cells. However, the changes, including dilated and ramifying spaces, some containing erythrocytes from the aspiraton procedure, and the atypical cytologic appearance of the follicular epithelial cells can be misinterpreted as a vascular neoplasm such as an angiosarcoma.

- In most instances and with some exceptions, surgical removal is the treatment of choice for a thyroid mass regardless of the diagnosis by FNA.
- The pathologist must be aware of the diversity of changes that can be induced by FNA in the thyroid gland.
- These post-FNA histologic changes occur in numerous lesions such as adenomatoid nodules, follicular adenoma and its variants, follicular carcinoma and its variants, papillary carcinoma and its variants, and hyperplastic lesions.
- The histologic alterations caused by FNA may lead to an erroneous diagnosis such as changing the interpretation from a benign process to a malignant one.
- Based on the type of reaction seen, post-FNA alterations may include acute or chronic changes.
- Acute changes are usually identified within 3 weeks from the FNA to surgical excision of a mass and may include the following:
  - Hemorrhage with hemosiderin-laden macrophages and granulation tissue (these are the most common findings).

- Localized follicular destruction.
- Capsular alterations.
- Atypical cytologic features with necrosis and mitoses; the nuclear atypia is reactive or reparative, typically occurs near the needle tract, and includes nuclear enlargement with clearing of the nuclear chromatin.
- Chronic changes are usually identified more than three weeks from the FNA to surgical excision of a mass and may include:
  - Metaplasia, squamous or oxyphilic.
  - Infarction.
  - Capsular alterations with foci of pseudoinvasive growth.
  - Vascular alterations, including (1) artifactual implantation or "invasion" of tumor cells—in this setting, the cells float within the vascular lumina and are not adherent to the vessel wall as in true vascular invasion; (2) dilated vascular spaces with thrombosis, organization, and papillary endothelial hyperplasia; and (3) endothelial cell atypia.
  - Cyst formation with papillary growth.
  - Fibrosis and calcification.
  - Random nuclear atypia.
  - Cholesterol granulomas.
- Oxyphilic cells occurring in all settings (metaplasia, follicular adenoma, follicular carcinoma, or papillary carcinoma) may be more sensitive to trauma because of the oxygen-sensitive mitochondria that predominate in these cells. Any compromise to the oxygen supply of the oxyphilic cells may result in degenerative changes that are not seen as readily in nonoxyphilic cells. Among these changes are hemorrhage, infarction, and papillary degeneration.
- The vascular alterations seen may suggest the presence of a vascular tumor such as a hemangioma or even an angiosarcoma. This possibility may be problematic, and the temporal sequence from the FNA to surgical removal is an important factor in the interpretation of these findings.

Bibliography

Thyroid Neoplasms—General Considerations

Bondeson L, Bengtsson A, Bondeson A-G, et al. Chromosome studies in thyroid neoplasia. Cancer 1989; 64:680–685.

Cady B, Sedgwick CE, Meissner WA, et al. Risk factor in differentiated thyroid cancer. Cancer 1979; 43:810–820.

Chen H, Nicol TL, Udelsman R. Follicular lesions of the thyroid: Does frozen section evaluation alter operative management? Ann Surg 1995; 222:1–6.

de Souza FM. Role of subtotal thyroidectomy in the management of the follicular neoplasm of the thyroid. Laryngoscope 1993; 103:477–493.

Ezaki H, Ebihara S, Fujimoto Y, et al. Analysis of thyroid carcinoma based on material registered in Japan during 1977–1986 with special reference to predominance of papillary type. Cancer 1992; 70:808–814.

Grossman RF, Tu SH, Siperstein AE, et al. Familial nonmedullary thyroid cancer: An emerging entity that warrants aggressive management. Arch Surg 1995; 130:892–897.

Harach HR, Williams GT, Williams ED. Familial adenomatous polyposis associated with thyroid carcinoma: A distinct type of follicular cell neoplasm. Histopathology 1994; 25:549–561.

Hedinger C, Williams ED, Sobin LH. The WHO histological classification of thyroid tumors: A commentary on the second edition. Cancer 1989; 63:908–911.

LiVolsi VA: Thyroid tumors. In: Surgical Pathology of the Thyroid: Major Problems in Pathology. Vol. 22. Philadelphia: WB Saunders, 1990, pp. 131–135.

Lote K, Andersen K, Nordal E, Brennhovd IO. Familial occurrence of papillary thyroid carcinoma. Cancer 1980; 46:1291–1297.

Mazzaferri EL. Treating differentiated thyroid carcinoma: Where do we draw the line? Mayo Clin Proc 1991; 66:105–111.

Mazzaferri EL. Carcinoma of follicular epithelium: Radioiodine and other treatment and outcomes. In: Braverman LE, Utiger RD, eds. Werner and Ingbar's The Thyroid: A Fundamental and Clinical Text, 6th ed. Philadelphia: JB Lippincott, 1991, pp. 1138–1165.

Plail RO, Bussey HJ, Glazer G, Thompson JP. Adenomatous polyposis: An association with carcinoma of the thyroid. Br J Surg 1987; 74:377–380.

Rosai J, Carcangiu ML, DeLellis RA: Thyroid tumors—general considerations. In: Rosai J, Sobin LH, eds. Tumors of the Thyroid Gland: Atlas of Tumor Pathology, Third series, Fascicle 5. Washington, DC: Armed Forces Institute of Pathology, 1992, pp. 327–338.

Schneider AB. Carcinoma of follicular epithelium: Pathogenesis. In: Braverman LE, Utiger RD, eds. Werner and Ingbar's The Thyroid: A Fundamental and Clinical Text, 6th ed. Philadelphia: JB Lippincott, 1991, pp. 1121–1129.

Siperstein AE, Clark OH. Carcinoma of follicular epithelium: Surgical therapy. In: Braverman LE, Utiger RD, eds. Werner and Ingbar's The Thyroid: A Fundamental and Clinical Text, 6th ed. Philadelphia: JB Lippincott, 1991, pp. 1129–1137.

Sridama V, Hara Y, Fauchet R, DeGroot LJ. Association of differentiated thyroid carcinoma and HLA-DR7. Cancer 1985; 56:1086–1088.

Sugenoya A, Shingu K, Kobayashi S, et al. Surgical strategies for differentiated carcinoma of the isthmus. Head Neck 1993; 15:158–160.

Benign Follicular Epithelial Neoplasms

Follicular Adenoma

Akslen LA, Myking AO. Differentiated thyroid carcinomas: The relevance of various pathological features for tumour classification and prediction of tumour progress. Virchows Arch [A] 1992; 421:17–23.

Böcker W, Raille H, Koch G, et al. Immunohistochemical and electron microscope analysis of adenomas of the thyroid gland: II. Adenomas with specific cytologic differentiation. Virchows Arch [A] 1978; 380:205–220.

Carcangiu ML, Sibly RK, Rosai J. Clear cell change in primary thyroid tumors: A study of 38 cases. Am J Surg Pathol 1985; 9:705–722.

Evans HL. Follicular neoplasms of the thyroid: A study of 44 cases followed for a minimum of 10 years, with emphasis on differential diagnosis. Cancer 1984; 54:535–540.

Greenebaum E, Koss LG, Elequin F, Silver CE. The diagnostic value of flow cytometric DNA measurements in follicular tumors of the thyroid gland. Cancer 1985; 56:2011–2018.

Hicks DG, LiVolsi VA, Neidich JA, et al. Clonal analysis of solitary follicular nodules in the thyroid. Am J Pathol 1990; 137:553–562.

Hostetter AL, Hrafnkelsson J, Winegren SO, et al. A comparative study of DNA cytometry methods for benign and malignant thyroid tissue. Am J Clin Pathol 1988; 89:760–763.

Hruban RH, Huvos AG, Traganos F, et al. Follicular neoplasms of the thyroid in men older than 50 years of age: A DNA flow cytometric study. Am J Clin Pathol 1990; 94:527–532.

Kini SR. Follicular adenoma and carcinoma. In: Kini SR, ed. Guides to Clinical Aspiration Biopsy. Thyroid. 2nd edition. New York: Igaku-Shoin, 1996, pp. 59–103.

Yamashina M. Follicular neoplasms of the thyroid: Total circumferential evaluation of the fibrous capsule. Am J Surg Pathol 1990; 16:392–400.

Follicular Adenoma with Atypical Features

Franssilla KO, Ackerman LV, Brown CL, Hedinger CE. Follicular carcinoma. Semin Diagn Pathol 1985; 2:101–122.

Hazard JB, Kenyon R. Atypical adenoma of the thyroid. Arch Pathol Lab Med 1954; 58:554–563.

Lang W, Georgi A, Stauch G, Kienzle E. The differentiation of atypical adenomas and encapsulated follicular carcinomas in the thyroid gland. Virchows Arch [A] 1980; 385:125–141.

Lang W, Georgi A. Minimally invasive cancer in the thyroid. Clin Oncol 1982; 1:527–537.

Hyalinizing Trabecular Adenoma

Bronner MP, LiVolsi VA, Jennings TA. PLAT: Paraganglioma-like adenomas of the thyroid. Surg Pathol 1988; 1:383–389.

Carney JA, Ryan J, Goellner JR: Hyalinizing trabecular adenoma of the thyroid gland. Am J Surg Pathol 1987; 11:583–591.

Chan JK, Tse CC, Chiu HS. Hyalinizing trabecular adenoma-like lesion in multinodular goitre. Histopathology 1990; 16:611–614.

Chetty R, Beydoun R, LiVolsi VA. Paraganglioma-like (hyalinizing trabecular) adenoma of the thyroid revisited. Pathology 1994; 26:429–431.

Goellner JR, Carney JA: Cytologic features of fine needle aspirates of hyalinizing trabecular adenoma of the thyroid gland. Am J Clin Pathol 1989; 91:115–119.

Katoh R, Jasani B, Williams ED. Hyalinizing trabecular adenoma of the thyroid: A report of three cases with immunohistochemical and ultrastructural studies. Histopathology 1989; 15:211–224.

Molberg K, Albores-Saavedra J. Hyalinizing trabecular carcinoma of the thyroid gland. Hum Pathol 1994; 25:192–197.

Scopa CD, Melachrinou M, Saradopoulou C, Merino MJ: The significance of the grooved nucleus in thyroid lesions. Mod Pathol 1993; 6:691–694.

Follicular Adenoma with Oxyphilia

Bondeson L, Bondeson A-G, Ljunberg O, Tibblin S. Oxyphil tumors of the thyroid: Follow-up of 42 surgical cases. Ann Surg 1981; 194:677–680.

Bronner MP, LiVolsi VA. Oxyphilic (Askanazy/Hürthle cell) tumors of the thyroid: Microscopic features predict biologic behavior. Surg Pathol 1988; 1:137–150.

Caplan RH, Abellera RM, Kisken WA. Hürthle cell tumors of the thyroid gland: A clinicopathologic review and long-term follow-up. JAMA 1984; 251:3114–3117.

Carcangiu ML, Bianchi S, Savino D, et al. Hürthle cell neoplasms of the thyroid gland: A study of 153 cases. Cancer 1991; 68:1944–1953.

Flint A, Lloyd RV. Hürthle cell neoplasms of the thyroid gland. Pathol Annu 1990; 25(Part 1):37–52.

Gosain AK, Clark OH. Hürthle cell neoplasms: Malignant potential. Arch Surg 1984; 119:515–519.

Johnson TL, Lloyd RV, Burney RE, Thompson NW. Hürthle cell thyroid tumors: An immunohistochemical study. Cancer 1987; 59:107–112.

Kendall CH, McCluskey E, Naylor J. Oxyphil cells in thyroid disease: A uniform change? J Clin Pathol 1986; 39:908–912.

Kini SR, Miller JM, Hamburger JI. Cytopathology of Hürthle cell lesions of the thyroid gland by fine needle aspiration. Acta Cytol 1981; 25:647–652.

McLeod MK, Thompson NW. Hürthle cell neoplasms of the thyroid. Otolaryngol Clin North Am 1990; 23:441–452.

Nesland JM, Sobrinho-Simões MA, Holm R, et al. Hürthle cell lesions of the thyroid: A combined study using transmission electron microscopy, scanning electron microscopy, and immunocytochemistry. Ultrastruct Pathol 1985; 8:269–290.

Follicular Adenoma with Clear Cells

Carcangiu ML, Sibley RK, Rosai J. Clear cell change in primary thyroid tumors: A study of 38 cases. Am J Surg Pathol 1985; 9:705–722.

Harach HR, Virgili E, Soler G, et al. Cytopathology of follicular tumours of the thyroid with clear cell change. Cytopathology 1991; 2:125–135.

Rosai J, Carcangiu ML, DeLellis RA: Tumors with clear cell features. In: Rosai J, Sobin LH, eds. Tumors of the Thyroid Gland: Atlas of Tumor Pathology, Third series, Fascicle 5. Washington, DC: Armed Forces Institute of Pathology, 1992, pp. 183–193.

Follicular Adenoma with Signet Ring Cells

Alsop JE, Yerbury PJ, O'Donnell PJ, Heydermann E. Signet ring cell microfollicular adenoma arising in a nodular ectopic thyroid: A case report. J Oral Pathol 1986; 15:518–519.

Brisigotti M, Lorenzini P, Alessi A, et al. Mucin-producing adenoma of the thyroid gland. Tumori 1986; 72:211–214.

Gherardi G. Signet ring cell "mucinous" thyroid adenoma: A follicle cell tumour with abnormal accumulation of thyroglobulin and a peculiar histochemical profile. Histopathology 1987; 11:317–326.

Mendelsohn G. Signet ring cell adenoma simulating microfollicular adenoma of the thyroid. Am J Surg Pathol 1984; 8:705–708.

Schröder S, Böcker W. Signet ring cell thyroid tumors: Follicle cell tumors with arrest of folliculogenesis. Am J Surg Pathol 1985; 9:619–629.

Rigaud C, Peltier F, Bogomoletz WV. Mucin-producing microfollicular adenoma of the thyroid. J Clin Pathol 1985; 38:277–280.

Rosai J, Carcangiu ML, DeLellis RA: Tumors with clear cell features. In: Rosai J, Sobin LH, eds. Tumors of the Thyroid Gland: Atlas of Tumor

Pathology. Third series, Fascicle 5. Washington, DC: Armed Forces Institute of Pathology, 1992, pp. 183–193.

Follicular Adenoma with Fat

Gnepp DR, Ogorzalek JM, Heffess CS. Fat-containing lesions of he thyroid gland. Am J Surg Pathol 1989; 13:605–612.

Schröder S, Böcker W. Adenolipoma (thyrolipoma) of the thyroid gland: Report of two cases and review of the literature. Virchows Arch [A] 1984; 404:99–103.

Schröder S, Hüsselmann H, Böcker W. Lipid-rich cell adenoma of the thyroid gland: Report of a peculiar thyroid tumour. Virchows Arch [A] 1984; 404:105–108.

Malignant Follicular Epithelial Neoplasms

Follicular Carcinoma

Akslen LA, Myking AO. Differentiated thyroid carcinomas: The relevance of various pathological features for tumour classification and prediction of tumour progress. Virchows Arch [A] 1992; 421:17–23.

Brennan MD, Bregstralh EJ, van Heerden JA, McConahey WM. Follicular thyroid cancer treated at the Mayo Clinic, 1946 through 1970: Initial manifestations, pathologic features, therapy, and outcome. Mayo Clin Proc 1991; 66:11–22.

Clark OH. Total thyroidectomy: The treatment of choice for patients with differentiated thyroid cancer. Ann Surg 1982; 196:361–370.

Emerick GT, Duh QY, Siperstein AE, et al. Diagnosis, treatment, and outcome of follicular thyroid carcinoma. Cancer 1993; 72:3287–3295.

Evans HL. Follicular neoplasms of the thyroid: A study of 44 cases followed for a minimum of 10 years, with emphasis on differential diagnosis. Cancer 1984; 54:535–540.

Fransilla KO, Ackerman LV, Brown CL, Hedinger CE. Follicular carcinoma. Semin Diagn Pathol 1985; 2:101–122.

Harness JK, Thompson NW, McLeod MK, et al. Follicular carcinoma of the thyroid gland: Trends and treatment. Surgery 1984; 96:972–980.

Hazard JB, Kenyon R. Atypical adenoma of the thyroid. Arch Pathol Lab Med 1954; 58:554–563.

Hazard JB, Kenyon R. Encapsulated angioinvasive carcinoma (angioinvasive adenoma) of the thyroid gland. Am J Clin Pathol 1954; 24:755–766.

Hruban RH, Huvos AG, Traganos F, et al. Follicular neoplasms of the thyroid in men older than 50 years of age: A DNA flow cytometric study. Am J Clin Pathol 1990; 94:527–532.

Kahn NF, Perzin KH. Follicular carcinoma of the thyroid: An evaluation of the histologic criteria used for diagnosis. Pathol Annu 1983; 18:221–253.

Kini SR. Follicular adenoma and carcinoma. In: Kini SR, ed. Guides to Clinical Aspiration Biopsy. Thyroid. 2nd edition. New York: Igaku-Shoin, 1996, pp. 59–103.

Lang W, Choritz H, Hundeshagen H. Risk factors in follicular thyroid carcinomas: A retrospective follow-up study covering a 14-year period with emphasis on morphological findings. Am J Surg Pathol 1986; 10:246–255.

Lang W, Georgi A, Stauch G, Kienzle E. The differentiation of atypical adenomas and encapsulated follicular carcinomas in the thyroid gland. Virchows Arch [A] 1980; 385:125–141.

Lang W, Georgi A. Minimally invasive cancer in the thyroid. Clin Oncol 1982; 1:527–537.

Paul SJ, Sisson JC. Thyrotoxicosis caused by thyroid cancer. Endocrinol Metab Clin North Am 1990; 19:593–612.

Schlumberger M, Tubiana M, De Vathaire F, et al. Long-term results of treatment in 283 patients with lung and bone metastases from differentiated thyroid carcinoma. J Clin Endocrinol Metab 1986; 63:960–967.

Schröder DM, Chambors A, Frances CJ. Operative strategy for thyroid cancer: Is total thyroidectomy worth the price? Cancer 1986; 58:2320–2328.

Segal K, Arad A, Lubin E, et al. Follicular carcinoma of the thyroid. Head Neck 1994; 16:533–538.

Starnes HF, Brooks DC, Pinkus GS, Brooks JR. Surgery for thyroid cancer. Cancer 1985; 55:1376–1381.

Warren S. Significance of invasion of blood vessels of the thyroid gland. Arch Pathol 1931; 11:255–257.

Warren S. Invasion of blood vessels in thyroid cancer. Am J Clin Pathol 1956; 26:64–65.

Yamashina M. Follicular neoplasms of the thyroid: Total circumferential evaluation of the fibrous capsule. Am J Surg Pathol 1990; 16:392–400.

Variants of Follicular Carcinoma

Carcangiu ML, Bianchi S, Savino D, et al. Hürthle cell neoplasms of the thyroid gland: A study of 153 cases. Cancer 1991; 68:1944–1953.

Carcangiu ML, Sibley RK, Rosai J. Clear cell change in primary thyroid tumors: A study of 38 cases. Am J Surg Pathol 1985; 9:705–722.

Civantos F, Albores-Saavedra J, Nadji M, Morales AR. Clear cell variant of thyroid carcinoma. Am J Surg Pathol 1984; 8:187–192.

Grant CS. Operative and postoperative management of the patient with follicular and Hürthle cell carcinoma. Do they differ? Surg Clin North Am 1995; 75:395–403.

Gundry SR, Burney RE, Thompson NW, Lloyd R. Total thyroidectomy for Hürthle cell neoplasm of the thyroid. Arch Surg 1983; 118:529–532.

McLeod MK, Thompson NW. Hürthle cell neoplasms of the thyroid. Otolaryngol Clin North Am 1990; 23:441–452.

Molberg K, Albores-Saavedra J. Hyalinizing trabecular carcinoma of the thyroid gland. Hum Pathol 1994; 25:192–197.

Schröder S, Böcker W. Clear cell carcinomas of the thyroid gland: A clinicopathological study of 13 cases. Histopathology 1986; 10:75–89.

Schröder S, Pfannschmidt N, Dralle H, et al. The encapsulated follicular adenoma of the thyroid. Virchows Arch [A] 1984; 402:259–273.

Watson RG, Brennan MD, Goellner JR, et al. Invasive Hürthle cell carcinoma of the thyroid: Natural history and management. Mayo Clin Proc 1984; 59:851–855.

Thyroid Papillary Carcinoma

Akslen LA, Myking AO. Differentiated thyroid carcinomas: The relevance of various pathological features for tumour classification and prediction of tumour progress. Virchows Arch [A] 1992; 421:17–23.

Carcangiu ML, Zampi G, Pupi A, et al. Papillary carcinoma of the thyroid: A clinicopathologic study of 241 cases treated at the University of Florence, Italy. Cancer 1985; 55:805–828.

Dinneen SF, Valimaki MJ, Bergstralh EJ, et al. Distant metastases in papillary thyroid cancer: 100 cases observed at one institution during 5 decades. J Clin Endocrinol Metab 1995; 80:2041–2045.

Francis IM, Das DK, Sheikh ZA, et al. Role of nuclear grooves in the diagnosis of papillary thyroid carcinoma: A quantitative assessment of fine needle aspiration smears. Acta Cytol 1995; 39:409–415.

Grossman RF, Tu SH, Siperstein AE, et al. Familial nonmedullary thyroid cancer: An emerging entity that warrants aggressive management. Arch Surg 1995; 130:892–897.

Hancock SL, McDougall IR, Constine LS. Thyroid abnormalities after therapeutic external radiation. Int J Radiat Oncol Biol Phys 1995; 31:1165–1170.

Hara H, Fulton N, Yashiro T, et al. N-*ras* mutation: An independent prognostic factor for aggressiveness of papillary thyroid carcinoma. Surgery 1994; 116:1010–1016.

Harach HR, Escalante DA, Oñativia A, et al. Thyroid carcinoma and thyroiditis in an endemic goitre region before and after iodine prophylaxis. Acta Endocrinol 1985; 108:55–60.

Harach HR, Williams ED. Childhood thyroid cancer in England and Wales. Br J Cancer 1995; 72:777–783.

Hay ID, Grant CS, Taylor WF, McConahey WM: Ipsilateral lobectomy versus bilateral lobar resection in papillary thyroid carcinoma: A retrospective analysis of surgical outcome using a novel prognostic scoring system. Surgery 1987; 102:1088–1095.

Hedman I, Tisell L-E. Associated hyperparathyroidism and nonmedullary thyroid carcinoma: The etiologic role of radiation. Surgery 1984; 95:392–397.

Hofstädter F. Frequency and morphology of malignant tumours of the thyroid before and after introduction of iodine-prophylaxis. Virchows Arch [A] 1980; 385:263–270.

Johannessen JV, Sobrinho-Simões M: The origin and significance of thyroid psammoma bodies. Lab Invest 1980; 43:287–296.

Kini SR. Papillary carinoma. In: Kini SR, ed. Guides to Clinical Aspiration Biopsy Thyroid. 2nd ed. New York: Igaku-Shoin, 1996; pp. 129–223.

LiVolsi VA: Papillary neoplasms of the thyroid: Pathologic and prognostic features. Am J Clin Pathol 1992; 97:426–434.

Lote K, Andersen K, Nordal E, Brennhovd IO. Familial occurrence of papillary thyroid carcinoma. Cancer 1980; 46:1291–1297.

Mazzaferri EL. Papillary thyroid carcinoma: Factors influencing prognosis and current therapy. Semin Oncol 1987; 14:315–332.

Mazzaferri EL, Young RL, Oertel JE, et al. Papillary thyroid carcinoma: The impact of therapy in 576 patients. Medicine 1977; 56:171–196.

McConahey WM, Hay ID, et al. Papillary thyroid cancer treated at the Mayo Clinic, 1946 through 1970: Initial manifestations, pathologic findings, therapy, and outcome. Mayo Clin Proc 1986; 61:978–996.

Moir CR, Telander RL. Papillary carcinoma of the thyroid in children. Semin Pediatr Surg 1994; 3:182–187.

Moreno-Egea A, Rodriguez-Gonzalez JM, Sola-Perz J, et al. Mutlivariate analysis of histopathological features as prognostic factors in patients with papillary thyroid carcinoma. Br J Surg 1995; 82:1092–1094.

Nikiforov YE, Heffess CS, Korzenko AV, et al. Characteristics of follicular tumors and non-neoplastic thyroid lesions in children and adolescents exposed to radiation as a result of the Chernobyl disaster. Cancer 1995; 76:900–909.

Patwardhan N, Cataldo T, Braverman LE. Surgical management of the patient with papillary cancer. Surg Clin North Am 1995; 75:449–464.

Plail RO, Bussey HJ, Glazer G, Thompson JP. Adenomatous polyposis: An association with carcinoma of the thyroid. Br J Surg 1987; 74:377–380.

Scopa CD, Melachrinou M, Saradopoulou C, Merino MJ. The significance of the grooved nucleus in thyroid lesions. Mod Pathol 1993; 6:691–694.

Sridama V, Hara Y, Fauchet R, DeGroot LJ. Association of differentiated thyroid carcinoma and HLA-DR7. Cancer 1985; 56:1086–1088.

Vickery AL, Wang C-A, Walker AM: Treatment of intrathyroidal papillary carcinoma of the thyroid. Cancer 1987; 60:2587–2595.

Vickery AL Jr: Thyroid papillary carcinoma: Pathological and philosophical controversies. Am J Surg Pathol 1983; 7:797–807.

Occult, Small, or Microscopic Papillary Carcinoma

Bondeson L, Ljungberg O. Occult papillary thyroid carcinoma in the young and the aged. Cancer 1984; 53:1790–1792.

Franssila KO, Harach HR. Occult papillary carcinoma of the thyroid in children and young adults: A systemic autopsy study in Finland. Cancer 1986; 58:715–719.

Gikas PW, Labow SS, DiGiulio W, Finger JE. Occult metastasis from occult papillary carcinoma of the thyroid. Cancer 1967; 20:2100–2104.

Harach HR, Franssila KO, Wasenius VM. Occult papillary carcinoma of the thyroid—a "normal" finding in Finland: A systematic autopsy study. Cancer 1985; 56:531–558.

Hazard JB. Small papillary carcinoma of the thyroid: A study with special reference to so-called nonencapsulated sclerosing tumor. Lab Invest 1960; 9:86–97.

Hubert JP Jr, Keirnan PD, Beahrs OH, et al. Occult papillary carcinoma of the thyroid. Arch Surg 1980; 115:394–398.

Kasai N, Sakamoto A. New subgrouping of small thyroid carcinoma. Cancer 1987; 60:1767–1770.

Klinck GH, Winship T. Occult sclerosing carcinoma of the thyroid. Cancer 1955; 8:701–706.

Lang W, Borrusch H, Bauer L. Occult carcinomas of the thyroid: Evaluation of 1020 sequential autopsies. Am J Clin Pathol 1988; 90:72–76.

Strate SM, Lee EL, Childers JH. Occult papillary carcinoma of the thyroid with distant metastases. Cancer 1984; 54:1093–1100.

Yamamoto Y, Maeda T, Izumi K, Otsuku H. Occult papillary carcinoma of the thyroid: A study of 408 autopsy cases. Cancer 1990; 65:1173–1179.

Encapsulated Type of Papillary Carcinoma

Evans HL. Encapsulated papillary neoplasms of the thyroid: A study of 14 cases followed for a minimum of 10 years. Am J Surg Pathol 1987; 11:592–597.

Schröder S, Böcker W, Dralle H, et al. The encapsulated papillary carcinoma of the thyroid: A morphologic subtype of the papillary thyroid carcinoma. Cancer 1984; 54:90–93.

Follicular Type of Papillary Carcinoma

Chen KT, Rosai J. Follicular variant of thyroid papillary carcinoma: A clinicopathologic study of six cases. Am J Surg Pathol 1986; 85:77–80.

Rosai J, Zampi G, Carcangiu ML. Papillary carcinoma of the thyroid: A discussion of its several morphologic expressions, with particular emphasis on the follicular variant. Am J Surg Pathol 1983; 7:809–817.

Tielens ET, Sherman SI, Hruban RH, Ladenson PW. Follicular variant of papillary thyroid carcinoma: A clinicopathologic study. Cancer 1994; 73:424–431.

Macrofollicular Type of Papillary Carcinoma

Albores-Saavedra J, Gould E, Vardaman C, Vuitch F. The macrofollicular variant of papillary thyroid carcinoma: A study of 17 cases. Am J Clin Pathol 1990; 94:442–445.

Oncocytic Papillary Carcinoma

Beckner M, Heffess CS, Oertel JE. Oxyphilic papillary thyroid carcinomas. Am J Clin Pathol 1995; 103:180–187.

Chen KTK. Fine-needle aspiration cytology of papillary Hürthle-cell tumors of thyroid: A report of three cases. Diagn Cytopathol 1991; 7:53–56.

Dickersin GR, Vickery AL Jr, Smith SB. Papillary carcinoma of the thyroid, oxyphil cell type, "clear cell" variant: A light and electron microscopic study. Am J Surg Pathol 1980; 4:501–509.

Herrera MF, Hay ID, Wu PS, et al. Hürthle cell (oxyphilic) papillary thyroid carcinoma: A variant with more aggressive biologic behavior. World J Surg 1992; 16:669–675.

Sobrinho-Simões MA, Nesland JM, Holm R, et al. Hürthle cell and mitochondrion-rich papillary carcinomas of the thyroid gland: An ultrastructural and immunocytochemical study. Ultrastruct Pathol 1985; 8:131–142.

Clear Cell Type of Papillary Carcinoma

Carcangiu ML, Sibley RK, Rosai J. Clear cell changes in primary thyroid tumors: A study of 38 cases. Am J Surg Pathol 1985; 9:705–722.

Graham LD, Roe SM. Metastatic papillary carcinoma presenting as a primary renal neoplasm. Am Surg 1995; 61:732–734.

Meissner WA, Adler A. Papillary carcinoma of the thyroid: A study of the pathology of two hundred twenty-six cases. Arch Pathol 1958; 66:518–525.

Variakojis D, Getz ML, Paloyan E, Straus FH. Papillary clear cell carcinoma of the thyroid gland. Hum Pathol 1975; 6:384–390.

Diffuse Sclerosing Type of Papillary Carcinoma

Carcangiu ML, Bianchi S. Diffuse sclerosing variant of papillary thyroid carcinoma: Clinicopathologic study of 15 cases. Am J Surg Pathol 1989; 13:1041–1049.

Chan JKC, Tsui MS, Tse CH. Diffuse sclerosing variant of papillary carcinoma of the thyroid: A histological and immunohistochemical study of three cases. Histopathology 1987; 11:191–201.

Fujimoto Y, Obara T, Ito Y, et al. Diffuse sclerosing variant of papillary carcinoma of the thyroid: Clinical importance, surgical treatment, and follow-up study. Cancer 1990; 66:2306–2312.

Gómez-Morales M, Alvaro T, Muñoz M, et al. Diffuse sclerosing papillary carcinoma of the thyroid gland: Immunohistochemical analysis of local host immune response. Histopathology 1991; 18:427–433.

Hayashi Y, Sasao T, Takeichi N, et al. Diffuse sclerosing variant of papillary carcinoma of the thyroid: A histopathological study of four cases. Acta Pathol Jpn 1990; 40:193–198.

Rousselet MC, Guyetant S, Croue A, et al. Diffuse sclerosing papillary carcinoma of the thyroid gland: Apropos of a pediatric case of association of an unilateral tumor with diffuse lymphocytic thyroiditis. Arch Anat Cytol Pathol 1994; 42:10–15.

Soares J, Limbert E, Sobrinho-Simões M. Diffuse sclerosing variant of papillary thyroid carcinoma: A clinicopathologic study of 10 cases. Pathol Res Pract 1989; 185:200–206.

Vickery AL Jr, Carcangiu ML, Johannessen JV, Sobrinho-Simões M. Papillary carcinoma. Semin Diagn Pathol 1985; 2:90–100.

Tall Cell Type of Papillary Carcinoma

Flint A, Davenport RD, Lloyd RV. The tall cell variant of papillary carcinoma of the thyroid gland: Comparison with the common form of papillary carcinoma by DNA and morphologic analysis. Arch Pathol Lab Med 1991; 115:169–171.

Harach HR, Zusman SB. Cytopathology of the tall cell variant of thyroid papillary carcinoma. Acta Cytol 1992; 36:895–899.

Hawk WA, Hazard JB. The many appearances of papillary carcinoma of the thyroid. Clev Clin Q 1976; 43:207–216.

Johnson TL, Lloyd RV, Thompson NW, et al. Prognostic implications of the tall cell variant of papillary thyroid carcinoma. Am J Surg Pathol 1988; 12:22–27.

Ostrowski ML, Merino MJ. Tall cell variant of papillary thyroid carcinoma: A reassessment and immunohistochemical study with comparison to the usual type of papillary carcinoma of the thyroid. Am J Surg Pathol 1996; 20:964–974.

Ozaki O, Ito K, Mimura T, et al. Papillary carcinoma of the thyroid: Tall cell variant with extensive lymphocyte infiltration. Am J Surg Pathol 1996; 20:695–698.

Tscholl-Ducommun J, Hedinger CE. Papillary thyroid carcinoma: Morphology and prognosis. Virchows Arch [A] 1982; 396:19–39.

Columnar Cell Type of Papillary Carcinoma

Akslen LA, Varhaug JE. Thyroid carcinoma with mixed tall cell and columnar cell features. Am J Clin Pathol 1990; 94:442–445.

Berends D, Mouthaan PJ. Columnar cell carcinoma of the thyroid. Histopathology 1992; 20:36–42.

Evans HL. Columnar cell carcinoma of the thyroid: A report of two cases of an aggressive variant of thyroid carcinoma. Am J Clin Pathol 1986; 85:77–80.

Evans HL. Encapsulated columnar cell neoplasms of the thyroid: A report of four cases suggesting a favorable prognosis. Am J Surg Pathol 1996; 20:1205–1211.

Ferreiro JA, Lloyd RV. Columnar cell carcinoma of the thyroid: Report of three additional cases. Hum Pathol 1996; 27:1156–1160.

Gaertner EM, Davidson M, Wenig BM. The columnar cell variant of thyroid papillary carcinoma: Case report and discussion of an unusually aggressive thyroid carcinoma. Am J Surg Pathol 1995; 19:940–947.

Hawk WA, Hazard JB. The many appearances of papillary carcinoma of the thyroid. Clev Clin Q 1976; 43:207–216.

Hui PH, Chan JKC, Cheung PSY, Gwi E. Columnar cell carcinoma of the thyroid: Fine needle aspiration findings in a case. Acta Cytol 1990; 34:355–358.

Mizukami Y, Nonomura A, Michigishi T, et al. Columnar cell carcinoma of the thyroid gland: A case report and review of the literature. Hum Pathol 1994; 25:1098–1101.

Sobrinho-Simões M, Nesland JM, Johannessen JV. Columnar cell carcinoma: Another variant of poorly differentiated carcinoma of the thyroid. Am J Clin Pathol 1988; 89:264–267.

Wenig BM, Thompson LDR, Adair CF, Heffess CS. Columnar cell variant of thyroid papillary carcinoma. Mod Pathol 1995; 8:56A.

Undifferentiated (Anaplastic) Carcinoma and Insular Carcinoma

Ashfaq R, Vuitch F, Delgado R, Albores-Saavedra J. Papillary and follicular thyroid carcinomas with an insular component. Cancer 1994; 73:416–423.

Ashfaq R, Vuitch F, Delgado R, Albores-Saavedra J. Author reply. Cancer 1995; 74:2599–2600.

Carcangiu ML, Steeper T, Zampi G, Rosai J. Anaplastic thyroid carcinoma: A study of 70 cases. Am J Clin Pathol 1985; 83:135–158.

Carcangiu ML, Zampi G, Rosai J. Poorly differentiated ("insular") thyroid carcinoma: A reinterpretation of Langhans' "wuchernde struma." Am J Surg Pathol 1984; 8:655–668.

Flynn SD, Forman BH, Stewart AF, Kinder BK. Poorly differentiated ("insular") carcinoma of the thyroid gland: An aggressive subset of differentiated thyroid neoplasms. Surgery 1988; 104:963–970.

LiVolsi VA. Undifferentiated or anaplastic carcinoma of the thyroid. In: Bennington JL, ed. Surgical Pathology of the Thyroid. Major Problems in Pathology. Vol. 22. Philadelphia: WB Saunders, 1990, pp. 253–274.

Ordóñez NG, El-Naggar AK, Hickey RC, Samaan NA: Anaplastic thyroid carcinoma: Immunocytochemical study of 32 cases. Am J Clin Pathol 1991; 96:15–24.

Papotti M, Botta Micca F, Favero A, et al. Poorly differentiated thyroid carcinomas with primordial cell component: A group of aggressive lesions sharing insular, trabecular, and solid patterns. Am J Surg Pathol 1993; 17:291–301.

Papotti M, Bussolati G. Papillary and follicular thyroid carcinomas with an insular component. Cancer 1994; 74:2599.

Rosai J, Carcangiu ML, DeLellis RA. Undifferentiated (anaplastic) carcinoma. In: Rosai J, Sobin LH, eds. Tumors of the Thyroid Gland: Atlas of Tumor Pathology. Third series, Fascicle 5. Washington, DC: Armed Forces Institute of Pathology, 1992, pp. 135–159.

Unusual Epithelial Tumors of the Thyroid Gland: Primary Thyroid Mucoepidermoid Carcinoma, Adenosquamous Carcinoma of the Thyroid, and Squamous Cell Carcinoma

Bakri K, Shimoaka K, Rao U, Tsukada Y. Adenosquamous carcinoma of the thyroid after radiotherapy for Hodgkin's disease. Cancer 1983; 52:465–470.

Harada T, Shimoaka K, Katagiri M, et al. Rarity of squamous cell carcinoma of the thyroid: Autopsy review. World J Surg 1994; 18:542–546.

Huang TY, Assor D. Primary squamous cell carcinoma of the thyroid gland: A report of four cases. Am J Surg Pathol 1971; 55:93–98.

Simpson WJ, Carruthers J. Squamous cell carcinoma of the thyroid gland. Am J Surg 1988; 156:44–46.

Wenig BM, Adair CF, Heffess CS. Primary mucoepidermoid carcinoma of the thyroid gland: A report of six cases and a review of the literature of a follicular epithelial-derived tumor. Hum Pathol 1995; 26:1099–1108.

C-Cell–Related Lesions: C-Cell Hyperplasia and Medullary Carcinoma

Albores-Saavedra J, Monforte H, Nadji M, Morales AR. C-cell hyperplasia in thyroid tissue adjacent to follicular cell tumors. Hum Pathol 1988; 19:795–799.

Barbot N, Calmettes C, Schuffenecker I, et al. Pentagastrin stimulation test and early diagnosis of medullary thyroid carcinoma using an immunoradiometric assay of calcitonin: Comparison with genetic screening in hereditary medullary thyroid carcinoma. J Clin Endocrinol Metab 1994; 78:114–120.

Biddinger PW, Ray M. Distribution of C cells in the normal and diseased thyroid gland. Pathol Annu 1993; 28(Part 1):205–229.

Bose S, Kapila K, Verma K. Medullary carcinoma of the thyroid: A cytological, immunocytochemical, and ultrastructural study. Diagn Cytopathol 1992; 8:28–32.

de Bustros AC, Baylin SB. Medullary carcinoma of the thyroid. In: Braverman LE, Utiger RD, eds. Werner and Ingbar's The Thyroid: A Fundamental and Clinical Text, 6th ed. Philadelphia: JB Lippincott, 1991, pp. 1167–1183.

DeLellis RA, Wolfe HJ. The pathobiology of the human calcitonin (C) cell: A review. Pathol Annu 1981; 16:25–52.

Dominguez-Malagon H, Delgado-Chavez R, Torres-Najera M, et al. Oxyphil and squamous variants of medullary carcinoma. Cancer 1989; 63:1183–1188.

Gagel RF, Tashijan AH Jr, Cummings T, et al. The clinical outcome of prospective screening for multiple endocrine neoplasia type 2a: An 18-year experience. N Engl J Med 1988; 318:478–484.

Gharib H, McConahey WM, Tiegs RD, et al. Medullary thyroid carcinoma: Clinicopathologic features and long-term follow-up patients treated during 1946 through 1970. Mayo Clin Proc 1992; 67:934–940.

Kini SR. Thyroid. In: Guides to Clinical Aspiration Biopsy. Vol. 3. New York: Igaku-Shoin, 1987.

Langle F, Soliman T, Neuhold N, et al. CD15 (LeuM1) immunoreactivity: Prognostic factor for sporadic and hereditary medullary thyroid cancer? Study group multiple endocrine neoplasia of Austria. World J Surg 1994; 18:583–587.

Ledger GA, Khosla S, Lindor NM, et al. Genetic testing in the diagnosis and management of multiple endocrine neoplasia type II. Ann Intern Med 1995; 122:118–124.

Marzano LA, Porcelli A, Biondi B, et al. Surgical management and follow-up of medullary thyroid carcinoma. J Surg Oncol 1995; 59:162–168.

Mendelsohn G, Wells SA, Baylin SB. Relationship of tissue carcinoembryonic antigen and calcitonin to tumor virulence in medullary thyroid carcinoma: An immunohistochemical study in early, localized and virulent disseminated stages of disease. Cancer 1984; 54:657–662.

Moley JF. Medullary thyroid cancer. Surg Clin North Am 1995; 75:405–420.

Normann T, Johannessen JV, Gautvik KM, et al. Medullary carcinoma of the thyroid: Diagnostic problems. Cancer 1976; 38:366–377.

Perry A, Molberg K, Albores-Saavedra J. Physiologic versus neoplastic C-cell hyperplasia of the thyroid. Cancer 1996; 77:750–756.

Rosai J, Carcangiu ML, DeLellis RA. Medullary carcinoma. In: Rosai J, Sobin LH, eds. Tumors of the Thyroid Gland: Atlas of Tumor Pathology. Third series, Fascicle 5. Washington, DC: Armed Forces Institute of Pathology, 1992, pp. 207–245.

Saad MF, Fritsche HA, Samaan NA. Diagnostic and prognostic value of carcinoembryonic antigen in medullary carcinoma of the thyroid. J Clin Endocrinol Metab 1984; 58:889–894.

Saad MF, Ordòñez NA, Guido JJ, Samaan NA. The prognostic value of calcitonin immunostaining in medullary carcinoma of the thyroid. J Clin Endocrinol Metab 1984; 59:850–856.

Saad MF, Ordòñez NA, Rashid RK, et al. Medullary carcinoma of the thyroid: A study of the clinical features and prognostic factors in 161 patients. Medicine 1984; 63:319–342.

Schröder S, Böcker W, Baisch H, et al. Prognostic factors in medullary thyroid carcinoma: Survival in relation to sex, stage, histology, immunocytochemistry, and DNA content. Cancer 1988; 61:806–816.

Telander RL, Moir CR. Medullary thyroid carcinoma in children. Semin Pediatr Surg 1994; 3:188–193.

Thomas CC, Cowan RJ, Albertson DA, Cooper MR. Detection of medullary carcinoma of the thyroid with I-131 MIBG. Clin Nucl Med 1994; 19:1066–1068.

Wells SA Jr, Dilley WG, Farndon JA, et al. Early diagnosis and treatment of medullary thyroid carcinoma. Arch Intern Med 1985; 145:1248–1252.

Lymphoproliferative Diseases of the Thyroid Gland

Langerhans' Cell Histiocytosis

Coode P, Shaikh MU. Histiocytosis X of the thyroid masquerading as thyroid carcinoma. Hum Pathol 1988; 19:239–241.

Thompson LDR. Langerhans cell histiocytosis of the thyroid gland. Eur Arch Otorhinolaryngol 1996; 253:62–65.

Thompson LDR, Wenig BM, Adair CF, et al. Langerhans cell histiocytosis of the thyroid gland. Mod Pathol 1996; 9:145–149.

Sinus Histiocytosis with Massive Lymphadenopathy (SHML)

Carpenter RJ III, Banks PM, McDonald RJ, Sanderson DR. Sinus histiocytosis with massive lymphadenopathy (Rosai-Dorfman disease): Report of a case with respiratory tract involvement. Laryngoscope 1978; 88:1963–1969.

Larkin DF, Dervan PA, Munnelly J, Finucane J. Sinus histiocytosis with massive lymphadenopathy simulating subacute thyroiditis. Hum Pathol 1986; 17:321–324.

Malignant Lymphoproliferative Disorders

Anscombe AM, Wright DH. Primary malignant lymphoma of the thyroid— a tumour of mucosa associated lymphoid tissue: Review of seventy-six cases. Histopathology 1985; 9:81–97.

Aosaza K, Inoue A, Tajima K, et al. Malignant lymphoma of the thyroid gland: Analysis of 79 patients with emphasis on histologic prognostic factors. Cancer 1986; 58:100–104.

Aozasa K, Ueda T, Katagiri S, et al. Immunologic and immunohistologic analysis of 27 cases with thyroid lymphoma. Cancer 1987; 60:969–973.

Ben-Ezra J, Wu A, Sheibani K. Hashimoto's thyroiditis lacks detectable clonal immunoglobulin and T-cell receptor gene rearrangements. Hum Pathol 1988; 19:1444–1448.

Chak LY, Hoppe RT, Burke JS, Kaplan HS. Non-Hodgkin's lymphoma presenting as thyroid enlargement. Cancer 1981; 48:2712–2716.

Compagno J, Oertel JE. Malignant lymphoma and other lymphoproliferative disorders of the thyroid gland: A clinicopathologic study of 245 cases. Am J Clin Pathol 1980; 74:1–11.

Devine RM, Edis AJ, Banks PM. Primary lymphoma of the thyroid: A review of the Mayo Clinic experience through 1978. World J Surg 1981; 5:33–38.

Doria R, Jekel JF, Cooper DL. Thyroid lymphoma: The case for combined modality therapy. Cancer 1995; 73:200–206.

Holm LE, Blomgren H, Löwagen T. Cancer risks in patients with chronic lymphocytic thyroiditis. N Engl J Med 1985; 312:601–604.

Hyjek E, Isaacson PG. Primary malignant lymphoma of the thyroid and its relationship to Hashimoto's thyroiditis. Hum Pathol 1988; 19:1315–1326.

Knowles DM, Athan E, Ubriaco A, et al. Extranodal noncutaneous lymphoid hyperplasias represent a continuous spectrum of B-cell neoplasia: Demonstration by molecular genetic analysis. Blood 1989; 73:1635–1645.

Matsuda M, Sone H, Koyama H, Ishiguro S. Fine needle aspiration cytology of malignant lymphoma of the thyroid. Diagn Cytopathol 1987; 3:244–249.

Mizukami Y, Matsubara F, Hashimoto T, et al. Primary T-cell lymphoma of the thyroid. Acta Pathol Jpn 1987; 37:1987–1995.

Mizukami Y, Michigishi T, Nonomura A, et al. Primary lymphoma of the thyroid: A clinical, histological and immunohistochemical study of 20 cases. Histopathology 1990; 17:210–219.

Oertel JE, Heffess CS. Lymphoma of the thyroid and related disorders. Semin Oncol 1987; 14:333–342.

Samaan NA, Ordòñez NG. Uncommon types of thyroid cancer. Endocrinol Metab Clin North Am 1990; 19:637–648.

Plasmacytoma

Alexanian R. Ten-year survival in multiple myeloma. Arch Intern Med 1985; 145:2073–2074.

Aozasa K, Inoue A, Yoshimura H, et al. Plasmacytoma of the thyroid gland. Cancer 1986; 58:105–110.

Holck S. Plasma cell granuloma of the thyroid. Cancer 1981; 48:830–832.

Mizukami Y, Ikuta N, Hashimoto T, et al. Pseudolymphoma of the thyroid. Acta Pathol Jpn 1988; 38:1329–1336.

Rubin J, Johnson JT, Killeen R, Barnes L. Extramedullary plasmacytoma of the thyroid associated with a serum monoclonal gammopathy. Arch Otolaryngol Head Neck Surg 1990; 116:855–859.

Yapp R, Lindner J, Schenken JR, Karrar FW. Plasma cell granuloma of the thyroid. Hum Pathol 1985; 16:848–850.

Hodgkin's Disease

Feigin GA, Buss DH, Paschal B, et al. Hodgkin's disease manifested as a thyroid nodule. Hum Pathol 1982; 13:774–776.

Nonepithelial Neoplasms of the Thyroid, Excluding Lymphoproliferative Disorders

Thyroid Paraganglioma

Banner B, Morecki R, Eviatar A. Chemodectoma in the mid-thyroid region. J Otolaryngol 1979; 8:271–273.

Buss DH, Marshall RB, Baird FG, Myers RT. Paraganglioma of the thyroid gland. Am J Surg Pathol 1980; 4:589–593.

Haeggert DG, Wang NS, Ferrar PA, et al. Non-chromaffin paragangliomatosis manifesting as a cold thyroid nodule. Am J Clin Pathol 1974; 61:561–570.

Heffess CS, Adair CF, Wenig BM. Paragangliomas of the thyroid gland. Int J Surg Pathol 1995; 2:188.

Kay S, Montague JW, Dodd RW. Nonchromaffin paraganglioma (chemodectoma) of thyroid region. Cancer 1975; 36:582–585.

Mitsudo SM, Grajower MD, Balbi H, Silver C. Malignant paraganglioma of the thyroid gland. Arch Pathol Lab Med 1987; 111:378–380.

Zak F, Lawson W. Glomic (paraganglionic) tissue in the larynx and capsule of the thyroid gland. Mt Sinai J Med 1972; 39:82–90.

Benign Mesenchymal Tumors

Andrion A, Bellis D, Delsemide L, et al. Leiomyoma and neurilemoma: Report of two unusual non-epithelial tumours of the thyroid gland. Virchows Arch [A] 1988; 413:367–372.

Gardner DR, Frable WJ. Primary lymphangioma of the thyroid gland. Arch Pathol Lab Med 1989; 113:1084–1085.

Pickleman JR, Lee JF, Straus FH II, Paloyan E. Thyroid hemangioma. Am J Surg 1975; 129:331–336.

Thompson LDR, Adair CF, Shmookler BM, et al. Primary smooth muscle tumors of the thyroid gland. Mod Pathol 1996; 9:52A.

Thompson LDR, Adair CF, Shmookler BM, et al. Peripheral nerve sheath tumors of the thyroid: A series of four cases and a review of the literature. Mod Pathol 1996; 9:52A.

Malignant Mesenchymal Tumors

Eusebi V, Carcangiu ML, Dina R, Rosai J. Keratin-positive epithelioid angiosarcoma of the thyroid: A report of four cases. Am J Surg Pathol 1990; 14:737–747.

Mills SE, Gaffey MJ, Watts JC, et al. Angiomatoid carcinoma and "angiosarcoma" of the thyroid gland: A spectrum of endothelial differentiation. Am J Clin Pathol 1994; 102:322–330.

Rosai J, Carcangiu ML, DeLellis RA. Sarcomas. In: Rosai J, Sobin LH, eds. Tumors of the Thyroid Gland: Atlas of Tumor Pathology. Third series, Fascicle 5. Washington, DC: Armed Forces Institute of Pathology, 1992, pp. 259–265.

Thompson LDR, Adair CF, Shmookler BM, et al. Primary smooth muscle tumors of the thyroid gland. Mod Pathol 1996; 9:52A.

Thompson LDR, Adair CF, Shmookler BM, et al. Peripheral nerve sheath tumors of the thyroid: A series of four cases and a review of the literature. Mod Pathol 1996; 9:52A.

Teratomas

Bale GF. Tertatomas of the neck in the region of the thyroid gland: A review of the literature and report of four cases. Am J Pathol 1950; 26:565–579.

Batsakis JG, El-Naggar AK, Luna MA. Teratomas of the neck with emphasis on malignancy. Ann Otol Rhinol Laryngol 1995; 104:496–500.

Bowker CM, Whittaker RS. Malignant teratoma of the thyroid: Case report and literature review of thyroid teratoma in adults. Histopathology 1992; 21:81–83.

Buckley NJ, Burch WM, Leight GS. Malignant teratoma of the thyroid gland in an adult: A case report and review of the literature. Surgery 1986; 100:932–937.

Fisher JE, Cooney DR, Voorhees ML, Jewett TC Jr. Teratoma of the thyroid gland in infancy: Review of the literature and two case reports. J Surg Oncol 1982; 21:135–140.

Kier R, Silverman PM, Korobkin M, et al. Malignant teratoma of the thyroid in an adult: CT appearance. J Comput Assist Tomogr 1985; 9:174–176.

Kimler SC, Muth WF. Primary malignant teratoma of the thyroid: Case report and literature review of cervical teratomas in adults. Cancer 1978; 42:311–317.

Kingsley DP, Elton A, Bennett MH. Malignant teratoma of thyroid: Case report and review of literature. Br J Cancer 1968; 22:7–11.

Murao T, Nakanishi M, Toda K, Konishi H. Malignant teratoma of the thyroid gland in an adolescent female. Acta Pathol Jpn 1979; 29:109–117.

Newstedt JR, Shirkey HC. Teratoma of the thyroid region. Am J Dis Child 1964; 107:88–95.

O'Higgins N, Taylor S. Malignant teratoma in the adult thyroid gland. Br J Clin Pract 1975; 29:237–238.

Rothschild MA, Catalano P, Urken M, et al. Evaluation of management of congenital cervical teratoma: Case report and review. Arch Otolaryngol Head Neck Surg 1994; 120:444–448.

Stone HH, Henderson WD, Guido FA. Teratomas of the neck. Am J Dis Child 1967; 113:222–224.

Weitzner S. Benign teratoma of the neck in an infant. Am J Dis Child 1964; 107:84–87.

Secondary or Metastatic Tumors to the Thyroid

Czech JM, Lichtor TR, Carney JA, van Heerden JA. Neoplasms metastatic to the thyroid gland. Surg Gynecol Obstet 1982; 155:503–505.

Elliot RH Jr, Kneeland FV. Metastatic carcinoma masquerading as primary thyroid cancer: A report of authors' 14 cases. Ann Surg 1960; 151:551–561.

Gherari G, Scherini P, Ambrosi S. Occult thyroid metastasis from untreated uveal melanoma. Arch Ophthalmol 1985; 103:689–691.

Graham LD, Roe SM. Metastatic papillary carcinoma presenting as a primary renal neoplasm. Am Surg 1995; 61:732–734.

Green LK, Ro JY, Mackay B, et al. Renal cell carcinoma metastatic to the thyroid. Cancer 1989; 63:1810–1815.

Halbauer M, Kardum-Skelin I, Vranesic D, Crepinko I. Aspiration cytology of renal cell carcinoma metastatic to the thyroid. Acta Cytol 1991; 35:443–446.

Ivy HK. Cancer metastatic to the thyroid: A diagnostic problem. Mayo Clin Proc 1984; 59:856–859.

McCabe DP, Farrar WB, Petkov TM, et al. Clinical and pathologic correlations in disease metastatic to the thyroid gland. Am J Surg 1985; 150:519–523.

Mizukami Y, Saito K, Nonomura A, et al. Lung carcinoma metastatic to microfollicular adenoma of the thyroid: A case report. Acta Pathol Jpn 1990; 40:602–608.

Rikabi AC, Young AE, Wilson C. Metastatic renal cell carcinoma in the thyroid gland diagnosed by fine needle aspiration cytology. Cytopathology 1991; 2:47–49.

Ro JY, Guerrieri C, El-Naggar A, et al. Carcinomas metastatic to follicular adenomas of the thyroid gland: Report of two cases. Arch Pathol Lab Med 1994; 118:551–556.

Schmid KW, Hittmair A, Ofner C, et al. Metastatic tumors in fine needle aspiration biopsy of the thyroid. Acta Cytol 1991; 35:722–724.

Shibutani Y, Inoue D, Yokota T, et al. Metastatic carcinoma of the sigmoid colon to the thyroid gland. Nippon Naibunpi Gakkai Zasshi (Jpn) 1992; 68:765–772.

Fine Needle Aspiration–Related Histologic Changes to the Thyroid Gland

Axiotis CA, Merino MJ, Ain K, Norton JA. Papillary endothelial hyperplasia in the thyroid following fine needle aspiration. Arch Pathol Lab Med 1991; 115:240–242.

Chan JKC, Tang SK, Tsang WYW, et al. Histologic changes induced by fine needle aspiration. Adv Anat Pathol 1996; 3:71–90.

Gordon DL, Gattuso P, Castelli M, et al. Effect of fine needle aspiration on the histology of thyroid neoplasms. Acta Cytol 1993; 37:651–654.

Hales MS, Hsu FSF. Needle tract implantation of papillary carcinoma of the thyroid following aspiration biopsy. Acta Cytol 1990; 34:801–804.

Layfield LJ, Jones MA. Necrosis in thyroid nodules after fine needle aspiration biopsy. Acta Cytol 1991; 35:427–430.

LiVolsi VA, Merino MJ. Worrisome histologic alterations following fine needle aspiration of the thyroid (WHAAFT). Pathol Annu 1994; 29(Part 2):99–120.

Tsang K, Duggan MA. Vascular proliferation of the thyroid: A complication of fine needle aspiration. Arch Pathol Lab Med 1992; 116:1040–1042.

CHAPTER 9

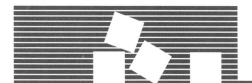

Non-Neoplastic Lesions of the Parathyroid Glands

A. CLASSIFICATION OF NON-NEOPLASTIC LESIONS OF THE PARATHYROID GLANDS

Table 9–1
NON-NEOPLASTIC LESIONS OF THE PARATHYROID GLANDS

Primary chief cell hyperplasia
Water-clear cell hyperplasia
Secondary hyperparathyroidism
Tertiary hyperparathyroidism
Parathyroiditis

B. PRIMARY CHIEF CELL HYPERPLASIA

Definition: Non-neoplastic increase in parenchymal cell mass of multiple parathyroid glands in the absence of a known clinical stimulus for increased secretion of parathyroid hormone.

Clinical

- An autopsy incidence of 7% has been reported.
- Affects females more often than males (ratio of 3:1); incidence increases with age.
- Sporadic cases represent 80% of patients with primary chief cell hyperplasia. Twenty percent have familial disease, usually associated with one of the multiple endocrine neoplasia (MEN) syndromes, although familial parathyroid hyperplasia without other endocrine abnormalities also occurs.
- This disorder is responsible for 15% of cases of hyperparathyroidism.
- Symptoms are related to the level and duration of serum calcium elevation. Patients are commonly asymptomatic or have vague complaints such as lethargy, weakness,

polyuria, polydipsia, arthralgia, constipation, and depression. This rather nonspecific presentation has been encountered more often in the past 2 decades because routine biochemical testing has resulted in an overall increase in the prevalence of primary hyperparathyroidism owing to detection of clinically silent cases.
- Advanced bone disease and recurrent nephrocalcinosis are uncommon compared with their incidence two to three decades ago. Diffuse osteopenia, with or without compression fractures, articular chondrocalcinosis, and other joint disorders such as pseudogout and true gout, are currently found more frequently.
- Other conditions associated with hyperparathyroidism include hypertension, peptic ulcer disease, and pancreatitis.
- Biochemical findings include:
  - Elevated serum calcium levels, which are most accurately reflected by the serum ionized calcium value because the regulated fraction of calcium is not bound to plasma proteins.
  - There is a decrease in serum inorganic phosphorus concentration resulting from increased urinary loss of phosphates induced by the action of parathyroid hormone at the renal tubular level; this leads to decreased tubular reabsorption of phosphate or increased renal phosphate clearance. A corresponding increase in urinary cyclic adenosine monophosphate (AMP) usually accompanies these parathormone-induced alterations in urinary phosphate metabolism.
  - Serum levels of parathyroid hormone vary depending on the type of assay used. The currently preferred assay quantitates the intact parathyroid hormone molecule rather than only a cleavage product, as was measured in earlier procedures. The normal serum value for intact parathyroid hormone is 210 to 310 pg/ml.
- Approximately 20% of patients with primary chief cell hyperplasia have one of the MEN syndromes. Of these, the association with chief cell hyperplasia is seen most frequently in Wermer's syndrome (MEN 1), in which 90% of patients have parathyroid hyperplasia or, less often, neoplasms. Parathyroid proliferative disease is seen in

160

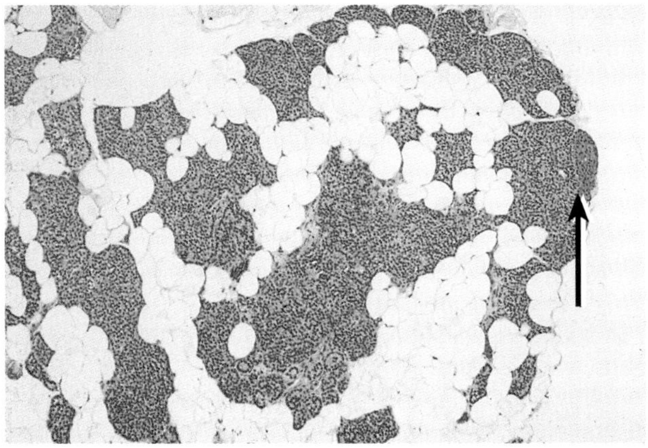

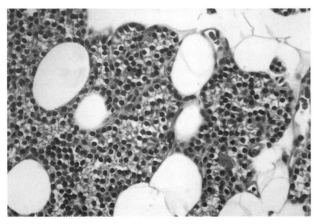

Figure 9–1. Normal parathyroid gland in a 40-year-old man. Distribution of lipocytes is variable in different areas of a single gland. Note a small group of oxyphilic cells *(arrow).*

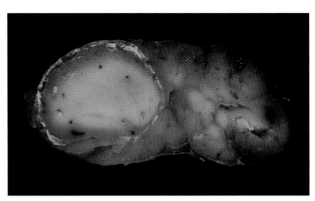

Figure 9–4. Parathyroid hyperplasia. This is one of three enlarged glands in a patient with primary hyperparathyroidism. The gland has a variegated nodular appearance.

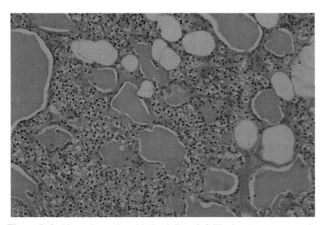

Figure 9–2. Normal parathyroid gland. Acinar groupings of chief cells are seen, admixed with lipocytes.

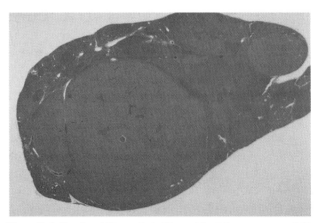

Figure 9–5. Parathyroid hyperplasia. The multinodular appearance of this gland is the result of proliferation of groups of cells with different cytologic features. The entire gland is affected by the proliferative process; no rim of normal parathyroid tissue is seen.

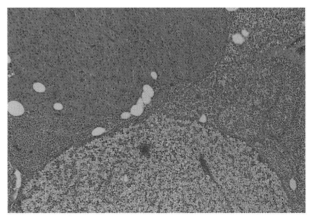

Figure 9–3. Normal parathyroid gland. Pseudofollicular structures may be prominent, as in this gland. The eosinophilic material, which resembles colloid, is periodic acid–Schiff (PAS) positive but fails to stain immunohistochemically for thyroglobulin.

Figure 9–6. Parathyroid hyperplasia. The nodules within the gland are composed of cell types with different cytologic features: some are typical chief cells, whereas others have more striking nuclear enlargement than normal chief cells or have prominent cytoplasmic oxyphilia.

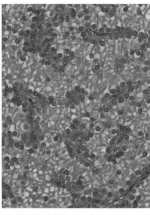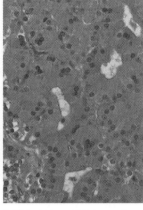

Figure 9–7. Parathyroid hyperplasia. Different areas of the same hyperplastic gland may contain predominantly chief cells (somewhat enlarged in this view) *(left)* or cells with cytoplasmic oxyphilia *(right)*.

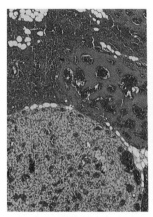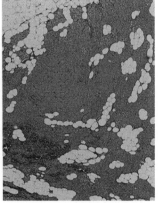

Figure 9–8. Parathyroid hyperplasia. The hyperplastic features may be unevenly distributed among the four glands or even within a single gland, as in this case. *Left,* Nodules and areas of solid growth with high cellularity. *Right,* Foci containing a higher percentage of lipocytes and scattered small cellular nodules.

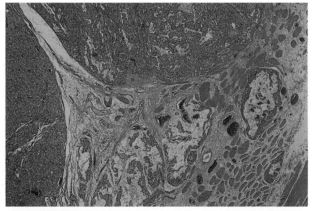

Figure 9–9. Recurrent parathyroid hyperplasia in a parathyroid gland that was autografted into the forearm. This patient had a history of chronic renal failure with secondary hyperparathyroidism. His hypercalcemia recurred several months after subtotal parathyroidectomy with autoimplantation of portions of parathyroid gland into the soft tissue of the forearm. The irregular islands of cellular parathyroid tissue may appear to be infiltrating skeletal muscle. This pattern, and even the presence of mitotic figures in the parathyroid tissue, do not necessarily indicate malignancy.

30% to 40% of patients with MEN 2A (Sipple's syndrome) but is quite rare in MEN 2B.
■ In Wermer's syndrome (MEN 1) the major findings are parathyroid hyperplasia (or neoplasia), islet cell hyperplasia or neoplasia, and gastrointestinal endocrine cell hyperplasia or neoplasia; some patients also develop pulmonary and thymic neuroendocrine neoplasms, adrenal cortical neoplasms, and thyroid follicular neoplasms. This syndrome is associated with a single locus on chromosome 11.

Radiology

■ Radiographic imaging techniques applied to the localization of hyperfunctioning parathyroid glands include retrograde phlebotomy with serum parathormone assays, CT scanning, ultrasonography, magnetic resonance imaging (MRI), thallium subtraction scanning, and, most recently, technetium-99m sestamibi imaging. Imaging procedures have been significantly less effective in localizing glands in patients with hyperplasia compared with those who have parathyroid adenomas or carcinomas. Technetium-99m sestamibi imaging has been effective in localizing up to 60% of hyperplastic glands. It has been more widely used in the evaluation of patients with recurrent hyperparathyroidism after parathyroid resection.

Pathology

Cytology

■ The cytologic findings in aspirate smears of parathyroid hyperplasia and parathyroid adenoma are indistinguishable and allow only documentation of "parathyroid proliferative disease." (For a discussion of the cytologic features of parathyroid lesions see Chapter 10B.)

Gross

■ Although all four glands may be enlarged, it is not uncommon for the enlargement to be somewhat asymmetric, with two or three glands much larger than the others. In some cases one gland is so much larger that the gross appearance suggests an adenoma, emphasizing the importance of sampling grossly "normal" glands to facilitate accurate discrimination between hyperplasia and adenoma; increased cellularity of the smaller glands may be the key to recognition of the multiglandular nature of the proliferation.
■ The glands may be diffusely enlarged or may be nodular, particularly as they increase in size.
■ Cystic changes may be present but are not common.
■ Total gland weight in primary chief cell hyperplasia is variable. Ranges of total weights in large series of patients show weights of less than 1 g in 54%, 1 to 5 g in 28%, and 5 to 10 g in 18%.
■ The glands are usually soft and are tan-brown in color. The distinction between hyperplastic and adenomatous glands cannot generally be made by gross examination.

Histology

■ Primary chief cell hyperplasia results from an increase in parenchymal cell mass, predominantly involving chief cell proliferation; however, oxyphilic cells may be present as well.

- Stromal fat cells are absent or markedly decreased in number in most areas, although foci of stromal fat cells may mimic those of the normal gland. Variations in the distribution of fat cells and in the density of chief cells, particularly in nodular hyperplasia, may produce a confusing histologic picture. Areas with residual fat may mimic a rim of "normal" gland, particularly when they are adjacent to large nodules, which generally lack fat cells. This picture may suggest a diagnosis of adenoma, again emphasizing the importance of microscopic examination of multiple glands and the need for processing multiple sections of larger glands.
- Although circumscribed by the delicate fibrous capsule of the gland, hyperplasia may also involve nests of parathyroid tissue in the soft tissue of the neck ("parathyromatosis"). This phenomenon may be the cause of recurrent disease after an apparently complete resection of glands that show grossly evident hyperplastic disease. This appearance should not be mistaken for "invasion" such as that characteristic of carcinoma; the lack of a fibroblastic reaction or infiltrative contour, the absence of an intravascular location of these nests, and the lack of other histologic features of carcinoma should help to exclude malignancy.
- A solid, follicular, or cordlike proliferation of predominantly chief cells is seen, with variable nodularity.
- Small follicular structures may contain periodic acid–Schiff (PAS)-positive material resembling dense colloid; this material is not immunoreactive for thyroglobulin.
- The hyperplastic cells usually contain less intracytoplasmic fat than normal or atrophic parathyroid tissue when demonstrated by oil red O or Sudan black stains; however, some hyperplastic parathyroid tissue may contain abundant intracytoplasmic fat. Intracytoplasmic fat may be more abundant in chief cells located between hyperplastic nodules, whereas it is usually absent in cells within the nodules.
- Hyperplastic cells generally contain more glycogen than normal or atrophic chief cells.
- Although mitotic figures may be seen, they usually number less than 1 per 10 high-power fields. In some cases mitotic rates of 1 to 5/10 HPF are seen; however, atypical mitoses are not present.
- *Immunohistochemistry:* Chief cells are positive for cytokeratin and chromogranin. Parathyroid hormone is difficult to demonstrate owing to small amounts of hormone stored in the cells; however, in situ hybridization to localize messenger RNA associated with production of parathyroid hormone has been more successful.
- *Electron microscopy:* Cells contain abundant mitochondria, endoplasmic reticulum, and large Golgi areas, as well as characteristic secretory granules. Interdigitating cell membranes are more complex than in normal parathyroid parenchymal cells.

Differential Diagnosis

- Parathyroid adenoma (Chapter 10B).

Treatment and Prognosis

- Subtotal parathyroidectomy with complete removal of three glands, leaving a remnant of the fourth, is the most

widely accepted therapy. Total parathyroidectomy with autotransplantation of remnants of parathyroid tissue in the forearm is also a common surgical procedure.
- The recurrence rate of hyperparathyroidism following subtotal parathyroidectomy is approximately 16%. Recurrences may not be evident for several years. They may be due to inadequate exploration of the neck, which may result from a diagnosis of "adenoma" in patients with asymmetric hyperplasia. Less frequent causes include failure to recognize supernumerary or ectopic glands, parathyromatosis, or surgical implantation of hyperplastic tissue in the soft tissue of the neck.

Additional Facts

- Lithium therapy for psychiatric disorders has been associated with a form of hyperparathyroidism similar to primary hyperparathyroidism; it produces hypercalcemia and elevated serum parathormone levels. Both chief cell hyperplasia and "adenomas" have been described in these patients. The hyperparathyroidism resolves after discontinuation of the lithium therapy; however, patients requiring lithium may be treated successfully with subtotal parathyroidectomy.
- Humoral hypercalcemia of malignancy (HHM) is an important clinical differential diagnostic consideration in patients in whom primary hyperparathyroidism is suspected. HHM is independent of the extent of metastatic disease involving bone and is characterized by hypercalcemia, hypophosphatemia, and elevated urinary cyclic AMP levels. Unlike hyperparathyroidism, HHM suppresses serum parathormone and 1,25-dihydroxyvitamin D levels. The mechanism for hypercalcemia appears to be increased bone resorption due to a humoral factor known as parathyroid hormone-related protein. This form of hypercalcemia is seen most frequently in patients with squamous cell carcinoma (lung, upper aerodigestive tract, and female genital tract), renal cell carcinoma, and transitional cell carcinoma.
- A second mechanism of hypercalcemia associated with malignancy is related directly to the osteolytic effect of bone metastases. This form of hypercalcemia is more common in patients with breast carcinoma and hematologic malignancies. These patients have suppressed levels of parathormone, but urinary cyclic AMP is not elevated, and parathyroid hormone-related protein has not been implicated.

C. WATER-CLEAR CELL HYPERPLASIA

Definition: Non-neoplastic increase in parenchymal cell mass of multiple parathyroid glands by proliferation of large cells with clear, vacuolated cytoplasm in the absence of a known clinical stimulus for increased secretion of parathyroid hormone.

Clinical

- Slightly more common in men (ratio 1.4:1; contrast this with the gender predilection seen in chief cell hyperplasia). It occurs most commonly in the fifth decade of life.

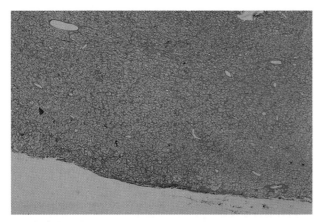

Figure 9–10. Water-clear cell hyperplasia. The glands are usually markedly enlarged and are replaced by a proliferation of clear cells with abundant cytoplasm and very distinct cell borders. There is usually little or no stromal fat in the glands.

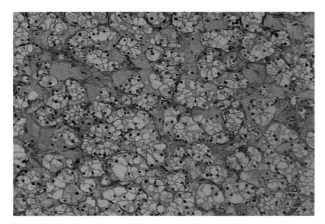

Figure 9–11. Water-clear cell hyperplasia. The clear cells are distinctively different from those of chief cell hyperplasia. The cytoplasm is much more abundant, and there is a much lower nucleus-to-cytoplasm ratio than is seen in primary chief cell hyperplasia; the cell membranes are very distinct.

- Very rare cause of hyperparathyroidism; most cases were identified prior to 1975.
- Hypercalcemia is usually more severe than in chief cell hyperplasia. The mean serum calcium level is 13.2 mg/100 ml compared with 11.7 mg/100 ml in cases of chief cell hyperplasia reported prior to 1975.
- Nephrolithiasis occurs in 90% of patients, in contrast to 53% in patients with chief cell hyperplasia during the same period.
- Overall incidence of bone disease is similar to that characteristic of chief cell hyperplasia; occasional patients present with osteitis fibrosa generalisata.
- No documented association with multiple endocrine neoplasia or other familial syndromes.

Pathology

Gross

- Usually all four glands are enlarged, although asymmetric enlargement is common, and the upper glands are often larger than the lower glands.

- Mean total gland weight is more than 10 g in 47% of cases; a combined weight of under 1 g has not been reported.
- Involved glands are dark brown and may show cystic change, areas of fibrosis, or hemorrhage; nodularity within the glands is uncommon, but the gland contour is often irregular.

Histology

- The glands are usually diffusely replaced by large clear cells and have little or no remaining stromal adipose tissue.
- The cells measure from 10 to 40 μm in diameter and have distinct cell borders. They are arranged in sheets, cords, or sometimes in acinar groups. Tubular or cystic spaces lined by clear cells may be seen, usually focally; they are filled with degenerated cells and faintly eosinophilic granular fluid.
- The cytoplasm appears clear but contains many small vacuoles, which produce a finely reticulated pattern in hematoxylin-eosin stained sections. The vacuoles are more readily apparent in plastic-embedded thin sections. The cell membranes are very distinct.
- The nuclei are small, round to ovoid, and rather hyperchromatic and are basally oriented in the polyhedral to slightly columnar cells.
- Scattered multinucleated cells and occasional large hyperchromatic nuclei may be observed.
- *Histochemistry:* Glycogen is demonstrable in the cytoplasm with PAS reagent, but neutral fat stains are negative.
- *Immunohistochemistry:* As in chief cell hyperplasia, the reaction with chromogranin and cytokeratin is positive.
- *Electron microscopy:* The clear cells contain numerous membrane-bound vacuoles, many of which appear "empty"; however, some contain electron-dense material similar to the smaller typical parathyroid secretory granules, which are also scattered through the cytoplasm.

Differential Diagnosis

- Primary chief cell hyperplasia (Chapter 9B).
- Parathyroid adenoma (particularly if only one gland has been sampled or if the hyperplasia is very asymmetric) (Chapter 10B).
- Metastatic renal cell carcinoma (biochemical findings of hyperparathyroidism and positive immunohistochemistry examination for chromogranin are helpful in confirming a diagnosis of parathyroid hyperplasia).
- Follicular thyroid neoplasm with clear cell features (thyroglobulin produces a positive reaction on immunohistochemistry examination).

Treatment and Prognosis

- Subtotal parathyroidectomy is the preferred therapy.
- Recurrent hyperparathyroidism occurs in approximately 45% of cases, probably because too large a remnant of parathyroid gland was preserved at the original operation.

Additional Facts

- The reason for the virtual disappearance of water-clear cell hyperplasia in the population is not known. Some suggest that it represents an advanced form of primary chief cell hyperplasia; the decreasing incidence and severity of chief cell hyperplasia as a result of routine biochemical screening of patients lends some support to this theory. Others believe that the electron-microscopic appearance of water-clear cell hyperplasia is so distinctive from primary chief cell hyperplasia that they doubt that it develops from pre-existing chief cell hyperplasia.

D. SECONDARY HYPERPARATHYROIDISM

Definition: An increase in parathyroid parenchymal cell mass of multiple glands in response to a known clinical stimulus for increased secretion of parathyroid hormone. These conditions are usually characterized by hypocalcemia and hyperphosphatemia.

Clinical

- Causes of secondary hyperparathyroidism include chronic renal failure (most common), dietary vitamin D deficiency or abnormalities of vitamin D metabolism, malabsorption, and pseudohypoparathyroidism.
- Occurs over a broad age range, reflecting the incidence of chronic renal failure, the most common cause of secondary hyperparathyroidism.
- Symptoms of secondary hyperparathyroidism are primarily related to parathyroid hormone-mediated bone resorption, which results in osteomalacia and osteitis fibrosa cystica.
- Abnormal calcium deposits in the soft tissues, particularly in a periarticular distribution, may be seen.
- Laboratory studies reveal elevation of parathyroid hormone levels with hypocalcemia and hyperphosphatemia.

Pathology

Gross

- The appearance is not significantly different from that of primary chief cell hyperplasia. There may be uniform enlargement of all glands, or the enlargement may be asymmetric.
- The glands are yellow-brown to gray, with weights ranging from 0.12 to 6 g.

Histology

- The proliferation includes chief cells, oxyphilic cells, and transitional cells.
- The increased parenchymal cell mass varies depending on the duration of disease, as does the number of residual stromal fat cells. In advanced disease the fat cells are absent.

- The parenchymal cells may grow in sheets, cords, or acinar structures. Nodular aggregates of chief cells or oxyphilic cells are common in very enlarged glands, and areas of fibrosis, cystic change, and calcification may be present. Some cases may exhibit a predominantly diffuse proliferation of chief cells.
- Oxyphilic cells seem to be a more common component of secondary hyperparathyroidism than of primary chief cell hyperplasia.

Differential Diagnosis

- Primary chief cell hyperplasia (Chapter 9B).
- Parathyroid adenoma (Chapter 10B).

Treatment and Prognosis

- Subtotal parathyroidectomy is the treatment of choice. The remnant of parathyroid gland may be left in situ or transplanted to the soft tissue of the forearm.
- Recurrence of hyperparathyroidism is a common problem in patients with chronic renal failure because the stimulus for hypersecretion of parathyroid hormone is frequently not correctable.

Additional Facts

- Autotransplantation of parathyroid tissue into the forearm musculature following total parathyroidectomy may be associated with graft failure and hypoparathyroidism, or with recurrent hyperparathyroidism due to hyperplasia of the transplanted remnant of parathyroid.
- Recurrent hyperplasia may be associated with a multifocal proliferation of islands of parathyroid tissue in the adipose tissue and skeletal muscle, sometimes rather widely separated from the original site of transplantation. The hyperplastic cells may be somewhat more pleomorphic than the original parathyroid proliferation and may even be mitotically active. These changes should not be interpreted as evidence of malignancy.

E. TERTIARY HYPERPARATHYROIDISM

Definition: An absolute increase in parathyroid parenchymal cell mass associated with autonomous hyperfunction and resultant hypercalcemia in a patient with previously known secondary hyperparathyroidism following implementation of dialysis or renal transplantation.

Clinical

- Tertiary hyperparathyroidism occurs in patients over a broad age range, reflecting the incidence of chronic renal failure.
- Hypercalcemia usually develops several years after the diagnosis of renal disease.
- Hypercalcemia due to tertiary hyperparathyroidism represents a serious threat to renal grafts and requires prompt surgical therapy.

■ Laboratory findings are similar to those described for primary hyperparathyroidism.

Pathology

Gross

■ The glands may be diffusely enlarged or nodular. Patients with nodular hyperplasia tend to have more striking but asymmetric gland enlargement.
■ Parathyroid glands with diffuse hyperplasia are 10 to 20 times the size of normal parathyroid glands; those with nodular hyperplasia are 20 to 40 times the normal size.

Histology

■ Ninety-five percent of patients with tertiary hyperparathyroidism have hyperplasia; only 5% have adenomas.
■ Chief cells predominate in hyperplasia due to tertiary hyperparathyroidism. However, oxyphilic and transitional cells may be seen in either diffuse or nodular hyperplasia. Rarely, areas with water-clear cells may be present.
■ Areas of hemorrhage, recent or remote, as well as fibrosis and calcification are common.
■ Mitotic figures are uncommon, as is nuclear pleomorphism.
■ Stromal fat cells are sparse but are more often present in areas between nodules. This distribution may suggest a diagnosis of "adenoma"; however, multinodularity is more consistent in patients with a hyperplastic process.

Differential Diagnosis

■ Parathyroid adenoma. The rare parathyroid adenomas responsible for tertiary hyperparathyroidism are indistinguishable from parathyroid adenomas associated with primary hyperparathyroidism (Chapter 10B). The distinction between parathyroid hyperplasia and adenoma is further discussed in Chapter 10 as well.

Treatment and Prognosis

■ Subtotal parathyroidectomy is the preferred therapy.
■ Recurrent hyperparathyroidism has been seen in approximately 8% of patients after surgery.

Additional Facts

■ The cause of autonomous hyperfunction of the parathyroids in patients with treated renal failure is not known. An elevation of the "set point" for serum calcium has been postulated; this would result in stimulation of parathyroid tissue despite normal serum calcium levels.
■ There is also evidence that the sheer mass of parathyroid tissue in patients with tertiary hyperparathyroidism may cause autonomous function. Removal of the bulk of the hyperplastic tissue results in a readily suppressible remnant.

F. PARATHYROIDITIS

Definition: Infiltration of the parathyroid gland by inflammatory cells, usually predominantly lymphocytes.

Clinical

■ Uncommon finding that may be seen in patients with hypoparathyroidism or, even more rarely, in those with primary chief cell hyperplasia.
■ Possible autoimmune etiology postulated.

Pathology

Gross

■ May be seen in grossly normal glands as an incidental finding or in enlarged glands with hyperplasia.

Histology

■ Scattered aggregates of lymphocytes may be found in otherwise normal glands as an incidental finding, or they may be seen in atrophic glands associated with hypoparathyroidism or primary chief cell hyperplasia.

Treatment and Prognosis

■ The significance of parathyroiditis is often unclear.
■ Clinical findings and treatment are based on the underlying disease process involving the parenchymal cells if clinically evident disease is present.

Bibliography

Primary Chief Cell Hyperplasia

Åkerström G, Rudberg C, Grimelius L, et al. Histologic parathyroid abnormalities in an autopsy series. Hum Pathol 1986; 17:520–527.

Bombi JA, Nadal A, Muñoz J, Cardesa A. Ultrastructural pathology of the parathyroid glands in hyperparathyroidism: A report of 69 cases. Ultrastruct Pathol 1993; 17:567–582.

Bondeson AG, Bondeson L, Ljungberg O, Tibblin S. Fat staining in parathyroid disease—diagnostic value and impact on surgical strategy: Clinicopathologic analysis of 191 cases. Hum Pathol 1985; 16:1255–1263.

Castleman B, Schantz A, Roth SI. Parathyroid hyperplasia in primary hyperparathyroidism: A review of 85 cases. Cancer 1976; 38:1668–1675.

Clark OH, Duh Q-Y. Primary hyperparathyroidism: A surgical perspective. Endocrinol Metab Clin North Am 1989; 18:701–714.

DeLellis RA. Primary chief cell hyperplasia. In: DeLellis RA, ed. Tumors of the Parathyroid Gland, Third series, Fascicle 6. Washington, DC: Armed Forces Institute of Pathology, 1991, pp. 65–78.

Fitco R, Roth SI, Hines JR, et al. Parathyromatosis in hyperparathyroidism. Hum Pathol 1991; 21:234–237.

Grimelius L, Åkerström G, Johansson H, et al. The parathyroid glands. In: Kovacs K, Asa SL, eds. Functional Endocrine Pathology, Vol 1. Boston: Blackwell Scientific, 1991, pp. 375–384.

Halbauer M, Črepinko I, Brzac HT, Simonović I. Fine needle aspiration cytology in the preoperative diagnosis of ultrasonically enlarged parathyroid glands. Acta Cytol 1991; 35:728–735.

Heath DA. Primary hyperparathyroidism: Clinical presentation and factors influencing clinical management. Endocrinol Metab Clin North Am 1989; 18:631–646.

Insogna K. Humoral hypercalcemia of malignancy: The role of parathyroid hormone-related protein. Endocrinol Metab Clin North Am 1989; 18:779–794.

Marcus R. Laboratory diagnosis of primary hyperparathyroidism. Endocrinol Metab Clin North Am 1989; 18:647–658.

McHenry CR, Rosen IB, Rotstein LE, et al. Lithiumogenic disorders of the parathyroid glands as surgical disease. Surgery 1990; 108:1001–1005.

Mundy G. Hypercalcemic factors other than parathyroid hormone-related protein. Endocrinol Metab Clin North Am 1989; 18:795–806.

Palmer M, Ljunghall S, Åkerström G, et al. Patients with primary hyperparathyroidism operated on over a 24-year period: Temporal trends of clinical and laboratory findings. J Chron Dis 1987; 40:121–130.

Snover DC, Foucar K. Mitotic activity in benign parathyroid disease. Am J Clin Pathol 1981; 775:345–347.

Water-Clear Cell Hyperplasia

Dawkins RL, Tashjian AH, Castleman B, Moore EW. Hyperparathyroidism due to clear cell hyperplasia. Serial determinations of serum ionized calcium, parathyroid hormone, and calcitonin. Am J Med 1973; 54:119–126.

DeLellis RA. Clear cell hyperplasia. In: DeLellis RA, ed. Tumors of the Parathyroid Gland, Third series, Fascicle 6. Washington, D.C.: Armed Forces Institute of Pathology, 1991, pp. 79–83.

Dorado AE, Hensley G, Castleman B. Water clear cell hyperplasia of parathyroid. Autopsy report of a case with supernumerary glands. Cancer 1976; 38:1676–1683.

Grimelius L, Åkerström G, Johansson H, et al. Water-clear cell hyperplasia. In: Kovacs K, Asa SL, eds. Functional Endocrine Pathology, Vol. 1. Boston: Blackwell Scientific, 1991, p. 384.

Roth SI. The ultrastructure of primary water-clear cell hyperplasia of the parathyroid glands. Am J Pathol 1970; 61:233–240.

Secondary Hyperparathyroidism

Grimelius L, Åkerström G, Johansson H, et al. Parathyroid glands in secondary and tertiary hyperparathyroidism. In: Kovacs K, Asa SL, eds. Functional Endocrine Pathology, Vol. 1. Boston: Blackwell Scientific, 1991, pp. 387–388.

Llach F, Massry SG. On the mechanism of secondary hyperparathyroidism in moderate renal insufficiency. J Clin Endocrinol Metab 1985; 61:601–606.

Tertiary Hyperparathyroidism

Grimelius L, Åkerström G, Johansson H, et al. Parathyroid glands in secondary and tertiary hyperparathyroidism. In: Kovacs K, Asa SL, eds. Functional Endocrine Pathology, Vol. 1. Boston: Blackwell Scientific, 1991, pp. 387–388.

Krause MW, Hedinger CE. Pathologic study of parathyroid glands in tertiary hyperparathyroidism. Hum Pathol 1985; 16: 772–784.

Parathyroiditis

Bondeson A-G, Bondeson L, Ljungberg O. Chronic parathyroiditis associated with parathyroid hyperplasia and hyperparathyroidism. Am J Surg Pathol 1984; 8:211–215.

Grimelius L, Åkerström G, Johansson H, et al. Parathyroiditis. In: Kovacs K, Asa SL, eds. Functional Endocrine Pathology, Vol. 1. Boston: Blackwell Scientific, 1991, p. 8.

CHAPTER 10

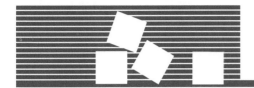

Neoplasms of the Parathyroid Glands

A. CLASSIFICATION OF NEOPLASTIC LESIONS OF THE PARATHYROID GLANDS

Table 10–1
NEOPLASMS OF THE PARATHYROID GLANDS

Parathyroid adenoma
Parathyroid cysts
Parathyroid carcinoma
Secondary neoplasms

B. PARATHYROID ADENOMA

Definition: Benign neoplasm of the parathyroid parenchyma.

Clinical

- More common in women than men (ratio of 3 to 4:1); tumors occur over a broad age range but are most frequently discovered in the fourth and fifth decades.
- Clinical findings are essentially the same as those associated with primary hyperparathyroidism due to hyperplasia (see Chapter 9). As in the latter condition, the symptomatology in patients with parathyroid adenomas is changing as a result of routine biochemical screening and early detection. Hypercalcemia may be incidentally discovered in asymptomatic patients, and many patients complain only of fatigue, weakness, or depression.
- Nephrolithiasis has been documented in 69% of men and 36% of women with adenomas overall, but the incidence has been decreasing in recent years to between 5% and 20%.
- Severe bone disease, once a common complication, is now rare; however, osteopenia is often present, and joint disease similar to that found in patients with parathyroid hyperplasia occurs.
- Serum calcium levels are generally higher than in patients with primary chief cell hyperplasia usually ranging from

12.5 to 13.5 mg/100 dL. Hypophosphatemia, hyperphosphaturia, and elevated serum parathormone levels are found.
- Rarely, parathyroid adenomas present as a palpable mass.

Radiology

- Several imaging methods have been used to localize hyperfunctioning parathyroid tissue, including retrograde phlebotomy (to determine serum parathormone levels), CT scanning, ultrasonography, magnetic resonance imaging (MRI), thallium subtraction scanning, and the more recent technetium-99m sestamibi imaging. The last-named technique appears to be the most useful; successful localization of over 90% of adenomas has been reported. It has been most widely used in patients with anatomic distortion due to previous surgery and in those who present a high surgical risk; however, more routine utilization has gained support.

Pathology

Cytology

- Occasionally enlarged parathyroid glands, either hyperplastic or, more commonly, adenomatous, have been serendipitously subjected to fine needle aspiration because they are thought to be a clinically suspicious "solitary thyroid nodule." More recently, several reports of ultrasonically guided fine needle aspiration for localization and confirmation of parathyroid proliferative disease have appeared.
- An awareness of the typical cytologic appearance of parathyroid tissue can be helpful during intraoperative examination of biopsies during a neck exploration for hyperparathyroidism, because examination of touch preparations provides a rapid means of confirming the presence of parathyroid tissue.
- Aspirates of parathyroid tissue typically contain numerous naked nuclei as well as as small sheets of cells, which sometimes form acinar or follicular structures. Small aggregates of dense colloid-like material may be seen but are not numerous.

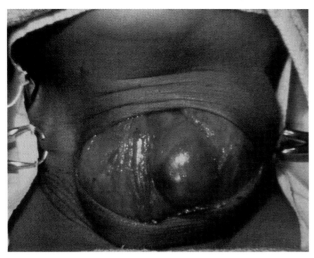

Figure 10–1. Parathyroid adenoma. This large encapsulated lesion bulges into the operative field. Parathyroid adenomas are typically easily dissected free of adjacent structures such as the thyroid gland. Difficulty in removing a parathyroid tumor should raise the suspicion of a parathyroid carcinoma.

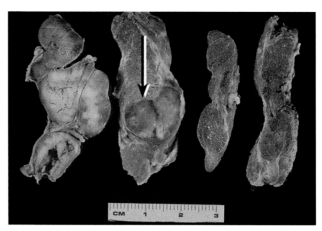

Figure 10–4. Intrathyroidal parathyroid adenoma. Occasionally parathyroid adenomas may be located within the thyroid parenchyma *(arrow)*. In such cases, confusion with a primary thyroid neoplasm can be a pitfall clinically as well as pathologically.

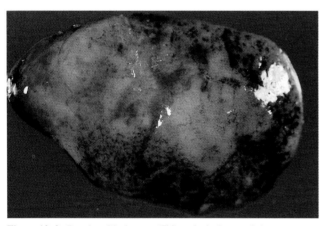

Figure 10–2. Parathyroid adenoma. This typical adenoma is homogeneous and light tan and has a delicate inconspicuous capsule. No remnant of uninvolved parathyroid tissue is visible.

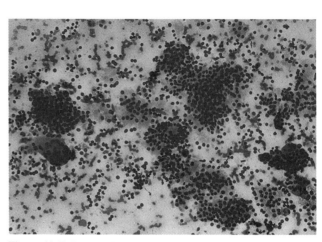

Figure 10–5. Parathyroid adenoma, fine needle aspirate. The cellular smear, which shows cohesive groups of small epithelial cells and fragments of pink colloid-like material, may suggest a follicular neoplasm of thyroid origin. The colloid-like material, however, is somewhat sparse (Diff-Quick stain).

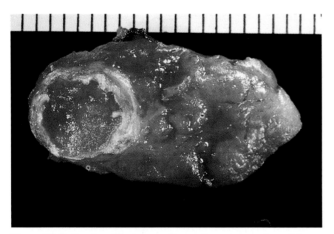

Figure 10–3. Parathyroid adenoma. Some adenomas contain nodular or cystic areas and may become partially calcified, as in this case.

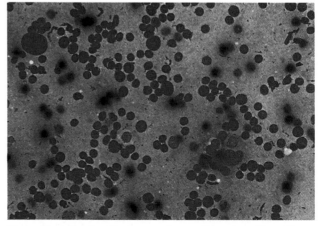

Figure 10–6. Parathyroid adenoma, fine needle aspirate. The cells are quite fragile, yielding smears with numerous naked nuclei, some of which are large and hyperchromatic. Scattered large atypical nuclei are common in parathyroid adenomas (Diff-Quick stain).

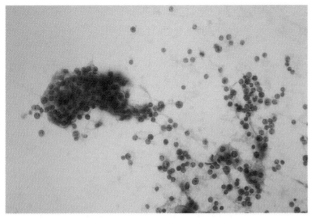

Figure 10–7. Parathyroid adenoma, fine needle aspirate. A Papanicolaou-stained smear reveals scattered compact clusters of quite small epithelial cells with distinct cell borders and a rim of clear cytoplasm. The nuclei are small and hyperchromatic.

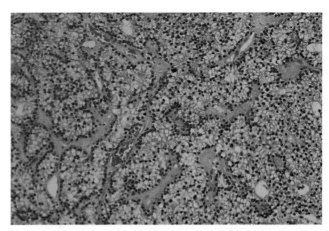

Figure 10–10. Parathyroid adenoma. This neoplasm displays a cordlike growth pattern. The chief cells have rather clear cytoplasm; however, the cells are much smaller and the cytoplasm is not so abundant or so distinctly clear as in the cells of water-clear cell hyperplasia.

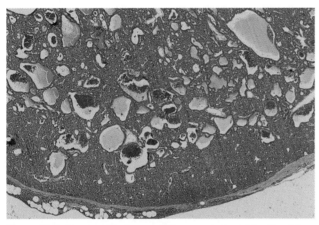

Figure 10–8. Parathyroid adenoma. This very cellular chief cell proliferation has a well-defined capsule and a thin rim of compressed normal parathyroid gland adjacent to the capsule *(bottom)*, findings that define it as a neoplasm rather than a hyperplastic lesion.

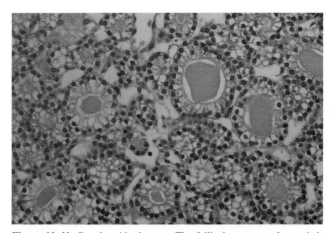

Figure 10–11. Parathyroid adenoma. The follicular pattern of growth is common in parathyroid adenomas and may cause confusion with follicular thyroid neoplasms. The eosinophilic material within the follicles here resembles colloid but is negative on immunostaining for thyroglobulin. The material is, however, PAS positive, as is colloid.

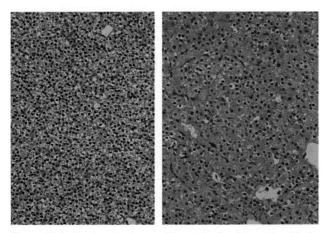

Figure 10–9. Parathyroid adenoma. The chief cells of a parathyroid adenoma resemble those of the normal gland but frequently have larger nuclei than the normal chief cells. *Left,* The cytoplasm may be clear to slightly eosinophilic or *(right)* may display some degree of oxyphilia.

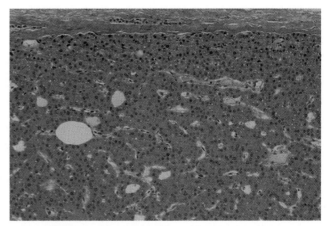

Figure 10–12. Parathyroid adenoma, oxyphilic. This tumor is composed of oxyphilic cells; such lesions have been referred to as oncocytic or oxyphilic adenomas. The epidemiology of such neoplasms does not differ significantly from that of the usual chief cell adenomas.

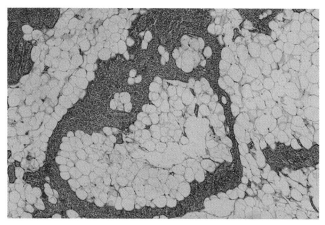

Figure 10–13. Lipoadenoma. Rarely, distinct tumors associated with hyperparathyroidism are composed of a proliferation of both parenchymal cells and stromal fat cells. They are encapsulated and may be associated with a rim of "normal" gland. They are difficult to distinguish from normal parathyroid gland in small biopsies.

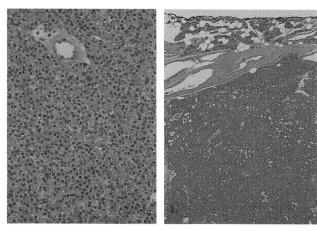

Figure 10–14. Parathyroid adenoma associated with osteitis fibrosa cystica. This adenoma is typical, with a distinct capsule and a rim of normal gland adjacent to it. The patient had a pathologic fracture of the humerus as well as generalized osteopenia with multiple lytic skeletal lesions. At the time of presentation he had hypercalcemia. The initial clinical impression was metastatic carcinoma with secondary hypercalcemia.

- The cells are generally small, with predominantly round nuclei; anisonucleosis in scattered cells and occasional large atypical naked nuclei are common.
- The cytoplasm is granular and may exhibit scattered large metachromatic granules with May-Grunwald-Giemsa's or Romanowsky's stain. Papanicolaou-stained cells have clear to finely granular cytoplasm.
- The nuclei are generally hyperchromatic and have the coarse chromatin typical of neuroendocrine cells.
- Distinction from follicular epithelium of the thyroid may be difficult, although the cells are usually smaller than those of the thyroid. Immunohistochemical staining for chromogranin and thyroglobulin may be helpful in this differential.

Gross

- Adenomas are almost always solitary. Most reports of "multiple adenomas" probably represent asymmetric or

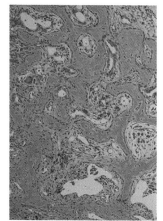 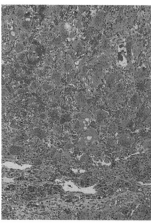

Figure 10–15. Osteitis fibrosa cystica. The humeral lesion from the patient shown in Figure 9–25. *Left,* Dissecting osteitis, with resorption of trabecular bone and replacement by fibrous tissue. The presence of hemosiderin indicates hemorrhage secondary to microfractures in the weakened bone. *Right,* Brown tumors develop after repeated cycles of bone resorption, microfractures, and hemorrhage lead to large areas of cystic degeneration with aggregates of osteoclast-like giant cells in a fibroblastic stroma containing hemosiderin.

nodular hyperplasia. The distinction between hyperplasia and adenoma may be extremely difficult and requires the pathologic examination of *more than a single gland.*
- Ninety percent of adenomas are found in parathyroid glands in their usual locations. The lower glands are more commonly involved. Adenomas may also occur in any location in which parathyroid tissue can be found, including the mediastinum, retroesophageal soft tissue, in the thyroid gland, or in thymic tissue. Adenomas in supernumerary glands have been reported, including tumors arising in the vagus nerve, pericardium, or other soft tissue sites in the neck.
- Adenomas have rounded borders and are firm and brown to tan in color; they are contained within a delicate capsule. They may be ovoid or lobulated. A remnant of uninvolved parathyroid tissue at the periphery of the tumor may be visible.
- Cystic change may be present; when marked, it may mask the neoplastic nature of the proliferation. Marked cystic degeneration is frequently associated with scarring and calcification.
- There is significant variation in weight, with most adenomas weighing between 0.3 and 1.0 g.

Histology

- Most parathyroid adenomas are composed predominantly of chief cells; however, oxyphilic cells may be present in variable numbers, either focally admixed with chief cells or as nodular aggregates. Some adenomas are composed entirely of oxyphilic cells and are referred to as oxyphilic or oncocytic adenomas.
- The cells of an adenoma may be arranged in sheets, cords, nests, or glandular structures. Glandular formations may contain eosinophilic "colloid-like" material. A distinct trabecular pattern is uncommon in adenomas.
- The chief cells of an adenoma are frequently somewhat larger than the non-neoplastic chief cells found in the unin-

volved rim of parathyroid tissue, if one is present. The cytoplasm is typically slightly eosinophilic but may be clear.

- The neoplastic cells usually have less intracellular fat than the cells in the uninvolved (or suppressed) parathyroid tissue, either in other glands or in a rim of non-neoplastic parathyroid tissue in an adenomatous gland.
- The nuclei are usually slightly larger than normal chief cells. They are usually round and have a central to slightly basal location within the cell. Nucleoli are not prominent.
- Cells with hyperchromatic enlarged nuclei, as well as multinucleated cells, are rather common. They may be scattered throughout the tumor or clustered in small foci. These scattered atypical nuclei are not an indicator of malignancy in the absence of other evidence of aggressive behavior.
- A rim of non-neoplastic parathyroid tissue is identified with only about half the adenomas. If present, this finding is very helpful in making a distinction between an adenoma and hyperplasia. The "rim" generally contains abundant stromal fat cells, unlike the very cellular adenoma, and the parenchymal cells of the rim are smaller than the tumor cells.
- Mitotic figures are identifiable in many adenomas but usually number fewer than 1/10 HPF. Mitotic rates of as high as 4/10 HPF have been described in occasional cases. Atypical mitoses are not present.
- *Immunohistochemistry:* Although the colloid-like material in glandular structures in the tumors is PAS-positive, like thyroglobulin, immunohistochemical stains are negative for thyroglobulin. Adenomas are also positive for cytokeratin, chromogranin (and other neuroendocrine markers), and parathormone. Immunohistochemical examination for parathormone has been less than satisfactory in many laboratories; in situ hybridization for messenger RNA for parathyroid hormone has been much more sensitive.
- *Electron microscopy:* Adenomas associated with very high serum calcium levels may have a large number of microvilli, which are thought to reflect a higher level of endocrine activity. Adenomas often have more abundant rough endoplasmic reticulum and a more prominent Golgi apparatus than non-neoplastic cells. Annulate lamellae may be seen.
- Flow cytometry has not been very useful in distinguishing parathyroid adenomas from carcinomas because aneuploidy has been found in up to 25% of histologically and clinically benign tumors.
- "Oxyphilic" adenomas were at one time thought to be nonfunctional; however, several reports have documented an association with primary hyperparathyroidism. They are composed of large cells with abundant eosinophilic granular cytoplasm and rather hyperchromatic nuclei. Scattered large atypical nuclei or multinucleated cells may be seen. The cytoplasm is stuffed with mitochondria on electron microscopic examination. The demographic features are similar to those of the more common adenomas composed of chief cells. An important differential consideration is the frequent presence of nodular oxyphilic changes seen in normal glands with increasing age.
- Lipoadenomas are rare benign neoplasms characterized by proliferation of parenchymal and stromal fat cells.

They are encapsulated and may be associated with a compressed rim of "normal" gland. They are difficult to recognize as "abnormal" parathyroid tissue in small biopsies, in which they are easily mistaken for normal parathyroid tissue or for normal adipose tissue because of the abundance of stromal fat. Grossly, these lesions resemble lipomas. The stromal fat often contains areas of fibrosis or myxoid alteration. Most are associated with hyperparathyroidism.

Differential Diagnosis

- Primary chief cell hyperplasia (Chapter 9).
- Parathyroid carcinoma (Chapter 10D).
- Follicular neoplasm of thyroid gland (Chapter 8B and C).

Treatment and Prognosis

- The most widely accepted therapy is excision of the adenomatous gland with biopsy of at least one additional gland that is "normal" in size.
- Some favor a full bilateral neck exploration with subtotal parathyroidectomy and have reported a lower incidence of recurrent hypercalcemia requiring reoperation. There is an increased incidence of postoperative hypoparathyroidism with this procedure.
- Recurrence rates vary significantly and may reflect problems in classification, particularly in cases of hyperplasia with nodules that may be designated adenomas erroneously.
- Although generalized osteopenia is now more common, *osteitis fibrosa cystica,* also known as "brown tumors," is occasionally seen. It may occur in patients with hyperparathyroidism of any cause but is related to the degree and duration of serum calcium elevation. The lesions are characterized by resorption of bone, which is replaced by fibrous tissue, probably as a response to microfractures. Hemorrhage within the fibrous tissue leads to the accumulation of hemosiderin and a proliferation of multinucleated giant cells in addition to the osteoclasts. With time, degenerative changes lead to the formation of cystic spaces. Osteitis fibrosa cystica cannot be distinguished histologically from the giant cell reparative granuloma of the jaw; clinical information is essential.

Additional Facts

- Recurrent hyperparathyroidism following surgery for an adenoma may result from incomplete excision, rupture of the tumor capsule with spillage into the operative field, or hyperfunction of autografted parathyroid tissue following subtotal parathyroidectomy.
- The uninvolved parathyroid glands in patients with adenomas are typically smaller and often have more stromal fat cells than glands in patients without hyperparathyroidism. They also have more cytoplasmic fat, often found as large droplets, than normally functioning parathyroid glands.
- There is considerable variation in the literature about the use of fat stains in the diagnosis of parathyroid proliferative diseases. Generally, hyperfunctioning cells have a sig-

nificantly decreased amount of intracellular fat (using Sudan black or oil red O) compared to normal or suppressed parenchymal cells. There is, however, variability in this finding. Fat stains, when used with adequate clinical information, intraoperative findings, and histologic examination, are useful if their limitations are kept in mind.

C. PARATHYROID CYSTS

Definition: Cystic lesions associated with a parathyroid parenchymal cell lining or associated parathyroid tissue in the cyst wall. These lesions may represent either hyperplasia or adenomas with cystic degeneration or developmental cysts (if they are not hyperfunctioning).

Clinical

- These rare lesions may be symptomatic or may be discovered incidentally during surgery or by radiographs (especially in the case of mediastinal parathyroid cysts).
- Patients may be either normocalcemic or hypercalcemic. Hypercalcemia is associated with the usual biochemical pattern of primary hyperparathyroidism.
- Symptoms may be caused by the presence of a mass lesion or by the hypercalcemia (as in other cases of primary hyperparathyroidism).

Pathology

Cytology

- Fine needle aspiration has been useful in the identification of some parathyroid cysts preoperatively, particularly palpable cervical lesions.
- Aspirated cyst fluid may contain clusters of cells in microacinar or papillary-like groups that have coarse chromatin and finely granular cytoplasm with poorly defined cell borders.
- The cellular component may be difficult to distinguish from follicular thyroid epithelium; immunohistochemistry for thyroglobulin and chromogranin may be helpful if adequate tissue is present.

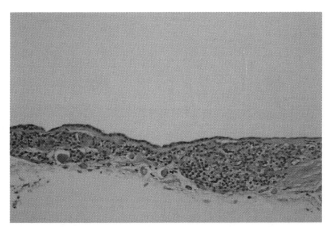

Figure 10–16. Parathyroid cyst. The cyst is lined by a thin layer of parathyroid parenchymal cells and is surrounded in some areas by a rim of parathyroid tissue.

- Assay of the cyst fluid for parathormone can be used to establish the diagnosis of a parathyroid cyst.

Gross

- Most cysts are located in the neck, but mediastinal cysts have been reported.
- Cysts vary in size. Although many smaller cysts obviously represent cystic change in a parathyroid adenoma, some as large as 10 cm have been described.
- The cyst wall may be represented by a rim of parathyroid tissue, or it may be quite thin and translucent. The cyst fluid is thin and colorless to yellow, although sometimes it is bloody. The capsule is typically well defined.

Histology

- The cyst may be lined by flattened epithelium or by recognizable chief cells.
- Islands of parathyroid tissue are present within or adjacent to the cyst wall. This parathyroid tissue may appear normal or may represent a parathyroid adenoma or a hyperplastic parathyroid gland.

Differential Diagnosis

- Cystic thyroid neoplasm or adenomatoid nodule.
- Lymphangioma.
- Thymic cyst.
- Bronchogenic, neurenteric, or esophageal foregut cysts.
- Pericardial or pleural cysts.

Treatment and Prognosis

- Preferred treatment is surgical removal.
- If hypercalcemia is present, the approach should include investigation of the status of other parathyroid glands—intraoperatively if the cyst is cervical or postoperatively if the lesion is intrathoracic.

D. PARATHYROID CARCINOMA

Definition: A malignant neoplasm of parathyroid parenchymal cells.

Clinical (Table 10–2)

- Rare neoplasm; responsible for less than 3% of cases of hyperparathyroidism.
- No gender predilection. It occurs most commonly in the fifth and sixth decades, but rare cases have been reported in children.

Table 10–2
CLINICAL FEATURES SUGGESTING MALIGNANCY IN PARATHYROID NEOPLASMS

Serum calcium level >14 mg/100 ml
Serum parathormone levels two to three times normal
Severe metabolic manifestations: nephrolithiasis, bone disease, etc.
Palpable neck mass
Difficulty in surgical dissection

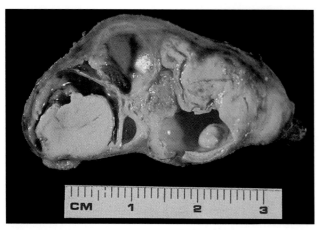

Figure 10–17. Parathyroid carcinoma. This large tumor has areas of cystic degeneration associated with large nodules of viable tumor. The capsule is grossly thickened.

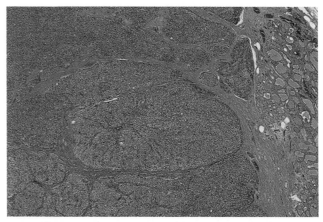

Figure 10–20. Parathyroid carcinoma. This neoplasm has the typical low-power appearance of carcinoma, with a thickened capsule, fibrous bands extending from the capsule and dissecting through the tumor, and adherence to the adjacent thyroid lobe *(extreme right).*

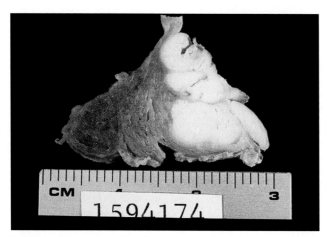

Figure 10–18. Parathyroid carcinoma. An irregular, infiltrative, indurated, white neoplasm, this carcinoma was adherent to the adjacent thyroid lobe *(left)* and could not readily be dissected free of it. Difficulty in dissecting parathyroid neoplasms free of adjacent tissues is very suggestive of malignancy.

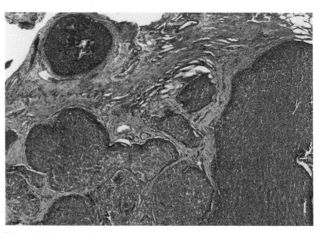

Figure 10–21. Parathyroid carcinoma. Multinodular growth and extensive fibrosis are clues to malignant behavior in parathyroid neoplasms. One nodule *(upper left)* is well outside the main contour of the tumor, indicating an infiltrative pattern (Movat stain).

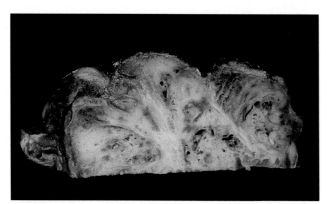

Figure 10–19. Parathyroid carcinoma. Some parathyroid carcinomas are more advanced and show extensive invasion of surrounding tissues. Cases such as this are rare today because of routine biochemical screening of most populations in developed countries.

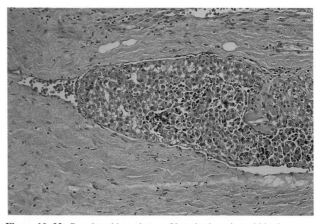

Figure 10–22. Parathyroid carcinoma. Vascular invasion within the capsular vessels. Vascular invasion is a definitive criterion for malignancy.

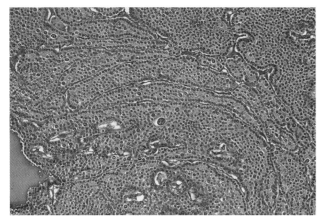

Figure 10–23. Parathyroid carcinoma. The intense cellularity and trabecular pattern are features that help distinguish parathyroid carcinoma from parathyroid adenoma. Trabecular growth is evident.

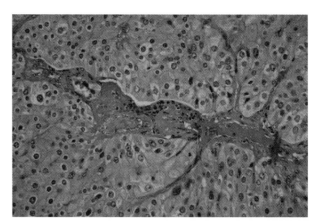

Figure 10–26. Parathyroid carcinoma. Nuclear pleomorphism is present throughout this neoplasm. Although pleomorphic nuclei are frequently seen in adenomas, they are not generally diffusely present but rather are scattered singly or in small foci within the tumor. A monotonous nuclear pattern is, surprisingly, more often seen in carcinomas than in adenomas.

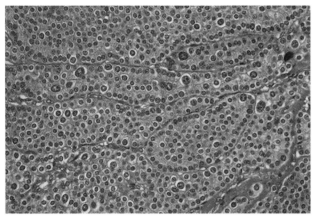

Figure 10–24. Parathyroid carcinoma. A prominent trabecular pattern is seen, with scattered large hyperchromatic nuclei. Such enlarged atypical nuclei are often seen in adenomas and are not definitive indicators of malignancy. They are, however, uncommon in hyperplasia. The otherwise monotonous nuclear pattern in this tumor is, however, frequently seen in carcinomas.

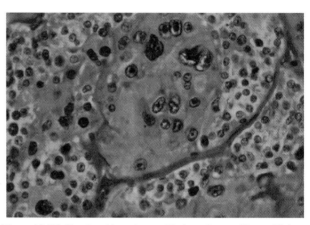

Figure 10–27. Parathyroid carcinoma. Nuclear pleomorphism, with large nuclei with prominent nucleoli and irregular chromatin distribution, is seen.

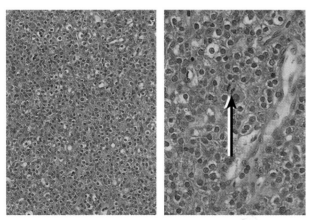

Figure 10–25. Parathyroid carcinoma. The cells in this neoplasm are crowded but are otherwise not greatly different from those of a typical adenoma. Mitotic figures are readily found *(right; arrow).* Mitoses are not by themselves accurate predictors of malignancy because they are seen in parathyroid hyperplasia and adenomas as well.

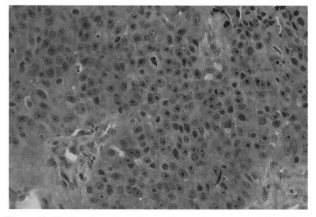

Figure 10–28. Parathyroid carcinoma. A monotonous crowded proliferation of cells with large nuclei and very large nucleoli is seen in many parathyroid carcinomas but not in benign parathyroid lesions. Mitoses were readily identified in this case (not shown).

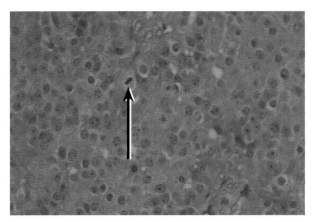

Figure 10–29. Parathyroid carcinoma. Another carcinoma, showing somewhat smaller but still prominent nucleoli as well as a mitotic figure *(arrow)*.

- Most patients have severe hypercalcemia (mean serum calcium 14.0 mg/100 ml; in contrast, the mean serum calcium in benign hyperparathyroidism is 12.0 mg/100 ml).
- Occasional normocalcemic patients have been reported.
- Symptoms are similar to those seen in patients with benign hyperparathyroidism but tend to be more severe because of the higher serum calcium levels in carcinoma. Presenting symptoms include fatigue and weakness, depression, bone disease (there was a high incidence in earlier series), nephrolithiasis (reported in up to two thirds of patients in earlier studies, but this is probably decreasing with routine biochemical screening and earlier detection), and peptic ulcer disease.
- Palpable neck masses are more common than in hyperplasia or adenoma.
- Some cases have been reported in patients with familial parathyroid proliferative diseases.

Radiology

- Imaging procedures are the same as those used for parathyroid adenomas. Technetium 99m sestamibi imaging is gaining wide acceptance.

Pathology (Table 10–3)

Gross

- Average tumor size is larger than that of parathyroid adenomas: mean weight 6.7 g (range 1.5 to 27 g), although smaller tumors are being identified more often in recent years.
- May be encapsulated or infiltrative.
- Brown to gray-white in color; carcinomas may have a smooth, firm cut surface that is indistinguishable from that of an adenoma, or they may be distinctly indurated.
- Difficulty in dissection of the tumor or adherence to the thyroid gland are common intraoperative observations.

Histology

- May be very difficult to distinguish from a parathyroid adenoma or may be obviously malignant.

Table 10–3

PATHOLOGIC FEATURES ASSOCIATED WITH MALIGNANCY IN PARATHYROID NEOPLASMS

Large size (mean weight, 6.7 g)
Adherence to thyroid tissue
Irregular contour, lack of distinct encapsulation
Thick capsule
Fibrous bands within tumor
Mitotic activity (especially >5–7/10 high-power fields [HPF])
Atypical mitoses (even if mitotic rate is low)
Capsular invasion, especially with extraglandular extension
Vascular invasion
Trabecular growth
Monotonous cytologic features
Spindling of tumor cells
Macronucleoli

- The tumor cells may have variable morphology, some being very similar to benign chief cells with a slightly eosinophilic to clear cytoplasm. Other areas may contain enlarged cells with a more distinctly eosinophilic cytoplasm and large nuclei with prominent nucleoli.
- The growth patterns also vary and include solid sheets, glandular or acinar formations, cords, rosettes, and, of particular differential diagnostic significance, trabeculae. Nuclear palisading may be prominent in trabecular areas. Spindling of cells is also a feature that is more often seen in carcinomas than in benign proliferations.
- Nuclear pleomorphism is, surprisingly, less common than in adenomas, which often contain scattered foci with enlarged atypical nuclei. Monotony of nuclear size and shape is frequently present in carcinomas; pleomorphism, when present, is usually more diffuse than in adenomas.
- Mitotic activity is identified in most, but not all, parathyroid carcinomas. Although a high mitotic rate is a helpful feature, the presence of mitotic activity exceeding 1/10 HPF has been reported in a minority of parathyroid adenomas and in parathyroid hyperplasia. This overlap makes mitotic activity a useful finding only when it is combined with other features of malignancy.
- Atypical mitoses are virtually diagnostic of malignancy.
- Many parathyroid carcinomas are encapsulated. Usually the capsule of a carcinoma is thicker than that seen in most adenomas. Some adenomas in which hemorrhage and degenerative changes have occurred have thick and uneven capsules; the presence of hemosiderin and other evidence of long-standing degenerative changes such as chronic inflammation and areas of cystic change is helpful in differentiating these adenomas from carcinomas.
- Capsular invasion may be obvious in some cases or may be represented only by irregular tongues or islands of parathyroid tissue protruding into the capsule. Invasion beyond the capsule is indicative of malignancy. Entrapped islands of parathyroid parenchymal cells in benign disease should be distinguished from these invasive foci by their rounded contours and lack of desmoplastic reaction.
- Fibrous bands, often contiguous with a thickened capsule, frequently divide the tumors into irregular compartments.
- Vascular invasion is diagnostic of carcinoma but is present in a minority of cases. It is usually found within ves-

sels in the thick tumor capsule. Artifactually displaced clumps of tumor cells in vascular spaces should be distinguished from true invasion by their frequently degenerated appearance and their lack of attachment to the vessel wall.

■ Perineural invasion, although rarely seen, is also virtually diagnostic of malignancy.

■ Although flow cytometric features of adenomas and carcinomas show significant overlap, with aneuploidy in some adenomas and diploidy in some carcinomas, there is some evidence that aneuploidy may be associated with a more aggressive course in parathyroid carcinomas.

Differential Diagnosis

■ Parathyroid adenoma (Table 10–4) (Chapter 10B).
■ Metastatic carcinoma from another site, particularly renal cell carcinoma.

Treatment and Prognosis

■ En bloc resection, including the ipsilateral thyroid lobe and the adjacent soft tissues and lymph nodes, at the time of initial surgery is the preferred therapy. Lymph node metastases are uncommon at the time of diagnosis; how-

Table 10–4
COMPARATIVE FEATURES OF PARATHYROID PROLIFERATIVE DISEASES

Features	Hyperplasia	Adenoma	Carcinoma
Gender, age	Slight female predilection; most common in 5th to 6th decades	More common in women; most common in 4th decade	Equal gender predilection; wide age range
Clinical	Asymptomatic or complaints of lethargy, weakness, polyuria, polydipsia, arthralgia, constipation, and depression	Similar to hyperplasia	Similar to hyperparathyroidism of benign etiology but more severe due to the higher serum calcium levels; higher proportion of renal disease (nephrolithiasis) and bone disease; peptic ulcer disease; palpable neck mass more common than in adenoma
Serum calcium	11.7 mg/10 ml (average)	12.5–13.5 mg/100 ml	Often >14 mg/100 ml
Intraoperative findings	Two or more glands enlarged, easily dissected. Enlargement may be very asymmetric	One gland enlarged; easily dissected; more frequent in lower glands or ectopic sites	One gland enlarged; often adherent to surrounding tissues
Weight	Total gland weight usually <1 g, but may be up to 5 g	0.3–1 g commonly, but may weigh several grams in patients with bone disease	>1.5 g (often much larger)
Capsule	Circumscribed by capsule of parathyroid gland; may be incomplete. No compressed rim of atrophic or normal parathyroid tissue	Thin tumor capsule, often surrounded by rim of uninvolved parathyroid, which may appear atrophic	Thickened capsule; rim of normal parathyroid rarely seen
Gross appearance	Gray-brown, soft. Cut surface may be homogeneous or nodular. Lacks fibrous bands	Red-brown, firm. Usually homogeneous, lacks fibrous bands	Gray-white, firm, often lobulated or irregular. Fibrous bands often produce coarse nodularity
Histologic growth pattern	Diffuse or nodular, sometimes pseudofollicular or acinar	Diffuse or nodular, frequently pseudofollicular or acinar	Diffuse, nodular, pseudofollicular, or acinar; often trabecular
Cytologic features	Chief cells predominate; transitional and oxyphilic cells often present	Chief cells predominate, but mixture of chief, transitional, and oxyphilic cells may be seen; rarely, purely oxyphilic	Cells usually resemble chief cells, but variable cytoplasmic oxyphilia may be seen; cell borders are often indistinct
Intracytoplasmic lipid	Decreased	Decreased in tumor; abundant in atrophic rim of parathyroid	Usually absent
Stromal fat cells	Scanty to absent	Usually absent in tumor; present in rim of atrophic parathyroid	Absent
Nuclear morphology	Normal to slightly increased N-to-C ratio; usually without nuclear pleomorphism	Nuclei enlarged, with variability in size; scattered groups of large pleomorphic, hyperchromatic nuclei, or multinucleated cells	Increased N-to-C ratio; enlarged atypical nuclei, often with a very monotonous pattern; prominent nucleoli
Nucleoli	Inconspicuous to small	Inconspicuous to small	Frequently prominent and enlarged

Table continued on following page

Table 10–4
COMPARATIVE FEATURES OF PARATHYROID PROLIFERATIVE DISEASES *(Continued)*

Features	Hyperplasia	Adenoma	Carcinoma
Mitoses	Usually rare	Usually rare (occasionally >1/ 10 HPF)	Usually present (80% of cases), may include atypical mitoses; may be numerous
Capsular and vascular invasion	Absent	Absent; entrapment of tumor cells may occur in capsule if degenerative changes present	Capsular invasion present in two thirds; may involve only capsule or extend into adjacent tissues; Vascular invasion present in 10–15%; usually in capsular vessels
Remainder of gland	Entire gland is abnormal	Normal or atrophic	Normal
Degenerative changes	May be seen in very large glands; includes hemorrhage, areas of fibrosis, and cystic change	Common, especially in larger adenomas; includes hemorrhage, fibrosis, hemosiderin-laden macrophages, and cystic change; sometimes calcification	Tumor cell necrosis; calcification and cystic changes may be present
Treatment	Subtotal parathyroidectomy with surgical removal of three glands leaving a remnant of the 4th or total parathyroidectomy* with autotransplantation of parathyroid tissue in forearm	Surgical removal of the enlarged gland	En bloc resection, including ipsilateral thyroid lobe and adjacent soft tissues and lymph nodes
Prognosis	Excellent	Excellent	Up to 50% of patients are cured by en bloc resection; considered an indolent malignancy, even in presence of recurrence or metastasis, with long survival even after recognition of tumor recurrence; morbidity and mortality correlate to complications of severe hypercalcemia
Recurrence and metastasis	Recurrence in approximately 16% of cases due to inadequate neck exploration and may not be evident for years	Absent	Recurrence in two thirds of patients usually within 3 years of the first surgery; metastasis in 35% is a late event usually preceded by local recurrence; most commonly to lung, cervical lymph nodes, and liver
Familial and/or MEN association	Yes, in approximately 20% of cases	Uncommon	Rare

*Particularly in cases of familial hyperparathyroidism.
MEN, multiple endocrine neoplasia syndrome; N-to-C, nuclear-to-cytoplasmic; HPF, high-power field.

ever, the presence of nodal disease is considered an indication for neck dissection.

■ The prognosis of parathyroid carcinoma appears to be changing as a result of earlier detection. The proportion of well-differentiated encapsulated lesions is increasing; risk of recurrence has been correlated with extraglandular invasiveness. Up to 50% of patients are cured by en bloc resection.

■ Recurrences generally become manifest within 3 years of the first surgery with locally recurrent disease.

■ Metastatic disease occurs rather late in the course of disease, usually several years after the primary diagnosis; it is found in 35% of patients.

■ Metastases most commonly involve the lung, cervical lymph nodes, and liver, in decreasing order.

■ Monitoring for recurrent disease is most effectively accomplished with serum calcium levels.

■ Surgical resection of metastatic or locally recurrent disease is frequently helpful owing to the rather indolent nature of parathyroid carcinoma. Patients usually survive for several years after tumor recurrence has been recognized.

■ The major difficulty in management of recurrent disease is severe hypercalcemia and its complications. Death is related to excessive hormonal product leading to subsequent hypercalcemia rather than directly to tumor burden.

Additional Facts

■ Recent evidence suggests that loss of the retinoblastoma tumor-suppressor gene may play an important role in the development of parathyroid carcinoma and that its absence may be helpful in distinguishing parathyroid adenomas from carcinomas.

- Immunoreactivity for Ki-67, a cell cycle-associated antigen, may also prove helpful in distinguishing adenomas from carcinomas; there have been recently reported increases in labeling indices for Ki-67 in parathyroid carcinomas.
- Occasional neoplasms may have some features that indicate malignancy but are inconclusive. Such features as mitoses (<5/10 HPF), capsular irregularities without infiltration of adjacent soft tissues, trabecular growth, and internal fibrosis without more conclusive features such as vascular invasion, extraglandular invasion, atypical mitoses, and macronucleoli are seen in a subset of clinically benign neoplasms that have been designated "atypical adenomas." These lesions, although not overtly malignant, require close patient follow-up because the possibility of aggressive behavior cannot be excluded.

E. SECONDARY NEOPLASMS

Definition: Contiguous involvement from tumors in adjacent structures or metastatic neoplasms from distant sites involving the parathyroid gland.

Clinical

- Usually asymptomatic, although rare cases have been associated with clinical hypoparathyroidism owing to massive replacement of multiple glands.
- May result from direct extension, especially from thyroid or laryngeal tumors, or from metastatic spread.
- Common primary malignancies include breast carcinoma (most common), hematologic malignancies, melanoma, and lung carcinoma.

Pathology

- Found in 11.9% of cancer patients in autopsy studies.
- May involve one or multiple glands.
- *Immunohistochemistry:* A variety of organ-specific markers may be helpful in the diagnosis of a metastatic tumor to the parathyroid gland. The presence of specific markers such as prostate-specific antigen or prostate-specific acid phosphatase, or the absence of the usual markers seen in parathyroid tissue, particularly chromogranin, can be helpful in distinguishing between primary and secondary neoplasms.

Differential Diagnosis

- Parathyroid carcinoma (Chapter 10D).

Treatment and Prognosis

- Treatment based on primary site of origin.
- Prognosis poor; related to dissemination of primary disease.

Bibliography

Parathyroid Adenoma

Abdul-Haj SK, Conklin H, Hewitt WC. Functioning lipoadenoma of the parathyroid gland: Report of a unique case. N Engl J Med 1962; 266:121–132.

Aguilar-Parada E, Gonzalez-Angulo A, Del Peon L, Mravko E. Functioning microvillous adenoma of the parathyroid gland containing nuclear pores and annulate lamellae. Hum Pathol 1985; 16:511–516.

Bedetti CD, Dekker A, Watson CG: Functioning oxyphil cell adenoma of the parathyroid gland: A clinicopathologic study of ten patients with hyperparathyroidism. Hum Pathol 1984; 15:1121–1126.

Bombi JA, Nadal A, Muñoz J, Cardesa A: Ultrastructural pathology of parathyroid glands in hyperparathyroidism: A report of 69 cases. Ultrastruct Pathol 1993; 17:567–582.

Bondeson A-G, Bondeson L, Ljungberg O, Tibblin S: Fat staining in parathyroid disease—diagnostic value and impact on surgical strategy. Hum Pathol 1985; 16:1255–1263.

Cinti S, Colussi G, Minola E, Dickersin GR: Parathyroid glands in primary hyperparathyroidism: An ultrastructural study of 50 cases. Hum Pathol 1986; 17:1036–1046.

Clark O, Duh Q-Y: Primary hyperparathyroidism: A surgical perspective. Endocrinol Metab Clin North Am 1989; 18:701–714.

DeLellis RA. Parathyroid adenoma. In: DeLellis RA, ed. Tumors of the Parathyroid Gland. Third series, Fascicle 6. Washington, DC: Armed Forces Institute of Pathology, 1991, pp. 25–51.

Fraker DL, Travis WD, Merendino JJ Jr, et al. Locally recurrent parathyroid neoplasms as a cause for recurrent and persistent primary hyperparathyroidism. Ann Surg 1991; 213:58–65.

Geelhoed GW. Parathyroid adenolipoma: Clinical and morphological features. Surgery 1982; 92:806–810.

Ghandur-Mnaymneh L, Kimura N. The parathyroid adenoma: A histopathologic definition with a study of 172 cases of primary hyperparathyroidism. Am J Pathol 1984; 115:70–83.

Grimelius L, Åkerström G, Johansson H, et al. Adenomas. In: Kovacs K, Asa SL, eds. Functional Endocrine Pathology. Vol. 1. Boston: Blackwell Scientific, 1991, pp. 380–383.

Lee VS, Wilkinson RH, Leight GS, et al. Hyperparathyroidism in high-risk surgical patients: Evaluation with double-phase technetium-99m sestamibi imaging. Radiology 1995; 197:627–623.

Palmer M, Ljunghall S, Åkerström G, et al. Patients with primary hyperparathyroidism operated on over a 24-year period: Temporal trends of clinical and laboratory findings. J Chron Dis 1987; 40:121–130.

Rudberg C, Åkerström G, Palmer M, et al. Late results of operation for primary hyperparathyroidism in 441 patients. Surgery 1986; 99:643–651.

Sasano H, Geelhoed GW, Silverberg SG. Intraoperative evaluation of lipid in the diagnosis of parathyroid adenoma. Am J Surg Pathol 1988; 12:282–286.

Snover DC, Foucar K. Mitotic activity in benign parathyroid disease. Am J Clin Pathol 1981; 75:345–347.

Wolpert HR, Vickery AL Jr, Wang CA: Functioning oxyphil cell adenomas of the parathyroid gland. A study of 15 cases. Am J Surg Pathol 1989; 13:500–504.

Parathyroid Cysts

Calandra DB, Shah KH, Prinz RA, et al. Parathyroid cysts: A report of 11 cases including two associated with hyperparathyroid crisis. Surgery 1983; 94:887–892.

Downey RJ, Cerfolio RJ, Deschamps C, et al. Mediastinal parathyroid cysts. Mayo Clin Proc 1995; 70:946–950.

Layfield LJ. Fine needle aspiration cytology of cystic parathyroid lesions. Acta Cytol 1991; 35:447–450.

Wang C, Vickery AL Jr, Maloof F. Large parathyroid cysts mimicking thyroid nodules. Ann Surg 1972; 175:448–453.

Wick MR. Mediastinal cysts and intrathoracic thyroid tumors. Semin Diagn Pathol 1990; 7:285–294.

Parathyroid Carcinoma

Bombi JA, Nadal A, Muñoz J, Cardesa A. Ultrastructural pathology of parathyroid glands in hyperparathyroidism: A report of 69 cases. Ultrastruct Pathol 1993; 17:567–582.

Bondeson L, Sandelin K, Grimelius L. Histopathological variables and DNA cytometry in parathyroid carcinoma. Am J Surg Pathol 1993; 17:820–829.

Cohn K, Silverman M, Corrado J, Sedgewick C. Parathyroid carcinoma: The Lahey Clinic experience. Surgery 1985; 98:1095–1100.

DeLellis RA. Parathyroid carcinoma. In: DeLellis RA, ed. Tumors of the Parathyroid Gland. Third series. Fascicle 6. Washington, DC: Armed Forces Institute of Pathology, 1991, pp. 53–63.

Cryns VL, Thor A, Xu H-J, et al. Loss of the retinoblastoma tumor-suppressor gene in parathyroid carcinoma. N Engl J Med 1994; 330:757–761.

Fitko R, Roth SI, Hines JR, et al. Parathyromatosis in hyperparathyroidism. Hum Pathol 1990; 21:234–237.

Fraker DL, Travis WD, Merendino JJ Jr, et al. Locally recurrent parathyroid neoplasms as a cause for recurrent and persistent primary hyperparathyroidism. Ann Surg 1991; 213:58–65.

Grimelius L, Åkerström G, Johansson, et al. Parathyroid carcinoma. In: Kovacs K, Asa SL, eds. Functional Endocrine Pathology. Vol. 1. Boston: Blackwell Scientific, 1991, pp. 384–387.

Harlow S, Roth SI, Bauer K, Marshall RB. Flow cytometric DNA analysis of normal and pathologic parathyroid glands. Mod Pathol 1991; 4:310–315.

Levin KE, Galante M, Clark OH. Parathyroid carcinoma versus parathyroid adenoma in patients with profound hypercalcemia. Surgery 1987; 101:640–660.

Lloyd RV, Carney JA, Ferreiro JA, et al. Immunohistochemical analysis of the cell cycle-associated antigens Ki-67 and retinoblastoma pro-tein in parathyroid carcinomas and adenoma. Endocr Pathol 1995; 6:279–287.

Schantz A, Castleman B. Parathyroid carcinoma: A study of 70 cases. Cancer 1973; 31:600–605.

Snover DC, Foucar K: Mitotic activity in benign parathyroid disease. Am J Clin Pathol 1981; 775:345–347.

Wang C, Gaz RD. Natural history of parathyroid carcinoma: Diagnosis, treatment, results. Am J Surg 1985; 149:522–527.

Wynne AG, van Heerden J, Carney JA, Fitzpatrick LA: Parathyroid carcinoma: Clinical and pathologic features in 43 patients. Medicine 1992; 71:197–205.

Secondary Neoplasms

DeLellis RA. Secondary tumors. In: DeLellis RA, ed. Tumors of the Parathyroid Gland, Third Series. Fascicle 6. Washington, DC: Armed Forces Institute of Pathology, 1991, p. 94.

Horwitz CA, Myers WP, Foote FW Jr: Secondary malignant tumors of the parathyroid glands: Report of two cases with associated hypoparathyroidism. Am J Med 1972; 52:797–808.

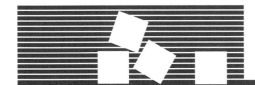

CHAPTER 11

Non-Neoplastic Lesions of the Pancreas

A. CLASSIFICATION OF NON-NEOPLASTIC LESIONS OF THE PANCREAS

Table 11–1

CLASSIFICATION OF NON-NEOPLASTIC LESIONS OF THE PANCREAS

Congenital Abnormalities of the Exocrine Pancreas

Aplasia and hypoplasia (congenital short pancreas)
Ductal abnormalities
Pancreas divisum
Annular pancreas
Congenital cysts
    Solitary
    Multiple
Choledochal cyst

Hereditary Diseases

Cystic fibrosis
Diabetes mellitus*
Shwachman-Diamond syndrome
Johanson-Blizzard syndrome
Sideroblastic anemia and exocrine pancreatic insufficiency
Enzymatic deficiencies
Hereditary pancreatitis

Infectious Diseases

Pancreatitis

Acute interstitial pancreatitis
Acute hemorrhagic pancreatitis
Chronic pancreatitis

Acquired Lesions/Diseases

Age-related alterations
Heterotopic pancreas
Pseudocysts
True (non-neoplastic) cysts
    Lymphoepithelial cyst
    Enterogenous cyst
    Endometrial cyst
    Parasitic cyst
Hamartoma
Inflammatory pseudotumor

*Not strictly a hereditary disease.

B. CONGENITAL ABNORMALITIES OF THE EXOCRINE PANCREAS

1. Aplasia, Hypoplasia, and Dysplasia

Definition: Agenesis—complete developmental absence of the pancreas. Aplasia or partial agenesis—the pancreas is histologically normal but defective in size and shape. Hypoplasia—the pancreas is of normal size and shape, but there is replacement of the normal epithelial structures with fatty tissue and reduction in the number of ducts and their terminal differentiation. Dysplasia—the pancreas is of normal size and shape, but the parenchyma is disorganized with dilated ducts surrounded by fibromuscular tissue.

Synonym: Congenital short pancreas.

Clinical

- Complete agenesis of the pancreas is rare and incompatible with life.
- Complete and partial agenesis result from a primary defect in early organogenesis.
- In partial agenesis, the pancreas is histologically normal but defective in size and shape owing to a failure of development of the dorsal bud segment.
- Pancreatic agenesis, hypoplasia, and dysplasia are often seen in association with other congenital pancreatic abnormalities and in syndromes involving a combination of hepatic, renal, and pancreatic dysplasia.
- Clinical features of malabsorption are present in those patients who retain minimally residual pancreatic exocrine function.
- Some patients with partial agenesis survive to adulthood and have presented with recurrent attacks of epigastric and back pain.
- The functional capacity of the pancreas can be assessed by direct measurement of pancreatic enzymes following secretin stimulation or indirectly by measurement of fecal fat analysis or circulating trypsinogen levels.

- The differentiation of partial agenesis, hypoplasia, or dysplasia cannot be made on the basis of pancreatic function testing; computed tomographic (CT) scan has proven to be effective in diagnosis based on the altered density owing to fatty replacement of pancreatic exocrine structures.
- Those patients with malabsorption require aggressive treatment with pancreatic enzyme therapy and nutritional supplementation.
- Those patients who also have endocrine insufficiency require insulin.
- Pancreatic agenesis is associated with severe intrauterine growth retardation and insulin-dependent hyperglycemia; patients generally die in the neonatal period.

2. Ductal Abnormalities

Definition: Anatomic variations in the normal distribution of the pancreatic duct system.

- The normal duct anatomy, including the main pancreatic duct of Wirsung and the accessory duct of Santorini, is found in approximately 60% to 70% of people; in the remaining people, any one of a number of common variations may occur.
- Two of the more common types of ductal abnormalities include pancreas divisum and common channel syndromes with choledochal cysts.
- Other ductal abnormalities include:
  - Regressive changes of either the accessory duct (from the dorsal anlage) or the main duct (from the ventral anlage).
  - Absence of communication of the accessory duct with the accessory duodenal papilla.
  - Persistent dorsal pancreatic duct which functions as the main duct and opens into the duodenum via the minor papilla; in such cases, the ventral duct, which maintains its communication with the common duct, may not communicate with the accessory duct; when there is complete separation of the respective pancreatic tissues, it is called pancreas divisum.
  - Variations in the pancreaticobiliary junction and ampulla of Vater, including complete separation of the orifices of the common duct and main pancreatic duct with formation of two papillae; entrance of the common bile duct into the pancreatic duct more than 2 cm proximal to the duodenum (implicated in the pathogenesis of choledochal cysts); long common channel, with the length of the intraduodenal segment being more than that of the opening into the duodenum; ductal stenosis of the distal common duct; and strictures of the more proximal segments of the duct.
- Some of the anatomic variations in the pancreatic duct system have been implicated in the development of chronic pancreatitis.

3. Pancreas Divisum

Definition: Separation of the pancreas resulting from incomplete fusion of the dorsal and ventral pancreatic ductal systems.

Clinical

- Represents the most common congenital anomaly of the pancreas with an incidence of from 3% to 10% of the population.
- No gender predilection; onset of symptoms is most common in the 3rd to 5th decades of life; considered uncommon but may occur in pediatric aged patients.
- Usually an incidental finding.
- Some patients present with recurrent attacks of epigastric pain and bouts of acute pancreatitis; the attacks tend not to be severe; the pancreatitis most often affects the dorsal derivative but the ventral derivative may also be affected.
- May be associated with the presence of pseudocysts at the time of presentation.
- The mechanism of pancreatitis in pancreas divisum remains unknown; there is no evidence of a causal relationship between pancreas divisum and pancreatitis (acute or chronic).

Radiology

- Endoscopic retrograde cholangiopancreatography (ERCP) with injection of contrast material is diagnostic and includes the presence of separate filling of the ventral and dorsal pancreatic ducts.
- The incidence of pancreas divisum increases to 50% among patients undergoing ERCP for evaluation of "idiopathic" pancreatitis.

Pathology

- The pathologist plays virtually no role in the diagnosis of pancreas divisum because this is a radiographic diagnosis.

Treatment and Prognosis

- Medical management of the pancreatitis is advocated for patients with less severe attacks.
- For patients with more severe attacks, various procedures, including endoscopic balloon dilatation, papillotomy, and stenting, have been used.
- In refractory cases, direct ductal drainage or distal resection with or without distal drainage into a Roux-en-Y loop has been performed.

4. Annular Pancreas

Definition: Embryologic abnormality in which the ventral primordium of the pancreas fails to rotate properly, resulting in complete or incomplete banding of pancreatic tissue around the second portion of the duodenum.

Clinical

- Rare lesion.
- Predominantly occurs in males; may occur from birth to adulthood.
- In the neonatal period, occurs in association with polyhydramnios presenting with failure to tolerate feedings, per-

sistent bile-stained vomiting, and distention of the upper abdomen.

- In adults, symptoms include epigastric or upper abdominal pain, nausea and vomiting, postprandial fullness and bloating, weight loss, and upper gastrointestinal bleeding.
- In adults, peptic ulcer, gastritis, and pancreatitis occurs in more than half the patients.
- High incidence in Down's syndrome suggesting a genetic etiology; familial occurrence also suggests genetic transmission.
- Occurs as an isolated finding or in association with other congenital anomalies of the gastrointestinal tract, including duodenal atresia or stenosis.
- Associated with a number of congenital malformations, including intestinal malrotation, cardiac defects, Meckel's diverticulum, imperforate anus, duodenal bands, spinal defects, and cryptorchidism.
- The proposed mechanisms for the development of annular pancreas include one or a combination of the following theories:
  • Hypertrophy of both the ventral and dorsal anlagen resulting in complete constriction around the duodenum.
  • Persistence and enlargement of the left bud of the paired ventral primordium.
  • Fixation of the ventral bud tip prior to rotation resulting in persistence of the ventral bud around the duodenum.

Radiology

- In neonates, plain abdominal film shows a "double bubble" sign indicative of duodenal obstruction.
  • This is not diagnostic of annular pancreas because there are other causes of duodenal obstruction such as atresia/stenosis, duodenal web, and volvulus due to intestinal malrotations.
  • Upper gastrointestinal contrast studies are not helpful in the diagnosis.
  • Laparoscopy confirms the diagnosis of annular pancreas.
- In older children and adults, upper gastrointestinal contrast studies show diagnostic features, including an annular filling defect across the second portion of the pancreas, symmetrical dilatation of the proximal duodenum, and reverse peristalsis of the duodenal segment proximal to the annulus.
- In older children and adults, plain abdominal films are not helpful in the diagnosis.

Pathology

Gross

- Flat band of pancreatic tissue encircling and constricting the duodenum.
- The duct system begins anteriorly and courses posteriorly from right to left moving over and behind the duodenum, passing near the common bile duct and uniting with the main pancreatic duct.

Histology

- The pancreatic tissue is essentially unchanged and includes normal exocrine and endocrine cellular components.

- Changes of pancreatitis may focally be seen.
- Given the origin from the ventral pancreatic bud, these lesions contain a large number of pancreatic polypeptide (PP) cells.

Treatment and Prognosis

- In the neonatal period, surgical bypass is required; the preferred surgery is complete bypass of the annulus by duodenoduodenostomy.
  • Division of the pancreatic ring and gastrojejunostomy are no longer advocated due to unacceptable high morbidity rates and high rates of stomal ulceration and other complications, including mortality.
- In adults, surgical bypass of the obstruction is the treatment of choice; similar surgical procedures used for neonates can be used for adults; gastric resection is reserved for those patients with documented peptic ulcer in association with annular pancreas.
- Prognosis is dependent on the age at onset of symptoms.
  • Highest mortality rates, reported as high as 43%, occur in infants owing to the frequency of associated severe anomalies in this age group.
  • In adults, the prognosis is excellent with low morbidity and mortality rates.

5. Choledochal Cysts

Definition: Cystic dilatation of the entire hepatic duct, saccular dilatation of a portion of the duct, or cystic dilatation of the intraduodenal duct.

Synonyms: Caroli's disease is designated for intrahepatic ductular dilatation; choledochocele represents cystic dilatation of the intraduodenal duct.

Clinical

- Rare.
- No gender predilection; the majority present in the first decade of life.
- Classic presentation includes right upper quadrant abdominal pain, jaundice, and a palpable right upper quadrant abdominal mass; other symptoms may include nausea, vomiting, and fever; sepsis due to cholangitis or peritonitis (secondary to cystic rupture) may be a complicating problem.
- Anomalous junctions of the common bile duct and main pancreatic duct are often found and have been implicated in the pathogenesis of choledochal cysts and pancreatitis; high amylase levels in choledochal cysts can be present at surgery and may also impact on pathogenesis with reflux of pancreatic fluid into the bile duct causing ductular dilatation.
- Abdominal ultrasonography assists in the diagnosis with dilatation of the extrapancreatic common bile duct or a cystic lesion in communication with the common bile duct.
- Treatment includes complete surgical resection of the extrapancreatic cyst with a Roux-en-Y hepatojejunostomy.
- A small but definitive risk of developing carcinoma exists.

6. Heterotopic Pancreas

Definition: The presence of pancreatic tissue lacking anatomic and vascular continuity to the main pancreas.

Synonyms: Ectopic, aberrant, or accessory pancreas.

Clinical

- The incidence is 0.55% to 15% of autopsy specimens.
- In approximately 70% of cases, the heterotopic pancreas is found in the upper gastrointestinal tract, including the duodenum > stomach (usually within 5 cm of the pylorus) > jejunum; other intra-abdominal sites of involvement include the liver, gallbladder and bile ducts, distal small intestine, appendix, colon, omentum, abdominal wall, Meckel's diverticulum, and spleen; extra-abdominal sites of involvement are rare and have included bronchogenic cyst, pulmonary sequestration, and umbilicus.
- Most patients with heterotopic pancreas are asymptomatic; discovery of the pancreatic heterotopia occurs incidentally, found during the work-up for unrelated (gastrointestinal) problems.

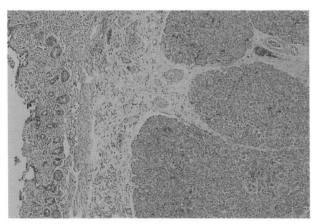

Figure 11–1. Heterotopic pancreas in the submucosa of the ileum entirely composed of exocrine pancreatic tissue.

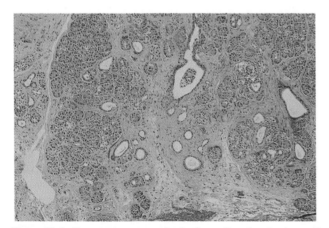

Figure 11–2. Heterotopic pancreas in the ileum. Ductal and acinar cell components are seen. Pancreatic islets were not present.

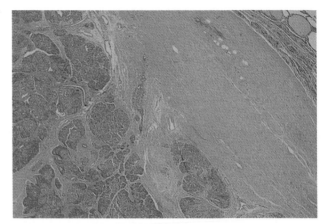

Figure 11–3. Thyroid teratoma that includes the presence of pancreatic tissue.

- Symptoms related to pancreatic heterotopia may include abdominal distention, epigastric pain, dyspepsia, nausea, and vomiting.
- Much less often secondary complications occur, including upper gastrointestinal bleeding, biliary obstruction, cholecystitis, pyloric obstruction, intussusception, intestinal obstruction, and atresia.
- Radiographic and endoscopic appearance include a well-defined dome-shaped filling defect with central umbilication usually measuring less than 1 cm in diameter; in the stomach, the usual location is along the greater curvature of the antrum or in a prepyloric position.
- Definitive diagnosis requires histologic confirmation; given the usual submucosal localization, deeper endoscopic biopsies are required to identify the pancreatic tissue, otherwise only normal host mucosa will be seen.

Gross

- Discrete, irregular, and firm yellow nodule or mass, measuring 0.2 to 4 cm in diameter.
- In the majority of cases, the heterotopic nodule or mass is submucosally situated but may be found in subserosal or intramuscular locations.

Histology

- Ductal and acinar cell components are seen in all cases; there may be ductal proliferation with decreased acini or a predominantly ductal proliferation.
- Endocrine (islets of Langerhans) are identified in only one third of cases; the endocrine cells include all cell types, but the numbers vary from case to case.
- All changes seen in the normally situated pancreas can occur in the heterotopic pancreatic tissue, including pancreatitis (acute or chronic), exocrine neoplasms, and endocrine neoplasms.

Differential Diagnosis (Clinical)

- Polyp.
- Leiomyoma.
- Lipoma.
- Carcinoma or lymphoma.

Treatment and Prognosis

- Incidental lesions can be left alone.
- In the presence of secondary complications, simple surgical resection of the heterotopic pancreas with treatment of the secondary problems are indicated.
- Additional criteria for simple resection include lesions found incidentally by laparoscopy, lesions larger than 1.5 cm in diameter, and lesions adjacent to or directly involving the mucosa of the involved site.

7. Pancreatic Congenital Cysts

Definition: Non-neoplastic solitary or multiple cysts.

Clinical

- Rare lesions.
- Primarily occur in infants and children younger than 2 years of age; rarely identified in adults.
- For a solitary congenital cyst, the most common clinical presentation is as an abdominal mass; other features may include prenatal polyhydramnios, biliary obstruction, gastroduodenal compression; rarely, other associated anomalies can occur.
- For multiple congenital cysts, most are diagnosed at autopsy as the severity of the associated anomalies often is incompatible with life; usually are associated with cysts of the kidneys, liver, lungs, and central nervous system.
- Associated anomalies seen in multiple congenital cysts include von Hippel-Lindau syndrome, Ivemark's syndrome (dysplasia of the kidneys, liver, and pancreas), and Gruber's syndrome (dysencephalia splanchnocystica).

Radiology

- Plain films of the abdomen may show displacement of the stomach, duodenum, or transverse colon.
- *Ultrasonography:* Cystic fluid-filled mass of the pancreas.

Pathology

Gross

- Solitary or multiple, unilocular to multilocular cysts.

Histology

- True cysts are lined by a single layer of cuboidal to columnar to flattened epithelium with a fibrous wall; stratified squamous epithelium may be present.
- Papillary tufting of the epithelial lining is uncommon.
- The epithelial cystic lining may be obliterated by associated inflammation or infection.
- Pancreatic acini and islets of Langerhans may occasionally be present in the cyst wall.
- *Histochemistry:* Epithelial mucin stains are usually negative.
- Cystic fluid content in uncomplicated cases is clear and may contain pancreatic enzymes; the latter would confirm the cyst as being of pancreatic origin, but pancreatic enzymes are not invariably present in the fluid content.
- Heterologous elements are not found in relationship to the cysts.

Differential Diagnosis

- Upper gastrointestinal duplication or neurenteric cysts.
- Pseudocysts (Chapter 11E, #1).

Treatment and Prognosis

- For solitary cysts, surgical excision is the treatment of choice.
  - Cysts in the pancreatic tail may be removed by partial pancreatectomy.
  - Cysts in the pancreatic head require more extensive surgery to completely excise the cyst, including cystenterostomy.
- For multiple cysts, no specific treatment is indicated unless the cysts become symptomatic, requiring surgical removal.

Additional Facts

- **Multiple pancreatic hamartoma** may represent a multicystic variation of congenital pancreatic cysts characterized by the following:
  - Abdominal pain and distention at presentation.
  - Encapsulated multicystic pancreatic lesion located near the pancreatic head.
  - Presence of a simple ductal epithelial lining, a fibrous wall containing pancreatic acini, and scattered endocrine cells (but not well-defined islets) within the exocrine tissue of the cyst wall.
  - Uninvolved pancreas is normal.
  - Unassociated with cysts of other organs, congenital anomalies, cytogenetic abnormalities, or familial association.

C. HEREDITARY DISEASES OF THE PANCREAS

1. The Pancreas in Cystic Fibrosis

Definition: Inherited multisystemic disease characterized by pancreatic insufficiency, chronic pulmonary disease, and failure to thrive.

Synonyms: Fibrocystic disease of the pancreas; mucoviscidosis; pancreatic fibrosis.

Clinical

- The most common inherited disease of the white population of North America and Europe.
  - Occurs in 1 per 2000 whites.
  - Occurs in 1 per 17,000 blacks.
- Believed to be an autosomal recessive disorder.
  - Chromosomal location on long arm of chromosome 7q31.

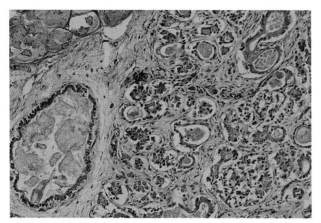

Figure 11–4. Pancreatic changes in cystic fibrosis include dilated (ectatic) ducts with intraluminal eosinophilic secretions. This finding represents one of the earliest alterations of cystic fibrosis. The eosinophilic secretions represent mucoprotein.

- Equal gender predilection.
- Hallmarks of disease are pancreatic insufficiency (steatorrhea), elevated sweat electrolytes (sodium and chloride), pulmonary involvement, increased viscosity of pancreatic and bronchial tree secretions, meconium ileus, and failure to thrive.

Pathology

Gross

- Small, hard, and nodular-appearing pancreas with increased fat and multiple cysts.

Histology

- The histologic changes are progressive, going through a variety of morphologic stages.
- Dilated (ectatic) ducts with intraluminal eosinophilic secretions/concretions are believed to represent the earliest alterations of disease.
  - The secretions represent mucoprotein and react with stains for acid mucopolysaccharide stains (but do not react with stains for neutral mucopolysaccharides).
  - Desquamated epithelial cells and inflammatory cells can be seen admixed with the intraluminal secretions.
  - The concretions are deeply eosinophilic and may be laminated or calcified.
- Additional changes in the course of the disease include intralobular fibrosis, interlobular fibrosis with associated ductular ectasia, microcysts, and exocrine (ductal and acinar cell) atrophy.
  - Acinar cells become flattened to form a thin epithelial cell wall.
  - An inflammatory cell infiltrate, including polymorphonuclear leukocytes, can be seen in the intralobular fibrous tissue in and around ducts and acini.
  - Marked interstitial lymphocytic infiltration is present.
  - Intraductal papillary hyperplasia and goblet cell metaplasia can be seen.
- With progression of disease, liposclerosis, ductal obliteration, and endocrine (islet cell) atrophy can be seen.

Table 11–2
MEDICAL CONDITIONS CAUSING PANCREATIC DYSFUNCTION

Diabetes mellitus
Cystic fibrosis
Hemosiderosis
Liver cirrhosis
Chronic ulcerative colitis
Uremia and dehydration
Amyloidosis
Others

Treatment (for pancreatic disease) and Prognosis

- Pancreatic enzyme replacement.
- Dietary management.
- Marked improved life expectancy as compared with several decades ago because of improved supportive therapy.

2. The Pancreas in Diabetes Mellitus

Definition: Diabetes mellitus is defined as a state of chronic hyperglycemia due to insulin deficiency (absolute or relative) as a consequence of severe loss of islet B cells and/or peripheral resistance to the effects of insulin.

Medical conditions associated with pancreatic dysfunction are listed in Table 11–2.

Clinical

- The classification of diabetes mellitus includes the following:
  - Type 1, or early-onset insulin-dependent diabetes, or juvenile diabetes.
  - Type 2, or insulin-independent diabetes, or mature-onset diabetes.
- **Type 1 diabetes:**
  - Classically occurs in children and juveniles.
  - Is prone to ketoacidosis.
  - Is associated with islet cell antibodies and certain HLA subtypes (autoimmunity and genetic predisposition).

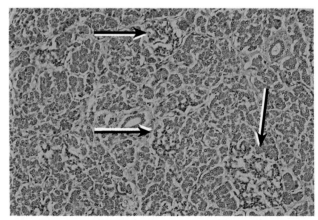

Figure 11–5. Type 1 diabetes mellitus showing scattered islets that vary in appearance from readily apparent to small and inconspicuous with irregular outlines *(arrows)*.

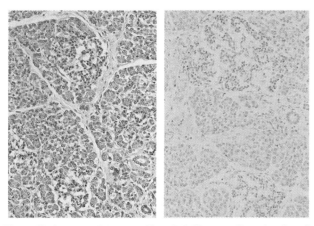

Figure 11–6. Type 1 diabetes mellitus. *Left,* Hematoxylin and eosin stain showing two small, ill-defined islets with irregular outlines at the top and bottom of the illustration. *Right,* Immunohistochemical staining with insulin showing absence of immunoreactivity signifying absence of islet B cells.

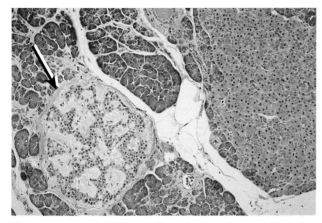

Figure 11–7. Type 2 diabetes mellitus showing islet amyloidosis (islet hyalinization) *(arrow),* a common and fairly distinctive feature for this type of diabetes, representing a form of localized amyloidosis that only occurs in islets that have B cells.

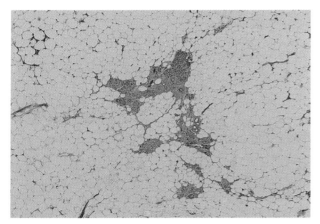

Figure 11–8. Type 2 diabetes mellitus showing pancreatic lipomatosis or fatty replacement of the pancreas.

- Is associated with severe loss of islet B cells.
- Is dependent on insulin therapy.
- Other possible pathogenetic considerations in the development of Type 1 diabetes include viral and toxic effects of drugs or chemicals.

■ **Type 2 diabetes:**
  - Classically occurs in adults.
  - Is associated with obesity, heredity (family history of diabetes), peripheral insulin resistance, and impaired B cell function.
  - Is not associated with islet cell antibodies or HLA subtypes.
  - Is not associated with severe loss of islet B cells; rather than a qualitative defect in B cells, in this form of diabetes there is a functional alteration or defect of islet B cells.
  - Is treated by diet and/or hypoglycemic medication.

■ Lack of insulin, absolute or relative, results in inadequate glucose utilization leading to the **diabetic syndrome,** which is characterized by the following:
  - Glucosuria accompanied by loss of water resulting in dehydration.
  - Weight loss due to loss of glucose and utilization of fat and protein energy reserves.
  - Increased breakdown of neutral fat leading to increased circulating free fatty acids (hyperlipidemia and hypercholesterolemia), which are oxidized by the liver into ketone bodies, potentially resulting in ketoacidosis.
  - The combination of these criteria may ultimately cause diabetic coma.

■ Sustained hyperglycemia impacts on virtually every organ (multisystemic effects), including
  - Macroangiopathy—atherosclerosis with increase risk of myocardial infarction, cerebral vascular accident (CVA or stroke), and gangrene of distal (lower) extremities.
  - Microangiopathy—diabetic glomerulosclerosis (Kimmelstiel-Wilson glomerulosclerosis), diabetic retinopathy, and diabetic polyneuropathy.
  - Susceptibility to infections (pyogenic and fungal) due to alterations in leukocyte function.

Pathology

Gross

■ In Type 1 diabetes, the pancreas shows little alteration if the disease is of recent onset (<1 year); long-standing disease may result in smaller pancreata with increased fibrosis due to progressive atrophy.

■ In Type 2 diabetes, there are little, if any, gross alterations of the pancreas.

Histology
a. Type 1 Diabetes

■ The islets show distinctive changes even in recent onset of disease.

■ The majority of islets are small and inconspicuous by conventional stains (hematoxylin and eosin).

■ The islets are composed of narrow cords of small cells in a fibrous stroma (islet fibrosis).

■ The outlines of the islets are irregular and there may be continuity between endocrine and acinar cells.

■ Inflammatory cell infiltration, predominantly mature lymphocytes, is present in some but not all islets and is termed "insulitis."
  • The inflammatory cell infiltration may be focal and limited (quantitatively), may be florid, or is extensive, obscuring the normal microanatomy of the involved islet(s).
  • Insulitis is restricted to islets still containing B cells.
  • Insulitis is more frequent in patients younger than 10 years of age.
  • Insulitis is transient and is generally not found in diabetics with disease of more than 1 year's duration.
■ Quantitative reduction of the islets to one third to one seventh of that of nondiabetics to loss of B cells.
■ Immunohistochemical evaluation shows loss of B cells but presence of A and D cells and, rarely, PP cells.
■ Hydropic change of B cells due to glycogen accumulation is no longer a common feature, probably the result of improved treatment of insulin-dependent diabetics.
■ Islet amyloidosis is a rare feature in Type 1 diabetes.
■ Exocrine pancreas alterations include acinar cell atrophy and interacinar and interlobular fibrosis.
■ Vascular changes include atherosclerosis of large arteries and diabetic microangiopathy of smaller arterioles.

b. Type 2 Diabetes

■ Qualitatively, the islets are essentially unchanged from those of nondiabetics.
■ Quantitative alterations vary, probably because of the heterogeneity of the disease, and include Type 2 diabetic patients in whom there is a reduction (50%) in islet cell mass due to a total decrease in total number of insulin-producing B cells and Type 2 diabetics in whom there are little quantitative alterations as compared with the islets in nondiabetic patients.
■ Islet amyloidosis (islet hyalinization) is a common feature in Type 2 diabetes.
  • Form of localized amyloidosis restricted to islets but occurs only in islets that have B cells.
  • Considered diagnostic of Type 2 diabetes but it is not specific for diabetes; it is much more common in Type 2 diabetics than in nondiabetics and is uncommon in the absence of a history of diabetes.
  • Related to patient age: more common in patients older than 50 years of age; uncommon in patients younger than 50 years of age and it affects approximately 50% of diabetic patients older than 70 years of age.
  • Stains with thioflavine T and weakly with Congo red.
■ Islet fibrosis.
■ Fatty infiltration.
■ Insulitis is a rare feature in Type 2 diabetes.

Treatment and Prognosis

■ Type 1 diabetes is managed by administration of insulin to counteract the effects of hyperglycemia.
■ Type 2 diabetes is controlled by diet and/or hypoglycemic medication.
■ Pancreas and islet cell transplantation have been selectively used in the treatment of Type 1 diabetic patients or patients made diabetic by total pancreatectomy.

■ The prognosis of diabetes is variable and is dependent on numerous factors, perhaps the most important being the type of diabetes and patient response to medical therapy; diabetes is a progressive multisystem disease with associated high morbidity and not insignificant mortality rates.

Additional Facts

■ **Secondary Diabetes**—another form of diabetes occurring secondary to or in association with the following:
  • Endocrine diseases: acromegaly, Cushing's syndrome, hyperthyroidism, pheochromocytoma, primary hyperaldosteronism, hyperprolactinemia, glucagonoma, carcinoid syndrome, and autoimmune polyendocrine syndromes.
  • Pancreatic diseases: pancreatectomy, pancreatitis (acute, chronic, hereditary), carcinoma, and hemochromatosis.
  • Medical disease: liver cirrhosis and others.
  • Drug induced: drugs impairing insulin secretion (α-adrenergic agents, diuretics, and phenytoin) and drugs that impair insulin action (glucocorticoids and oral contraceptive agents).
  • Genetic syndromes associated with impaired glucose intolerance, including cystic fibrosis and many others.

3. Other Hereditary Diseases of the Pancreas

■ Generalized pancreatic insufficiency occurs in both primary and developmental varieties.
■ Believed to be transmitted as an autosomal recessive mode of inheritance.

a. Shwachman-Diamond Syndrome (Lipomatous Atrophy)

■ Second most common cause (after cystic fibrosis) of pancreatic insufficiency; associated with increased spontaneous chromosomal breakage.
■ Characterized by pancreatic insufficiency, cyclic neutropenia, recurrent infections, metaphyseal dysostosis, and growth retardation.
■ Equal gender predilection.
■ Pancreas is atrophic and characterized histologically by the presence of marked fatty infiltration with little acinar tissue, normal-appearing islets, and minimal fibrosis or inflammatory cell infiltration; the duct system is intact.

b. Johanson-Blizzard Syndrome

■ Characterized by congenital aplasia of the alae nasi, deafness, hypothyroidism, dwarfism, microcephaly, absence of permanent teeth, and malabsorption.
■ Pancreatic insufficiency is the most consistent feature of this syndrome; trypsinogen secretion is especially low.
■ No gender predilection.

c. Sideroblastic Anemia and Exocrine Pancreatic Insufficiency (Pearson's Marrow-Pancreas Syndrome)

- Pancreatic insufficiency includes low bicarbonate, lipase, and amylase secretion.
- Acinar atrophy with fibrosis but absent liposis is found.
- Pathogenesis may correlate with defect in mitochondrial respiratory enzyme.

d. Developmental Deficiencies of Pancreatic Function

- Transient physiologic pancreatic insufficiency, characterized by low or absent amylase concentrations and minimal lipase concentrations, occurs in term newborns and persists for months, with maturation around 1 year of age.
- Developmental deficiencies of pancreatic function include isolated enzyme disorders as follows:
  - Congenital lipase deficiency.
  - Combined lipase-colipase deficiency.
  - Isolated colipase deficiency.
  - Congenital amylase deficiency.
  - Congenital trypsinogen deficiency.
  - Congenital enterokinase deficiency.
- Rare disorders.
- Clinical presentations vary on the deficient enzyme and include steatorrhea, malabsorption, failure to thrive, diarrhea, edema, anemia, and hypoproteinemia.
- Treatment includes replacement of deficient enzyme with pancreatic enzyme preparations.

e. Hereditary Pancreatitis

Definition: Pancreatic inflammation, usually recurrent, occurring in genetically related individuals over two or more generations.

Clinical

- Autosomal dominant inheritance; chromosomal abnormality has not been definitively identified.
- Equal gender predilection; characteristically, symptoms occur at an early age, usually within the first decade of life.
- Clinical presentation is similar to those of pancreatitis of other causes and includes:
  - Abdominal pain—characteristic of the acute attack; pain is prolonged and severe, typically epigastric in location, and it may radiate to the back.
  - Nausea and vomiting.
- With increasing age, the attacks become less severe.
- Physical examination shows epigastric tenderness, decreased bowel sounds, and abdominal distention.
- Laboratory findings include elevated serum pancreatic amylase and lipase with increased amylase creatinine clearance ratio.
- Associated abnormalities may include hyperlipemia, hypercalcemia, increased serum immunoglobulin concentrations, and increased frequency of HLA types B-12, B-13, and BW-40.

- Precise mechanism causing disease remains unknown; inherited pancreatic ductal anatomic defects causing obstruction has been considered.

Radiology (in acute stages)

- *Plain abdominal films:* may show increased gastrocolic separation, left upper quadrant sentinel loops of distended bowel, or compression of the duodenal sweep.
- *Ultrasonography:* pancreatic edema.
- *Plain abdominal films and ultrasonography:* calcifications are common.
- *CT scan or ERCP:* dilatation of the duct of Wirsung (not a constant finding).

Pathology

- Histologic features are indistinguishable from other causes of chronic pancreatitis.
- No pathognomonic features.

Treatment and Prognosis

- Treatment of acute attacks is similar to that of chronic pancreatitis due to other causes, including analgesics to control pain, minimize pancreatic exocrine secretion by stopping enteral intake and nasogastric drainage with suction to limit gastric secretions into the duodenum.
- Management of patients in chronic stage of disease is similar to that of chronic pancreatitis due to other causes, including correction of steatorrhea with pancreatic enzyme supplements; patients who develop diabetes are treated by diet control, oral antidiabetic agents, or insulin.
- Surgical drainage is indicated in the presence of pancreatic abscess formation.
- Complications include pancreatic calcification, diabetes mellitus, exocrine pancreatic insufficiency, pseudocysts, abscess formation, and pancreatic carcinoma; less frequently, portal or splenic vein thrombosis, jaundice, and pancreatic ascites may occur.

D. ACQUIRED LESIONS/DISEASES

1. Age-Related Alterations of the Pancreas

- With age, the adult pancreas decreases in weight.
- Histologic alterations with increasing age may include the following:
  - Fatty replacement, also referred to as **lipomatosis** of the pancreas which increases the weight of the gland; pancreatic lipomatosis contrasts with **lipomatous atrophy** (or **Shwachman-Diamond syndrome**); fatty replacement of the pancreas also occurs in obesity and/or adult onset diabetes mellitus.
  - Focal and/or diffuse fibrosis of unknown etiology or a component of diabetes.
  - Focal chronic inflammation.
- Acinar cell changes may include decreased or absent basophilia, decrease in zymogen granules, reduction in cell size, alterations of nuclear size and shape (enlargement,

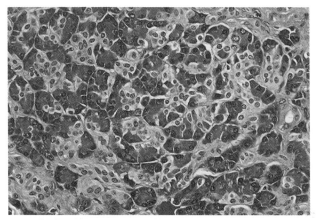

Figure 11–9. Centroacinar cell changes related to aging include increase numbers of centroacinar cells. These centroacinar cell changes can also be seen in metabolic disturbances such as uremia and dehydration, as well as in hypergastrinemia, in insulin-producing pancreatic endocrine neoplasms, and following obstruction of major pancreatic ducts.

pyknosis, variations in shape), cytoplasmic vacuoles, and acinar dilatation (ectasia).

• These acinar cell changes can also be seen in association with acute ductal destruction, heavy cigarette smoking, excessive alcohol use, chronic renal failure (uremia), dehydration and other metabolic disturbances, in children treated with chemotherapy for cancer, and severe bacterial infection, as well as intrapancreatic lesions such as pancreatic endocrine neoplasms, especially in untreated Zollinger-Ellison syndrome.

■ Ductal changes related to aging include dilatation of major and small peripheral ducts with inspissated secretions, periductal fibrosis, enlargement of duct epithelial cells that includes mucus-cell hyperplasia (also known as mucoid transformation, mucinous hyperplasia, goblet cell metaplasia, and nonpapillary hyperplasia), and other metaplastic changes, including squamous metaplasia, papillary hyperplasia, pyloric gland metaplasia (periodic acid–Schiff positive, Alcian blue negative at low pH indicative of sialomucin rather than sulfomucin).

• These ductal changes can also be seen in chronic pancreatitis, following administration of large doses of adrenal steroids, in association with pancreatic ductal carcinoma, ductal obstruction, and diabetes mellitus.

• These ductal changes are most often found in the pancreatic head as compared with the tail and body.

• Squamous metaplasia is uncommon.

• Atypical cytologic changes, including nuclear pleomorphism, nuclear stratification, increased nuclear:cytoplasmic ratio, and prominent nucleoli and mitoses, rarely occur unless associated with pancreatic ductal carcinoma; the presence of cytologic atypia may indicate intraductal carcinoma, the presence of frank carcinoma nearby to the atypical foci, or the evolution to carcinoma (Chapter 12D, #1).

■ Centroacinar cell and intercalated duct changes related to aging include dilatation of centroacinar cells, and increased numbers of centroacinar cells and intercalated ducts.

• These centroacinar cell and intercalated duct changes can also be seen in metabolic disturbances such as ure-

mia and dehydration, in hypergastrinemia, in insulin-producing pancreatic endocrine neoplasms, and following obstruction of major pancreatic ducts.

Additional Facts

■ Lipomatosis of the pancreas can also occur in severe generalized lipomatosis, Type 2 diabetes mellitus, and obesity.

E. NON-NEOPLASTIC CYSTIC LESIONS OF THE PANCREAS

1. Pseudocysts

Definition: The presence of a cystic lesion devoid of an epithelial cell lining.

Clinical

■ Occur in relation to pancreatitis (acute or chronic) and trauma; rarely, may be seen in association with a neo-

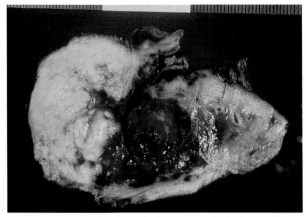

Figure 11–10. Pancreatic pseudocyst appearing as a unilocular cystic lesion. The inner lining consisted of a ragged surface with a thick fibrotic wall. Adherent to the cyst is hemorrhagic and amorphous tissue with hemorrhage extending into the adjacent pancreatic tissue.

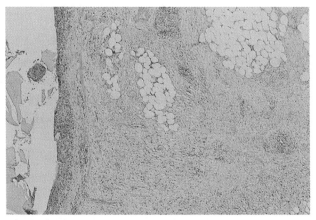

Figure 11–11. Pancreatic pseudocyst (left side of illustration) is characterized by the absence of an epithelial lining. The cyst lining is composed of granulation tissue and inflammatory cells.

plasm as a secondary process to neoplastic ductal obstruction.
- No gender predilection; usually occurs in adults but may occur in children, particularly when resulting from trauma.
- May attain large sizes presenting as an extrapancreatic abdominal mass; common extrapancreatic sites of involvement includes the lesser sac of the peritoneum; may be multiple.
- Pseudocysts attaining large sizes may compress the gastric pylorus and the duodenum; uncommonly, compression of the common bile duct, portal vein, or colon may occur.
- Most patients with pseudocysts present with abdominal pain; other symptoms may include nausea, vomiting, jaundice, and weight loss.
- A palpable abdominal mass may be present.
- May occur in any portion of the pancreas.
- In patients recovering from an attack of acute pancreatitis, pseudocyst can be suspected when the patient again develops pain, nausea, fever, an abdominal mass, or elevated serum amylase levels.

Pathogenesis

- In acute pancreatitis, pseudocysts develop when inflammation (pancreatitis) disrupts pancreatic duct integrity and pancreatic secretions accumulate in the pancreatic interstitium.
- In chronic pancreatitis and/or neoplastic ductal obstruction, pseudocysts develop when ductal strictures, inspissated secretory protein or intrapancreatic calcifications obstruct the duct, producing localized dilatations that coalesce, loose their epithelial lining, and enlarge to produce a pseudocyst.
- Pseudocysts may or may not communicate with the duct system.

Radiology

- *CT scan:*
  - In early stages appear as ill-defined, fluid-filled, low-density lesions without definable walls.
  - In later stages appear as better-defined cystic lesion with smooth walls, fibrous capsules, and low-density fluid centers.
- May extend beyond the confines of the pancreas into adjacent spaces and/or viscera.
- *Ultrasonography:* cystic lesions with mixed internal echoes due to septations, necrotic tissue, and blood.

Pathology

Fine Needle Aspiration

- Scanty cellularity.
- Inflammatory cells, including neutrophils, lymphocytes, histiocytes, and plasma cells, and granulation tissue.
- Granular debris and lipid droplets; calcifications may be present.

Gross

- Usually unilocular with an inner ragged surface and a thick fibrotic wall.

- Cyst content may include thick or thin, turbid and milky, or clear or blood-tinged fluid; fluid content has a high amylase content, measuring from 200 to 1000 ml; rarely, the fluid may measure as much as 3 liters.

Histology

- Absence of an epithelial lining.
- Lining is composed of granulation tissue and inflammatory cells.
- Thickened fibrotic wall with prominent vascularity; with time, the wall of the pseudocyst becomes more fibrotic and less vascular.
- Atrophic pancreatic parenchyma can be seen in or adjacent to the fibrous wall of the pseudocyst.
- Liquefaction necrosis is absent, a feature that separates a pseudocyst from a pancreatic abscess.

Differential Diagnosis

- True (epithelial-lined) cystic neoplasms of the pancreas (Table 11–3).
- Congenital cysts (Chapter 11B, #7).
- Pancreatic abscess.

Treatment and Prognosis

- The therapy for pancreatic pseudocysts includes medical management, surgery or surgical drainage, percutaneous external drainage, or endoscopic internal drainage.
- Small (<6 cm in diameter) asymptomatic pseudocysts may resolve spontaneously so that these patients can be vigilantly monitored (clinically and radiographically) without additional therapeutic intervention.
- Surgery may include the following:
  - Resection—preferred method of treatment, but possible only when the cyst is in the pancreatic tail and the head and body are normal or minimally changed.
  - External drainage—preferred when the cyst wall is not thick enough to allow for anastomosis.
  - Internal drainage—Roux-en-Y anastomosis to the jejunum (cystojejunostomy) or to the posterior wall of the stomach (cystogastrostomy) or to the duodenum (cystoduodenostomy).
- Complications of pancreatic pseudocyst include hemorrhage, rupture, and infection.
  - Hemorrhage results from erosion of the pseudocyst into vascular structures and is associated with increased morbidity and mortality.
  - Acute rupture (perforation) is uncommon; if it occurs into the abdomen, signs and symptoms of acute peritonitis result; rupture into the gastrointestinal tract produces vomiting and diarrhea and is associated with high morbidity—if it occurs with hemorrhage, it is associated with increased mortality rates; splenic artery involvement may result in massive hemorrhage and sudden death.
  - Infected pseudocysts and development of sepsis are not uncommon complications.

Table 11–3
CYSTIC LESIONS OF THE PANCREAS

Features	Pseudocysts	Microcystic Adenoma	Mucinous Cystic Neoplasms
Gender/age	M > F; wide age range	F > M; 5th–7th decades	F > M; middle age
Clinical	Generally found in patients with chronic pancreatitis often associated with biliary tract disease, alcoholism	Found incidentally at autopsy or presents as an abdominal mass with or without associated pain; tumors in pancreatic head may cause biliary tract or gastrointestinal obstruction, resulting in jaundice	Intermittent or continuous abdominal pain or discomfort; enlarging abdominal mass
Radiology	Well-defined fibrous capsule; low-density fluid centers	Multicystic, honeycomb-appearing mass; most cysts <2 cm in diameter; small calcifications and central stellate scar common	Large, multicystic masses, may be unilocular, without honeycomb appearance; cysts measure >2 cm in diameter; prominent internal septations; absent central scar; enhancement of solid components after contrast; peripheral calcifications
Location in pancreas	Anywhere	Anywhere (even distribution)	More common in body and tail
Gross	Thick-walled; adherent to surrounding structures; hemorrhagic fluid contents rich in pancreatic enzymes	Well-circumscribed; spongy and honeycomb appearance; central, often calcified, scar; clear, watery fluid contents, occasionally hemorrhagic	Encapsulated mass with smooth surface; uni- or multilocular with smooth cyst lining, but papillary excrescences are common; occasional calcifications at periphery; thick, mucoid or gelatinous fluid content; necrosis and hemorrhage can be seen
Histology	Absence of epithelial lining; fibrous wall with chronic inflammation and necrotic debris	Cysts lined by cuboidal to flattened cells with round nuclei, inconspicuous nucleoli, and clear to occasionally eosinophilic cytoplasm; tiny papillae may be present; hypocellular stroma	Cysts lined by columnar, mucus-producing cells aligned in a single row but may form papillae; cellular atypia, including nuclear pleomorphism, nuclear stratification can be seen; hypercellular "ovarian-type" stroma is present
Histochemistry	Absence of mucus production	Glycogen is present in epithelial cells (PAS +; DPAS−)	Epithelial cells are mucin positive (mucicarmine, PAS+; DPAS+)
Adjacent pancreas	Healing pancreatitis common	Normal appearance; atrophic changes secondary to tumor compression or to obstruction uncommon	Normal appearance; atrophic changes secondary to obstruction occasionally seen
Treatment and prognosis	Pain medications; pancreatic enzyme replacement; surgery as last resort; morbidity high but mortality is low	Surgery is generally curative	Surgical resection; generally has an indolent course with cure following resection; due to metastatic capability of all histologic types, considered a low- or intermediate-grade malignant neoplasm

PAS, Periodic acid–Schiff without diastase digestion; DPAS, periodic acid–Schiff with diastase digestion.

2. Non-Neoplastic, Noncongenital True Cysts of the Pancreas

a. Lymphoepithelial Cyst

Definition: Benign pancreatic cyst with features of cutaneous epidermal inclusion cysts.

Clinical

- Uncommon lesion.
- Predominantly affects adult men.
- May be asymptomatic, discovered incidentally for other intra-abdominal complaints or at autopsy; symptoms related to this cyst may include vague, intermittent abdominal pain, persistent diarrhea, weight loss, intermittent nausea and vomiting, and an abdominal mass.
- Located in all pancreatic sites (head, body, and tail), within the pancreas, connected to the pancreas by a stalk of normal pancreatic tissue, or closely associated with the pancreas with protrusion onto the surface of the pancreas.

- Histogenesis remains unresolved; possible origin includes derivation from a branchial cleft cyst misplaced and fused with the pancreas during embryogenesis or benign epithelial inclusions in a peripancreatic lymph node.

Radiology

- Cystic to solid pancreatic or extrapancreatic mass.

Pathology

Fine Needle Aspiration

- Squamous epithelial cells, lymphocytes, foam cells (histiocytes), and cholesterol crystals.

Gross

- Well-demarcated to encapsulated spherical to egg-shaped lesion measuring 2 to 17 cm in diameter.
- Cut section shows a unilocular to multilocular cyst with smooth, thin walls and septa, semisolid, gray-white to

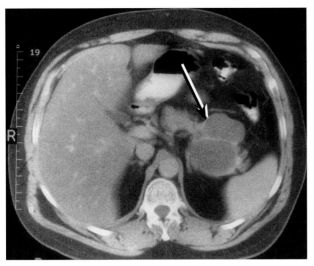

Figure 11–12. CT scan of a lymphoepithelial cyst showing the presence of a multicystic lesion in the tail of the pancreas *(arrow).*

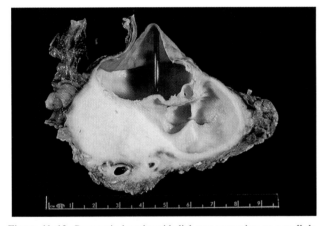

Figure 11–13. Pancreatic lymphoepithelial cyst appearing as a well-demarcated to encapsulated spherical to egg-shaped lesion consisting of a multilocular cyst with smooth thin walls and septa.

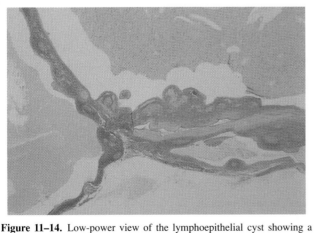

Figure 11–14. Low-power view of the lymphoepithelial cyst showing a multicystic lesion with an epithelial lining and a lymphocytic cell infiltrate in the cyst wall, including lymphoid aggregates. Amorphous pink material can be seen within the cystic spaces.

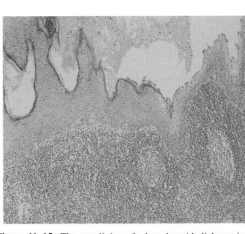

Figure 11–15. The cyst lining of a lymphoepithelial cyst is a keratinizing squamous epithelium, including a focal granular layer.

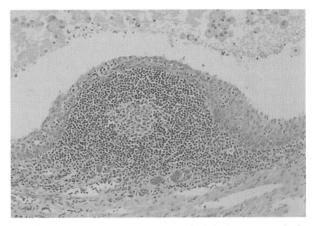

Figure 11–16. Other areas of the cyst lining include the presence of a flattened, cuboidal-appearing epithelium and a mature lymphocytic cell infiltrate in the cyst wall with an associated lymphoid aggregate.

tan; somewhat laminated material is present within the cyst.

Histology

- Cyst lining includes a flattened, cuboidal-appearing epithelium to keratinizing squamous epithelium; the latter may include a focal granular layer.
- Epidermal appendages are not present.
- Mature lymphocytes are found in the cyst wall; lymphoid aggregates or germinal centers may be present.
- A thin rim of pancreatic tissue, including ducts, acini, and islets, may lie immediately outside the lymphocytic layer; this pancreatic parenchyma may show atrophic changes; the remainder of the uninvolved pancreas is unremarkable.

Differential Diagnosis

- Cystic teratoma (dermoid cyst) (Chapter 12C, #2).

Treatment and Prognosis

- Surgical resection is curative.

3. Other Pancreatic Cysts

■ Enterogenous or enteric duplication cyst:
  • Occurs early in life.
  • Presents with symptoms of gastric acid secretion or pancreatitis; may be asymptomatic.
  • Usually of gastric origin.
  • Characteristically includes the presence of well-developed bilayered muscular wall.
  • Lining epithelium varies to include gastric type; intestinal type; and serous, mucous, or ciliated epithelium.
  • May originate from midgut or foregut.
■ Endometrial cyst:
  • Rare occurrence of endometrial tissue in the pancreas.

F. INFECTIOUS DISEASES

■ Infectious diseases of the pancreas with associated clinical symptomatology are rare.
■ Bacterial and other microorganisms may complicate acute pancreatitis in the form of infected necrosis, infected acute pseudocyst, and/or abscess formation.
■ Pancreatic infections may be a complication seen in immunosuppressed patients, including patients with human immunodeficiency virus (HIV) infection and acquired immunodeficiency syndrome (AIDS) (see Chapter 16).
■ Microorganisms implicated in pancreatic infections include *Escherichia coli*, enterococcus, *Staphylococcus*, *Klebsiella*, *Proteus*, *Candida albicans*, parasites (e.g., *Ascaris lumbricoides*, *Clonorchis sinensis*) and others; parasites recovered from the pancreatic duct in patients with pancreatitis may obstruct the pancreatic duct, causing episodes of acute pancreatitis.
■ Presenting symptomatology in patients with pancreatic infections include fever, abdominal pain, abdominal tenderness, palpable mass, nausea and vomiting, abdominal distention, jaundice, sepsis, pulmonary failure, or gastrointestinal bleeding.
■ Rarely, parasitic infestation of the pancreas may result in infectious cyst formation.
  • Organisms implicated in infectious pancreatic cysts may include *Echinococcus*.
  • The cysts associated with *Echinococcus* do not have an epithelial lining (pseudocysts).
  • Parasitic cysts require surgical removal.

G. NONINFECTIOUS PANCREATITIS

■ Pancreatitis is divided into acute and chronic disease.
■ Acute pancreatitis is further divided into acute interstitial pancreatitis and acute hemorrhagic pancreatitis.

1. Acute Pancreatitis

Definition: Noninfectious acute inflammation of the pancreas associated with abdominal pain and raised pancreatic enzymes in blood and/or urine.

Acute interstitial pancreatitis includes the presence of acute intrapancreatic inflammation associated at times with peripancreatic inflammation but without disruption of the

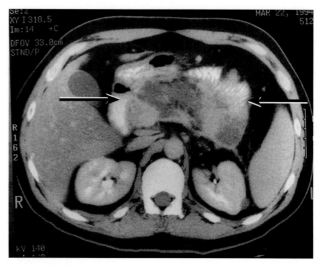

Figure 11–17. CT scan of acute pancreatitis showing generalized enlargement of the pancreas *(arrows)*.

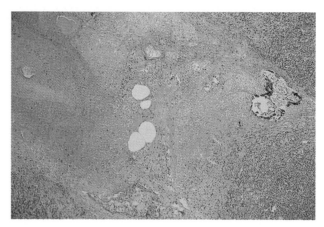

Figure 11–18. Acute pancreatitis. The remnant of the pancreas is seen to the right of this illustration and is infiltrated by inflammatory cells. The remainder of the pancreatic tissue is necrotic with an acute inflammatory cell infiltrate and focal calcifications.

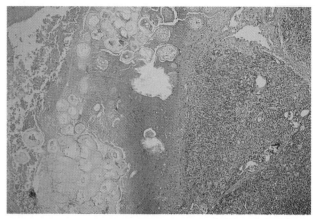

Figure 11–19. Acute pancreatitis with associated necrosis and fat necrosis.

pancreatic microvasculature (pancreas remains well perfused).

- Acute interstitial pancreatitis generally is considered to be the clinically "mild" form of pancreatitis, unassociated with local or systemic complications, successfully managed medically, and associated with an excellent prognosis with extremely low mortality rates.

Acute hemorrhagic pancreatitis includes the presence of disruption of the pancreatic microcirculation resulting in necrotizing pancreatitis.

- Acute hemorrhagic pancreatitis generally is considered to be the clinically "severe" form of pancreatitis, more often associated with local and/or systemic complications, more often requiring surgical intervention, and having higher morbidity and mortality rates.

Clinical

- Acute pancreatitis is considered to be an uncommon condition; the incidence is difficult to state because:
  - The distinction between acute and chronic pancreatitis is not always possible on clinical grounds.
  - Patients with mild to moderate forms of the disease may not be identifiable.
  - Nonpancreatic diseases may be clinically indistinguishable from acute pancreatitis unless tissue is available for histologic study.
- The causes of acute pancreatitis are listed in Table 11–4.
  - Together, biliary tract disease and alcoholism account for 80% to 90% of cases of acute pancreatitis.
  - Most acute episodes of alcohol-induced pancreatitis represent acute manifestations of chronic pancreatitis; therefore, biliary tract disease represents the single most associated cause of acute pancreatitis.
  - Acute pancreatitis may represent the initial clinical manifestations of a periampullary tumor originating in the duodenum, distal bile duct, or the head of the pancreas.
- Overall, approximately 80% of patients develop acute interstitial pancreatitis, and 20% develop acute hemorrhagic pancreatitis; factors governing the severity of response are unknown.

Table 11–4
ETIOLOGY OF ACUTE PANCREATITIS

Biliary tract stones
Ethanol abuse
Tumors
Infections:
   Mumps
   Viral
   Ascariasis
   Mycoplasma
Drug-associated
Metabolic
   Hyperlipidemia
   Hyperparathyroidism
   Renal failure
Trauma
Metabolic
Miscellaneous
Idiopathic

- Acute pancreatitis secondary to biliary tract disease is more common in women than in men, whereas acute pancreatitis secondary to alcoholism is more common in men than in women.
- Acute pancreatitis most frequently occurs in adults older than 40 years of age and is rare in childhood or adolescence.
- An important clinical parameter in a patient suspected of having acute pancreatitis is the past history; acute attacks of pancreatitis tend to be recurrent, and a history of past attacks is perhaps the most important parameter suggesting a diagnosis of pancreatitis.
- The most frequent clinical complaints are abdominal pain and epigastric tenderness; each independently occurs in more than 95% of patients:
  - The pain is usually epigastric in location and may radiate to the back or to the right and/or left upper quadrants; lower quadrant pain may occur hours after the onset of the attack.
  - Radiation of abdominal pain to the back is suggestive of pancreatic origin; left upper quadrant pain as a major component of abdominal pain suggests acute pancreatitis; severe right upper quadrant pain in a patient with acute pancreatitis is indicative of gallstone origin.
  - The pain varies in onset from gradual to sudden; peak intensity is reached in 30 minutes to 6 hours.
  - The pain is characteristically steady and dull in quality, ranging from minor to unbearable in intensity.
  - Patients are typically restless, searching for the most comfortable position; the pain may be eased by lying on one's side with knees pulled up or sitting with the upper torso bent forward; these features contrast with those associated with perforated peptic ulcer (a major clinical entity in the differential diagnosis of acute pancreatitis), which is characterized by the patient remaining motionless and increasing intensity of pain while lying on one's back.
- Other common associated signs and symptoms include nausea and vomiting and low-grade fever; less frequently, patients present with hypotension, mental aberrations (confusion, coma, delirium tremens), pleuritic chest pain, and subcutaneous fat necrosis (leakage of lipase into the circulation); gastrointestinal bleeding (varices or gastritis) may occur in acute pancreatitis secondary to alcoholism.
- In severe hemorrhagic pancreatitis, blood may dissect from the retroperitoneal space to the flanks or periumbilical areas, resulting in a bluish discoloration termed "Grey Turner's sign" or "Cullen's sign," respectively; these findings occur a few days after the onset of disease rather than at presentation.
- Laboratory studies include the following:
  - Elevated serum amylase (hyperamylasemia) and lipase levels; sampling of serum amylase several days after the onset of abdominal pain may show return to normal levels.
  - Hyperglycemia, typically transient with disappearance in days; the presence of hyperglycemia in patients with abdominal pain and no past history of diabetes is strongly suggestive of pancreatitis; persistent hyperglycemia in a nondiabetic patient is indicative of extensive destruction of the pancreatic parenchyma.

- Hypertriglyceridemia (but normal or near-normal serum cholesterol levels): because of the elevated serum triglyceride levels, the sera of patients with acute pancreatitis may be lactescent.
- Hypocalcemia occurs in approximately 25% of cases, and its pathogenesis is not completely understood.
- Hypovolemia and hypotension: extravasation of pancreatic enzymes out of the pancreas causes widespread chemical inflammation of tissues, resulting in loss of protein-rich fluid from injured surfaces ("third space losses"), leading to hypovolemia and hypotension.
- Mild abnormalities of liver function tests are common, including mild elevations of serum bilirubin, serum glutamine oxaloacetic transaminase (SGOT), and gamma-glutamyl transaminase (GGT) and alkaline phosphatase levels.

■ The mechanism by which common duct stones cause acute pancreatitis remains uncertain.

Radiology

■ *Abdominal radiographs:* findings on plain films of patients with acute pancreatitis may include extension of pancreatic exudate beyond the confines of the pancreas, loss of peritoneal fat, ascites, ileus, and displacement of the transverse colon from the stomach due to fluid distention of the lesser sac; these findings are not necessarily diagnostic of acute pancreatitis, but abdominal films are important in patients with severe acute abdominal pain to exclude other causes of acute abdomen (e.g., bowel perforation and bowel infarction).

■ *Ultrasonography and CT scan:* enlargement of the pancreas, which is usually generalized but may be localized, irregular or diffuse distention of the pancreatic duct, and extrapancreatic fluid collections (mostly occur in the lesser sac, left anterior renal space and inferior to the pancreas).

■ Radiographic (CT scan) differentiation can be made between interstitial pancreatitis and hemorrhagic pancreatitis.

- Following an intravenous contrast agent using bolus techniques, there is uniform enhancement of the gland in acute interstitial pancreatitis, indicating an intact microcirculation, whereas in acute hemorrhagic pancreatitis there is diminished to absent enhancement of the gland corresponding to areas of fluid and necrosis and indicative of microcirculatory compromise.

Pathology

Fine Needle Aspiration

■ Moderate to marked cellularity predominantly composed of neutrophils, with degenerative cellular debris, foam cells, and a dirty background.

■ Ductal epithelial cells may be seen with associated reparative atypia.

Gross

■ The pancreas is swollen, pale appearing, and indurated.

■ Cut section shows lobules separated by edematous interstitial tissue; purulent material may be present.

■ Fat necrosis appears as white opaque areas within peripancreatic tissue.

■ Hemorrhage is generally not a feature that is present unless associated with acute hemorrhagic pancreatitis.

■ In hemorrhagic pancreatitis, sharply defined areas of relatively normal appearing pancreas may persist in between areas of red to reddish-black necrotic tissue.

Histology

■ In general, acute pancreatitis is a clinical diagnosis, and biopsy material from patients with acute pancreatitis seldom is obtained.

■ The inflammatory process appears to take origin in acinar cells; acinar cell injury causes leakage of enzymes; if the injury is mild, the process is termed **interstitial pancreatitis;** if the process is severe, there may be frank necrosis and the process is termed **necrotizing pancreatitis;** the necrosis may involve a small part of the gland, most of the gland, or rarely, all of the gland.

■ In **acute interstitial pancreatitis:**

- There is diffuse acute inflammatory cell infiltrate consisting of polymorphonuclear leukocytes in the interstitial tissues, as well as edematous change and fibrinous exudate.
- Focal or diffuse ductular dilatation may be present; with resolution, secondary metaplastic changes can be seen, including mucus cell metaplasia and hyperplasia, and squamous metaplasia.
- Vascular thrombosis and acute necrotizing arteritis are not found.

■ In **acute hemorrhagic pancreatitis:**

- The essential feature is necrosis involving all of the components of the pancreas, including acini and ducts, interstitial tissues, vascular structures, nerves, islets of Langerhans, and fat; the necrosis is patchy and seldom involves the entire gland.
- The necrosis may be in a periductal and/or perilobular distribution.
- The degree of inflammation varies depending on the duration of illness; in early stages of disease and/or when survival is short, there is a relatively minimal amount of (acute) inflammatory reaction; with time, the amount of polymorphonuclear leukocyte infiltration becomes more marked, especially in the interlobular septa.
- Vascular thrombosis and acute necrotizing arteritis are present.

■ Acute pancreatitis may be associated with fat necrosis, pseudocyst formation, and pancreatic abscess, all related to release of digestive enzymes from the pancreas.

- Release of lipase results in injury to adipose tissue and fat necrosis in peripancreatic tissues or distantly, in subcutaneous fat.
- Pseudocysts represent extrapancreatic collections of pancreatic juice resulting from ductal rupture.
- Pancreatic abscesses are composed of necrotic pancreatic connective tissue containing activated digestive enzymes and mixed bacterial flora; this complication is associated with significant morbidity and mortality.

■ From the pathologic standpoint, complete restitution of the pancreatic parenchyma occurs when the episode of acute pancreatitis subsides or resolves.

Differential Diagnosis

■ Chronic pancreatitis with superimposed acute inflammation (Chapter 11G, #2).

Treatment and Prognosis

■ Patients with acute pancreatitis usually are treated by medical management, including supportive care with fluid replacement, relief of pain with parenteral injections of meperidine, and reduction of pancreatic secretion by avoidance of oral alimentation until the acute pancreatic inflammation has subsided; at the present time, there is no therapy shown to reduce pancreatic inflammation.
■ Metabolic complications, such as hyperglycemia and hypocalcemia, are treated accordingly.
■ Pancreatic infection, seen much more frequently in acute hemorrhagic pancreatitis than in acute interstitial pancreatitis, requires appropriate antibiotic therapy; infection may take the form of infected necrosis, infected pseudocyst, or an abscess; antibiotics alone are not sufficient in the treatment of infected necrosis, which requires surgical debridement, too; prophylactic antibiotic therapy in acute necrotizing pancreatitis remains unproven, but recent experimental studies may prove beneficial in improving survival in these patients.
■ Surgical intervention for acute pancreatitis may be necessary to establish the diagnosis or to treat complications such as pancreatic abscess formation, pseudocyst formation, or necrosis.
■ Mortality rates associated with acute interstitial pancreatitis is less than 2%.
■ Mortality in acute necrotizing pancreatitis varies depending on whether the necrosis is sterile ("sterile necrosis") or infected ("infected necrosis").
  • Overall mortality in sterile necrosis is approximately 10%; in the absence of systemic complications, this mortality rate is lower, but when present they are higher.
  • Overall mortality in infected necrosis is approximately 30%; in the absence of systemic complications, this mortality rate is lower, but when present the mortality rates may exceed 50%; in infected necrosis treated by antibiotics without surgical debridement, mortality rates are virtually 100%.
■ Systemic complications of acute pancreatitis, seen more often with acute hemorrhagic pancreatitis rather than in acute interstitial pancreatitis, occur when the pancreatic enzymes gain access to the systemic circulation; these complications may include the following:
  • Cardiovascular collapse—systolic blood pressure lower than 80 mm Hg for at least 15 minutes.
  • Respiratory failure—Po_2 less than 60 mm Hg, requiring oxygen therapy for more than 24 hours.
  • Renal failure—serum creatinine higher than 1.4 mg/dl; sepsis-like picture: high temperature (>38.5°C) and leukocytosis (white blood count >20,000/mm^3).

Additional Facts

■ Drugs associated with acute pancreatitis include the following:

  • Thiazide diuretics, furosemide, estrogens, azathioprine, L-asparaginase, 6-mercaptopurine, methyldopa, sulfonamides, tetracycline, pentamidine, procainamide, nitrofurantoin, dideoxyinosine, valproic acid, and metronidazole.
■ Lipid disorders associated with acute pancreatitis include Types I and V familial hyperlipoproteinemia and chylomicronemia syndrome (hyperlipidemia and severely elevated levels of triglycerides and cholesterol).
■ Measurement of serum amylase and lipase are not helpful in distinguishing interstitial from necrotizing pancreatitis.
■ Prognostic predictors of severity in acute pancreatitis include Acute Physiology and Chronic Health Evaluation (APACHE-II) scores and Ranson's signs.
  • APACHE-II illness grading system assesses severity points of disease on the basis of a quantitative measurement of abnormalities of multiple parameters, including vital signs and specific laboratory values, plus severity points based on age and chronic health status; APACHE-II scores of 9 or lower in the first 48 hours are predictive of survival, whereas scores of 13 and higher are associated with a high likelihood of fatal outcome.
  • Ranson's criteria of severity include those measured at admission and those measured during the initial 48 hours and include the following:
    • At admission: age >55 years; white blood cell count >16,000/mm^3; glucose >200 mg/dl; lactate dehydrogenase >350 IU/L; aspartate aminotransferase >250 U/L.
    • During the initial 48 hours: hematocrit >10; blood urea nitrogen increase of >5 mg/dl; calcium <8 mg/dl; Pao_2 <60 mm Hg; base deficit >4 mEq/L; fluid sequestration >6 L.
    • In general, mortality increases with an increasing number of Ranson's signs: when 2 or fewer Ranson's signs are positive, mortality is nil; with 3 to 5 positive signs, mortality is 10% to 20%; when more than 6 signs are positive, mortality is 50%; patients with more than 3 Ranson's signs have a high incidence of systemic complications and pancreatic necrosis; patient's with more than 6 positive signs have infected necrosis.

2. Chronic Pancreatitis

Definition: Chronic progressive disease with persistent pancreatic damage both morphologic and functional in nature characterized by the clinical triad of diabetes, steatorrhea, and radiographic evidence of calcification. Chronic pancreatitis may clinically and histopathologically simulate a malignant neoplasm; changes of chronic pancreatitis may accompany a pancreatic neoplasm.

Clinical

■ Considered to be an uncommon condition; the incidence may be geographic.
■ The causes of chronic pancreatitis are listed in Table 11–5.
■ In urban areas of the United States, Europe, and South Africa, chronic pancreatitis is most often caused by alco-

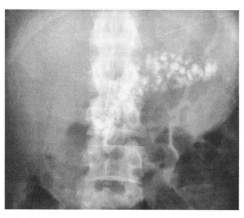
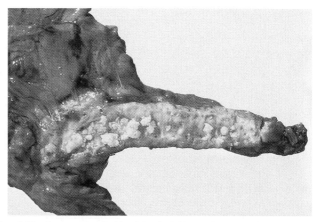

Figure 11–20. Chronic pancreatitis. *Left,* In the presence of pancreatic calcifications, as seen in this abdominal film, a diagnosis of chronic pancreatitis can be made. *Right,* Grossly, this patient's pancreas shows an identical distribution of the calcifications seen in the abdominal film, as well as other alterations of chronic pancreatitis, including a shrunken gland with fibrous tissue replacement.

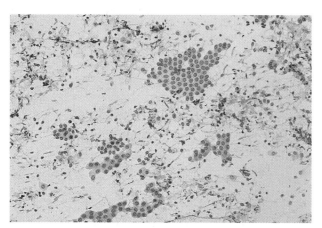

Figure 11–21. Fine needle aspiration in chronic pancreatitis showing relatively low cellularity, including mixed inflammatory cells, and granular debris. Sheets of benign ductal epithelial cells are seen.

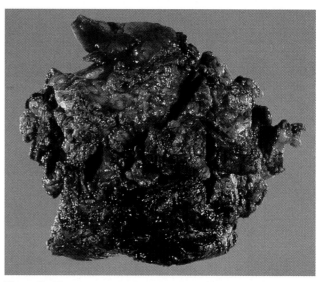

Figure 11–23. Advance chronic pancreatitis as depicted by this shrunken pancreas with marked reduction in pancreatic tissue.

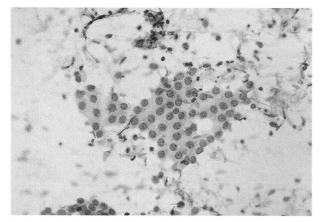

Figure 11–22. Fine needle aspiration in chronic pancreatitis showing benign ductal epithelial cells. The background includes mixed inflammatory cells and cellular debris.

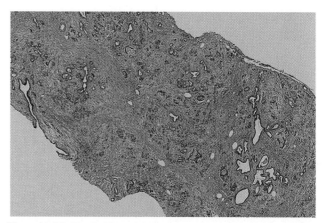

Figure 11–24. Needle biopsy in chronic pancreatitis showing the retention of the normal lobular architecture of the gland, a key feature seen in chronic pancreatitis assisting in differentiating it from adenocarcinoma. Additional features include loss of acinar and ductal tissue, focal ductal dilatation with inspissated secretions, and fibrosis.

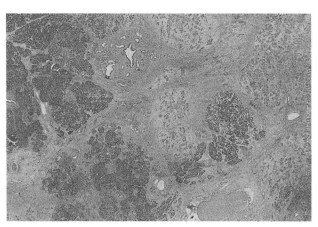

Figure 11–25. Resected pancreas showing similar features to those described in the previous illustration, including preservation of the lobular architecture, areas in which there is loss of acinar and ductal tissue, focal ductal dilatation, and fibrosis. Fibrosis is another common feature in chronic pancreatitis and is irregular or uneven in distribution and seen in periductal, intralobular, and interlobular areas.

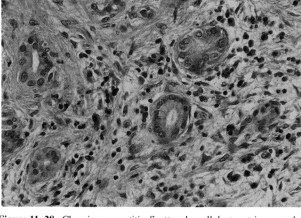

Figure 11–28. Chronic pancreatitis. Scattered small ducts retain a rounded configuration composed of enlarged but regular-appearing nuclei with a linear arrangement along the basal area of the cells. The background includes a mixed inflammatory infiltrate within an edematous stroma.

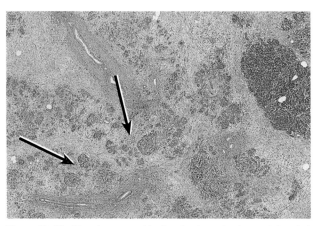

Figure 11–26. Chronic pancreatitis showing loss of acinar and ductal tissue with replacement by granulation tissue. The loss of exocrine pancreatic tissues results in relatively prominent appearing islets of Langerhans *(arrows)*. Periductal fibrosis is present and includes the presence of dense eosinophilic hyalinized material.

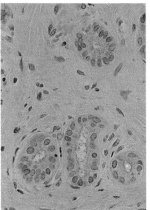

Figure 11–29. Chronic pancreatitis versus ductal adenocarcinoma. *Left,* Chronic pancreatitis showing small round ducts composed of enlarged but uniform nuclei without significant pleomorphism or increased nuclear-to-cytoplasmic ratio, and with relative linear arrangement along the basal portion of the cell. In contrast, the malignant ducts in adenocarcinoma are composed of irregularly shaped ducts with enlarged, pleomorphic nuclei with increased nuclear-to-cytoplasmic ratio, prominent nucleoli, and haphazard arrangement in the cell.

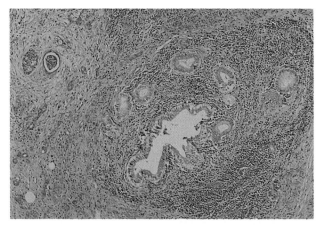

Figure 11–27. A variable degree of chronic inflammation is present in chronic pancreatitis. The chronic inflammatory cell infiltrate is usually a minor component of the process but occasionally, as illustrated in this figure, the chronic inflammation may dominate the histologic picture.

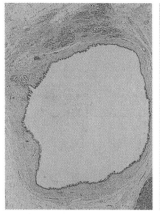
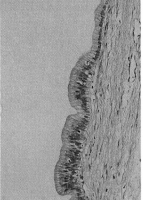

Figure 11–30. Ductal epithelial alterations are commonly found in chronic pancreatitis. *Left,* Ductal dilatation (ectasia) is seen. *Right,* The ductal epithelial cells include columnar, mucin-producing cells with basally located nuclei.

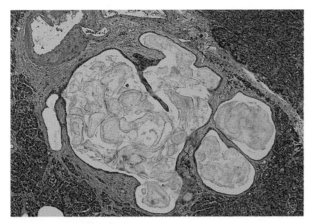

Figure 11–31. Chronic pancreatitis with duct ectasia. The ducts contain amorphous eosinophilic and somewhat laminated secretions.

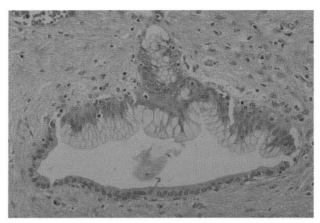

Figure 11–34. Mucus cell metaplasia and hyperplasia showing a transition from the cuboidal-appearing epithelium in the lower portion of the duct to tall columnar cells containing mucin (mucus-rich cells) in the upper portion of the duct. The nuclei in the mucus-rich cells are aligned toward the basal aspect of the cells and are without atypical features.

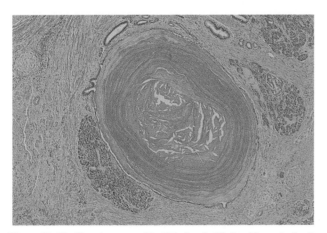

Figure 11–32. Chronic pancreatitis. This duct is filled and is markedly dilated by inspissated eosinophilic and laminated material.

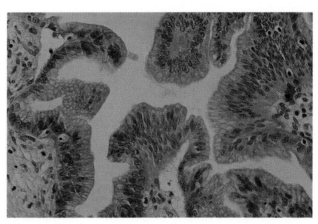

Figure 11–35. Chronic pancreatitis. This duct with mucus cell metaplasia and pseudopapillary hyperplasia shows minimal cytologic atypia, including nuclear crowding, nuclear stratification, increased nuclear-to-cytoplasmic ratio, and nucleoli. Although atypical, the features fall short of severe dysplasia or carcinoma in situ.

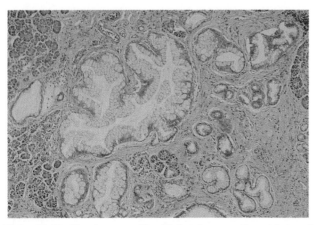

Figure 11–33. Chronic pancreatitis with ductal mucus cell metaplasia and hyperplasia.

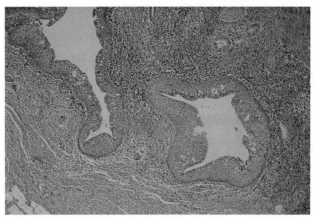

Figure 11–36. Chronic pancreatitis with squamous metaplasia.

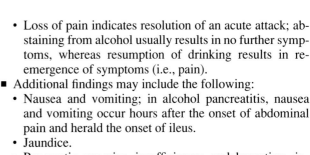

Figure 11–37. The endocrine pancreas is the most resistant component to the effects of chronic pancreatitis. As seen here, due to exocrine pancreatic "drop-out," the unaffected islets of Langerhans may stand out in chronic pancreatitis, possibly resulting in the interpretation of a pancreatic endocrine neoplasm. It is not until the advanced stages of chronic pancreatitis that morphologic alterations of the islets occur, including reduction in number and progressive atrophy with preferential loss of insulin cells. At that point, clinical manifestations of diabetes may occur.

hol abuse; in conjunction with alcohol abuse, tobacco smoking may be an additive factor in chronic pancreatitis, because smoking increases the risk of chronic pancreatitis almost tenfold; preexisting gallstones are present in a very small percentage of cases (approximately 4%).
- Chronic pancreatitis is more common in men than in women; most frequent in the 4th to 6th decades.
- Patients generally present with abdominal pain (>80%) and weight loss.
  - Most often the pain is chronic, but a minority of patients have intermittent attacks.
  - When present, the pain is continuous, lasting for more than 24 hours.
  - Pain is most frequently epigastric, often radiates to the back, but can radiate to either the upper quadrant or into the left lower quadrant; less frequently, pain may radiate to the shoulders, and substernal pain may radiate to the arms.
  - Positionally, during pain patients assume a stooped or "jackknife" posture.
  - Typically, in patients who abuse alcohol, the pain in chronic pancreatitis begins 12 to 48 hours after cessation of alcohol ingestion, frequently without nausea and vomiting.

Table 11–5
ETIOLOGY OF CHRONIC PANCREATITIS

Alcohol
Idiopathic
Nutritional
Hereditary
Cystic fibrosis
Trauma
Hypercalcemia
Chronic renal failure
Vascular disease
Hyperlipidemia
Gallstones
Others

- Loss of pain indicates resolution of an acute attack; abstaining from alcohol usually results in no further symptoms, whereas resumption of drinking results in reemergence of symptoms (i.e., pain).
- Additional findings may include the following:
  - Nausea and vomiting; in alcohol pancreatitis, nausea and vomiting occur hours after the onset of abdominal pain and herald the onset of ileus.
  - Jaundice.
  - Pancreatic exocrine insufficiency: malabsorption, including steatorrhea and azotorrhea; however, with rare exceptions, steatorrhea and azotorrhea do not occur until there is a 90% reduction in pancreatic enzyme secretion (lipase and trypsin, respectively); in chronic pancreatitis secondary to alcoholism, it may take decades for severe exocrine insufficiency to develop; lipase secretion decreases more rapidly than secretion of proteolytic enzymes, so steatorrhea is often an earlier and more severe problem than azotorrhea.
  - Pancreatic endocrine insufficiency: diabetes is common in pancreatitis but usually does not occur until advanced disease; in early alcoholic pancreatitis, diabetes does not occur except transiently after an episode of acute pancreatitis; the cause of pancreatitis has no relationship to the likelihood of developing diabetes, but the time period is influenced by the cause as diabetes appears with shorter time periods to the development of diabetes seen in alcohol-related chronic pancreatitis than with nonalcoholic disease.
  - Pancreatic mass (pseudocyst or abscess).
  - Ascites and pleural effusion both occur secondary to leakage of pancreatic juice from a ruptured pancreatic duct or cyst; the ascitic fluid has elevated amylase concentration.
  - Miscellaneous clinical features include gastrointestinal bleeding, peptic ulceration, metastatic fat necrosis (leakage of lipase into the circulation), and cirrhosis in alcoholic pancreatitis.
- Occurs anywhere in the pancreas as focal, segmental, or diffuse involvement.
- Laboratory studies measuring pancreatic exocrine function:
  - Noninvasive—in contrast with acute pancreatitis, serum amylase and lipase levels are usually not elevated.
    - Fecal fat: represents the "gold standard" test for malabsorption; normally, 7% or less of ingested fat appears in stool; in malabsorption of all causes, there is an abnormal amount of fecal fat (ingesting 100 g fat diet with fecal fat excretion >7 g/24 hours is abnormal); as such, as a test of pancreatic function, quantitative fecal fat is insensitive and nonspecific.
    - Fecal chymotrypsin: very sensitive in advanced disease.
    - Triolein breath test: measurement of fat malabsorption; like fecal fat, this test result is abnormal in patients with chronic pancreatic disease when there is advanced pancreatic insufficiency.
  - Invasive—requires oroduodenal intubation.
    - Measures pancreatic secretion in response to intraluminal stimuli or in response to exogenous hormones (e.g., secretin and cholecystokinin).
  - Invasive tests are more sensitive and specific than noninvasive tests.

- Additional laboratory findings may include impaired glucose tolerance and elevated fasting blood glucose levels; slight elevation of serum bilirubin and alkaline phosphatase levels may indicate cholestasis secondary to chronic inflammation around the common bile duct.
- Elevated serum levels of CA 19–9, considered highly specific for pancreatic cancer (see Pancreatic Cancer—General Considerations, Chapter 12B) can occur in patients with chronic pancreatitis in the absence of a pancreatic adenocarcinoma.

Radiology

- *Conventional abdominal films:* in the presence of calcifications on abdominal films, a diagnosis of chronic pancreatitis can be made with 90% confidence and no further tests are needed.
  - The presence of calcifications in the pancreas in a patient with abdominal pain strongly suggests the presence of acute exacerbation of chronic pancreatitis; pancreatic calcifications may be present in 30% to 70% of patients at clinical presentation.
  - In alcoholic pancreatitis, pancreatic calcifications occur a mean of approximately 1 decade after the onset of alcoholism; in idiopathic pancreatitis, pancreatic calcifications develop over two decades after diagnosis.
  - Secondary radiographic changes seen may include sentinel loop, colon cutoff sign, and "soap bubble sign," indicative of pancreatic abscess.
  - Conventional chest radiograph may include pleural effusions.
- *Ultrasonography:* in chronic pancreatitis, the echo pattern is coarse, hyperechoic, and more intense than that of the liver (normal pancreas has uniform, bright echo pattern with the same or slightly greater intensity than that of the liver); ultrasonography is less sensitive and specific than CT scan but is less expensive and does not expose the patient to ionizing radiation; if ultrasonography fails to result in diagnostic features of chronic pancreatitis, then CT scan can be performed.
- *CT scan:* primary findings include alteration of the gland size and dilatation of the pancreatic duct, which may contain stones; ductal dilatation is usually beaded ("chain-of-lakes" effect) but can be smooth; the sensitivity and specificity of CT for the diagnosis of chronic pancreatitis are high (75–90% and 94–100%, respectively).

Pathology

Fine Needle Aspiration

- Relatively low cellularity, including mixed inflammatory cells, and granular and calcified debris.
- Ductal epithelial cells may be seen with reparative or inflammatory atypia, including altered cell polarity, large nuclei, and prominent nucleoli; flat sheets with reduced cohesion may be present.

Gross

- The distribution of the lesions include focal, segmental, or diffuse.

- The involved pancreas is enlarged (either in part or in toto) and is indurated with associated sclerosis.
- With progression of disease, the gland shrinks.
- Lesions of chronic calcific pancreatitis are irregularly distributed; some lobules are essentially normal, whereas others are severely damaged.
- Cysts may be present.

Histology

- In the absence of confirmatory radiographic findings or blood and urine analysis, tissue sampling (needle biopsy) may be indicated.
- The essential histologic features of chronic pancreatitis are the same irrespective of the etiology of chronic pancreatitis, except that obstructive causes (stones, fibrosis, or tumor) result in a less severe and more uniform process than the more severe and diffuse changes that occur with alcohol-related chronic pancreatitis.
- In contrast with acute pancreatitis in which there is complete restitution of the pancreatic parenchyma following resolution of the acute attack, in chronic pancreatitis, the morphologic alterations are permanent.
- Irregular loss of acinar and ductal tissue with various ductal alterations, including dilatation, cyst formation, and presence of inspissated secretions or calculi.
- Ductal epithelial alterations can also be seen and may include atrophy, hyperplasia, or metaplasia (mucus cell or squamous); tiny ducts may be ectatic, and rare ones are filled with secretions.
- In mucus cell hyperplasia:
  - Ducts may be lined by tall columnar cells containing mucin (mucus-rich cells) in the apical region of the cell; nuclei are aligned along the basal aspect of the cells and are small and uniform.
  - Atypical cytologic features, including nuclear pleomorphism, nuclear crowding, nuclear stratification, increased nuclear:cytoplasmic ratio, prominent nucleoli, and mitotic figures, are not present; *minimal* ductal epithelial atypia can be seen, but intraductal epithelial hyperplasia with cytologic atypia is not a feature of pancreatitis and more likely represents a premalignant alteration or de novo malignancy (Chapter 12D, #1).
  - Papillary growth may or may not be present; obstructed ducts may contain pseudopapillae.
- Characteristically, there is preservation of the pancreatic lobular architecture; this is perhaps the most important feature and represents a cardinal feature in differentiating chronic pancreatitis from ductal adenocarcinoma; the individual lobules range from normal to quite atrophic.
- A variable degree of chronic inflammation is present; typically, the chronic inflammatory cell infiltrate is a minor component of the process, but occasionally chronic inflammation may dominate the histologic picture.
- Fibrosis is another common feature; the fibrosis is irregular or uneven in distribution and can be seen in periductal, intralobular, and interlobular areas.
- Perineural and intraneural inflammation, followed by perineural fibrosis, can be seen in chronic pancreatitis.
- In the early stages of chronic pancreatitis, most of the islets are normal or show only minimal distortional alterations; in the more advanced stages of disease, abnormal

islet alterations include a reduction in number and progressive atrophy; insulin cells tend to be lost preferentially; occasionally, islet cell hyperplasia may be seen.

■ Pseudocyst formation—pseudocysts are characterized by the absence of an epithelial lining and the presence of fibrosis, inflammation, and granulation tissue.

■ In acute exacerbation, a prominent polymorphonuclear leukocyte infiltrate can be seen, as well as necrosis (intraparenchymal and in peripancreatic adipose tissue).

Differential Diagnosis

■ Ductal adenocarcinoma (Table 11–6) (Chapter 12E, #1).
■ Acute pancreatitis (Chapter 11G, #1).

Treatment and Prognosis

■ Medical treatment includes analgesics for pain (aspirin, acetaminophen with codeine), abstinence from alcohol, eating frequent, small meals in an attempt to decrease the magnitude of prandial pancreatic secretion.

■ Treatment for severe exocrine pancreatic insufficiency (malabsorption) includes enzyme replacement therapy (Viokase and others).

■ Surgery is recommended as a last resort and only after medical measures fail to relieve the symptoms, specifically for relief from intractable pain; intractable pain is the most common reason for surgery in chronic pancreatitis; surgery is also performed for complications of pancreatitis, including bile duct obstruction or pseudocyst formation; surgical exploration may also be indicated when it is not possible based on the clinical features to differentiate chronic pancreatitis from pancreatic cancer.

■ The mortality rate secondary to chronic pancreatitis is low, especially for idiopathic and alcohol-related disease; for the latter, patient deaths do not generally result from chronic pancreatitis or its complications.

■ The incidence of pancreatic cancer in chronic pancreatitis varies from 0% to 30%; multiple interrelated factors associated with chronic pancreatitis, including alcohol and smoking, probably increase the risk for pancreatic cancer.

Additional Facts

■ The irregularity of the process is most characteristic of chronic pancreatitis secondary to ethanol abuse or the presence of poorly defined dietary and/or environmental factors; the process tends to be more uniform and with greater dilatation of the larger ducts when secondary to obstruction of the major ducts (for example, a calculus from chronic biliary tract disease or a stricture of the ampulla of Vater).

■ Alcoholic chronic pancreatitis and "tropical" chronic pancreatitis are irregular in distribution, have inspissated secretions in the ducts, show considerable loss of acinar tissue, and have irregular fibrosis: intralobular, interlobular, and periductal; calcification in the ducts may be marked; varying numbers of chronic inflammatory cells are present. Some ducts are dilated; others disappear; ductal epithelium may be atrophic, metaplastic, or hyperplastic.

Table 11–6
CHRONIC PANCREATITIS VERSUS DUCTAL ADENOCARCINOMA

Features	Chronic Pancreatitis	Ductal Adenocarcinoma
Gender/age	More common in men than women; most frequent in the 4th–6th decades of life	More common in men than in women; incidence increases with age; peak incidence in the 7th–8th decades; uncommon below 40 years of age
Clinical	Abdominal pain (>80%) and weight loss	Jaundice, epigastric pain, weight loss
Etiology	Alcohol, idiopathic, nutritional, hereditary, biliary tract disease (gallstones), others	Tobacco, alcoholism, dietary, coffee, occupational factors, radiation exposure, preexisting medical conditions (diabetes, pancreatitis [acquired, hereditary], genetic and familial factors
Radiology	Calcifications on abdominal films	Mass deforming contours of gland; severe ductal abnormalities (strictures longer than 10 mm and duct irregularities), with pancreatitis; cancers in head may obstruct pancreatic and common bile ducts, resulting in "double duct sign" on ERCP; abrupt cut-off to the main pancreatic duct seen on ERCP
Location	Occurs anywhere in the pancreas as focal, segmental, or diffuse involvement	Occurs in head more often than in body and tail
Gross	Involved pancreas is enlarged (in either part or in toto), indurated with associated sclerosis; fibrous strand in end-stage	Mass lesion, solitary and poorly demarcated
Histology	Preservation of lobular architecture; irregular loss of acinar and ductal tissue with ductal dilatation, cyst formation; inspissated secretions or calculi; ductal epithelial alterations (atrophy, hyperplasia or metaplasia) with minimal atypia; variable inflammation; fibrosis; islets are not altered in early stages but are abnormal in later stages of disease (reduction in number and progressive atrophy)	Loss of lobular architecture; invasive growth by neoplastic ducts or individual tumor cells with desmoplastic reaction; ducts or glands composed of atypical columnar or cuboidal cells with enlarged, irregular nuclei, prominent nucleoli, and mitoses; neurotropism; variable mucin production; minor alterations of islets
Treatment and prognosis	Analgesics for pain; enzyme replacement for exocrine insufficiency; surgery for pain as a last resort; mortality rate secondary to chronic pancreatitis is low	Surgery; adjuvant therapy of limited assistance; poor prognosis: >95% of patients die of their disease

ERCP, endoscopic retrograde cholangiopancreatography.

Bibliography

Classification

Chen J, Baithun SI. Morphological study of 391 cases of exocrine pancreatic tumours with special reference to the classification of exocrine pancreatic carcinoma. J Pathol 1985; 146:17–29.

Morohoshi T, Held G, Klöppel G. Exocrine pancreatic tumours and their histological classification: A study based on 167 autopsy and 97 surgical cases. Histopathology 1983; 7:645–661.

Congenital Abnormalities

Aplasia, Hypoplasia, and Dysplasia

Bernstein J, Chandra M, Creswal J, et al. Renal-hepatic-pancreatic dysplasia: A syndrome reconsidered. Am J Med Genet 1987; 26:391–403.

Gilinsky NH, Del Favero G, Cotton PB, Lees WR. Congenital short pancreas: A report of two cases. Gut 1985; 26:304–310.

Hill ID, Lebenthal E. Congenital abnormalities of the exocrine pancreas. In: Go VLW, DiMagno EP, Gardner JD, et al, eds. The pancreas: Biology, Pathobiology and Disease. 2nd edition. New York: Raven Press, 1993, pp. 1029–1040.

Lemons JA, Ridenour R, Orsini EN. Congenital absence of the pancreas and intrauterine growth retardation. Pediatrics 1979; 64:255–257.

Madrazo-de la Garza JA, Gotthold M, Lu RB, Hill ID, Lebenthal E. A new direct pancreatic function test in pediatrics. J Pediatr Gastroenterol Nutr 1991; 12:356–360.

Ductal Abnormalities

Berman LG, Prior JT, Abramow SM, Ziegler DD. A study of the pancreatic duct system in man by the use of vinyl acetate casts of postmortem preparations. Surg Gynecol Obstet 1960; 110:391–403.

Hill ID. Lebenthal E. Congenital abnormalities of the exocrine pancreas. In: Go VLW, DiMagno EP, Gardner JD, et al, eds. The Pancreas: Biology, Pathobiology and Disease. 2nd edition. New York: Raven Press, 1993, pp. 1029–1040.

Skandalakis JE, Gray SW, Rowe JS, Skandalakis LJ. Surgical anatomy of the pancreas. Contemp Surg 1979; 10:1–31.

Pancreas Divisum

Bernard JP, Sahel J, Giovannini M, Sarles H. Pancreas divisum is a probable cause of acute pancreatitis: A report of 137 cases. Pancreas 1990; 5:248–254.

Blair AJ, Russel CG, Cotton PB. Resection for pancreatitis in patients with pancreas divisum. Ann Surg 1984; 200:590–594.

Brenner P, Duncombe V, Ham JM. Pancreatitis and pancreas divisum: Aetiological and surgical considerations. Aust NZ J Surg 1990; 60:899–903.

Cotton PB. Congenital anomaly of pancreas divisum as a cause of obstructive pain and pancreatitis. Gut 1980; 21:105–114.

Cotton PB, Kizu M. Malfusion of dorsal and ventral pancreas: A cause of pancreatitis? Gut 1977; 18:400A.

Gregg JA. Pancreas divisum: Its association with pancreatitis. Am J Surg 1977; 134:539–543.

Hill ID. Lebenthal E. Congenital abnormalities of the exocrine pancreas. In: Go VLW, DiMagno EP, Gardner JD, et al, eds. The Pancreas: Biology, Pathobiology and Disease. 2nd edition. New York: Raven Press, 1993, pp. 1029–1040.

Oertel JE, Oertel YC, Heffess CS. Pancreas. In: Sternberg SS, ed. Diagnostic Surgical Pathology. 2nd edition. New York: Raven Press, 1994, pp. 1419–1457.

Rosch W, Koch H, Schnaffner O, Demling L. The clinical significance of the pancreas divisum. Gastrointest Endosc 1976; 22:206–207.

Saltzberg DM, Schreiber JB, Smith K, Cameron JL. Isolated ventral pancreatitis in a patient with pancreas divisum. Am J Gastroenterol 1990; 85:1407–1410.

Annular Pancreas

Kiernan PD, ReMine SG, Kiernan PC, ReMine WH. Annular pancreas: Mayo clinic experience from 1957 to 1976 with review of the literature. Arch Surg 1980; 115:46–50.

Levy J. The gastrointestinal tract in Down syndrome. Prog Clin Biol Res 1991; 373:245–256.

Ravitch MM, Woods AC. Annular pancreas. Ann Surg 1950; 132:1116–1127.

Sessa F, Fiocca R, Tenti P, et al. Pancreatic polypeptide rich tissue in annular pancreas: A distinctive feature of ventral primordium derivatives. Virch Arch [A] 1983; 339:227–232.

Suda K. Immunohistochemical and gross dissection studies of annular pancreas. Acta Pathol Jpn 1990; 40:505–508.

Choledochal Cysts

Alonso-Lej F, Rever WB, Pessagno DJ. Congenital choledochal cyst, with a report of 2 cases, and an analysis of 94 cases. Int Abstr Surg 1959; 108:1–30.

Flanigan DP. Biliary carcinoma associated with biliary cysts. Cancer 1977; 40:880–883.

Miyano T, Suruga K, Chen SC. A clinicopathologic study of choledochal cysts. World J Surg 1980; 4:231–238.

Sparks AK, Connor DH, Neafie RC. *Echinococcus*. In: Binford CH, Connor DH. Pathology of Tropical and Extraordinary Disease: An Atlas. Washington, DC: Armed Forces Institute of Pathology, 1976, pp. 530–533.

Todani T, Urushihara N, Morotomi Y, et al. Characteristics of choledochal cysts in neonates and early infants. Eur J Pediatr Surg 1995; 5:143–145.

Voyles CR, Smadja C, Shands C, Blumgart LH. Carcinoma in choledochal cysts. Arch Surg 1983; 118:986–988.

Heterotopic Pancreas

Armstrong CP, King PM, Dixon JM, MacLeod IB. The clinical significance of heterotopic pancreas in the gastrointestinal tract. Br J Surg 1981; 68:384–387.

Busard JM, Walters W. Heterotopic pancreatic tissue. Arch Surg 1950; 60:674–682.

Brotman SJ, Pan W, Pozner J, et al. Ductal adenocarcinoma arising in duodenopyloric heterotopic pancreas. Int J Surg Pathol 1994; 2:37–42.

Carp NZ, Paul AR, Kowalshyn MJ, et al. Heterotopic mucinous cystadenoma of the pancreas. Dig Dis Sci 1992; 37:1297–1301.

DeBord JR, Majarakis JD, Nyhus LM. An unusual case of heterotopic pancreas of the stomach. Am J Surg 1981; 141:269–273.

Dolan RV, ReMine WH, Dockerty MB. The fate of heterotopic pancreatic tissue: A study of 212 cases. Arch Surg 1974; 109:762–765.

Pearson S. Aberrant pancreas: Review of the literature and report of 3 cases, one of which produced common and pancreatic duct obstruction. Arch Surg 1951; 63:168–184.

Sapino A, Pietribiasi F, Papotti M, Bussolati G. Ectopic endocrine pancreatic tumour simulating splenic angiosarcoma. Pathol Res Pract 1989; 184:292–296.

Shim YT, Kim SY. Heterotopic gastric mucosa and pancreatic tissue in the skin of the abdominal wall. J Pediatr Surg 1992; 27:1539–1540.

Tanaka K, Tsunoda T, Eto T, et al. Diagnosis and management of heterotopic pancreas. Int Surg 1993; 78:32–35.

Tanigawa K, Yamashita S, Tezuka H, et al. Diagnostic difficulty in a case of heterotopic pancreatic tissue of the ileum. Am J Gastroenterol 1993; 88:451–453.

Pancreatic Congenital Cysts

DeLange C, Janssen TAE. Large solitary pancreatic cyst and other developmental errors in a premature infant. Am J Dis Child 1948; 75:587–594.

Flaherty MJ, Benjamin DR. Multicystic pancreatic hamartoma: A distinctive lesion with immunohistochemical and ultrastructural study. Hum Pathol 1992; 23:1309–1312.

Hill ID. Lebenthal E. Congenital abnormalities of the exocrine pancreas. In: Go VLW, DiMagno EP, Gardner JD, et al, eds. The Pancreas: Biology, Pathobiology and Disease. 2nd edition. New York: Raven Press, 1993, pp. 1029–1040.

Kalani BP, Broadhead RL, Bhargav RK. Giant congenital pancreatic cyst in a child. Ann Trop Pediatr 1982; 2:47–49.

Mares AJ, Hirsch M. Congenital cysts of the head of the pancreas. J Pediatr Surg 1977; 12:547–552.

Miles RM. Pancreatic cyst of the newborn. Ann Surg 1959; 149:576–581.

Norris RF, Tyson RM. The pathogenesis of congenital polycystic lung and its relationship with polycystic disease of other epithelial organs. Am J Pathol 1947; 23:1075–1087.

Hereditary Diseases of the Pancreas

Cystic Fibrosis

Agrons GA, Corse WR, Markowitz RI, et al. Gastrointestinal manifestations of cystic fibrosis: Radiologic-pathologic correlation. Radiographics 1996; 16:871–893.

Andersen DH. Cystic fibrosis of the pancreas and its relation to celiac disease. Am J Dis Child 1938; 56:344–399.

Andersen DH. Pathology of cystic fibrosis. Ann NY Acad Sci 1962; 95:500–517.

Cruickshank AH. Effects upon the pancreas of disease in various organs and systems. In: Pathology of the Pancreas. Berlin, Springer-Verlag, 1986, pp. 45–63.

Farber S. Pancreatic function and disease in early life: V. Pathologic changes associated with pancreatic insufficiency in early life. Arch Pathol Lab Med 1944; 37:238–250.

Lebenthal E, Lerner A, Rolston DDK. The pancreas in cystic fibrosis. In: Go VLW, DiMagno EP, Gardner JD, et al, eds. The Pancreas: Biology, Pathobiology and Disease. 2nd edition. New York: Raven Press, 1993, pp. 1041–1081.

Vawter GF, Shwachman H. Cystic fibrosis in adults: An autopsy study. Pathol Annu 1979; 14:357–382.

Diabetes Mellitus

Catanese VM, Kahn CR. Secondary forms of diabetes mellitus. In: Becker KL, ed. Principles and Practice of Endocrinology and Metabolism. 2nd edition. Philadelphia: JB Lippincott, 1995, pp. 1220–1228.

Clark A, de Koning EJ, Hattersely AT, et al. Pancreatic pathology in non-insulin dependent diabetes mellitus (NIDDM). Diabetes Res Clin Pract 1995; 28:S39–S47.

Farney AC, Sutherland DE. Pancreas and islet transplantation. In: Go VLW, DiMagno EP, Gardner JD, et al, eds. The Pancreas: Biology, Pathobiology and Disease. 2nd edition. New York: Raven Press, 1993, pp. 815–835.

Foulis K, Stewart JA. The pancreas in recent-onset type I (insulin-dependent) diabetes mellitus: Insulin content of islets, insulitis and associated changes in the exocrine acinar tissues. Diabetologia 1984; 26:456–461.

Gepts W. Pathologic anatomy of the pancreas in juvenile diabetes mellitus. Diabetes 1965; 14:619–633.

Gepts W, Schofield JB. The pancreas and diabetes. In: Lewis PD, ed. Systemic Pathology: The Endocrine System. 3rd edition. New York: Churchill Livingstone, 1996, pp. 221–254.

Klöppel G, Drenck CR, Oberholzer MR, Heitz PU. Morphometric evidence for a striking B-cell reduction at the clinical onset of type 1 diabetes. Virchows Arch [A] Pathol Anat 1984; 403:441–452.

Klöppel G, Löhr M, Habich K, et al. Islet pathology and the pathogenesis of type 1 and type 2 diabetes mellitus revisited. Surv Synth Pathol Res 1985; 4:110–125.

Stefan Y, Orci L, Malaisse-Lagae F, Perrelet, et al. Quantitation of endocrine cell content in the pancreas of non-diabetic and diabetic humans. Diabetes 1982; 31:694–700.

Other Hereditary Diseases

Comfort MW, Steinberg AG. Pedigree of a family with hereditary chronic relapsing pancreatitis. Gastroenterology 1952; 21:54–63.

Cormier V, Rotig A, Quartino AR, et al. Widespread multitissue deletions of mitochondrial genome in the Pearson marrow-pancreas syndrome. J Pediatr 1990; 117:599–602.

Gershoni-Baruch R, Lerner A, Braun J, et al. Johanson-Blizzard syndrome: Clinical spectrum and further delineation of the syndrome. Am J Med Genet 1990; 35:546–551.

Lerner A, Lebenthal E. Hereditary disease of the pancreas: Congenital abnormalities of the exocrine pancreas. In: Go VLW, DiMagno EP, Gardner JD, et al, eds. The Pancreas: Biology, Pathobiology and Disease. 2nd edition. New York: Raven Press, 1993, pp. 1083–1094.

Lynch HY, Smyrk T, Kern SE, et al. Familial pancreatic cancer: A review. Semin Oncol 1996; 23:251–275.

Madrazo de la Garza JA, Hill ID, Lebenthal E. Hereditary pancreatitis. In: Go VLW, DiMagno EP, Gardner JD, et al, eds. The Pancreas: Biology, Pathobiology and Disease. 2nd edition. New York: Raven Press, 1993, pp. 1095–1101.

Pearson HA, Lobel JS, Kocoshis SA, et al. A new syndrome of refractory sideroblastic anemia with vacuolization of marrow precursors and exocrine pancreatic insufficiency. J Pediatr 1979; 95:976–984.

Robberecht E, Nachtegaele P, Van Rattinghe R, et al. Pancreatic lipomatosis in Shwachman-Diamond syndrome: Identification by sonography and CT scan. Pediatr Radiol 1985; 15:348–9.

Rotig A, Colonna M, Bonnefont JP, et al. Mitochondrial DNA deletion in Pearson's marrow/pancreas syndrome. Lancet 1989; 1:902–903.

Shwachman H, Diamond LK, Oski FA, Khaw Kon T. The syndrome of pancreatic insufficiency and bone marrow dysfunction. J Pediatr 1964; 65:645–663.

Tada H, Ri T, Yoshida H, et al. A case report of Shwachman syndrome with increased spontaneous chromosome breakage. Hum Genet 1987; 77:289–291.

Acquired Lesions/Diseases

Age-Related Alterations of the Pancreas

Allen-Mersh TG. What is the significance of pancreatic ductal mucinous hyperplasia. Gut 1985; 26:825–833.

Oertel JE. The pancreas: Nonneoplastic alterations. Am J Surg Pathol 1989; 13(Supp 1):50–65.

Oertel JE, Oertel YC, Heffess CS. Pancreas. In: Sternberg SS, ed. Diagnostic Surgical Pathology. 2nd edition. New York: Raven Press, 1994, pp. 1419–1457.

Non-Neoplastic Cystic Lesions of the Pancreas

Pseudocysts

D'Egidio A, Schein M. Pancreatic pseudocysts: A proposed classification and its management implications. Br J Surg 1991; 78:981–984.

Klöppel G, Maillet B. Pseudocysts in chronic pancreatitis: A morphological analysis of 57 resection specimens and 9 autopsy pancreata. Pancreas 1991; 6:266–274.

MacCarty RL, Ward EM, Charboneau JW, et al. Imaging of the pancreas. In: Go VLW, DiMagno EP, Gardner JD, et al, eds. The Pancreas: Biology, Pathobiology and Disease. 2nd edition. New York: Raven Press, 1993, pp. 1103–1135.

Oertel JE, Oertel YC, Heffess CS. Pancreas. In: Sternberg SS, ed. Diagnostic Surgical Pathology. 2nd edition. New York: Raven Press, 1994, pp. 1419–1457.

Young NA, Villani MA, Khoury P, Naryshkin S. Differential diagnosis of cystic neoplasms of the pancreas by fine-needle aspiration. Arch Pathol Lab Med 1991; 115:571–577.

Lymphoepithelial Cysts

Adair C, Thompson L, Wenig B, Heffess C. The lymphoepithelial cyst (LEC) of the pancreas: A lesion of uncertain etiology. Mod Pathol 1995; 8:127A.

Cappellari JO. Fine needle aspiration cytology of a pancreatic lymphoepithelial cyst. Diagn Cytopathol 1993; 9:77–81.

Hisaoka M, Haratake J, Horie A, et al. Lymphoepithelial cyst of the pancreas in a 65-year-old man. Hum Pathol 1991; 22:924–926.

Lüchtrath H, Schriefers KH. Pankreazyste unter dem Bild einer sogenannten brachiogenen Zyste. Pathologe 1985; 6:217–219.

Mockli GC, Stein RM. Cystic lymphoepithelial lesion of the pancreas. Arch Pathol Lab Med 1990; 114:885–887.

Ramsden KL, Newman J. Lymphoepithelial cyst of the pancreas. Histopathology 1991; 18:267–268.

Truong LD, Rangdaeng S, Jordan PH Jr. Lymphoepithelial cyst of the pancreas. Am J Surg Pathol 1987; 11:899–903.

Other Pancreatic Cysts

Howard JM. Cystic neoplasms and true cysts of the pancreas. Surg Clin North Am 1989; 69:651–665.

Pins MR, Compton CC, Southern JF, et al. Ciliated enteric duplication cyst presenting as a pancreatic neoplasm: Report of a case with cyst fluid analysis. Clin Chem 1992; 38:1309–1312.

Infectious Diseases

Bradley EL, Warshaw AI. Pancreatic abscess. In: Go VLW, DiMagno EP, Gardner JD, et al, eds. The Pancreas: Biology, Pathobiology and Disease. 2nd edition. New York: Raven Press, 1993, pp. 649–663.

Acute Pancreatitis

Aho HJ, Nevalainen TJ, Havia VT, et al. Human acute pancreatitis: A light and electron microscopic study. Acta Pathol Microbiol Immunol Scand [A] 1982; 90:367–373.

Baluvelt H. A case of acute pancreatitis with subcutaneous fat necrosis. Br J Surg 1946; 34:207.

Banks PA. Medical management of acute pancreatitis and complications. In: Go VLW, DiMagno EP, Gardner JD, et al, eds. The Pancreas: Biology, Pathobiology and Disease. 2nd edition. New York: Raven Press, 1993, pp. 593–611.

Cameron JL, Crisler C, Margolis S, et al. Acute pancreatitis with hyperlipemia. Surgery 1971; 70:53–61.

de Jongh FE, Ottervanger JP, Stuiver PC. Acute pancreatitis caused by metronidazole. Ned Tijdschr Geneeskd (Netherlands) 1996; 140:37–38.

Cruickshank AH. Non-infective acute pancreatitis. In: Diseases of the Pancreas. Berlin: Springer-Verlag, 1986, pp. 195–232.

Graham DF, Wylie FJ. Prediction of gallstone pancreatitis by computer. Br Med J [Clin Res] 1979; 1:515–517.

Kessler JI, Miller M, Barza D, Mishkin S. Hyperlipidemia in acute pancreatitis. Am J Med 1967; 42:968–976.

Lawson TL. Acute pancreatitis and its complications. Radiol Clin North Am 1983; 21:495–513.

Minguez M, Garcia A, Boix V. Acute pancreatitis: A prospective epidemiological study in the province of Alicante. Rv Esp Enferm Dig (Spain) 1995; 87:869–873.

Mithofer K, Fernandez-del Castillo C, Ferraro MJ, et al. Antibiotic treatment improves survival in experimental acute necrotizing pancreatitis. Gastroenterolgy 1996; 110:232–240.

Olsen H. Pancreatitis: A prospective clinical evaluation of 100 cases and review of the literature. Dig Dis Sci 1974; 19:1077–1090.

Opie EL. The etiology of acute hemorrhagic pancreatitis. Bull Johns Hopkins Hosp 1901; 12:182–188.

Shuster MM, Iber FL. Psychosis with pancreatitis. Arch Intern Med 1965; 116:228–233.

Silverman JF, Geisinger KR. Pancreas. In: Fine needle aspiration cytology of the thorax and abdomen. New York: Churchill Livingstone, 1996, pp. 135–170.

Steer ML. Etiology and pathophysiology of acute pancreatitis. In: Go VLW, DiMagno EP, Gardner JD, et al, eds. The Pancreas: Biology, Pathobiology and Disease. 2nd edition. New York: Raven Press, 1993, pp. 581–591.

van de Vrie W, Baggen MG, Janssen IM, Ouwendijk RJ. Acute pancreatitis caused by chylomicronemia syndrome. Ned Tijdschr Geneeskd (Netherlands) 1996; 140:34–36.

Willemer S, Adler G. Mechanism of acute pancreatitis. Int J Pancreatol 1991; 9:21–30.

CHAPTER 12

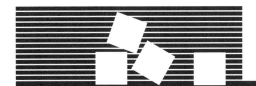

Neoplasms of the Pancreas

A. CLASSIFICATION OF PANCREATIC NEOPLASMS

Table 12–1
CLASSIFICATION OF PANCREATIC AND AMPULLARY NEOPLASMS

Exocrine Pancreas

Benign

Microcystic adenoma
Cystic teratoma

Intermediate Biologic Potential

Intraductal proliferative processes
Mucinous cystic neoplasms
Solid and papillary epithelial carcinoma

Malignant

Ductal adenocarcinoma
Variants of ductal adenocarcinoma:
   Adenosquamous carcinoma
   Mucinous adenocarcinoma
   Microglandular adenocarcinoma
   Oncocytic adenocarcinoma
Acinar cell carcinoma
Pancreatoblastoma
Anaplastic carcinoma

Endocrine Pancreas

Pancreatic endocrine neoplasms
Nesidioblastosis
Carcinoid tumor
Mixed exocrine and endocrine neoplasms

Mesenchymal Tumors

Lymphoproliferative Malignancies

Secondary Tumors

Duodenal Ampullary Tumors

Adenoma
Adenocarcinoma

B. GENERAL CONSIDERATIONS

- The incidence of pancreatic cancer has remained stable for approximately the past quarter of a century, with about 25,000 cases reported annually. In the United States, the incidence (age-adjusted) is approximately 10 per 100,000 person-years among males and 7.5 per 100,000 among females.
- Pancreatic cancer is one of the most lethal human neoplasms, ranking fourth as a cause of cancer deaths in the United States. The 5-year survival rate for pancreatic adenocarcinoma in the United States is 1.3%, and the median survival is 4.1 months; this cancer is virtually 100% lethal over short time periods.
- In the United States pancreatic cancer ranks second among gastrointestinal tumors in terms of incidence and cancer mortality.
- Worldwide, approximately 185,000 new cases of pancreatic cancer occurred in 1985 (the last year for which comprehensive figures were tabulated). Pancreatic cancer ranks fifth worldwide among gastrointestinal tumors in incidence and in cancer mortality.
- Pancreatic cancer is slightly more common in men than in women.
- The incidence of pancreatic cancer increases with age. Approximately 80% of cases of pancreatic cancer occur between the 7th and 9th decades of life; peak incidence occurs in the seventh to 8th decades. Pancreatic cancer in patients younger than 40 years of age is uncommon.
- The overall incidence of pancreatic cancer is 30% to 40% higher in African Americans than in whites. The incidence among native African populations is low. Koreans in the Los Angeles region also have an increased incidence of pancreatic cancer.
- Worldwide, pancreatic cancer is primarily a disease of developed countries; the one exception occurs in the native Maori population of New Zealand. In developed countries, urban populations appear to have a higher incidence of pancreatic cancer than rural populations. There are conflicting data about the relationship between socioeconomic status and pancreatic cancer; lower socioeconomic groups appear to have a higher incidence, but this has not been uniformly reported. Similarly, data about the incidence of pancreatic cancer according to religion are conflicting, also.
- Cancer arising in the head of the pancreas is more common than that in the body and tail combined.
- Because of its proximity to the biliary tract, carcinoma of the pancreatic head is associated with jaundice and pruri-

tus; the majority of patients have symptoms for less than 2 months.

- Most cancers of the pancreatic head result in the characteristic triad of jaundice, epigastric pain, and weight loss; however, these features are not pathognomonic of pancreatic cancer and can occur with other cancers.
- The median weight loss is about 25 pounds. Weight loss is higher in patients with unresectable tumors and liver metastases. Cancers in the body and tail of the pancreas produce more weight loss and pain than do proximally located tumors.
- Additional symptoms may include nausea and vomiting (more commonly associated with the presence of liver metastases), constipation, and food intolerance.
- Diabetes is present in about one third of patients with advanced disease, but up to 15% of patients present with de novo diabetes shortly before the diagnosis of cancer is made.
- Physical examination reveals the presence of an abdominal mass in up to 28% of cases, ankle edema in 17%, fever in 16%, abdominal distention in 12%, palpable gallbladder (Courvoisier's sign associated with cancer in the head of the pancreas) in 10%, and thrombophlebitis (Trousseau's sign) in 2%.
- **Laboratory findings** are nonspecific and include hyperbilirubinemia (direct), elevated alkaline phosphatase, aminotransferase, 5'-nucleotidase, anemia, and hypoalbuminemia.
  - Pancreatic function tests are at present rarely performed in the diagnosis of pancreatic cancer.

Tumor Markers

- **Pancreatic mucins.** Mucins are glycoprotein components of mucus that consist of water, electrolytes, lipids, proteins, and degradative products of the microbial and cellular environment of epithelial cells in addition to glycoproteins.
  - Mucins are characteristically produced by ductal epithelial cells, submucosal gland cells, and adenocarcinomas.
  - Mucus found in pancreatic ducts is composed of a mixture of mucins derived from different cell types from distinct portions of the pancreatic duct system.
  - Several different mucin cDNAs and genes coding for core proteins have been described; however, to date in only one mucin gene, Muc1, has the complete genomic and protein sequence been identified.
  - The Muc1 gene has been shown to be expressed by both acinar and ductal cells of the pancreas.
  - A pancreatic adenocarcinoma cell line produces and secretes a highly glycosylated form of Muc1 containing a large biantenarry carbohydrate structure that has an epitope recognized by the monoclonal antibody DUPAN-2.
- **DUPAN-2 antibody** is strongly reactive with the cytoplasm and apical portions of the pancreatic ductal epithelial cells but is nonreactive with acinar cells.
- **CA 19-9** is another monoclonal antibody that reacts with carbohydrate epitopes on pancreatic mucins.
  - Antibody CA 19-9 has been elicited to a colon carcinoma cell line and is reactive with the sialylated Lewis A blood group antigen; patients who are Lewis A blood group negative (approximately 5% of the general population) cannot synthesize CA 19-9 antigen.
  - CA 19-9 is considered a tumor-associated but not tumor-specific antigen. The sensitivity of CA 19-9 is increased in patients with larger tumors and advanced disease, and the sensitivity is the same for pancreatic cancers in all locations (head, body, tail). However, only about half of patients with tumors measuring 2 cm or less in diameter have increased CA 19-9 levels, thus limiting its use as a screening test.
- Another mucin-related carbohydrate epitope is **SPan-1.**
- Mucin epitopes can be evaluated as serum tumor markers in pancreatic adenocarcinoma.
  - Serologic measurements of serum mucin levels (by radioimmunoassay [RIA] and enzyme-linked immunosorbent assay [ELISA]) have shown that they are elevated in patients with pancreatic (ductal) adenocarcinoma.
  - The combination of two or more serum markers (e.g., DUPAN-2 and CA 19-9) increases the sensitivity to 90% or more in pancreatic cancer patients; however, a significant percentage of patients with benign disease of the pancreas and liver may also have elevated serum mucin levels of DUPAN-2 and CA 19-9.
  - The combination of a serum tumor marker and a single imaging study has a higher sensitivity than that of a tumor marker alone.
  - The resectability of pancreatic cancer decreases with increasing serum CA 19-9 levels. Serum levels of CA 19-9 have also been used as a postoperative marker and provide help in the early detection of recurrent tumor. Normalization of elevated serum CA 19-9 levels after pancreatectomy is associated with improved prognosis.
  - In addition to DUPAN-2 and CA 19-9, there is increasing evidence of the presence of truncated oligosaccharide structures on mucins produced by human pancreatic tumors. Presently, the best example is reactivity with the monoclonal antibody **B72.3** with pancreatic tumor cells and secreted products but not with normal human pancreatic tissue. The **B72.3** antibody recognizes an epitope that is not detected on normal pancreatic ductal epithelial tissue but is reactive with a high percentage of pancreatic adenocarcinoma cells. Carcinoembryonic antigen (CEA) is another putative tumor marker, but it is too nonspecific to be of diagnostic use.

Etiology of Pancreatic Cancer

- Among the contributing factors or etiologic agents with a suspected link to the development of pancreatic ductal adenocarcinoma are:

1. Tobacco. Cigarette smoking is considered a significant risk factor for pancreatic cancer, and there appears to be a dose relationship to the quantity of cigarettes smoked. Further, there appears to be an increased risk of pancreatic cancer as a second malignancy in patients with a cigarette-related malignancy in mucosal sites of the head and neck, lung, and bladder.

2. Alcohol. Evidence relating pancreatic cancer to alcohol consumption is inconsistent, and based on current data it appears that increased risk of pancreatic cancer from alcoholism is fairly small. Alcoholics who develop chronic pancreatitis have not been shown to have an increased risk of pancreatic cancer; however, heavy alcohol users also tend to be cigarette smokers, a known etiologic factor in pancreatic cancer.

3. Diet. Increased risk of pancreatic cancer has been correlated with increased consumption of dietary fat (total and saturated). Chemicals used in meat preservation and preparation, such as N-nitroso compounds, have been shown to induce pancreatic cancer in laboratory animals; although they have been suggested as a possible contributor to the development of pancreatic cancer, direct evidence is lacking. A significant protective effect has been found with the consumption of fruits and juices, beans and lentils, vegetarian protein sources, and wine (due to the antioxidative effects of various compounds extracted during fermentation).

4. Coffee. An association between coffee consumption (caffeinated and decaffeinated) and pancreatic cancer has been suggested; however, the number of studies linking coffee to pancreatic cancer have been surpassed by the numerous large prospective studies showing no clear association. Similarly, there is no clear link between tea consumption and pancreatic cancer.

5. Occupational factors, including industrial carcinogens, chemical exposure. Animal studies have shown the development of pancreatic cancer in laboratory animals following exposure to various chemicals, including n-nitrosurea, diisopropanol-nitrosamine, aflatoxin B_1, azaserine, acetaminofluorene, p-dimethylaminoazobenzene, methylcholanthrene, 2,2-dihydroxy-di-N-propylnitrosamine (DHPN), and N-nitrosobis (2-hydroxypropylamine, BHP). In humans, several occupations have been associated with increased risk for pancreatic cancer, including chemists, chemical and coke plant workers, mine workers, metal workers and aluminum millers, sawmill workers, dry cleaning workers, and electrical equipment manufacturers. However, significant risk has not been definitively proved between occupational factors and pancreatic cancer.

6. Radiation. Evidence that exposure to radiation increases the risk of pancreatic cancer has not been conclusively found, although an increased incidence of pancreatic cancer has been reported in patients receiving therapeutic abdominal irradiation. In animal models, islet cell tumors have been found in irradiated rats, but an animal model for radiation-induced pancreatic adenocarcinoma has not been found.

7. Predisposing medical conditions. (a) Diabetes: Diabetes has been suggested as a risk factor for pancreatic cancer, but this association is highly debatable, and it is unlikely that a causative relationship exists. (b) Chronic (nonfamilial) pancreatitis: Acute and chronic pancreatitis correlate with alcoholism, but a relationship between pancreatitis and pancreatic cancer remains questionable at best. (c) Hereditary chronic relapsing pancreatitis: In contrast to acquired nonfamilial pancreatitis, the hereditary form of pancreatitis, representing an autosomal dominant trait with probable complete penetrance, has been shown to increase the risk of pancreatic cancer significantly. (d) Pancreatic cancer after partial gastrectomy: Regardless of the reasons for surgery, there appears to be an increased risk of pancreatic cancer in patients who have undergone partial gastrectomy.

8. Familial and genetic factors. Pancreatic cancer has been associated with familial adenomatous polyposis and Gardner's syndrome, von Hippel-Lindau disease, neurofibromatosis, immunodeficiency syndromes including ataxia-telangiectasia, multiple endocrine neoplasia type 1 (Wermer's syndrome), hereditary nonpolyposis colorectal cancer (Lynch syndrome II), familial atypical multiple mole melanoma syndrome (FAMMM), and hereditary chronic relapsing pancreatitis. Familial occurrence of pancreatic cancer is rare but appears to be real because the numerous strong family clusters of disease cannot be explained solely on the basis of chance.

Diagnosis
Imaging Studies
- **Percutaneous ultrasound (US)** has the advantage of being the most available and least expensive imaging modality of the upper abdominal region. It also has high patient acceptance and no complications.
  - US may establish the diagnosis of pancreatic cancer in up to 90% of patients if the pancreas is well defined.
  - US has a sensitivity of 87% when its findings are correlated with intraoperative and pathologic findings; its sensitivity decreases in cases with nodal and vascular involvement and in those with peritoneal carcinomatosis.
  - The diagnostic accuracy of US is greatest for cancers in the pancreatic head and lowest for cancers in the tail.
  - US is very accurate in predicting the unresectability of a given tumor (see the later list of criteria for unresectability in the section on Treatment of Pancreatic Cancer, Surgery) but is less accurate at predicting resectability.
- **Angiography** is a valuable tool in the preoperative management of patients with pancreatic cancer.
  - It is most useful when combined with other imaging studies.
  - It has a 95% accuracy rate in predicting unresectability (see the list of criteria for unresectability in the later section Treatment of Pancreatic Cancer, Surgery) but is less accurate at predicting resectability.
- **Computed tomography (CT)** is most useful in detecting mass lesions of over 2 cm in the pancreatic head and less useful in detecting smaller tumors that are more distally located.
  - CT is fairly accurate in differentiating pancreatic cancer from chronic pancreatitis, for which it has a reported 77% accuracy rate.
  - CT, like US, is very accurate in predicting the unresectability of a given tumor (see later section on Criteria

for Unresectability) but is less accurate at predicting resectability.

- **Endoscopic retrograde cholangiopancreatography (ERCP)** is an imaging study that is very successful in making a diagnosis of pancreatic cancer and in differentiating cancer from chronic pancreatitis.
  - On ERCP, the presence of moderate to severe ductal abnormalities, including strictures longer than 10 mm, and duct irregularities, accompanied by moderate to severe pancreatitis, is highly suggestive of a diagnosis of pancreatic cancer.
  - Cancers located in the head of the pancreas may result in obstruction of both the pancreatic and common bile ducts, resulting in the characteristic "double duct sign" on ERCP.
  - Another highly suggestive ERCP finding for pancreatic cancer is an abrupt cut-off to the main pancreatic duct.
- **Magnetic resonance imaging (MRI)** is comparable or even superior to CT in the diagnosis of pancreatic cancer.

Laparoscopy

- Laparoscopy is valuable in assessing the resectability of pancreatic cancer and detecting the presence of tumor implants in the liver and peritoneum.
- Laparoscopy, combined with CT scan and angiography, is highly accurate (in more than 85% of cases) in predicting unresectability (see the later list of criteria for unresectability in the section, Treatment of Pancreatic Cancer, Surgery).

Fine Needle Aspiration (FNA)

- CT or US-guided FNA, using a 23-gauge needle, is extremely useful in the diagnosis of pancreatic cancer and in differentiating cancer from chronic pancreatitis.
- The sensitivity of FNA in the diagnosis of pancreatic cancer is high, ranging from 75% to 100%.
- The specificity of FNA in the diagnosis of pancreatic cancer is 100%.
- FNA is simple, safe, rapid, and accurate; however, a potential complication of FNA in patients with pancreatic cancer is the possibility of tumor seeding in the needle tract.
- In pancreatic cancer causing biliary obstruction, brush cytology of the common bile duct may be positive for malignant cells in approximately half of the patients.

Pathology

- Adenocarcinoma of pancreatic ductal origin is the most common pancreatic malignant neoplasm and represents 80% to 90% of all pancreatic cancers.
- Premalignant intraductal alterations include papillary duct hyperplasia with or without cytologic atypia, supporting a possible sequence of progression that is analogous to similar pathologic processes in other organs such as colorectal cancer (this will be discussed later in the section on Pancreatic Neoplasms of Intermediate Biologic Potential).

Molecular Biology of Pancreatic Cancer

- Flow cytometry studies have shown that from 15% to 90% of ductal adenocarcinomas show DNA aneuploidy.

- Chromosomal alterations in pancreatic cancer include loss of chromosomes 18 (the most frequent), 13, 12, 17, and 6, chromosomal break points (involving 6q, 1p, 3p, 11p, 17p, 1q, 8p, and 19q), and a high frequency of allelic loss (at chromosomes 17p, 18q, 9p, 1p, 3p, 6p, 6q, 8p, 10q, 12q, 13q, 18p, 21q, and 22q). Given these findings, the possible genes involved in the pathogenesis of pancreatic cancer may reside on chromosomes 18q, 17p, 6p, 1p, 8p, 12q, 13q, and/or 9p.
- Many of the chromosomes cited above contain known tumor-suppressor genes, including p53 tumor suppressor gene on chromosome 17p, the deleted colon cancer (DCC) tumor suppressor gene on 18q, the multiple tumor suppressor-1 (MTS1) gene on 9p, and the p16 gene (CDKN2) on 9p (this gene is lost in 90% of patients with pancreatic cancer, whereas a mutated p53 suppressor gene is present in approximately 60% of cases).
- Oncogenes may play a role in the development of pancreatic cancer. The most widely implicated oncogene is K-ras; 75% to 95% of pancreatic cancer studies have shown point mutations in codon 12 of the K-ras oncogene. These mutations in K-ras appear to represent an early event in the development of pancreatic cancer. Point mutations in codon 12 of K-ras have also been identified in hyperplastic alterations (papillary and nonpapillary) of pancreatic ducts in the absence of carcinoma, suggesting that these duct alterations are also neoplastic.

Treatment of Pancreatic Cancer
Surgery

- Surgical resection remains the best therapeutic option for pancreatic cancer, even though few patients are ultimately cured.
- Only about 10% of pancreatic cancers located in the pancreatic head are resectable; as such, nonresectable pancreatic cancers predominate, making surgery a purely palliative procedure.
- **Criteria for unresectability of a pancreatic cancer include:** distant metastases (to the liver, peritoneal surfaces, distant lymph nodes), adenopathy proved by needle aspiration, obstruction or invasion of the portal or mesenteric veins, and/or encasement of the celiac or superior mesenteric arteries by cancer.
- Among the surgical procedures performed for pancreatic cancer are the following:

1. **Pancreaticoduodenectomy** or the **Whipple procedure** remains the procedure of choice for pancreatic head and periampullary tumors. This procedure includes resection of the distal stomach, gallbladder, distal common bile duct, head of pancreas, duodenum, proximal jejunum, and regional lymphatics with restoration of gastrointestinal continuity by pancreaticojejunostomy, choledochojejunostomy, and gastrojejunostomy.
2. **Pylorus-sparing pancreaticoduodenectomy (PSPD)** is a modified Whipple procedure in which the stomach and pylorus are preserved.
3. Total pancreatectomy.
4. Regional pancreatectomy includes total pancreatectomy, splenectomy, and resection of portions of the

portal and superior mesenteric artery and the celiac axis if involved by tumor.

- Cancers of the body and tail of the pancreas are almost never resectable because they present late in the disease course as advanced-stage tumors. In patients who do have resectable tumors, total pancreatectomy and splenectomy are performed.
- The operative mortality rate of pancreaticoduodenal resection is now less than 5%, compared to previous rates of as high as 20%.
- Complications of pancreaticoduodenal resection include pancreatic fistula, gastric outlet obstruction with delayed gastric emptying, gastrointestinal or intra-abdominal hemorrhage, abscess, wound infection, sepsis, biliary fistula, and others. Diabetes is unusual in patients after pancreaticoduodenal resection, but brittle diabetes is a complication of total pancreatectomy.

Adjuvant Therapy
- Radiotherapy is used to control local disease following surgery.
- Chemotherapy is used to treat systemic disease.
- Neither radiotherapy nor chemotherapy alone appears to have a significant impact on patient survival. Used in combination, either after surgery or in patients with unresectable tumor, radiotherapy and chemotherapy have resulted in longer survival periods, but even so, survival rates are poor.

Palliative Management
- Pancreatic cancer can be highly painful, producing unremitting, intractable pain. Treatment of pain in patients with pancreatic cancer includes pharmacotherapy, invasive anesthetics, and surgery.
- Patients with pancreatic cancer have higher rates of depressive symptoms, which can be independent of pain. Treatment includes pharmacotherapy for depression and supportive psychotherapy for emotional problems.
- Pancreatic cancer often produces distal obstruction of the biliary tree. Endoscopic surgery as an alternative to surgery can be used to relieve distal common bile duct obstruction.

Prognosis of Pancreatic Cancer
- The prognosis associated with pancreatic ductal adenocarcinoma is poor.
- More than 95% of patients with pancreatic ductal adenocarcinoma die from their disease.
- At the time of diagnosis, 10% of patients have disease confined to the pancreas, 40% have locally advanced disease, and more than 50% have distant spread of disease.
- The median length of survival is 18 to 20 months, and the 5-year survival rate is 5% to 18%; the 5-year survival rate of patients with pancreatic adenocarcinoma in the United States is 1.3%, and the median survival is 4.1 months.
- Tumor size appears to be a strong predictor of prognosis. Five-year patient survival is nil in tumors measuring more than 5 cm in diameter; tumors measuring 2.5 cm or smaller are associated with an overall better mean survival rate than larger tumors.

Table 12–2A
TNM CLASSIFICATION OF PANCREATIC CARCINOMA (AMERICAN JOINT COMMITTEE ON CANCER STAGING)

T1	No direct extension of primary tumor beyond the pancreas
T2	Limited direct extension to duodenum, bile duct, or stomach
T3	Advanced direct extension, incompatible with surgical resection
TX	Direct extension not assessed
N0	Regional lymph nodes not involved
N1	Regional lymph nodes involved
NX	Regional lymph nodes not assessed
M0	No distant metastasis
M1	Distant metastasis present
MX	Distant metastasis not assessed

Table 12–2B
STAGING OF PANCREATIC CARCINOMA (AMERICAN JOINT COMMITTEE ON CANCER STAGING)

Stage I	T1–T2, N0, M0; no direct extension with no regional node involvement
Stage II	T3, N0, M0; direct extension into adjacent tissue with no lymph node involvement
Stage III	T1–T3, N1, M0; regional lymph node involvement with or without direct tumor extension
Stage IV	T1–T3, N1, M1; distant metastatic disease present

Staging of Pancreatic Cancer
- See Table 12–2*A* and *B*.

C. BENIGN EXOCRINE NEOPLASMS

1. Serous Microcystic Adenoma

Definition: Benign tumor of uncertain histogenesis but possibly of centroacinar cell origin.

Synonyms: Glycogen-rich cystadenomas; serous cystadenoma.

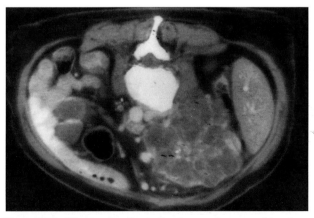

Figure 12–1. CT scan of a microcystic adenoma shows a multicystic tumor. Cystic spaces are relatively small and appear as tiny septated compartments, creating a honeycomb appearance. In addition to the cysts, solid portions of the tumor can be seen as well as a central scar area.

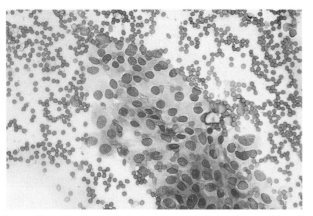

Figure 12–2. Fine needle aspiration of a microcystic adenoma. The cells appear monotonous and include round to oval uniform nuclei, inconspicuous nucleoli, and a moderate amount of granular cytoplasm.

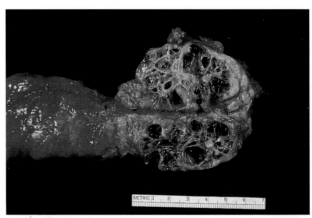

Figure 12–5. Microcystic adenoma appearing as a circumscribed, pseudoencapsulated or partly encapsulated, lobulated multiloculated lesion composed of numerous variably sized cysts that create a spongelike or honeycomb appearance. A central stellate scarlike area is seen.

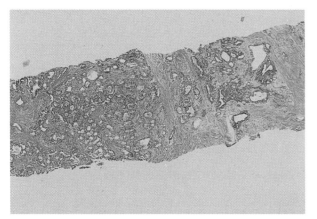

Figure 12–3. Needle biopsy of a microcystic adenoma showing variably sized microcysts in a fibrous stroma.

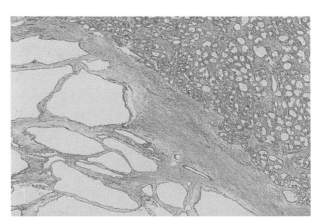

Figure 12–6. In this microcystic adenoma, variably sized cysts are seen, including smaller uniform-appearing cysts at the top and right, and larger dilated epithelial-lined cystic spaces toward the lower and left sides of the illustration.

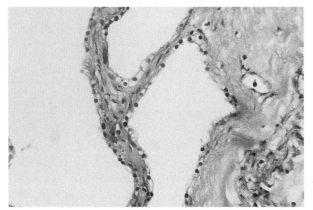

Figure 12–4. Microcystic adenoma. Higher magnification of Figure 12–3 shows the epithelial cells lining the cysts composed of cuboidal to flat cells with compact small, rounded nuclei and clear cytoplasm.

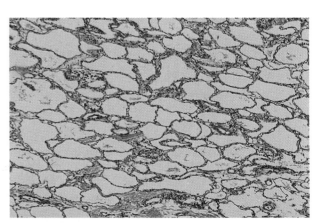

Figure 12–7. Microcystic adenoma characterized by groups of small regular cysts lined by cuboidal to low-cuboidal cells.

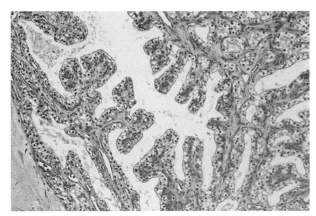

Figure 12–8. Occasionally, microcystic adenomas may show branching papillary growth.

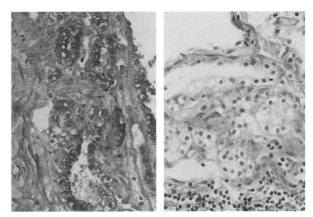

Figure 12–10. Histochemical evaluation of microcystic adenomas includes the presence of intracytoplasmic glycogen as seen by *(left)* periodic acid-Schiff (PAS)-positive material that is washed away (sensitive) to diastase digestion *(right)*.

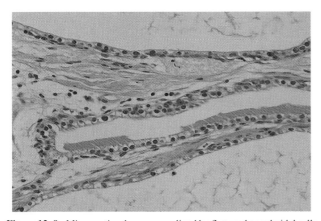

Figure 12–9. Microcystic adenomas are lined by flattened or cuboidal cells with small round to oval nuclei, inconspicuous nucleoli, and clear cytoplasm. In this example, there is focal nuclear pleomorphism.

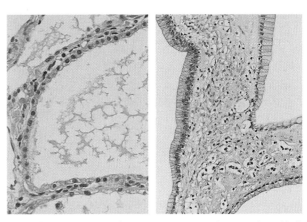

Figure 12–11. This illustration shows the contrast between the epithelial lining of a microcystic adenoma *(left)*, composed of flattened or cuboidal cells with small round to oval nuclei, inconspicuous nucleoli, and eosinophilic to clear cytoplasm, with that of a mucinous cystic neoplasm *(right)* that includes tall columnar, mucin-producing cells. In addition, mucinous cystic neoplasms have a cellular "ovarian-type" stroma as seen here.

Clinical

- Represents approximately 1% of all exocrine pancreatic tumors and 4% to 10% of all cystic pancreatic tumors.
- Slightly more common in women than in men; occurs most commonly in elderly people in the sixth to seventh decades of life.
- May be found incidentally at autopsy, or patients may present with an abdominal mass with or without associated pain. Tumors located in the head of the pancreas may cause biliary tract or gastrointestinal tract obstruction, resulting in jaundice.
- Generally presents as a single mass that may arise in any portion of the pancreas (no site predilection).
- May coexist with pancreatic ductal adenocarcinoma.
- May be associated with diabetes mellitus and extrapancreatic malignancies.
- Increased frequency of association with von Hippel-Lindau syndrome; in patients with von Hippel-Lindau syndrome, microcystic adenomas may be multiple and multifocal.

Radiology

- CT scan and ultrasound: Multicystic tumor; cysts are usually under 2 cm in diameter, and the small cysts appear as tiny septated compartments, creating a honeycomb appearance. In addition, solid portions of the tumor can be seen.
- MRI: Cystic and lobulated, high-intensity masses on T2-weighted imaging.
- Angiography: Highly vascular lesion that demonstrates large feeding arteries, occasional neovascularity, and prominent draining veins; occasional arteriovenous shunting can be seen.
- Small calcifications are common, and a stellate scar can be seen.

Pathology

Fine Needle Aspiration

- Variable cellularity; generally, cellularity is limited.
- Flat sheets with a honeycomb pattern or individually dispersed cells.

- Cuboidal, flattened, or low columnar epithelial cells that have a single round to oval, uniform nucleus, inconspicuous nucleoli, and a moderate amount of cytoplasm. Cytoplasm is often vacuolated owing to glycogen deposition.
- Overall appearance of cells may resemble that of mesothelial cells.

Gross

- Circumscribed, pseudoencapsulated or partly encapsulated, lobulated mass varying in size from as small as 1 cm to as large as 25 cm.
- Cut section shows a multiloculated lesion composed of innumerable cysts, creating a spongelike appearance. Most of the locules are less than 1.0 cm in diameter, but they may measure up to 2 cm in diameter.
- A central stellate scar can be seen. Occasionally, calcifications are present that may have a "sunburst" appearance.
- The cystic fluid is clear and watery and has a colorless to yellow to blood-stained appearance.
- The tumor is well vascularized. Prominent vascularity is seen on the surface of the tumor; hemorrhagic foci within the parenchyma are common.

Histology

- Typically, groups of small variably sized cysts are seen, but other patterns include larger, more irregular-appearing cysts as well as macrocysts. Solid growth composed of small acini arranged in nests, sheets or trabeculae may be present. There may be an admixture of patterns in any one tumor. The smaller cysts tend to be more centrally located.
- The cystic lining cells vary from cuboidal to low-cuboidal to flat. The cytoplasm ranges from clear to occasionally eosinophilic. Compact small rounded nuclei are present with inconspicuous nucleoli; irregular and enlarged nuclei are rare.
- Occasionally, tiny branching papillae, formed by the cuboidal cells, are present.
- There is a hypocellular stroma.
- Secondary hemorrhagic change may occur.
- Islands of Langerhans and other pancreatic structures may be trapped within the tumors. The adjacent pancreas is generally unremarkable, but atrophic changes secondary to obstruction can be present.
- Histochemistry: Intracytoplasmic glycogen is present as seen by diastase-sensitive, periodic acid-Schiff (PAS)-positive material. Mucin stains are negative. Rarely, these tumors may not be PAS positive (so-called nonmucinous, glycogen-poor cystadenoma).
- *Immunohistochemistry:* Cells are keratin and CA 19-9 positive; CEA negative.
- *Electron microscopy:* There are prominent intracytoplasmic collections of glycogen, junctional complexes (desmosomes), and short microvilli on the apical surfaces of the cells. Myoepithelial cells have been identified lying beneath the epithelial cells.

Differential Diagnosis

- Pseudocysts (Table 12–3) (Chapter 11E, #1).
- Pancreatic mucinous cystic neoplasm (see Table 12–3) (Chapter 12D, #2).

- Lymphangioma (Chapter 12G, #1).
- Metastatic renal cell carcinoma.

Treatment and Prognosis

- Complete surgical excision is the treatment of choice. Depending on the location of the tumor, surgical resection can be conservative or more radical.
- Surgical resection is usually curative.
- Very rare malignant examples (see later) have occurred in which the tumor has metastasized to the stomach and liver and invaded the splenic vein.

Additional Facts

Serous Cystadenocarcinoma

- Extraordinarily rare tumor, if it exists.
- Diagnosis is predicated on the presence of metastasis or invasive growth, including metastasis to the stomach and liver and neurotropism and invasion into the splenic vein.
- Histologically, this tumor may show cytologic atypia, including nuclear atypia, or it may be essentially identical to conventional microcystic adenoma with no significant cytologic atypical features.
- DNA aneuploidy may be present, but benign microcystic adenomas may also be DNA aneuploid.

von Hippel-Lindau Disease

- Autosomal dominant disorder with variable expression.
- The tumor suppressor gene for von Hippel-Lindau disease has been identified at chromosome 3p25–p26.
- Individuals with von Hippel-Lindau disease are predisposed to the development of numerous tumors of the central nervous system and abdominal viscera.
- The tumors and cysts that can occur in association with von Hippel-Lindau syndrome include:

1. Retinal angiomas.
2. Cerebellar and spinal hemangioblastomas.
3. Endolymphatic sac aggressive papillary cystadenomas.
4. Renal cysts and renal cell carcinomas.
5. Epididymal cysts and cystadenomas.
6. Pancreatic microcystic adenomas.
7. Pancreatic endocrine neoplasms.
8. Pheochromocytomas.

2. Pancreatic Cystic Teratoma

Definition: Benign neoplasm composed of tissues derived from all three germ layers.

Synonym: Dermoid cyst.

Clinical

- Rare pancreatic tumor.
- No gender predilection; occurs primarily (but not exclusively) in the first two decades of life.

Table 12–3
CYSTIC LESIONS OF THE PANCREAS

Features	Pseudocysts	Microcystic Adenoma	Mucinous Cystic Neoplasm
Gender/age	M > F; wide age range	F > M; 5th–7th decades	F > M; middle age
Clinical	Generally found in the setting of chronic pancreatitis often associated with biliary tract disease, alcoholism	Found incidentally at autopsy or presents as an abdominal mass with or without associated pain; tumors in pancreatic head may cause biliary tract or gastrointestinal obstruction resulting in jaundice	Intermittent or continuous abdominal pain or discomfort; enlarging abdominal mass
Radiology	Well-defined fibrous capsule; low-density fluid centers	Multicystic, honeycomb-appearing mass; most cysts <2 cm in diameter; small calcifications and central stellate scar common	Large, multicystic mass; may be unilocular, without honeycomb appearance; cysts measure >2 cm in diameter; prominent internal septations; absent central scar; enhancement of solid components after contrast
Location in pancreas	Anywhere	Anywhere (even distribution)	More common in tail and body
Gross	Thick-walled; adherent to surrounding structures; hemorrhagic fluid contents rich in pancreatic enzymes	Well-circumscribed; spongy, honeycomb appearance; central, often calcified, scar; clear, watery fluid contents, occasionally hemorrhagic	Encapsulated mass with smooth surface; uni- or multilocular with smooth cyst lining but papillary excrescences are common; occasional calcifications at periphery; thick, mucoid, or gelatinous fluid content; necrosis and hemorrhage can be seen
Histology	Absent epithelial lining; fibrous wall with chronic inflammation and necrotic debris	Cysts lined by cuboidal to flattened cells with round nuclei, inconspicuous nucleoli, and clear to occasionally eosinophilic cystoplasm; tiny papillae may be present; hypocellular stroma	Cysts lined by columnar, mucus-producing cells aligned in a single row but may form papillae; cellular atypia, including nuclear pleomorphism and nuclear stratification can be seen; cellular "ovarian-type" stroma
Histochemistry	Absent mucus production	Glycogen is present in epithelial cells (PAS+; DPAS−)	Epithelial cells are mucin positive (mucicarmine; PAS+; DPAS+)
Adjacent pancreas	Healing pancreatitis common	Normal appearance; atrophic changes secondary to tumor compression or to obstruction uncommon	Normal appearance; atrophic changes secondary to obstruction occasionally seen
Treatment and prognosis	Pain medications; pancreatic enzyme replacement; surgery as last resort; morbidity high but mortality is low	Surgery generally curative	Complete surgical resection; generally has an indolent course with cure following resection; due to metastatic capability of all histologic types, this is considered a malignant neoplasm

PAS, Periodic acid–Schiff without diastase digestion; DPAS, periodic acid–Schiff with diastase digestion.

- Presentation includes abdominal pain, nausea, vomiting or constipation; may be asymptomatic.
- May originate from any pancreatic site.

Radiology

- Plain abdominal films may show a cystic and solid lesion.
- Calcifications may be seen within the cyst wall.

Pathology

Gross

- Solid and cystic tumor; may contain hair and/or cheesy and foul-smelling (sebaceous) material.

Histology

- Elements of all three germ layers are present, including:

  1. Epithelial: simple ciliated epithelium, squamous epithelium, adnexal structures, seromucous glands.
  2. Mesenchymal: fat, smooth muscle, cartilage, bone.
  3. Neuroectodermal: neural and glial tissue.

Differential Diagnosis

- Cystic neoplasms: This is more of a clinical differential diagnosis.

Treatment and Prognosis

- Surgical removal is curative.

D. PANCREATIC NEOPLASMS OF INTERMEDIATE BIOLOGIC POTENTIAL

1. Intraductal Epithelial Proliferative Processes

Definition: Spectrum of intraductal pancreatic epithelial proliferations that are possibly associated with and/or possibly represent a premalignant alteration with subsequent progression to carcinoma (in situ or invasive) or are definitely malignant and will become invasive cancer if left untreated.

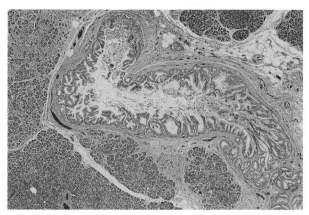

Figure 12–12. Atypical ductal epithelial hyperplasia. Dilated and irregularly shaped duct with intraductal papillary epithelial proliferation showing a complex (arborizing) growth pattern.

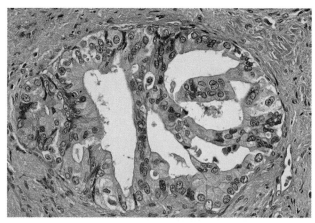

Figure 12–15. Atypical ductal epithelial hyperplasia. The cytologic changes in this pancreatic duct are those of an intraductal carcinoma, including a cribriform architecture with severe cytologic atypia.

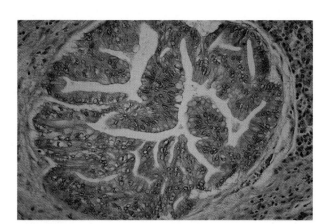

Figure 12–13. Atypical ductal epithelial hyperplasia in which there is mild cytologic atypia.

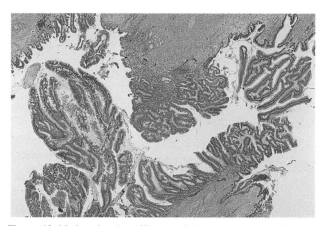

Figure 12–16. Intraductal papillary mucin-hypersecretory neoplasm. In contrast with the atypical ductal epithelial hyperplasia, which is an incidentally found feature usually seen in association with an invasive adenocarcinoma (or less often in chronic pancreatitis), the intraductal papillary mucin-hypersecreting neoplasm presents as a mass lesion. As seen in this illustration, the involved duct is cystically dilated and includes the presence of a complex papillary epithelial proliferation projecting into and filling the duct lumen. The papillae include the presence of fibrovascular core.

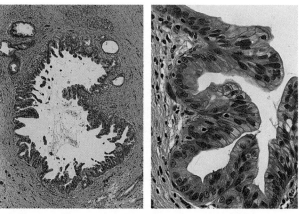

Figure 12–14. Atypical ductal epithelial hyperplasia. *Left,* This duct is dilated and shows the presence of papillary epithelial hyperplasia. *Right,* The epithelial cells show mild to moderate cytologic atypia. A chronic inflammatory cell infiltrate is seen in association with the hyperplastic duct as well as in the surrounding pancreatic tissue. Atypical ductal epithelial hyperplasia can be seen in association with chronic pancreatitis and/or in association with a concomitant pancreatic adenocarcinoma.

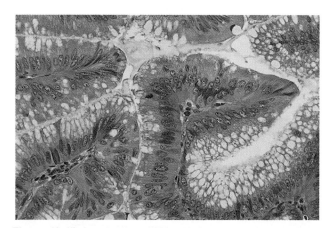

Figure 12–17. Intraductal papillary mucin-hypersecretory neoplasm. Higher magnification of Figure 12–16 showing the presence of enlarged nuclei with increased nuclear-to-cytoplasmic ratio, prominent nucleoli, and mitotic figures. The mucinous differentiation of the cells is readily apparent.

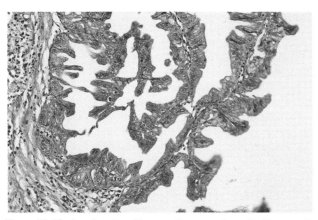

Figure 12–18. Intraductal papillary mucinous neoplasm. In this example, there is bridging architecture, papillary fronds with fibrovascular core, and pleomorphic nuclei with scattered mitotic figures.

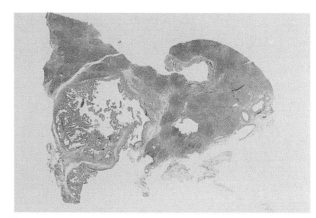

Figure 12–21. Intraductal papillary oncocytic neoplasm. Cystically dilated and ramifying duct is lined by a papillary epithelial cell proliferation.

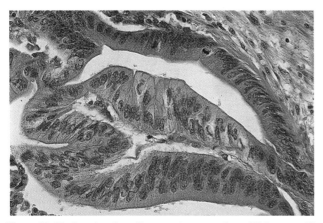

Figure 12–19. Intraductal papillary mucinous neoplasm. Higher magnification of Figure 12–18 showing markedly enlarged nuclei with increased nuclear-to-cytoplasmic ratio, nuclear stratification with loss of nuclear basal polarity, and mitotic figures. Despite the cytologic atypia, the cells retain mucinous differentiation.

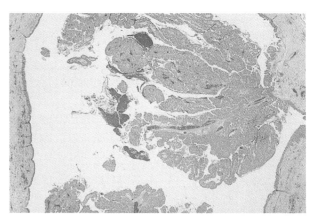

Figure 12–22. Intraductal papillary oncocytic neoplasm characterized by cells with a prominent eosinophilic cytoplasm. Transitional areas can be seen from a relatively flat-appearing epithelium to an obvious papillary epithelial cell proliferation growing into and filling the duct lumen.

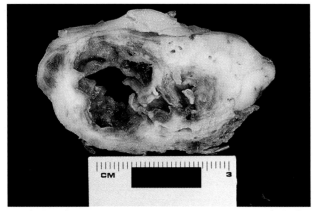

Figure 12–20. Intraductal papillary oncocytic neoplasm. Resection specimen showing marked dilatation of the pancreatic duct system. Papillary growths and associated mucoid material can be seen within the ectatic pancreatic ducts.

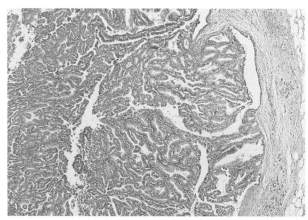

Figure 12–23. Intraductal papillary oncocytic neoplasm. The duct is virtually filled and expanded by the oncocytic epithelial cell proliferation, which demonstrates a complex papillary growth.

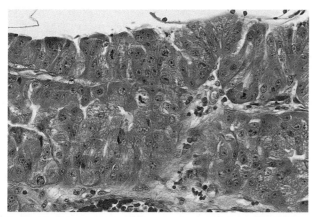

Figure 12–24. Intraductal papillary oncocytic neoplasm showing severe dysplasia (intraductal carcinoma) characterized by the presence of cells with prominent granular eosinophilic cytoplasm (oncocytes) with nuclear pleomorphism and hyperchromasia, nuclear crowding, nuclear stratification with loss of nuclear basal polarity and haphazard arrangement within the cells, loss of cellular differentiation (mucin production), increased nuclear-to-cytoplasmic ratio, prominent nucleoli, and mitotic figures.

Synonyms: Intraductal atypical papillary hyperplasia; intraductal papillary (adeno)carcinoma; in situ intraductal carcinoma; intraductal mucus-hypersecreting tumor; intraductal mucin-hypersecreting neoplasm; intraductal papillary-mucinous neoplasm; mucinous ductal ectasia; intraductal papillary oncocytic neoplasm.

NOTE: This discussion includes intraductal epithelial changes *with* cytologic atypia. For intraductal epithelial alterations without atypia, see the sections on chronic pancreatitis and age-related alterations (Chapter 11G, #2 and 11D, #1).

■ As shown by the numerous synonyms used for the spectrum of pancreatic intraductal epithelial proliferations, there is much confusion in the terminology and, perhaps more important, in the clinical significance of these alterations.

Clinical

■ These lesions are considered uncommon, but descriptions of them are increasing, perhaps reflecting an increased awareness of their significance in Japan (where much of the literature describing these lesions originated) as well as in western countries (Europe and North America).
■ They are slightly more common in men than in women and occur mainly in older individuals (these demographics are similar to those described for pancreatic ductal adenocarcinoma).
■ Due to the extensive involvement of the pancreatic duct system by intraductal papillary proliferations or the production of massive amounts of (sticky) mucin, patients present with a pancreatitis-like picture (chronic relapsing pancreatitis) caused by obstruction of the main pancreatic duct. Pancreatitis-like symptoms may be present for years before the diagnosis is made.
■ Lesions may be focal or diffuse; they tend to involve the more proximal portions of the pancreatic duct system but can spread to involve the entire duct system, even extending to the ampulla of Vater.

Radiology

• Ultrasound, CT scan, MRI, and ERCP: Focal or diffuse ectasia of the pancreatic duct system with or without identification of intraductal mucus.
• ERCP: Visualization of thick tenacious mucus within the involved duct or from the orifice of the ampulla of Vater.
• The cysts communicate with the main pancreatic duct system and, following injection with retrograde contrast material, can be filled, a finding that differs from that seen with mucinous cystic neoplasms.

Pathology

Gross

• Marked dilatation of the main pancreatic duct or tributaries of the major duct system.
• Multicentric intraductal papillary growth(s) can be seen.
• Thick, tenacious mucus may or may not be present within the ectatic pancreatic ducts.
• Atrophy and fibrosis of the pancreatic parenchyma may be present.

Histology

■ In the presence of papillary proliferations, exophytic epithelial proliferations with a complex (arborizing) growth pattern and fibrovascular cores are seen; cribriform patterns may also be present independent of or in association with the complex papillary architecture.
■ Mucinous hyperplasia is seen; this involves the presence of tall columnar epithelial cells containing mucin (mucus-rich cells) in the apical region of the cells lining the ducts.
■ Cytologic atypia (dysplasia) is always present in varying degrees of severity. The atypical features include the presence of nuclear pleomorphism, hyperchromasia, nuclear stratification with loss of nuclear basal polarity and a haphazard arrangement within the cells, increased nucleus-to-cytoplasm ratio, prominent nucleoli, absence of intracytoplasmic mucin (loss of differentiation), and presence of mitoses.
■ The atypia may be limited in extent and degree, or it may be sufficiently widespread to reach the status of intraductal (in situ) carcinoma. The latter includes marked cellular pleomorphism, loss of cellular differentiation (mucin production), and the presence of atypical mitotic figures.
■ Another alteration included within the spectrum of intraductal pancreatic proliferative lesions is the **intraductal oncocytic papillary neoplasm** characterized by a complex architecture and the presence of cells with prominent granular eosinophilic cytoplasm (oncocytes). The complexity of the architecture, including papillary, cribriform, and solid growth patterns, justifies inclusion of these lesions in the spectrum of intraductal neoplasms despite the cytologic changes, which fall short of severe dysplasia but include nuclear stratification and pseudostratification. Evidence of intracellular and intraluminal mucin production can be seen.
■ By definition, invasive cancer is not present. However, the presence of atypical intraductal hyperplastic and/or papillary proliferations may signal the presence of frank invasive carcinoma near the atypical foci or the evolution to

carcinoma. The presence of extraductal, extracellular mucin pools without associated neoplastic cells is extremely suggestive of invasive cancer and should prompt extensive tissue sampling and serial sections in order to identify the presence of associated neoplastic cells that would confirm a diagnosis of invasive carcinoma.

■ Histochemistry: Presence of epithelial mucin is readily apparent by light microscopy, and confirmation with histochemical stains is aesthetically pleasing but unnecessary. Argyrophilic and argentaffin positive cells can be seen admixed within the hyperplastic ductal epithelium representing scattered neuroendocrine cells. Oncocytic lesions stain positively with phosphotungstic acid–hematoxylin (PTAH) and Novelli's stain for mitochondria (the latter typically with a purple coloration).

■ *Immunohistochemistry:* As expected, epithelial markers (cytokeratin, EMA) produce positive reactions, as do CEA, CA 19-9, and B72.3 (TAG 72). The presence of cytokeratin and CEA reactivity in the cells floating in the mucin pools would be confirmatory of carcinoma.

■ *Molecular biology*
  • K-ras point mutations occur in the ducts of patients with papillary and nonpapillary hyperplasia, indicating that these duct lesions are truly neoplastic and that the K-ras mutations appear to occur early in the development of pancreatic cancer while the lesions are still confined to the pancreatic ducts.
  • Progression from an intraductal lesion to invasive carcinoma is associated with mutations and/or deletions of K-ras, p53, and the DCC gene.
  • c-erb-2 oncogene product overexpression also occurs.

Treatment and Prognosis

■ Surgery is the treatment of choice; because of the extent of involvement and/or the tendency to multifocality, total pancreatectomy is advocated.

■ Evaluation of the ductal margins of resection are critical to exclude involvement that would necessitate additional surgical extirpation.

■ Prognosis is considered good as long as the pathologic proliferation is entirely confined in the duct system and is completely removed by surgical resection; long-term survival of 10 or more years occurs if these criteria are met.

■ These intraductal lesions appear to progress slowly, evolving over extended periods of time prior to the development of invasive growth or metastatic disease.

■ In the presence of invasive growth and metastatic disease (nodal or visceral), these lesions are classified as invasive ductal adenocarcinomas and carry the dire prognosis associated with that neoplastic category.

2. Mucinous Cystic Neoplasms

Definition: Distinctive cystic pancreatic neoplasm, probably of ductal epithelial cell origin and generally with an indolent clinical course, but the biologic behavior cannot always be predicted on the basis of the histologic appearance.

Synonyms: Mucinous cystic tumor of borderline or indeterminate malignant behavior; mucinous cystadenocarcinoma.

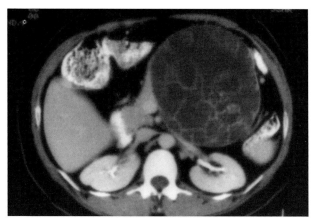

Figure 12–25. Mucinous cystic neoplasm. CT scan shows a sharply circumscribed (encapsulated) multicystic tumor in the distal pancreas. The cysts are relatively large, measuring more than 2 cm in diameter, which is noticeably larger than the cysts seen in a microcystic adenoma. The internal septations are prominent with thick-walled cysts. The honeycomb appearance characteristic of microcystic adenomas is not a feature of this tumor.

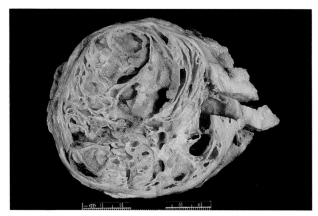

Figure 12–26. Mucinous cystic neoplasm. Large encapsulated tumor measures more than 10 cm in diameter. Cut section shows a multiloculated tumor with thick fibrous walls and cysts of varying size separated by gray-white solid tissue of varying thickness. The cyst wall lining also shows variability, including smooth areas and foci with papillary excrescences; mucoid material is present.

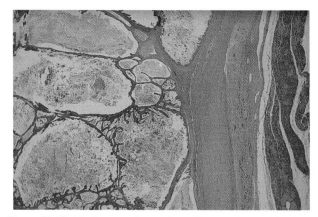

Figure 12–27. Mucinous cystic neoplasm. The cysts are widely dilated and filled with mucinous material and are lined by epithelium with a papillary architecture. The wall of the cyst includes thickened hyalinized or sclerotic fibrous tissue. Immediately to the right of the fibrous capsule is a layer of compressed and atrophic pancreatic parenchyma, to the extreme right of which is relatively unremarkable pancreatic tissue.

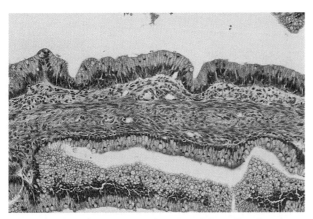

Figure 12–28. Cystic spaces are lined by tall (nonciliated), columnar, mucin-producing cells with basally located single nuclei. A cellular "ovarian-type" stroma is present, characterized by oval to spindle-shaped cells with mild pleomorphism.

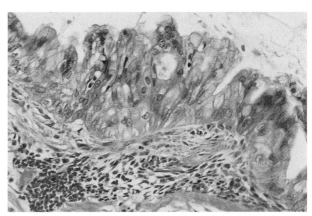

Figure 12–31. Compared to Figure 12–30, this mucinous cystic neoplasm shows a more complex growth with focal cribriform growth.

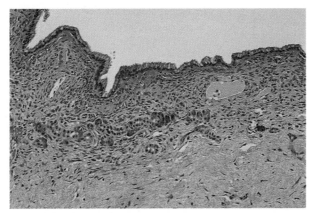

Figure 12–29. This mucinous cystic tumor, located in the tail of the pancreas occurred in an adult man, shows the presence of an "ovarian-type" stroma. This stromal component is generally a feature of tumors occurring in women and is considered an unusual finding in male patients. Atrophic pancreatic parenchyma is present in the cyst wall.

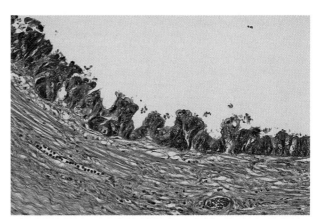

Figure 12–32. Mucinous cystic neoplasm with severe cytologic atypia (tantamount to carcinoma in situ) characterized by loss of cellular differentiation (mucin production), with enlarged and markedly pleomorphic nuclei.

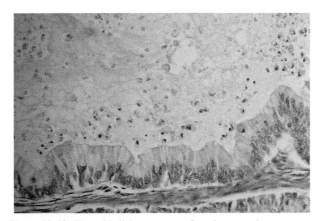

Figure 12–30. The epithelial component of mucinous cystic tumors may vary from case to case or even within a single case. In this example, there is mild cytologic atypia.

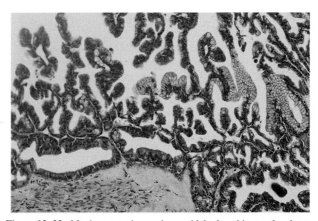

Figure 12–33. Mucinous cystic neoplasm with both architectural and cytomorphologic atypia. The changes were confined to the cystic epithelial spaces and there was no invasive growth.

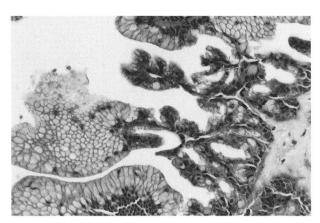

Figure 12–34. Higher magnification of Figure 12–33 shows the complex papillary growth with associated cytologic atypia.

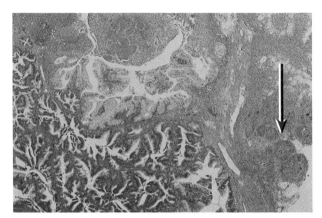

Figure 12–35. Mucinous cystic neoplasm showing transition from columnar epithelium to an epithelium with complex papillary architecture. Although difficult to appreciate at this magnification, squamous metaplastic foci were present *(arrow)*.

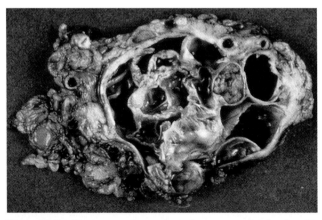

Figure 12–36. Mucinous cystic neoplasm. Large encapsulated and multiloculated tumor with thick fibrous walls and cysts of varying size separated by gray-white solid tissue of varying thickness. Focally, the tumor showed more cellular (solid) foci, in which invasive carcinoma was found.

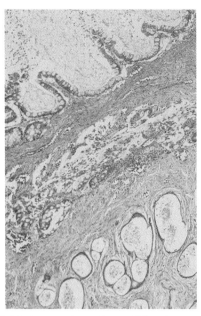

Figure 12–37. Mucinous cystic neoplasm with invasive tumor (cystadenocarcinoma). The invasive foci are seen in the lower portion of the illustration and are characterized by irregularly shaped infiltrative glands with an associated desmoplastic stromal reaction. While invasive carcinoma is present, the epithelium lining the cyst is not atypical.

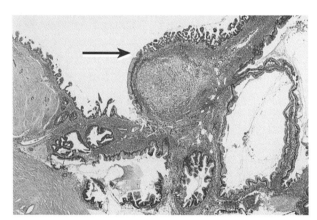

Figure 12–38. In this mucinous cystic neoplasm with invasive tumor (cystadenocarcinoma), the invasive glands are characterized by complex glandular growth with incomplete glandular lumina, seen in the lower portion of the illustration. There is a transition in the cyst epithelial lining from tall columnar cells to epithelium with a variably complex architecture *(arrow)*.

Clinical

- Uncommon tumor accounting for approximately 2% of all exocrine pancreatic neoplasms.
- Much more common in women than in men, with a female-to-male ratio of approximately 6:1; most occur between 30 and 60 years of age.
- Clinical presentation includes abdominal pain (intermittent or continuous) and an enlarging (left-sided) abdominal mass. Other findings may include weight loss, weakness, anorexia, nausea and vomiting. Symptoms may be nonspecific and may be present for many years.
- Occasionally, a mass is identified on physical examination or radiographic imaging for unrelated problems.

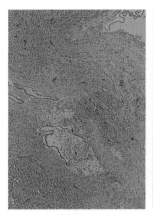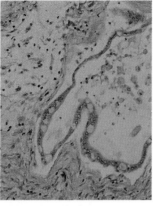

Figure 12–39. Mucinous cystic neoplasm (remnants of which are not shown) with invasive carcinoma. *Left,* In the central aspect of the panel there is an invasive adenocarcinoma in which a gland with an incomplete epithelium-lined lumen is invading the stroma, causing an associated desmoplastic reaction. Acellular mucin pools can be seen. *Right,* Higher magnification shows that the invasive glandular epithelium has malignant cytomorphologic features.

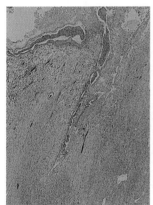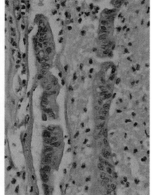

Figure 12–40. Another example of mucinous cystic neoplasm with invasive carcinoma showing *(left)* the invasive adenocarcinoma invading the stromal tissue, which includes the "ovarian-type" stroma, and *(right)* the malignant cytomorphologic appearance of the invasive glandular component.

- Most tumors occur in the tail of the pancreas; they also may occur in the body of the pancreas; rarely, they may occur in the head of the pancreas.
- There are no known etiologic factors.

Radiology

- CT scan and ultrasound: Multicystic tumor; cysts are usually large, measuring more than 2 cm in diameter. The honeycomb appearance characteristic of microcystic adenomas is not a feature of this tumor. Internal septations are often prominent with thick-walled cysts. Solid portions of the tumor can be seen.
- MRI: Cystic and lobulated, high-intensity masses on T2-weighted imaging are evident.
- Calcifications located in the periphery of the tumor are seen; no stellate scar is seen.
- The cysts are not found to communicate with the main pancreatic duct system and will not fill following injec-

tion with retrograde contrast material, a finding that differs from that of intraductal hyperplastic (papillary or nonpapillary) proliferative lesions.

Pathology

Fine Needle Aspiration

- Moderately cellular aspirates; abundant extracellular mucin.
- Tumor cells occur in a sheetlike or honeycomb arrangement, lie singly, or appear in three-dimensional aggregates.
- Neoplastic cells have a clear to vacuolated to foamy cytoplasm with round nuclei, a finely granular chromatin pattern, and inconspicuous nucleoli.
- Atypical cytologic features include the presence of large, round nuclei with variations in nuclear size and conspicuous nucleoli.
- Malignant cytologic features may include the presence of cells with large nuclei, marked variations in nuclear size and shape with an increased nucleus-to-cytoplasm ratio, a coarse chromatin pattern, and disordered arrangement.

Gross

- Usually large encapsulated tumors are seen, often measuring over 10 cm in diameter.
- External surface is smooth and glistening; an irregular external surface may be seen when the tumor has extended through the capsule.
- Cut section shows a multiloculated tumor with thick fibrous walls. Cysts vary in size and may measure several centimeters in diameter and contain thick mucoid material. The inner cyst wall lining may also vary from smooth and pink to foci with papillary excrescences.
- Unilocular tumors can occur.
- Cysts are separated by gray-white solid tissue of varying thickness.
- Extension and adherence to adjacent (extrapancreatic) structures can be seen.
- Calcifications occur in the cyst wall. Hemorrhage and other degenerative changes can be seen.

Histology

- Histologic classification similar to that used for ovarian mucinous cystic neoplasms has been proposed for pancreatic mucinous cystic neoplasms, including mucinous cystadenoma, typical or borderline mucinous cystic neoplasm, and mucinous cystadenocarcinoma. However, a strict distinction between cystadenoma and cystadenocarcinoma is not always possible.
- Cystic spaces are lined by tall (nonciliated) columnar, mucin-producing cells with basally located single nuclei. Papillary structures are commonly seen and are also lined by mucin-producing, tall columnar epithelial cells. The histologic appearance of the columnar epithelial cells is similar to that of cells of the major pancreatic ducts. Glandular components resemble colonic and/or prepyloric glands.
- In addition to the tall columnar epithelial cells, cuboidal or flattened epithelial cells devoid of mucin can be seen.

Transitional areas from the tall mucin-producing columnar epithelium to low-cuboidal appearing epithelium can be seen.

■ Endocrine cells and Paneth's cells are interspersed among the mucus cells.

■ The epithelial component may vary from case to case or even within a single case to include atypical cytomorphologic features, including nuclear stratification or pseudostratification with loss of the basal polarity or orientation of the nuclei, enlarged nuclei with marked pleomorphism, increased nucleus-to-cytoplasm ratio, and prominent nucleoli. A transition from benign to atypical or malignant epithelium can be seen. The presence of atypical features suggests the possibility of malignancy and requires extensive sectioning of the tumor to exclude the presence of invasive growth into the stroma. The presence of malignant cytologic features within the cystic epithelial component, even in the absence of unequivocal invasive growth, would be sufficient for a diagnosis of carcinoma.

■ A cellular "ovarian-type" stroma is usually conspicuously present beneath the epithelial component in the cyst wall; this stromal component is generally a feature of tumors occurring in women but may rarely be found in men. The cellular stroma includes oval to spindle-shaped cells with mild pleomorphism but no features of malignancy. Exceptional cases of mucinous cystic neoplasms with sarcomatous stroma may occur.

■ A hyalinized or sclerotic fibrous tissue is found deep to the ovarian-type stroma or below the surface epithelium in cases that lack the cellular stroma. Sclerosis may be a degenerative change.

■ Invasive growth unequivocally defines malignancy. In some instances, invasion may be difficult to identify definitively because glands may ramify below the surface epithelium, giving the impression of neoplastic foci within the stroma. Features of invasive growth similar to those seen in "conventional" pancreatic adenocarcinoma are present, including stromal desmoplasia associated with complex glandular (cribriform) growth with extreme cellular pleomorphism and increased mitotic activity, neural invasion, vascular space invasion, invasion into peripancreatic soft tissues, and metastatic tumor. Additional features that may indicate malignancy include the presence of incomplete glandular lumina, intraluminal necrotic material or neutrophilic infiltrate, and mucin pools with or without associated malignant cells.

■ Metastatic deposits may include foci with obviously cytologic features of malignancy as well as foci with cytologic benign-appearing epithelium. The latter finding supports consideration of the entire cytomorphologic spectrum of mucinous cystic neoplasms as potentially malignant; hence the classification of this tumor type in the category of indeterminate biologic behavior.

■ Histochemistry: Stains for epithelial mucin (mucicarmine, PAS with diastase, Alcian blue) are positive (intracytoplasmic and extracellular.)

■ *Immunohistochemistry*
   • The epithelial component is reactive with epithelial markers, including cytokeratin, EMA, CEA, and pan-

creatic mucin markers, including CA 19-9 and DUPAN-2.
   • Pancreatic endocrine peptide markers can be identified in interspersed endocrine cells but not in the epithelial component of the mucinous cystic neoplasm.
   • Cellular "ovarian-type" stroma is reactive with vimentin and may be reactive with estrogen or progesterone markers.

Differential Diagnosis

■ Pseudocyst (Table 12–4) (Chapter 11).
■ Microcystic adenoma (see Table 12–4) (Chapter 12C, #1).
■ Premalignant intraductal alterations (Chapter 12D, #1).
■ Conventional pancreatic ductal adenocarcinoma (Chapter 12E, #1).

Treatment and Prognosis

■ Complete surgical resection is the treatment of choice. The type of surgery depends on the location of the tumor. Because most tumors are located in the tail of the pancreas, subtotal (conservative) pancreatectomy can be performed. Surgical marsupialization is contraindicated; this type of surgery will not eradicate the tumor and may result in the spillage of the cyst content; spillage of cyst content may result in peritoneal implants, disseminated disease, and patient deaths.

■ The majority of patients (more than 50%) are cured following complete resection of the tumor. However, the biology of these tumors is unpredictable, and late recurrence and metastasis years after resection may occur. Recurrent tumor may include definitive foci of cystadenocarcinoma.

■ The histologic picture is not predictive of prognosis because tumors with bland, benign epithelium may have metastasis composed of similar benign epithelium. This may be a function of sampling in that mucinous cystic tumors often are large, and inadequate sampling may not identify cytomorphologically malignant foci or invasive carcinoma. Alternatively, given the presence of metastatic foci composed of benign epithelium, the true malignant potential of these tumors may not be reliably correlated with their histologic picture; hence the suggestion that this entire neoplastic group be considered potentially malignant and collectively designated mucinous cystic tumors (unless unequivocally malignant foci, appropriately termed mucinous cystadenocarcinoma, are identified).

■ Metastases occur to the regional lymph nodes and liver.

■ Even in the presence of malignant transformation, the prognosis is guarded, but it is thought to be better than that for conventional ductal adenocarcinoma.

■ Patients who present with metastatic disease at the time of diagnosis may have the poor prognosis ascribed to conventional ductal adenocarcinoma.

Additional Facts

■ Unusual examples of pancreatic mucinous cystic neoplasms with osteoclastic giant cells or associated with

Table 12–4
CYSTIC LESIONS OF THE PANCREAS

Features	Pseudocysts	Microcystic Adenoma	Mucinous Cystic Neoplasm
Gender/age	M > F; wide age range	F > M; 5th–7th decades	F > M; middle age
Clinical	Generally found in patients with chronic pancreatitis often associated with biliary tract disease, alcoholism	Found incidentally at autopsy or presents as an abdominal mass with or without associated pain; tumors in pancreatic head may cause biliary tract or gastrointestinal obstruction resulting in jaundice	Intermittent or continuous abdominal pain or discomfort; enlarging abdominal mass
Radiology	Well-defined fibrous capsule; low-density fluid centers	Multicystic, honeycomb-appearing mass; most cysts <2 cm in diameter; small calcifications and central stellate scar are common	Large, multicystic masses, may be unilocular, without honeycomb appearance; cysts measure >2 cm in diameter; prominent internal septations; absent central scar; enhancement of solid components after contrast
Location in pancreas	Anywhere	Anywhere (even distribution)	More common in tail and body
Gross	Thick-walled; adherent to surrounding structures; hemorrhagic fluid contents rich in pancreatic enzymes	Well-circumscribed; spongy, honeycomb appearance; central, often calcified, scar; clear, watery fluid contents, occasionally hemorrhagic	Encapsulated mass with smooth surface; uni- or multilocular with smooth cyst lining but papillary excrescences are common; occasional calcifications at periphery; thick, mucoid, or gelatinous fluid content; necrosis and hemorrhage can be seen
Histology	Absence of an epithelial lining; fibrous wall with chronic inflammation and necrotic debris	Cysts lined by cuboidal to flattened cells with round nuclei, inconspicuous nucleoli, and clear to occasionally eosinophilic cytoplasm; tiny papillae may be present; hypocellular stroma	Cysts lined by columnar, mucus-producing cells aligned in a single row but may form papillae; cellular atypia, including nuclear pleomorphism, nuclear stratification can be seen; cellular "ovarian-type" stroma
Histochemistry	Absence of mucus production	Glycogen is present in epithelial cells (PAS+; DPAS−)	Epithelial cells are mucin positive (mucicarmine; PAS+; DPAS+)
Adjacent pancreas	Healing pancreatitis common	Normal appearance; atrophic changes secondary to tumor compression or to obstruction uncommon	Normal appearance; atrophic changes secondary to obstruction occasionally seen
Treatment and prognosis	Pain medications; pancreatic enzyme replacement; surgery as last resort; morbidity high but mortality is low	Surgery is generally curative	Complete surgical resection; generally has an indolent course with cure following resection; due to metastatic capability of all histologic types, this is considered a malignant neoplasm

PAS, Periodic acid–Schiff without diastase digestion; DPAS, periodic acid–Schiff with diastase digestion.

pancreatic giant cell tumors occur; rare recurrences may include unusual features such as foci of choriocarcinoma and osteoclastic-like giant cells.

■ Cyst fluid content may be helpful in differentiating benign from malignant mucinous cystic neoplasms: high levels of CA 125 (>200 U/ml), CEA (>350 ng/ml), CA 15-3 (>100 ng/ml), and CA 72-4 or TAG 72 (>750 U/ml) in the cystic fluid may indicate a mucinous cystadenocarcinoma; however, although it is potentially helpful, cyst fluid content is not diagnostic of malignancy.

3. Solid and Papillary Epithelial Carcinoma

Definition: Low-grade malignant epithelial neoplasm of uncertain histogenesis.

Synonyms: Solid, cystic, papillary epithelial neoplasm; papillary-cystic tumor.

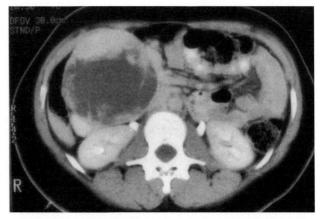

Figure 12–41. CT scan of a solid and papillary epithelial carcinoma of the pancreas showing water density and soft tissue areas that correspond with the more central cystic area and rim of the solid tumor, respectively.

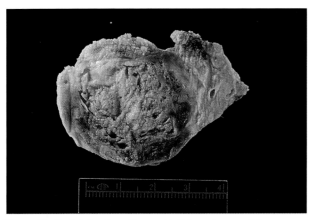

Figure 12–42. Solid and papillary epithelial carcinoma of the pancreas. This tumor has a predominantly solid and papillary appearance. These tumors are encapsulated and vary in size from as small as 3 cm to as large as 20 cm in diameter; the average size is approximately 8 cm in diameter.

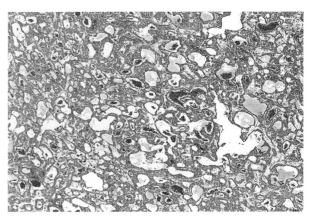

Figure 12–45. A microcystic pattern is seen in this solid and papillary epithelial carcinoma of the pancreas.

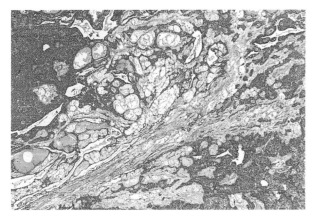

Figure 12–43. Solid and papillary epithelial carcinoma of the pancreas. This tumor has a predominantly solid and papillary cystic appearance with hemorrhagic changes.

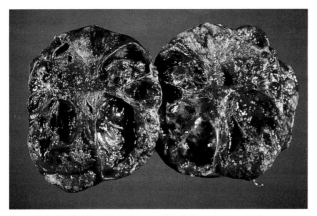

Figure 12–46. Papillary frond with a fibrovascular connective tissue core. The neoplastic cells are rather uniform, polygonal to elongated in shape, and have ovoid nuclei, vesicular chromatin, inconspicuous nucleoli, and eosinophilic cytoplasm.

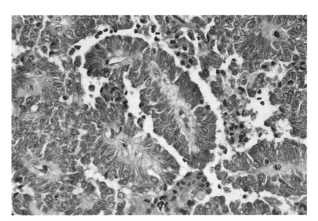

Figure 12–44. Solid and papillary epithelial carcinoma of the pancreas. Histologically, this tumor shows solid and cystic growth patterns.

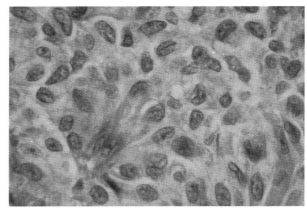

Figure 12–47. Higher magnification of the neoplastic cells of the solid and papillary epithelial carcinoma showing characteristic nuclear grooves or indentations, which create a "coffee-bean" appearance.

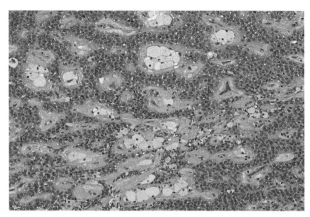

Figure 12–48. Solid and papillary epithelial carcinoma showing trabecular growth and clusters of foamy macrophages.

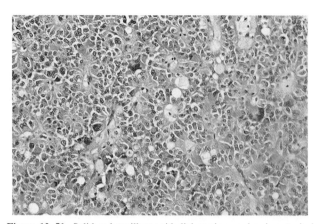

Figure 12–51. Solid and papillary epithelial carcinoma showing atypical cytomorphologic features, including nuclear pleomorphism and hyperchromasia, are seen.

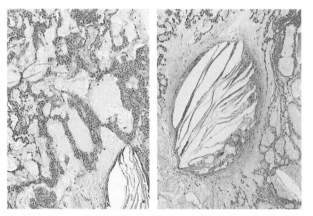

Figure 12–49. Additional changes seen in solid and papillary epithelial carcinoma of the pancreas include *(left)* myxoid changes and *(right)* cholesterol clefts and granulomas. The myxoid change often is seen around small vascular spaces, creating a pseudomicrocystic pattern.

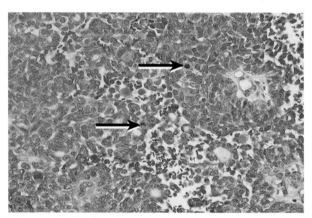

Figure 12–52. Occasionally, increased mitotic activity *(arrows)* can be seen in solid and papillary epithelial carcinoma, but this is considered an uncommon feature of this tumor.

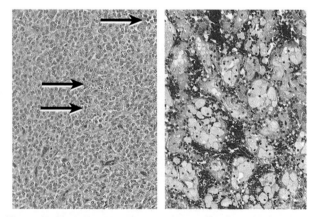

Figure 12–50. Solid and papillary epithelial carcinoma. *Left,* Clusters of small eosinophilic or hyaline cytoplasmic globules or droplets are seen *(arrows)*. These globules are α_1-antitrypsin positive *(not shown)*. *Right,* Collections of lipid-laden macrophages are common.

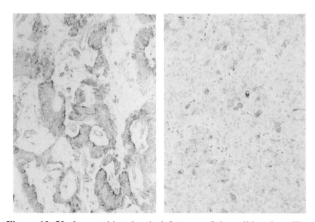

Figure 12–53. Immunohistochemical features of the solid and papillary epithelial neoplasm include consistent diffuse reactivity with *(left)* vimentin, and sporadic reactivity with *(right)* cytokeratin. Most other immunostains are sporadically reactive at best. Neuroendocrine markers are absent, but occasionally entrapped endocrine cells within the tumor react with neuroendocrine and/or pancreatic peptide hormone markers. These scattered endocrine cells admixed within the neoplastic (exocrine) cells should not be considered a cellular component of this tumor.

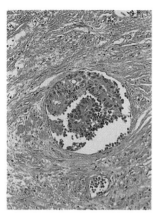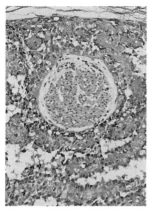

Figure 12–54. Solid and papillary epithelial carcinoma showing *(left)* vascular space invasion and *(right)* perineural invasion. Although the majority of these tumors have an indolent biology, they are fully malignant and are capable of invasive growth into the capsule or the adjacent pancreatic parenchyma and outside the pancreas, and they can metastasize as well.

Clinical

- Considered an uncommon neoplasm; Armed Forces Institute of Pathology (AFIP) files contain approximately 200 cases.
- More common in women than in men; typically occurs in adolescent and young women who have an average age of 30 and a median age of 29 years. Occasionally, the tumor occurs in men and older women.
- Not infrequently, these tumors are incidentally identified on routine physical examination or imaging studies. Clinical manifestations may include abdominal discomfort or pain or an abdominal mass. Hemorrhagic changes occurring spontaneously or secondary to abdominal trauma may result in abdominal pain.
- In order of decreasing frequency, the localization of this tumor in the pancreas is (1) tail, (2) head, (3) body, and (4) tail and body.
- Etiology is unknown; common occurrence in younger women suggests the possibility of a hormonal relationship, but a hormonal or endocrine pathogenesis has not been definitively identified.

Radiology

- Large, encapsulated masses demonstrating variable degrees of internal hemorrhage and cystic degeneration are found.
- On CT scan, hyperdense, soft tissue-dense, and water-dense areas are seen corresponding with cystic, solid hemorrhagic, and solid nonhemorrhagic regions of the tumor. Calcifications can also be seen on CT, including dense peripheral and punctate peripheral appearances.
- On ultrasound, a variable echo texture is found, most tumors appearing hyperechoic (greater than hypoechoic or isoechoic); these variations correspond to solid, cystic, or hemorrhagic foci.
- On MRI, water intensity signals on T1- and T2-weighted images correspond to cystic foci; areas of increased signal on T1- and T2-weighted images represent extracellular

hemorrhagic material. A high T2 signal also corresponds to solid areas of the tumor without gross hemorrhage.
- Fluid-debris levels can be seen on all imaging studies. On CT and ultrasound, the fluid-debris levels correspond to the cystic cavities of the tumor; on MRI, they correspond to cystic hemorrhagic cavities and hemorrhagic degeneration.

Pathology

Fine Needle Aspiration

- Cellular smears with papillary clusters, small aggregates, and individual cells are found.
- Papillary fronds may be straight or branched, have connective tissue cores, and are lined by one or more layers of uniform cells with small, regular, isomorphic nuclei, nuclear grooves, inconspicuous nucleoli, and eosinophilic to vacuolated cytoplasm; the nucleus-to-cytoplasm ratio is increased.
- Eosinophilic globules may be present.

Gross

- These tumors are encapsulated and vary in size from as small as 3 cm to as large as 20 cm in diameter; the average size is approximately 8 cm in diameter.
- Cut sections show a solid and cystic lesion with a soft to rubbery consistency, with hemorrhage and necrotic changes.

Histology

- The neoplasm appears to begin as a solid mass traversed by many tiny blood vessels; degeneration of the cells farthest from the vessels leads to a pseudopapillary pattern and the development of cystic spaces.
- The tumors may or may not have a capsule; regardless, infiltration into the capsule or into surrounding pancreas is common.
- The cells are rather monomorphous, small to medium sized, polygonal to elongated, with ovoid nuclei that have characteristic nuclear grooves or indentations that create a "coffee-bean" appearance. Nucleoli are often inconspicuous. The cytoplasm is clear to eosinophilic, and cell borders are rather poorly defined. Occasionally, nuclear pleomorphism or hyperchromasia is seen.
- Small eosinophilic or hyaline cytoplasmic globules or droplets are seen.
- Mitotic figures are rare.
- Accumulation of connective tissue around small blood vessels, often myxoid in character, is fairly characteristic. This feature may create a pseudomicrocystic pattern.
- Collagen deposition occurs along vascular spaces, resulting in a trabecular pattern of the epithelial cells.
- Hemorrhage and collections of lipid-laden macrophages are common. Foreign body giant cells, cholesterol clefts, and granulomas can be seen.
- Occasionally the tumor is reduced to a hemorrhagic cyst; rarely, extensive fibrosis and calcification may be present.
- Invasive growth may be seen, including growth into the capsule, into the adjacent pancreatic parenchyma, into the vascular space, and outside the pancreas.
- Histochemistry: Stains for glycogen and mucin are negative; the eosinophilic globules are PAS positive.

■ *Immunohistochemistry:* Neoplastic cells are consistently vimentin positive. Focal α_1-antitrypsin reactivity can be seen, and cytokeratin and amylase are sporadically positive. Endocrine and pancreatic enzyme markers are absent. Immunoreactivity with endocrine or pancreatic enzyme markers may be due to entrapped (non-neoplastic) endocrine or exocrine pancreas cells rather than to the neoplastic cells. Eosinophilic or hyaline globules are α_1-antitrypsin positive.

Differential Diagnosis

■ Pancreatic endocrine neoplasm (Chapter 12F, #1).

Treatment and Prognosis

■ Complete surgical resection is the treatment of choice. Depending on the location of the tumor, the surgical resection can be conservative or more radical.
■ The prognosis is favorable following complete surgical excision.
■ Complications include local recurrence, and the possibility of metastatic disease to the liver, peritoneum, or regional lymph nodes.
■ Even in the presence of metastatic disease, these tumors generally follow an indolent course; however, death directly attributable to disseminated disease does occur.

Additional Facts

■ The histogenesis of this tumor remains elusive. At present, the cell of origin can be considered an uncommitted cell, possibly derived from intercalated duct cells or centroacinar cells.

E. MALIGNANT EXOCRINE NEOPLASMS

1. Pancreatic Ductal Adenocarcinoma

Definition: Malignant neoplasm of the exocrine pancreas arising from ductal epithelial cells.

Clinical

NOTE: See earlier section (Chapter 12B) under General Considerations for more details about demographics, clinical data, tumor markers, etiology, pathogenesis, and imaging of pancreatic adenocarcinoma.

■ Most common pancreatic malignant neoplasm, representing 80% to 90% of all pancreatic cancers.
■ Is the fourth leading cause of cancer deaths, and is second only to colon cancer among gastrointestinal tract neoplasms as a cause of death.
■ More common in men than in women.
■ Incidence increases with age. Approximately 80% of pancreatic cancers occur between the seventh and ninth decades of life. Peak incidence occurs in the seventh to eighth decades; less than 5% of cases occur in patients under 45 years of age.

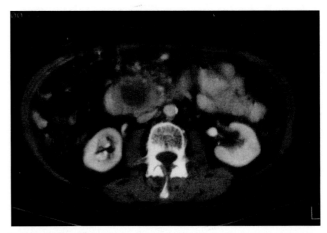

Figure 12–55. CT scan of a pancreatic ductal adenocarcinoma appearing as a large solid mass in the head of pancreas.

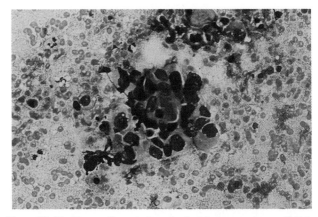

Figure 12–56. Fine needle aspiration of a ductal adenocarcinoma. Cellular aspirate (tumor cellularity) with irregular, three-dimensional pleomorphism with enlarged nuclei, coarse chromatin, increased nuclear-to-cytoplasmic ratio, and eosinophilic to focally vacuolated cytoplasm.

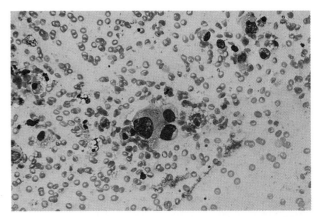

Figure 12–57. Fine needle aspiration of a ductal adenocarcinoma. In this aspirate, dyscohesive or single cells with nuclear pleomorphism are seen, as well as enlarged nuclei, nucleoli, coarse chromatin, an increased nuclear-to-cytoplasmic ratio, and eosinophilic to vacuolated-appearing cytoplasm.

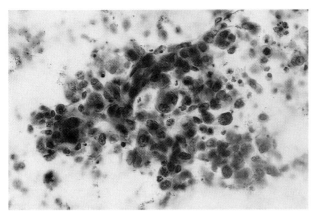

Figure 12–58. Fine needle aspiration of a ductal adenocarcinoma. Cellular arrangement includes a three-dimensional arrangement of cohesive cells with nuclear crowding and pleomorphism, enlarged nuclei, prominent nucleoli, coarse chromatin, increased nuclear-to-cytoplasmic ratio, and relatively scanty cytoplasm.

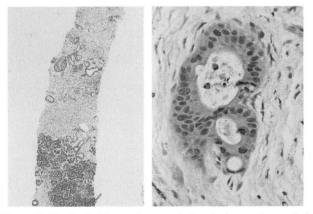

Figure 12–59. Needle biopsy of pancreatic ductal adenocarcinoma. *Left,* In the lower portion of the illustration the pancreatic tissue is relatively normal. However, in the upper portion of the illustration, there is disorganized duct distribution. *Right,* Higher magnification shows a gland-in-gland growth pattern composed of cells with enlarged, hyperchromatic nuclei, prominent eosinophilic nucleoli, mitotic figures, intraluminal necrotic material and neutrophilic infiltrate. The features in this illustration are diagnostic of adenocarcinoma.

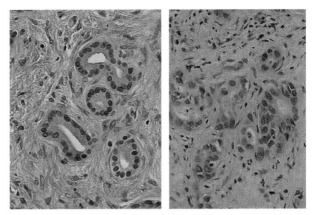

Figure 12–60. Separate needle biopsies comparing *(left)* non-neoplastic ducts in chronic pancreatitis with *(right)* ductal adenocarcinoma. The ducts in chronic pancreatitis have uniform nuclei without pleomorphism or increased nuclear-to-cytoplasmic ratio, and there is a linear arrangement along the basal portion of the cell. In contrast, the malignant duct cells in adenocarcinoma are composed of enlarged, pleomorphic nuclei with an increased nuclear-to-cytoplasmic ratio and a haphazard arrangement in the cell (loss of basilar polarity).

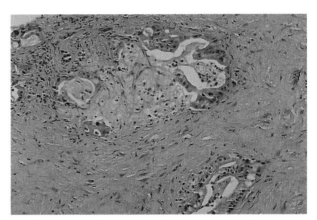

Figure 12–61. Needle biopsy from a pancreatic adenocarcinoma shows the presence of incomplete glandular lumina and mucin pools with associated neoplastic cells.

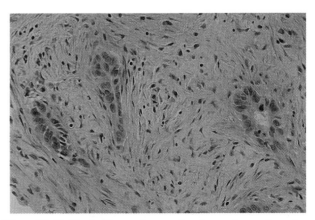

Figure 12–62. Needle biopsy of pancreatic adenocarcinoma shows haphazardly arranged glands invading the stroma, causing an associated desmoplastic stromal reaction.

■ Due to its proximity to the biliary tract, carcinoma of the pancreatic head is associated with jaundice and pruritus; the majority of patients have symptoms for less than 2 months prior to diagnosis.

■ Most cancers of the pancreatic head lead to the characteristic triad of jaundice, epigastric pain, and weight loss; however, these features are not pathognomonic of pancreatic cancer and can occur in other cancers as well.

• Weight loss is greater in patients with unresectable tumors and liver metastases.

• Cancers in the pancreatic body and tail produce more weight loss and pain than proximally located tumors.

■ With pancreatic duct obstruction, pancreatic insufficiency and malabsorption occur.

■ Additional symptoms may include nausea and vomiting (more commonly associated with the presence of liver metastases), constipation, and food intolerance.

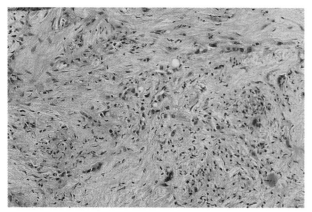

Figure 12–63. Needle biopsy of pancreatic adenocarcinoma shows malignant cells infiltrating the stroma as dyscohesive or single cells without obvious gland formation. Intracytoplasmic mucin was found with epithelial mucin stains.

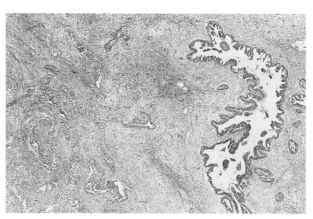

Figure 12–66. Pancreatic adenocarcinoma including intraductal adenocarcinoma is seen at the right side of the illustration and invasive carcinoma occupies most of the remainder. The normal pancreatic parenchyma is lost owing to replacement and invasion by adenocarcinoma, which causes an associated desmoplastic stromal reaction.

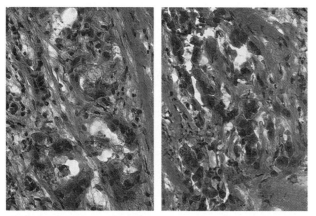

Figure 12–64. *Left* and *right,* Frozen section of pancreatic ductal adenocarcinoma characterized by disorganized duct distribution, incomplete glandular lumens, and neoplastic cells with increased nuclear size of 4:1 or greater between duct epithelial cells. The combination of these features is diagnostic for a ductal adenocarcinoma.

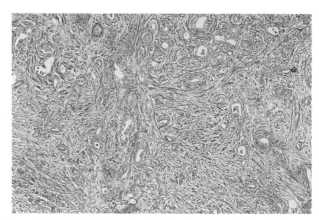

Figure 12–67. Well-differentiated infiltrating pancreatic ductal adenocarcinoma composed of medium to small glands with stromal desmoplasia.

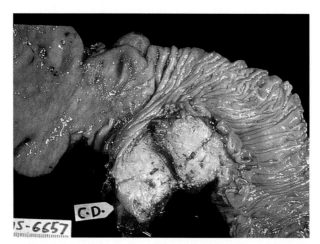

Figure 12–65. Pancreatic adenocarcinoma located at the head of the pancreas, obstructing and causing dilatation of the common duct (CD) and composed of a solitary firm to hard, tan-yellow large mass.

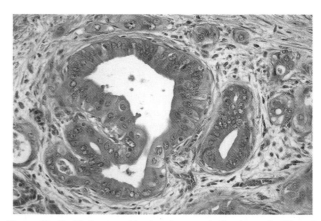

Figure 12–68. Higher magnification shows an infiltrative well-differentiated ductal adenocarcinoma. The glands are variable in size and composed of cells with enlarged, pleomorphic nuclei and prominent nucleoli. Necrotic debris is focally present within glandular lumens. Outside the glands, individual neoplastic cells can be seen infiltrating the surrounding stroma.

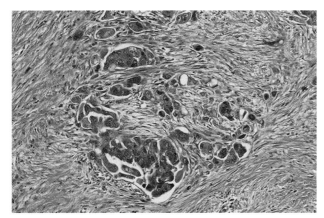

Figure 12–69. Infiltrative poorly differentiated ductal adenocarcinoma. The neoplastic cells are infiltrative as small clusters or individual cells composed of hyperchromatic and pleomorphic nuclei.

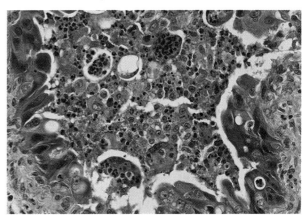

Figure 12–72. Infiltrative, moderately well differentiated pancreatic ductal adenocarcinoma shows intraluminal necrotic material and neutrophilic infiltrate, features generally associated with ductal malignancies.

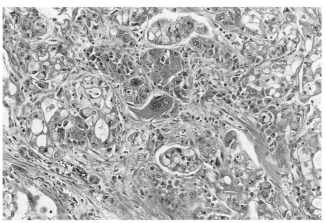

Figure 12–70. Another example of a poorly differentiated ductal adenocarcinoma. Numerous cells with markedly pleomorphic and bizarre nuclei, including multinucleated cells with prominent eosinophilic nucleoli, and eosinophilic, clear, and vacuolated cytoplasm, are seen. The cytoplasmic changes are those of mucin-producing cells, and mucin stains *(not shown)* were intensely positive in these cells.

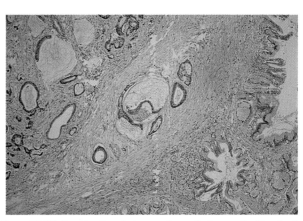

Figure 12–73. Invasive ductal adenocarcinoma is characterized by glandular lumina with an incomplete epithelial lining and mucin pools. In the center of the illustration the neoplastic infiltrate is neurotropic.

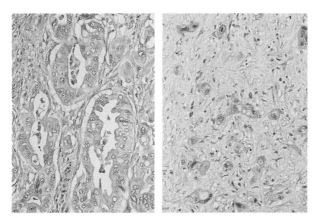

Figure 12–71. This illustration contrasts a well-differentiated, gland-forming, invasive ductal adenocarcinoma *(left)* with an invasive, poorly differentiated ductal adenocarcinoma *(right)*, which is characterized by small clusters of individually invasive neoplastic cells. Although gland formation in the poorly differentiated tumor is not present, some of the cells suggest mucin production (center and bottom of illustration). Mucin stains *(not shown)* would be helpful in determining the presence of intracytoplasmic epithelial mucin within neoplastic cells and could confirm ductal origin.

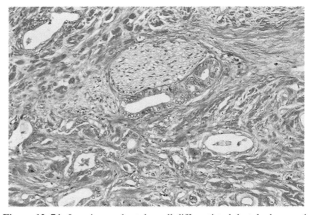

Figure 12–74. Invasive moderately well differentiated ductal adenocarcinoma shows perineural invasion, a characteristic feature of pancreatic adenocarcinoma.

■ Diabetes generally occurs in patients with advanced disease in about one-third of patients, but a smaller percentage (up to 15%) have de novo diabetes around the time of diagnosis.

■ Physical examination reveals the presence of an abdominal mass, ankle edema, fever, abdominal distention, palpable gallbladder (Courvoisier's sign associated with cancer in the head of the pancreas), and thrombophlebitis (Trousseau's sign).

■ Any portion of the pancreas can be affected, but the most common site of involvement (60% to 70% of cases) is the head of the pancreas; 10% to 15% of tumors are localized to the body, and 5% to 10% are localized to the tail.

■ **Laboratory findings** are nonspecific and may include hyperbilirubinemia (direct), elevated alkaline phosphatase, aminotransferase, and 5′-nucleotidase levels, anemia, and hypoalbuminemia. Pancreatic function tests are at present rarely performed in the diagnosis of pancreatic cancer.

■ **Tumor markers:** Pancreatic mucin epitopes can be evaluated as serum tumor markers in pancreatic adenocarcinoma. These include DUPAN-2, CA 19-9, SPan-1 and B72.3.

  • The combination of two or more serum markers (e.g., DUPAN-2 and CA 19-9) increases the sensitivity to cover more than 90% of pancreatic cancer patients. However, a significant percentage of patients with benign diseases of the pancreas and liver may also have elevated serum mucin levels of DUPAN-2 and CA 19-9.

  • The combination of a serum tumor marker and a single positive imaging study achieves a higher sensitivity than that of a tumor marker alone.

  • The resectability of pancreatic cancer decreases with increasing serum CA 19-9 levels. Serum levels of CA 19-9 have also been used as a postoperative marker as well as a means of early detection of recurrent tumor. Normalization of elevated serum CA 19-9 levels after pancreatectomy is associated with an improved prognosis.

■ **Etiology of pancreatic cancer:** Among the contributing factors or etiologic agents with a suspected link to the development of pancreatic ductal adenocarcinoma are tobacco, alcohol, diet, coffee, occupational factors, radiation, predisposing medical conditions (including diabetes), chronic (nonfamilial) pancreatitis, hereditary chronic relapsing pancreatitis, partial gastrectomy, and familial and genetic factors.

Radiology

Radiographic Studies

■ Invasive and noninvasive techniques have been used in the detection and diagnosis of pancreatic adenocarcinoma. Among the procedures used are percutaneous ultrasound, endoscopic ultrasonography, angiography, CT scan, endoscopic retrograde cholangiopancreatography (ERCP), and MRI. These procedures vary in sensitivity and specificity for detecting a neoplasm.

  • On ERCP, the presence of moderate to severe ductal strictures (longer than 10 mm) and duct irregularities accompanied by moderate to severe pancreatitis is highly suggestive of a diagnosis of pancreatic cancer.

  • Cancers located at the head of the pancreas may result in obstruction of both the pancreatic and common bile ducts, resulting in the characteristic "double duct sign" on ERCP.

  • Another highly suggestive ERCP finding for pancreatic cancer is an abrupt cut-off to the main pancreatic duct.

Laparoscopy

■ Laparoscopy is valuable for assessing the resectability of pancreatic cancer and detecting the presence of tumor implants in the liver and peritoneum.

■ Laparoscopy combined with CT scan and angiography is highly accurate (in more than 85% of cases) in predicting unresectability (see the criteria for unresectability listed under Treatment and Prognosis, later).

Pathology

Fine Needle Aspiration

■ Highly cellular aspirate (tumor cellularity).

■ Cellular arrangement includes irregular tight, three-dimensional arrangement ranging from sheets and cohesive groups (well and moderately differentiated adenocarcinoma) to dyscohesive or single cells (moderately and poorly differentiated adenocarcinoma).

■ Nuclear crowding and pleomorphism with enlarged nuclei, inconspicuous to prominent nucleoli, coarse chromatin, and relatively scanty to abundant clear, pale, and vacuolated cytoplasm (indicative of mucin secretion), and naked nuclei may be seen.

■ The less differentiated the tumor, the more cytologic atypia is present, including bizarre cells, and mitotic activity will be present as well.

■ Fine needle aspiration (FNA) (under CT or ultrasound guidance) has a sensitivity of 75% to 100% and a specificity of 100%.

Frozen Section

■ Frozen section diagnosis of pancreatic adenocarcinoma can be extremely difficult because of the fact that many tumors are well differentiated.

■ **Major criteria** for a diagnosis of carcinoma include the following:
  • Nuclear size variation of 4:1 or greater between ductal epithelial cells.
  • Incomplete glandular lumina.
  • Disorganized duct distribution.

■ **Minor criteria** for a diagnosis of carcinoma include the following:
  • Prominent nucleoli (huge and irregular).
  • Intraluminal necrosis and neutrophilic infiltrate.
  • Glandular mitoses, including atypical forms.
  • Neurotropism.
  • Glands unaccompanied by stroma in smooth muscle fascicles.

■ These combined features are not found in benign pancreatic lesions; combined application of both major and minor criteria in frozen sections maximizes accuracy of the diagnostic interpretation.

Gross

- Solitary firm to hard, poorly demarcated mass of varying size.
- Occasionally appears as a scar.

Histology

- Pancreatic lobular architecture is lost.
- Neoplastic ducts or glands formed by atypical columnar to cuboidal cells may be present, showing loss of polarity; a cribriform (microglandular) growth pattern may be present.
- Cytomorphology is characterized by the presence of large irregular nuclei, conspicuous nucleoli, and mitoses, including atypical mitotic figures. The neoplastic cells and their nuclei are much larger than the cells of the normal ducts.
- Cellular components may include mucus-producing columnar cells, goblet cells, signet ring cells, clear cells, and others.
- An intraductal component may or may not be present.
- Incomplete glandular lumina characterized by an incomplete epithelial lining and intraluminal necrotic material and/or neutrophilic infiltrate may be seen. The presence of incomplete glandular lumina with intraluminal necrotic material and/or neutrophilic infiltrate raises concern about a carcinoma in the absence of more definitive features (i.e., cytomorphologic features, invasive growth, or neurotropism).
- Invasive growth with desmoplasia and neurotropism (perineural and intraneural) is present. Because carcinomas themselves are often desmoplastic, fibrosis and inflammation are additional microscopic features. Pancreatic adenocarcinomas spread along nerves and in lymphatic vessels, so a careful search for carcinoma cells in these locations is often rewarding.
- Variable production of mucin, either intracytoplasmic or in the form of extracellular mucin pools, is seen. "Naked" mucin pools (without associated malignant neoplastic cells) within the stroma are another worrisome feature for invasive carcinoma and require extensive evaluation to exclude the presence of intraductal or definitively invasive carcinoma.
- Secondary chronic pancreatitis is seen. Evidence of chronic pancreatitis often accompanies the cancer, largely because of ductal obstruction.
- The islets of Langerhans are preserved.

- Histologic grading of pancreatic ductal adenocarcinoma (see Table 12–5).
- *Histochemistry:* Epithelial mucin staining (mucicarmine, PAS with diastase digestion) may be helpful in determining the presence of an infiltrating tumor.
- *Immunohistochemistry:* Immunoreactivity is seen with epithelial markers, including cytokeratin, CEA, and others. Ductal adenocarcinoma will also react with pancreatic mucin markers such as CA 19-9, DUPAN-2, and SPan-1. However, these markers are not specific for pancreatic ductal adenocarcinoma and also react with other mucin-producing adenocarcinomas.
- *Molecular biology*
  - Flow cytometry studies have shown that from 15% to 90% of ductal adenocarcinomas are DNA aneuploid.
  - Point mutations at codon 12 of the K-ras oncogene occurs in 75% to 95% of tumors, and a mutated p53 suppressor gene is seen in approximately 60% of cases. K-ras mutations appear to happen early in the development of pancreatic cancer. Point mutations in codon 12 of K-ras have also been identified in hyperplastic alterations (papillary and nonpapillary) of pancreatic ducts in the absence of carcinoma, suggesting that these duct alterations are also neoplastic.

Differential Diagnosis

- Chronic pancreatitis (Table 12–6) (Chapter 11G, #2).
- Pancreatic endocrine (islet cell) neoplasm (Chapter 12F, #1).

Treatment and Prognosis

- Surgical resection is the only treatment that offers a chance of long-term disease-free survival. Surgery includes pancreaticoduodenectomy (Whipple procedure) or total pancreatectomy.
- Even after surgical resection, the prognosis is poor, with 3- and 5-year survival rates reported to be 13% and 8%, respectively.
  - Only about 10% of cancers located in the pancreatic head are resectable; therefore, nonresectable pancreatic cancer predominates, making surgery a purely palliative procedure.

Table 12–5
HISTOLOGIC GRADING OF PANCREATIC DUCTAL ADENOCARCINOMA

Tumor Grade	Glandular Differentiation	Mucin Production	Mitoses (Per 10 High-Power Fields)	Nuclear Anaplasia
1	Well-differentiated ductlike glands	Prominent	1–5 (<5)	Minimal pleomorphism and loss of nuclear polarity
2	Moderately differentiated ductlike and tubular glands	Focal	6–10	Moderate pleomorphism and loss of nuclear polarity
3	Poorly differentiated glands; single malignant cells with pleomorphic nuclei	Little to absent	>10	Marked

Table 12–6
CHRONIC PANCREATITIS VERSUS DUCTAL ADENOCARCINOMA

Features	Chronic Pancreatitis	Ductal Adenocarcinoma
Gender/age	More common in men than in women; most frequent in the 4th–6th decades of life	More common in men than in women; incidence increases with age; peak incidence occurs in 7th–8th decades; uncommon below 40 years of age
Clinical	Abdominal pain (>80% of cases) and weight loss	Jaundice, epigastric pain, weight loss
Etiology	Alcohol, idiopathic, nutritional, hereditary, biliary tract disease (gallstones), others	Tobacco, alcoholism, diet, coffee, occupational factors, radiation exposure, preexisting medical conditions (diabetes), pancreatitis (acquired, hereditary), genetic and familial factors
Radiology	Calcifications on abdominal films	Mass deforms contours of gland; severe ductal abnormalities (strictures longer than 10 mm and duct irregularities) with pancreatitis; cancers in pancreatic head may obstruct pancreatic and common bile ducts, resulting in "double duct sign" on ERCP; abrupt cut-off to main pancreatic duct seen by ERCP
Location	Occurs anywhere in the pancreas as focal, segmental, or diffuse involvement	In head more often than in body and tail
Gross	Involved pancreas is enlarged (in part or in toto) and indurated with associated sclerosis	Mass lesion, solitary and poorly demarcated
Histology	Preservation of lobular architecture; irregular loss of acinar and ductal tissue with ductal dilatation, cyst formation; inspissated secretions or calculi; ductal epithelial alterations (atrophy, hyperplasia, or metaplasia) with minimal atypia; variable inflammation; fibrosis; islets are not altered in early stages but are abnormal in later stages of disease (reduction in number and progressive atrophy)	Loss of lobular architecture; invasive growth by neoplastic ducts and/or individual tumor cells with desmoplastic reaction; ducts or glands composed of atypical columnar or cuboidal cells with enlarged, irregular nuclei, prominent nucleoli, and mitoses; neurotropism; variable mucin production; minor alterations of islets
Treatment and prognosis	Analgesics for pain; enzyme replacement for exocrine insufficiency; surgery for pain as a last resort; mortality rate secondary to chronic pancreatitis is low	Surgery; adjuvant therapy of limited assistance; poor prognosis: >95% of patients die of their disease

- Criteria for unresectability of a pancreatic cancer include distant metastases (to the liver, peritoneal surfaces, distant lymph nodes), adenopathy proved by needle aspiration, obstruction or invasion of the portal or mesenteric veins, and/or encasement of the celiac or superior mesenteric arteries by cancer.
■ Among the surgical procedures performed are the following:
  - Pancreaticoduodenectomy, or the Whipple procedure, which is the procedure of choice for pancreatic head and periampullary tumors. The operative mortality rate of pancreaticoduodenal resection is now less than 5%, compared with previous rates, which were as high as 20%.
  - Pylorus-sparing pancreaticoduodenectomy (PSPD), which is a modified Whipple procedure in which the stomach and pylorus are preserved.
  - Total pancreatectomy.
■ Cancers of the body and tail of the pancreas are almost never resectable because they present late in the disease course as advanced stage tumors. In patients who have unresectable tumors, total pancreatectomy and splenectomy are performed.
■ Complications of pancreaticoduodenal resection include pancreatic fistula, gastric outlet obstruction with delayed gastric emptying, gastrointestinal and/or intra-abdominal hemorrhage, abscess, wound infection, sepsis, biliary fistula, and others. Diabetes is unusual in patients after pancreaticoduodenal resection, but brittle diabetes is a complication of total pancreatectomy.
■ Adjuvant therapy: Radiotherapy is used to control local disease following surgery. Chemotherapy is used to treat systemic disease.

- Neither radiotherapy nor chemotherapy alone appears to have a significant impact on patient survival. Used in combination either after surgery or in patients with unresectable tumor, radiotherapy and chemotherapy have resulted in longer survival periods, but even so, survival rates are poor.
■ Palliative management includes the treatment of:
  - Pain, with pharmacotherapy, invasive anesthetics, and surgery.
  - Depression and emotional problems, with pharmacotherapy and supportive psychotherapy.
  - Biliary obstruction via endoscopic surgery, as an alternative to surgery to relieve distal common bile duct obstruction.
■ Prognosis associated with pancreatic ductal adenocarcinoma is poor.
  - More than 95% of patients with pancreatic ductal adenocarcinoma die of their disease.
  - At the time of diagnosis, 10% of patients have disease confined to the pancreas, 40% have locally advanced disease, and more than 50% have distant spread of disease.
  - The median length of survival is 18 to 20 months.
  - The 5-year survival rate is 5% to 18%. The 5-year survival rate of patients with pancreatic adenocarcinoma in the United States is 1.3%, and the median survival is 4.1 months.
  - Tumor size appears to be a strong predictor of prognosis. The 5-year patient survival is nil in tumors measuring more than 5 cm in diameter, but patients with tumors measuring 2.5 cm or smaller have an overall better mean survival than patients with larger tumors.

- Periampullary pancreatic tumors have a better prognosis, with 3- and 5-year survival rates reported to be 32% and 18%, respectively.
- Metastatic tumor is often encountered at surgery; favored metastatic sites include the regional lymph nodes, liver, pleura, and lungs.

Additional Facts

- Histologic variants of "conventional" ductal adenocarcinoma include adenosquamous carcinoma, squamous cell carcinoma, mucinous adenocarcinoma, clear cell carcinoma, oncocytic adenocarcinoma, and microglandular carcinoma.
- Histologic variants do not represent distinct clinicopathologic entities separate from conventional types of ductal adenocarcinoma.
- The clinical parameters relative to these histologic variants, including gender, age, clinical presentation, treatment and prognosis, are essentially the same as those described for conventional pancreatic ductal adenocarcinoma, and these tumors are just as lethal as conventional ductal adenocarcinoma.

2. Adenosquamous Carcinoma

Synonyms: Mucoepidermoid carcinoma.

- Characterized by the presence of glandular (adenocarcinomatous) and squamous cell carcinoma components.
- The squamous component probably originates from foci of squamous metaplasia, but in contrast to squamous metaplasia, squamous carcinoma has cytologic features of malignancy and is invasive.
- Ionizing radiation may be an etiologic factor in the development of this type of pancreatic cancer.
- May be associated with hypercalcemia.
- The proportion of glandular and squamous elements varies, but both components are readily apparent and intimately associated.
- Squamous cell carcinoma includes keratinization (keratin pearls or individual cell keratinization) and intercellular bridges, but the identification of these elements varies from case to case and by the degree of cellular differentiation.

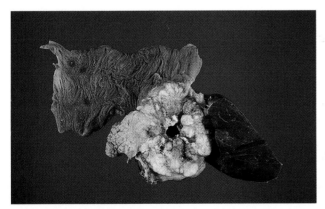

Figure 12–75. Pancreatic adenosquamous carcinoma appears as a large, white mass with extension into the spleen.

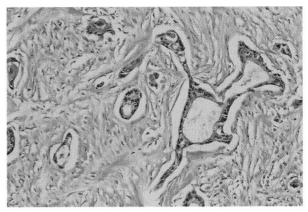

Figure 12–76. Pancreatic adenosquamous carcinoma. In this portion of the tumor, glandular differentiation is seen.

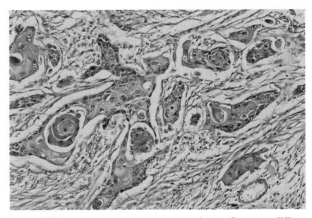

Figure 12–77. Pancreatic adenosquamous carcinoma. Squamous differentiation is evident in this portion of the tumor, with keratinization (keratin pearls or individual cell keratinization).

- Invasive growth patterns, including desmoplasia and neurotropism, are similar to those of conventional pancreatic adenocarcinoma.
- The adenocarcinomatous component generally predominates over the squamous cell carcinoma in metastatic foci or represents the only component in the metastases.
- Metastases occurs primarily to the regional lymph nodes, liver, and peritoneum.

3. Squamous Cell Carcinoma

- The existence of pure pancreatic squamous cell carcinoma remains questionable and is an extraordinarily rare variant of pancreatic ductal adenocarcinoma.
- In the presence of pure squamous cell carcinoma, many tissue sections may ultimately reveal a malignant glandular component consistent with a diagnosis of adenosquamous carcinoma.
- Squamous cell carcinoma of the pancreas probably originates from foci of squamous metaplasia.
- Ionizing radiation may be an etiologic factor in the development of this type of pancreatic cancer.

4. Mucous or Mucinous Adenocarcinoma

Synonyms: Colloid carcinoma; gelatinous carcinoma.

■ Tumor is characterized by the presence of excessive amounts of mucin in the form of mucin pools in which malignant neoplastic cells are floating, forming glands or solid nests, or they may appear as single cells.
■ Cellular constituents may include signet ring cells and columnar epithelial cells.
■ Mucin pools may be devoid of cellular components. Deeper sectioning may reveal a neoplastic cellular infiltrate. In the absence of cells, benign mucous "squirts" can simulate invasive cancer.
■ This tumor is not synonymous with or related to mucinous cystic neoplasms (mucinous cystadenocarcinoma) because:
  • It has neither a cyst wall nor a complete epithelial lining characteristic of a cystic lesion; absence of cellular "ovarian-type" stroma.
  • Its behavior is that of a "conventional" ductal adenocarcinoma.

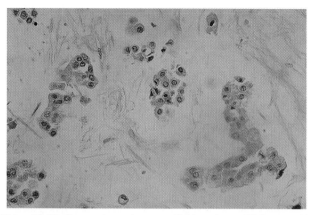

Figure 12–80. Pancreatic mucinous or colloid carcinoma. Higher magnification shows that the neoplastic cells "floating" in the mucin pools are malignant epithelial cells.

■ Fine needle aspiration shows large mucin pools with or without groups of malignant epithelial cells; thin smears may be difficult to achieve owing to the abundant mucus.

5. Clear Cell Carcinoma

■ Clear cells may represent a small cellular component of an otherwise conventional ductal adenocarcinoma. To be classified as a clear cell carcinoma, the clear cell component should be the dominant cell type.
■ The cellular component is characterized by cells with clear cytoplasm. The nuclei are enlarged, irregular in size and shape, and hyperchromatic with or without prominent nucleoli. Cell borders may be distinct.
■ Must be differentiated from a metastatic renal cell carcinoma. The presence of intracytoplasmic mucin will exclude a diagnosis of metastatic renal cell carcinoma but will not exclude the presence of other primary malignant neoplasms arising from other organ sites (e.g., lung) that metastasize to the pancreas. In this situation, the presence of a pancreatic intraductal carcinoma will confirm the pancreas as the site of origin of the tumor.

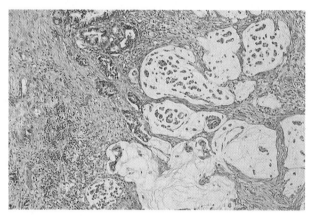

Figure 12–78. Pancreatic mucinous or colloid carcinoma is characterized by the presence of excessive amounts of mucin in the form of mucin pools, in which malignant neoplastic cells are floating or form glands. Toward the top of the illustration, conventional adenocarcinomatous foci can be seen.

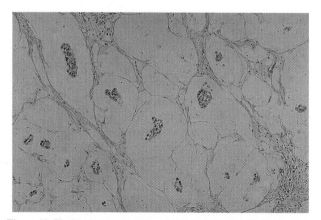

Figure 12–79. Pancreatic mucinous or colloid carcinoma. In this example, there were no foci of conventional adenocarcinoma, but the tumor included mucin pools within which the neoplastic infiltrate appeared to be "floating."

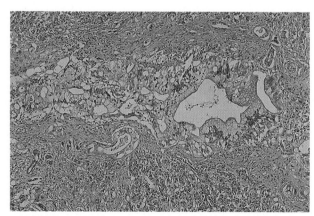

Figure 12–81. Invasive pancreatic adenocarcinoma predominantly composed of cells with a clear cytoplasm (clear cell adenocarcinoma.)

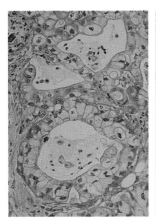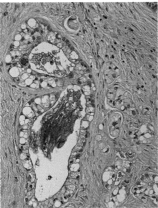

Figure 12–82. Pancreatic adenocarcinoma with clear cells. *Left,* Complex glandular growth composed of cells with pleomorphic, hyperchromatic nuclei with clear cytoplasm and distinct cell membranes. Mitotic figures are present. *Right,* Mucin stain shows the presence of intracytoplasmic and intraluminal mucin-positive material.

6. Oncocytic Carcinoma

- Characterized by mitochondria-rich cells with a prominent granular, eosinophilic cytoplasm.
- Must be differentiated from other pancreatic tumors that can have oncocytic cells, including pancreatic endocrine neoplasm and solid and papillary epithelial carcinoma.

7. Microglandular Carcinoma

Synonym: Microadenocarcinoma.

- Carcinoma characterized by small microglandular or solid cribriform pattern of growth.
- Must be differentiated from other pancreatic tumors that can have a cribriform (microglandular) growth, including pancreatic endocrine neoplasms and acinar cell carcinoma.
- Some authorities believe that the microglandular carcinoma (microadenocarcinoma) represents a distinct clinicopathologic entity. More likely, a pancreatic carcinoma with microglandular or solid cribriform features represents a pattern of growth seen in a ductal adenocarcinoma. Alternatively, a pancreatic carcinoma with microglandu-

lar or solid cribriform growth represents another type of pancreatic malignancy, such as an acinar cell carcinoma or a pancreatic endocrine neoplasm, that requires immunohistochemical studies to confirm the diagnosis.

8. Anaplastic Carcinoma

Definition: Aggressive undifferentiated malignant pancreatic neoplasm of ductal epithelial cell origin with varied morphologic features and evidence of epithelial differentiation by light microscopy, immunohistochemistry, or ultrastructural analysis. It merits separate classification from ductal adenocarcinoma based on its distinctive histology and highly aggressive clinical behavior.

Synonyms: Pleomorphic, sarcomatoid, spindle cell, giant cell, and undifferentiated carcinoma.

Clinical

- Uncommon tumor representing approximately 5% to 7% of all pancreatic exocrine neoplasms.
- More common in men than in women; age distribution is similar to that of ductal adenocarcinoma, occurring most commonly in patients between the seventh and ninth decades of life.

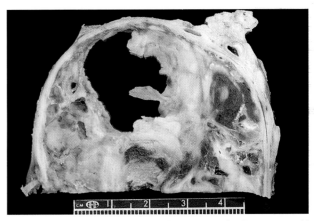

Figure 12–84. Anaplastic carcinoma of the pancreas is a large tumor with a mottled appearance, including areas of gray, yellow, red, and brown coloration, and cystic degenerative change.

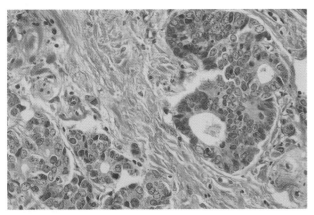

Figure 12–83. Pancreatic adenocarcinoma characterized by small microglandular or cribriform pattern of growth.

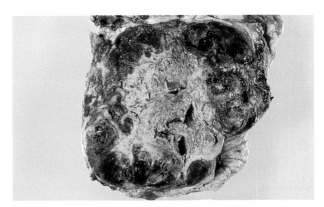

Figure 12–85. Anaplastic carcinoma of the pancreas shows necrosis, hemorrhage, and cystic degenerative changes.

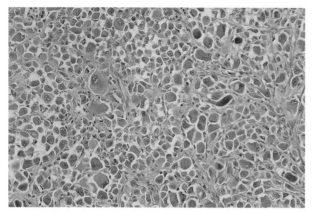

Figure 12–86. Anaplastic carcinoma of the pancreas, giant or pleomorphic cell type. The tumor is predominantly composed of giant or pleomorphic cells, including bizarre, odd-shaped, medium-sized to large cells with one or more nuclei. Nuclei are markedly enlarged and hyperchromatic with prominent eosinophilic cytoplasm.

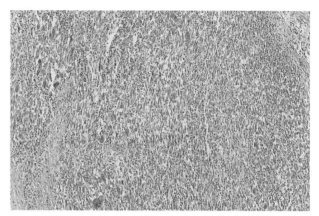

Figure 12–89. Anaplastic carcinoma of the pancreas, spindle cell type. The tumor is characterized by a fascicular growth pattern and is predominantly composed of spindle-shaped neoplastic cells.

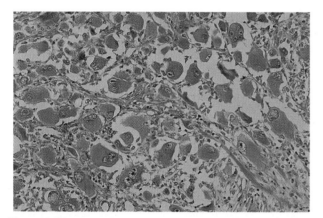

Figure 12–87. Anaplastic carcinoma of the pancreas, giant or pleomorphic cell type. Higher magnification shows the multinucleated (nonosteoclast-like) giant (pleomorphic) cells with prominent eosinophilic nucleoli.

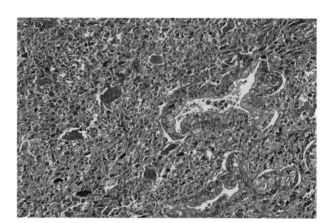

Figure 12–90. Anaplastic carcinoma of the pancreas, osteoclastic giant cell type. This tumor is characterized by the presence of two cell types, benign appearing osteoclast-like giant cells and smaller malignant, round to spindle-shaped cells. A differentiated malignant gland (ductal adenocarcinoma) is seen from which the anaplastic component has originated.

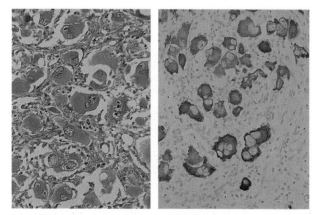

Figure 12–88. Anaplastic carcinoma of the pancreas, giant or pleomorphic cell type. *Left,* Conventional light microscopic staining and appearance of the neoplastic cells. *Right,* Epithelial histogenesis of the giant or pleomorphic cells is confirmed by the presence of cytokeratin immunoreactivity.

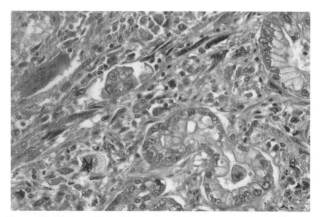

Figure 12–91. Anaplastic carcinoma of the pancreas, osteoclastic giant cell type. Higher magnification shows the combination of differentiated ductal adenocarcinoma, "undifferentiated" malignant, round to spindle-shaped cellular infiltrate, and osteoclastic giant cells.

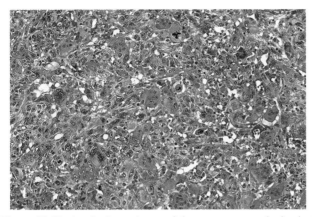

Figure 12–92. Anaplastic carcinoma of the pancreas, osteoclastic giant cell type. Osteoclast-like giant cells are enlarged, multinucleated giant cells with uniform small nuclei clustered in the central portion of the cell. The nuclei are fairly uniform in size and have an oval shape, vesicular chromatin, and abundant eosinophilic cytoplasm. The osteoclastic giant cells are admixed with a smaller malignant cellular infiltrate that includes bizarre cells with atypical nuclei and increased mitotic activity, including atypical forms.

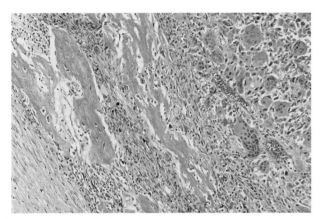

Figure 12–93. Anaplastic carcinoma of the pancreas, osteoclastic giant cell type. Focally, osteoid can be seen.

- May arise in any part of the pancreas. Occurs roughly equally in the pancreatic head and tail. It may occur less frequently in the head than the usual ductal adenocarcinomas.
- Signs and symptoms are similar to those of ductal adenocarcinoma. Depending on the site of occurrence, the clinical presentation may include jaundice, epigastric pain, and weight loss; with pancreatic duct obstruction, pancreatic insufficiency and malabsorption occur.

Pathology

Fine Needle Aspiration
- Highly cellular; isolated and poorly cohesive cells.
- Marked cellular pleomorphism, large nuclei with coarse chromatin and prominent nucleoli.
- Cytoplasm varies; cytophagocytosis, including neutrophils, is present.
- Depending on the cytologic make-up of the tumor (see section on histology later), mononuclear and bizarre

multinucleated giant cells, spindle cells, and osteoclastic giant cells can be seen.

Gross
- Tumors tend to be large (not infrequently measuring more than 10 cm in diameter) and have a mottled appearance, with gray, yellow, red, and brown coloration and a solid to soft consistency.
- Necrosis, hemorrhage, and cystic degeneration may be conspicuous features.

Histology
- Pancreatic anaplastic carcinoma is a single neoplastic entity that may include several morphologic types, including giant cell (pleomorphic), spindle cell, and osteoclastic giant cell type. One morphologic type may predominate to the exclusion of the others, or these types may occur in combination, the proportion of each component varying.
- There is no difference in the treatment or prognosis of these tumors based on the morphologic type, so the morphologic subdivisions in anaplastic pancreatic carcinoma are artificial relative to their biology.
- Diligent sectioning of the tumor often reveals foci of ductal adenocarcinoma, or the anaplastic component may arise from a larger pancreatic duct or from dysplastic ductal epithelial cells.
- Typically, there is an absence of stroma in anaplastic carcinoma.
- Osseous or chondroid metaplasia may be seen.
- Histochemistry: Scattered neoplastic cells may show intracytoplasmic epithelial mucin (mucicarmine, PAS with diastase).
- *Immunohistochemistry:* Focal cytokeratin reactivity is seen in various cellular components (e.g., pleomorphic and spindle cells).

a. Giant Cell or Pleomorphic
- Composed of bizarre, odd-shaped, medium-sized to large cells with one or more nuclei.
- Nuclei are markedly enlarged and hyperchromatic with prominent eosinophilic nucleoli.
- Multinucleated (nonosteoclast-like) giant cells often show phagocytosis of mononuclear cells.
- Numerous mitoses, including atypical forms, are seen.

b. Spindle Cell
- May show a storiform or fascicular growth pattern.
- Neoplastic cells are elongated with enlarged, elongated, and hyperchromatic nuclei with prominent eosinophilic nucleoli.
- Numerous mitoses, including atypical forms, are seen.

c. Osteoclast-Like Giant Cells
- Composed of two cell types: benign appearing osteoclast-like giant cells and smaller malignant round to spindle-shaped cells.
- Osteoclast-like giant cells are enlarged, multinucleated giant cells with uniform small nuclei clustered in the central

portion of the cell. The number of nuclei vary in any cell, but multiple nuclei are present and can include 100 (or more) nuclei per giant cell.

- Nuclei are fairly uniform in size and have an oval shape, vesicular chromatin, and abundant eosinophilic cytoplasm.
- Bizarre giant cells, atypical nuclei, and mitotic activity are features not found in association with the osteoclastic giant cells.
- Histogenesis of the osteoclast giant cells remains the subject of debate (epithelial versus mesenchymal). The osteoclast-like giant cell is probably of macrophage or histiomonocytic origin and represents a reactive (non-neoplastic) component rather than an epithelial neoplastic cell. Support for this interpretation includes the following facts:
  - Histochemical studies may show the presence of acid phosphatase.
  - Immunohistochemical reactivity includes vimentin, α_1-antitrypsin, α_1-antichymotrypsin, leukocyte common antigen (LCA), CD68, and MB2, with absence of epithelial markers such as cytokeratin.
  - Localization to regions of hemorrhage, calcification, or osseous metaplasia is seen.
  - The origin of these cells may be similar to that of giant cell tumor of bone.
- Smaller cells, composed of round to spindle-shaped cells, are neoplastic and show cytologic abnormalities of malignancy, including hyperchromasia and mitotic activity with atypical forms.

Differential Diagnosis

- Sarcomas, including leiomyosarcoma, malignant fibrous histiocytoma, others (Chapter 12G, #1).
- Lymphoma (Chapter 12G, #2).
- Metastatic carcinoma (Chapter 12H).

Treatment and Prognosis

- Surgery and adjuvant therapies have been used in the treatment of pancreatic anaplastic carcinoma.
- Regardless of therapeutic intervention, these tumors are lethal over very short periods of time (months); the poor prognosis is also true for the osteoclast-like giant cell tumor although some investigators claim that among this group of neoplasms, this tumor type has a better prognosis.
- Dissemination occurs early and is widespread, involving regional lymph nodes as well as many viscera.

Additional Facts

- A **small cell variant** has been described and is included in the morphologic spectrum of anaplastic carcinoma. This purported small cell type is characterized by a solid growth pattern of small monotonous cells with round, hyperchromatic nuclei and a scant amount of cytoplasm.
  - This variant is so rare that it may not exist as a definitive subtype of anaplastic carcinoma but may simply be part

of the pleomorphic morphologic spectrum, or it may not be a primary pancreatic epithelial malignancy but a metastasis from another site, or it may not be an epithelial malignancy at all.

9. Acinar Cell Carcinoma

Definition: Malignant pancreatic tumor of acinous cells.

Clinical

- Represents approximately 1% of all exocrine pancreatic tumors and less than 5% of all pancreatic malignant tumors.
- More common in men than in women; generally occurs in older individuals (older than the seventh decade of life). It may also occur in children.
- Clinical presentation may be nonspecific, with symptoms including weight loss, abdominal pain, nausea and vomiting. Jaundice is uncommon, even in patients in whom the tumor occurs in the head of the pancreas.
- In order of decreasing frequency, the sites of occurrence include the head, tail, and body.

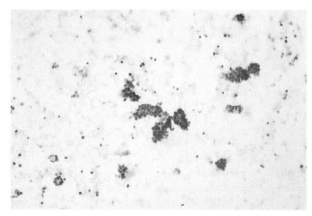

Figure 12–94. Acinar cell carcinoma—fine needle aspiration. Cellular aggregates with cellular cohesion and complex acinar structures are seen.

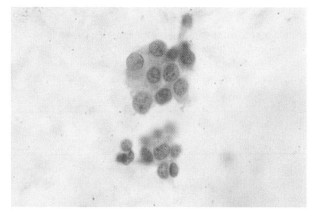

Figure 12–95. Acinar cell carcinoma—fine needle aspiration. Cell nests composed of round and hyperchromatic nuclei with prominent nucleoli and eosinophilic, granular cytoplasm are seen.

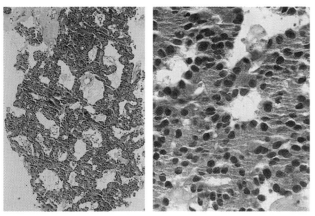

Figure 12–96. Needle biopsy of an acinar cell carcinoma. *Left,* The tumor has acinar and trabecular growth. *Right,* Higher magnification shows the acinar configuration of the tumor consisting of cells with a fine to coarse, eosinophilic granular eosinophilic cytoplasm (corresponding to zymogen granules), and hyperchromatic nuclei with prominent nucleoli.

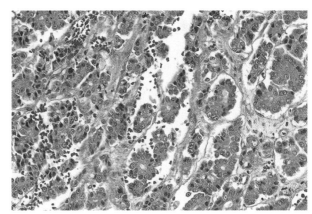

Figure 12–99. Acinar cell carcinoma, showing an acinar growth pattern, which is the most distinctive pattern of growth. Well-formed acini composed of small lumina with delineated borders are seen.

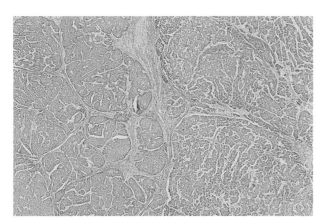

Figure 12–97. Acinar cell carcinoma in a resected pancreas with solid, cribriform (microglandular) and acinar growth patterns.

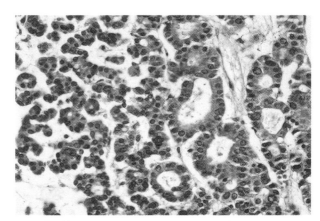

Figure 12–100. Acinar cell carcinoma. In this part of the tumor, a glandular pattern predominated, composed of larger lumina than those seen in the acinar pattern.

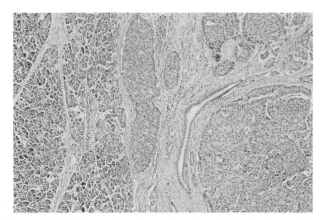

Figure 12–98. Acinar cell carcinoma, showing an infiltrative tumor with a predominantly solid growth pattern juxtaposed with the non-neoplastic acini (left side of illustration) from which this tumor originates.

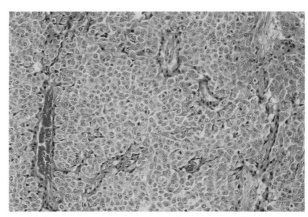

Figure 12–101. Acinar cell carcinoma, characterized by a predominantly solid growth.

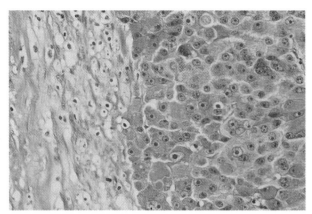

Figure 12–102. Acinar cell carcinoma. These tumors tend to be well circumscribed to encapsulated (partly or completely) cellular tumors. Typically, tumors that are encapsulated nearly always show evidence of tumor invasion into the capsule. Neoplastic cells show the presence of prominent eosinophilic nucleoli.

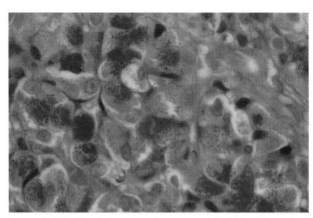

Figure 12–105. Acinar cell carcinoma. Histochemical reactivity includes the presence of diastase-resistant, PAS-positive intracytoplasmic granules, as depicted in this illustration.

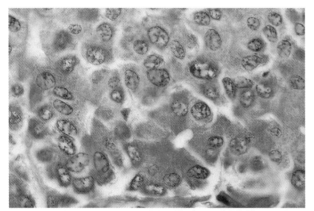

Figure 12–103. Acinar cell carcinoma, showing the presence of acini. The cytomorphology includes round to polyhedral to triangular cells with round to oval, uniform-appearing nuclei, chromatin clumping toward the periphery of the nuclei, a single prominent nucleolus, and the presence of a fine to coarse, eosinophilic granular cytoplasm. The latter corresponds to the presence of zymogen granules.

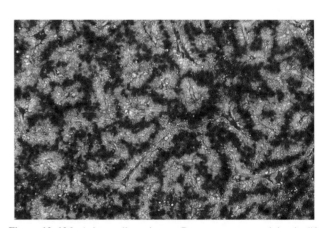

Figure 12–106. Acinar cell carcinoma. Butyrate esterase staining is diffuse, indicating the presence of lipase.

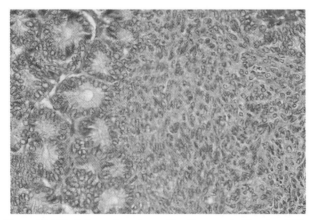

Figure 12–104. Acinar cell carcinoma. Readily recognizable acinar differentiation is seen to the left, but there is a transition to a dedifferentiated cellular infiltrate in the center and right portions of the illustration.

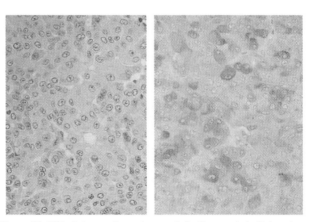

Figure 12–107. Acinar cell carcinoma. *Left,* Characteristic light microscopic features. *Right,* Trypsin immunoreactivity is seen, confirming the acinar cell differentiation.

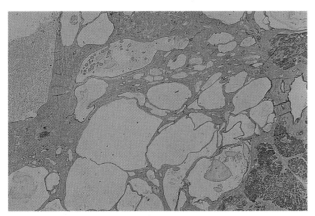

Figure 12–108. Acinar cell cystadenocarcinoma represents an unusual morphologic variant of acinar cell carcinoma and is characterized by the presence of acinar cell epithelium-lined cysts of variable size and shape.

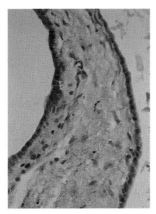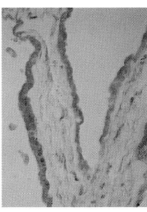

Figure 12–111. Acinar cell cystadenocarcinoma. *Left,* Cystic epithelial lining composed of a single layer of cuboidal epithelial cells with no acinar growth. *Right,* The epithelial component demonstrates the presence of trypsin immunoreactivity, confirming acinar cell differentiation.

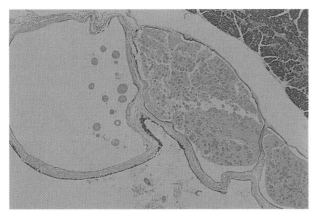

Figure 12–109. Acinar cell cystadenocarcinoma, showing the epithelial lining, including acinar growth. Inspissated eosinophilic material is present within the cystic spaces.

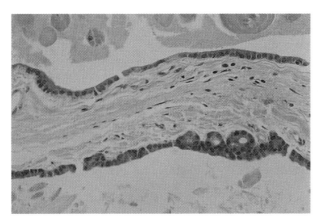

Figure 12–110. Acinar cell cystadenocarcinoma. At higher magnification, the acinar growth pattern of the cyst epithelial cell lining becomes more apparent.

- Laboratory findings include elevated serum lipase and alpha-fetoprotein levels. The consequences of elevated serum lipase may include:

  1. Subcutaneous fat or marrow necrosis.
  2. Panniculitis.
  3. Polyarthralgia.
  4. Nonbacterial thrombotic endocarditis.
  5. Peripheral eosinophilia may be present in as many as 10% of cases.

- There are no known etiologic factors.

Radiology

- Large solid tumors, generally larger than ductal adenocarcinomas.

Pathology

Fine Needle Aspiration

- Cellular smears with numerous cellular aggregates are seen; cellular cohesion is relatively well maintained.
- Lobulated acini may be seen; nuclei are round and hyperchromatic with prominent nucleoli and abundant eosinophilic granular cytoplasm. Nuclear polarity is altered with overlapping and displaced nuclei.

Gross

- Large, circumscribed to encapsulated, fleshy mass measures on average more than 10 cm in diameter.
- Invasion into adjacent structures can be seen.
- Necrosis and hemorrhage commonly are present, and cystic changes are occasionally present; calcifications are unusual.

Histology

- Well-circumscribed to encapsulated (partly or completely) cellular tumor; tumors that are encapsulated nearly always show evidence of tumor invasion into the capsule.

■ Four architectural growth patterns occur, often in combination.

- Frequent patterns:
  - **Acinar:** Most distinctive pattern in which the cells grow in well-formed acini with small lumina having delineated borders.
  - **Solid:** Sheets and cords of cells separated by fibrovascular stroma.
- Less frequent patterns:
  - **Glandular:** Larger lumina than are seen in the acinar pattern.
  - **Trabecular:** Long strands or cords of cells with double rows of nuclei; may include gyriform growth.
  - **Cribriform or microglandular:** Composed of back-to-back glands or acini.

■ The cytomorphologic features include round to polyhedral to triangular cells with round to oval, uniform nuclei, chromatin clumping toward the periphery of the nuclei, and a single prominent nucleolus.

■ Aside from the acinar growth, the most characteristic feature is the appearance of the cytoplasm, which includes the presence of fine to coarse, eosinophilic granules corresponding to zymogen granules.

■ Mitotic activity varies and ranges from rare mitotic figures to cases in which more than 50 mitoses per 10 high-power fields are seen. Atypical mitosis may be present.

■ Necrosis may be conspicuous.

■ Squamoid corpuscles (as seen in pancreatoblastomas) are not present.

■ Histochemistry: Diastase-resistant, PAS-positive intracytoplasmic granules are present in the great majority (more than 90%) of cases. Butyrate esterase stains for lipase are present in the majority of cases (more than 70%). Staining is localized to the apical regions of the cell. In a small percentage of cases, mucin positive staining may be seen in the apical surfaces of cells lining acini or glandular spaces.

■ *Immunohistochemistry:* Trypsin immunoreactivity is invariably present. In a majority of cases (more than 75%) cytokeratin or lipase immunoreactivity is seen. Less frequently, immunoreactivity with chymotrypsin and amylase is seen. Reactivity with epithelial membrane antigen, CEA, alpha-fetoprotein, chromogranin, and pancreatic endocrine peptide markers is absent.

■ *Electron microscopy:* Features of acinar cell differentiation are seen, including apically situated, electron-dense, membrane-bound zymogen granules measuring from 125 to 1000 nm in diameter and apical lumina lined by short microvilli. A second population of granules characterized by a haphazard distribution of pleomorphic elongated cytoplasmic granules measuring from 250 to 800 nm up to 3500 nm, and containing parallel arrays of electron-dense filamentous material have been described. These granules resemble the zymogen granules in the fetal pancreas and may represent a diagnostic feature of acinar cell carcinoma.

Differential Diagnosis

■ Pancreatic endocrine neoplasm (Chapter 12F, #1).
■ Pancreatoblastoma (Chapter 12E, #10).

■ Solid and papillary epithelial carcinoma (Chapter 12D, #3).
■ Ductal adenocarcinoma (Chapter 12E, #1).

Treatment and Prognosis

■ Complete surgical resection is the treatment of choice; however, because of the presence of invasive disease, complete surgical extirpation of the tumor may not always be possible.

■ The role of adjuvant radiotherapy or chemotherapy remains speculative, but prolonged survival may be achieved with these forms of supplemental therapy.

■ Acinar cell carcinoma is a highly aggressive tumor. Five-year survival rates are less than 6%, and mean survival is 18 months; however, the overall survival is better than that for pancreatic ductal adenocarcinoma. Acinar cell carcinoma in children may have a better prognosis than that in adults.

■ Metastatic disease commonly occurs either at presentation or subsequently; metastatic sites may include the liver, regional lymph nodes, gastrointestinal tract, mesentery, omentum, peritoneum, lung or chest wall, adrenal glands, abdominal wall or intra-abdominal dissemination, and spleen.

■ Patients treated by surgical resection have a slightly better mean survival as compared with patients treated by biopsy and bypass surgery or bypass surgery alone.

■ There is little statistical correlation between prognosis and any pathologic parameters except the size of the tumor. Patients with tumors of more than 10 cm have shorter mean survival times than those with tumors measuring less than 10 cm.

Additional Facts

■ A rare cystic variant or subtype termed **acinar cell cystadenocarcinoma** may be characterized by the following features:

1. Multiloculated tumor.
2. Cysts lined by acinar cells.
3. Solid nests or glands within the septa between the cysts.
4. Histochemistry, immunohistochemistry, and ultrastructural features similar to those of conventional types of acinar cell carcinoma.
5. Treatment and prognosis similar to that of conventional acinar cell carcinoma.

■ Given the presence of prominent acinar cell differentiation in pancreatoblastomas as well as the occurrence of acinar cell carcinomas in childhood, acinar cell carcinomas and pancreatoblastomas may represent a continuum in the spectrum of differentiation from a common progenitor cell.

■ Acinar cell adenoma is a dubious entity and in all probability is a small acinar cell carcinoma or a small islet cell tumor.

10. Pancreatoblastoma

Definition: Primitive pancreatic tumor showing multidirectional differentiation along epithelial, endocrine, and mesenchymal cell lines.

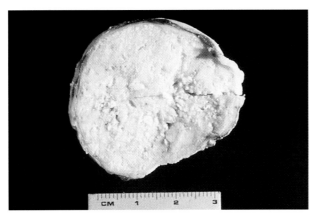

Figure 12–112. Pancreatoblastoma appears as a tan to yellow, delineated tumor with a soft to fleshy to firm consistency.

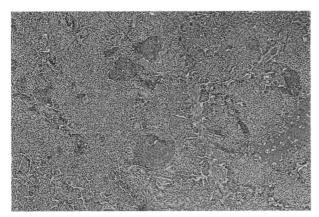

Figure 12–113. Pancreatoblastoma, showing solid and acinar growth patterns with scattered squamoid corpuscles.

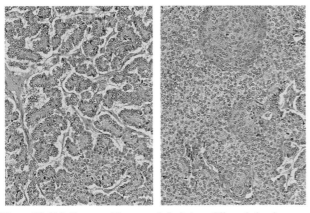

Figure 12–114. Pancreatoblastoma. *Left,* Acinar differentiation is apparent. *Right,* Squamoid corpuscles include whorled nests of cells with squamous differentiation, including keratinization.

Synonyms: Pancreatic carcinoma in childhood; infantile pancreatic carcinoma.

Clinical

- Rare.
- Slightly more common in men than in women; occurs most commonly in infancy and early childhood, with the

majority of cases occurring in the first decade of life (mean age, 4.1 years). It may involve older children in the second decade of life and rarely may occur in adults.
- Most patients present with an incidental abdominal mass. In addition, pain, weight loss, diarrhea, and obstructive jaundice may occur but are uncommon.
- In order of decreasing frequency, the sites of occurrence include the pancreatic head, body, and/or tail.
- Laboratory findings are nonspecific. Elevated serum alpha-fetoprotein levels may be present. Other tumor markers are not typically found. Serum levels of alpha-fetoprotein may be used as a marker of tumor recurrence.
- There are no known etiologic factors. Limited cases have been associated with Beckwith-Wiedemann syndrome (exophthalmos, macroglossia, and gigantism associated with an increased risk of malignant neoplasms), Cushing's syndrome, and inappropriate antidiuretic hormone secretion (SIADH).

Radiology

- Large solid tumors with associated hemorrhage.
- Metastatic tumor may be seen at presentation (liver, regional lymph nodes).

Pathology

Gross

- Partially encapsulated tumors measure from 1.5 to 20 cm in greatest dimension (mean, 10.6 cm).
- On cut section the tumors show prominent lobulation with a tan to yellow appearance and a soft to fleshy to firm consistency.
- Necrosis, cystic change, and calcifications may be present.

Histology

- Partially or unencapsulated tumors typically are associated with invasive growth into the surrounding pancreas and extrapancreatic region (duodenum, adjacent soft tissues) and with vascular and perineural invasion.
- The tumors are composed of a combination of epithelial and stromal components.
- The **epithelial** component predominates; it is cellular and has a lobulated, nested, organoid, and solid growth pattern. Lobules are separated by a fibrovascular stroma; the epithelial elements include the following:
  - **Acinar** differentiation—identical to that of acinar cell carcinoma.
  - **Endocrine** differentiation—often confirmed solely on immunohistochemical features (see later).
  - **Squamoid corpuscles**—vary from ill-defined whorled nests of cells to sharply delineated foci of well-developed squamous differentiation, including keratinization and a granular cell layer.
  - **Ductal** differentiation—occasionally found focally; it includes foci of tall columnar cells with abundant apical cytoplasm containing intracellular mucin and ectatic lumina.
- The **stromal** components are distinct from the epithelial components but are quite variable and include (acellular)

fibrous bands, hypercellular areas with plump fibroblasts or elongated, serpiginous nuclei. Metaplastic osteoid and chondroid may be present.

■ Mitotic activity is present and varies from as few as 1 in 10 high-power fields to as many as 42 in 10 high-power fields.

■ Foci of necrosis are invariably present and may show associated calcification.

■ *Histochemistry*
  • Acinar component: Diastase resistant, PAS positive, mucin positive, butyrate esterase positive.
  • Ductal component: Mucin positive.

■ *Immunohistochemistry*
  • Acinar component: Reacts with cytokeratin, epithelial membrane antigen, CEA, trypsin, chymotrypsin, lipase, CA 19-9, DUPAN-2, and alpha-fetoprotein. Endocrine component: Reacts with chromogranin, synaptophysin, and neuron-specific enolase. Peptide hormone stains may show the presence of rare positive cells for glucagon and vasoactive intestinal polypeptide (VIP). Insulin, gastrin, somatostatin, and pancreatic peptide are negative.
  • Squamoid corpuscles: CEA reactive.

■ *Electron microscopy:* Acini are arranged around central lumina, and there are numerous electron-dense zymogen granules measuring from 400–800 nm. Rare neurosecretory granules and mucigen granules may be present.

Differential Diagnosis

■ Acinar cell carcinoma (Chapter 12E, #9).
■ Mixed acinar-endocrine carcinoma (Chapter 12F, #4).
■ Solid and papillary epithelial carcinoma (Chapter 12D, #3).
■ Pancreatic endocrine neoplasm (Chapter 12G, #1).

Treatment and Prognosis

■ Surgical resection is the treatment of choice. Some tumors may be unresectable owing to extensive invasive growth or metastatic disease.

■ Adjunctive radiotherapy and chemotherapy may be beneficial, but their efficacy in controlling disease remains questionable.

■ Pancreatoblastomas are malignant tumors that have a tendency to recur locally, invade locally, or metastasize. Metastases usually occur to the liver, regional lymph nodes, and lung, with less frequent spread occurring to bone and the posterior mediastinum.

■ The prognosis is generally considered poor; the mean survival rate from the time of diagnosis to death is approximately 17 months. However, these tumors are potentially curable.
  • Long-term survival may occur, and death does not generally occur in patients who survive more than 3.5 years after diagnosis.
  • Pediatric patients who present with a palpable asymptomatic mass may have a good prognosis in that the tumors are detected early in the disease course (in a more localized stage) and are therefore more amenable to complete excision.

■ Adverse prognostic findings include the presence of metastatic disease, and occurrence in adults.

Additional Facts

■ Classification schemes based on tumor location have been proposed; these include:
  • Ventral pancreatoblastoma—tumors arising from the head or ventral pancreatic anlage, which are thought to have a better prognosis.
  • Dorsal pancreatoblastoma—tumors arising from the body or tail or dorsal pancreatic anlage, which are thought to have a worse prognosis.
  • This histologic classification scheme cannot be confirmed.

■ Given the presence of prominent acinar cell differentiation in pancreatoblastomas as well as the occurrence of acinar cell carcinomas in childhood, acinar cell carcinomas and pancreatoblastomas may represent a continuum in the spectrum of differentiation from a common progenitor cell.

F. PANCREATIC ENDOCRINE LESIONS

1. Pancreatic Endocrine Neoplasms (PEN)

Definition: Neoplastic proliferation arising from the pancreatic endocrine cells (islets of Langerhans) associated with a variety of clinical presentations, production of excessive pancreatic hormone(s), and unpredictable biologic behavior.

Synonyms: Islet cell tumor; islet cell carcinoma; insulinoma; gastrinoma; glucagonoma; VIPoma; somatostatinoma; PPoma; nesidioblastoma.

Clinical

■ Uncommon; represent less than 2% of all pancreatic neoplasms.

■ Approximately 1% of pancreata examined at autopsy have an incidental (microscopic) PEN.

Text continued on page 251

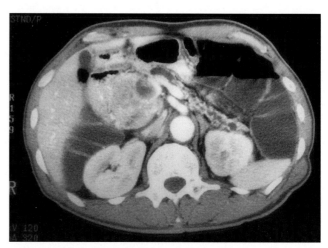

Figure 12–115. Pancreatic endocrine neoplasm. CT scan shows a large delineated predominantly solid tumor in the head of the pancreas.

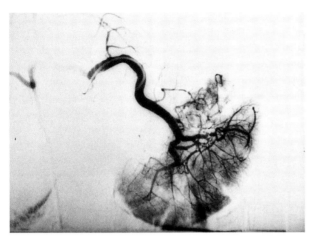

Figure 12–116. Angiography shows prominent vascularization of a pancreatic endocrine neoplasm that proved to be a vasoactive intestinal peptide-secreting tumor (VIPoma).

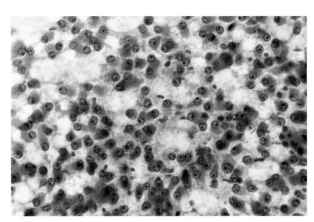

Figure 12–119. Pancreatic endocrine neoplasm, fine needle aspiration. The tumor is composed of small and uniform cells with small, round, often eccentrically located nuclei and abundant cytoplasm.

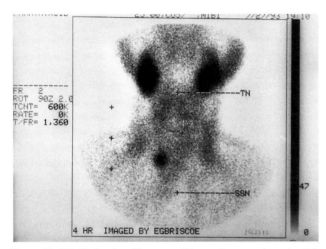

Figure 12–117. Technetium-99m sestamibi scan shows uptake to the right and above the substernal notch (SSN). This increased uptake represented metastasis to a supraclavicular lymph node from a pancreatic endocrine neoplasm (VIPoma—same tumor as shown in Figure 12–116). In addition, the patient had parathyroid hyperplasia as seen by the increased uptake of the parathyroid glands above the thyroid notch (TN) area, bilaterally.

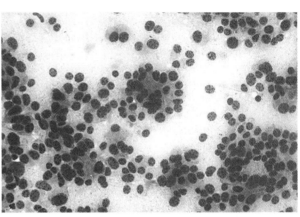

Figure 12–120. Pancreatic endocrine neoplasm, fine needle aspiration. Cells that resemble plasma cells are seen, including small and uniform cells with small, round, often eccentrically located nuclei, inconspicuous nucleoli, and a limited amount of eosinophilic cytoplasm.

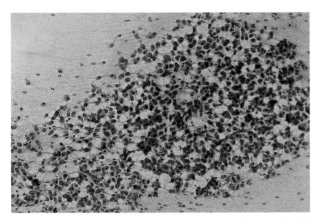

Figure 12–118. Pancreatic endocrine neoplasm, fine needle aspiration. Extremely cellular aspirate; smear background may have granular green tint on Diff-Quik stain.

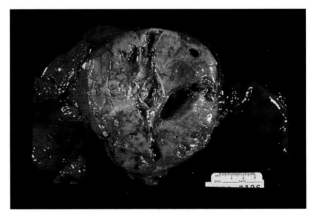

Figure 12–121. Pancreatic endocrine neoplasm, nonfunctioning, insulin-producing, appears as a well delineated, predominantly solid, tan-yellow tumor.

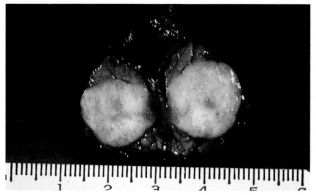

Figure 12–122. Pancreatic endocrine neoplasm, functioning, insulin-producing. This tumor is smaller (<2 cm) than the tumor illustrated in Figure 12–121. It is well circumscribed, firm, and tan-white in appearance.

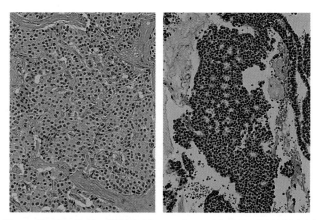

Figure 12–125. Pancreatic endocrine neoplasm with *(left)* solid and *(right)* microglandular (cribriform) patterns.

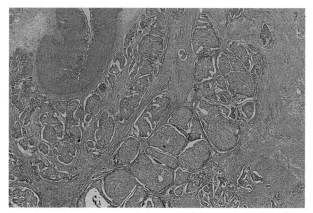

Figure 12–123. Pancreatic endocrine neoplasms are characterized by variability in growth patterns, including an organoid or lobular pattern, as seen in this illustration. This tumor is invasive.

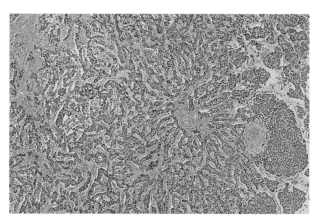

Figure 12–126. Pancreatic endocrine neoplasm with a trabecular ("hepatoid") appearance.

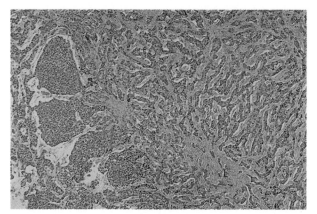

Figure 12–124. Pancreatic endocrine neoplasm with a predominantly trabecular or ribbon-like growth pattern; more lobular nests are seen to the left of the illustration.

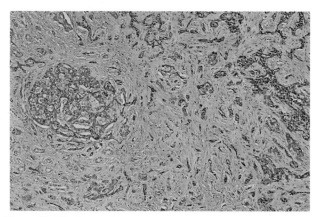

Figure 12–127. Pancreatic endocrine neoplasm with acini and strands of cells in dense fibrous tissue.

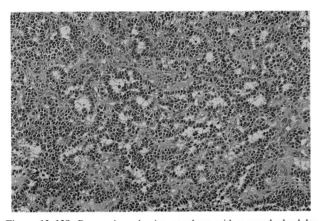

Figure 12–128. Pancreatic endocrine neoplasm with a pseudoglandular appearance.

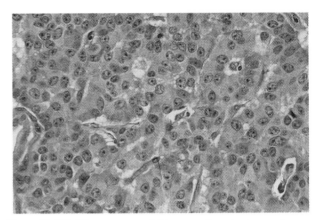

Figure 12–131. The appearance of this pancreatic endocrine neoplasm on high magnification, including foci of acinar-like growth and prominent eosinophilic nucleoli, can be confused with an acinar cell carcinoma.

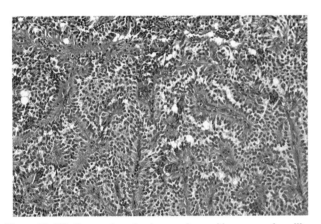

Figure 12–129. Pancreatic endocrine neoplasm with an unusual papillary pattern simulating the appearance of a solid and papillary epithelial carcinoma of the pancreas.

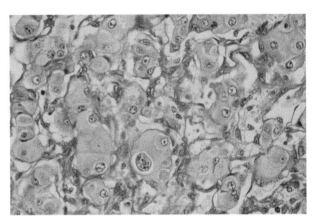

Figure 12–132. Occasionally, the cells in pancreatic endocrine neoplasms may be large, even giant sized, creating variations in the usual cytoplasmic appearance.

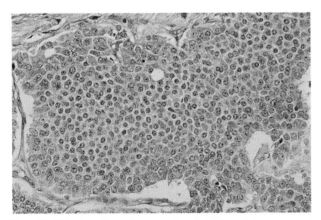

Figure 12–130. Regardless of the growth pattern, the cellular components of pancreatic endocrine neoplasms remain essentially the same. They include small to medium-sized, isomorphic neoplastic cells with uniform round to ovoid nuclei, abundant finely granular, eosinophilic cytoplasm, distinct nucleoli, and a stippled chromatin pattern.

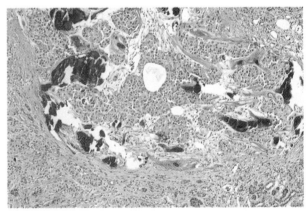

Figure 12–133. Stromal alterations associated with pancreatic endocrine neoplasms may include prominent calcifications, a finding that may suggest the possibility of a somatostatin-producing tumor.

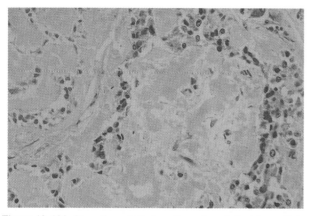

Figure 12–134. Stromal amyloid deposition, characterized by acellular, eosinophilic extracellular material, is seen in association with this pancreatic endocrine neoplasm.

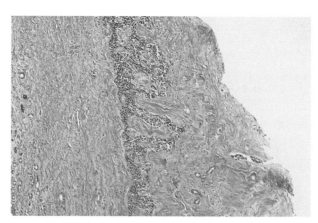

Figure 12–137. Pancreatic endocrine neoplasm with degenerative changes, including cyst formation and prominent fibrosis.

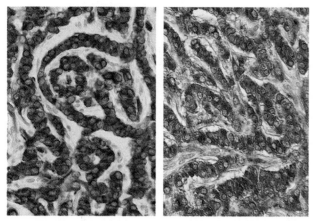

Figure 12–135. Immunohistochemical reactivity of pancreatic endocrine neoplasms invariably includes the presence of cytokeratin *(left)* and a neuroendocrine marker, such as chromogranin or synaptophysin *(right)*. The presence of pancreatic peptide hormone reactivity varies for any given tumor.

Figure 12–138. This pancreatic endocrine neoplasm shows an unusual sarcomatoid growth pattern. At the left, the tumor retains a typical architectural appearance that includes a trabecular and solid growth pattern; however, the majority of the tumor shows a fascicular or storiform growth pattern composed of spindle-shaped cells.

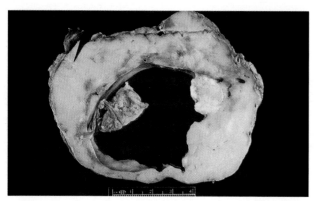

Figure 12–136. Pancreatic endocrine neoplasm with cystic change.

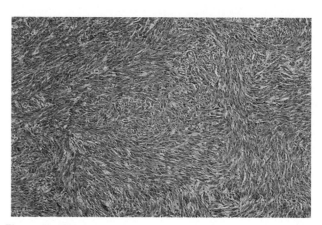

Figure 12–139. Sarcomatoid-appearing pancreatic endocrine neoplasm shows fascicular growth.

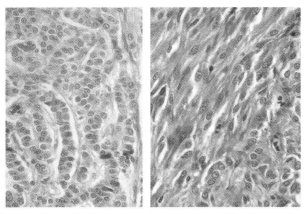

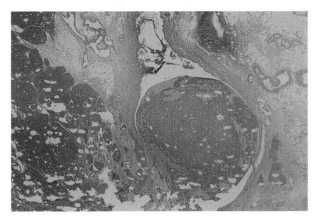

Figure 12–140. Sarcomatoid-appearing pancreatic endocrine neoplasm, showing the typical architectural and cytomorphologic appearance of this tumor *(left),* which contrasts with other areas of the tumor that demonstrate the unusual fascicular growth with spindle-shaped cells. It still retains the characteristic nuclear morphology that includes dispersed ("salt and pepper") nuclear chromatin.

Figure 12–143. Pancreatic endocrine neoplasm, showing invasion of a large-caliber vascular space.

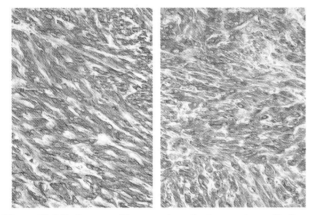

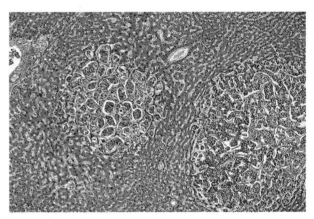

Figure 12–144. Pancreatic endocrine neoplasm metastatic to the liver.

Figure 12–141. Sarcomatoid pancreatic endocrine neoplasm. Confirmation of pancreatic endocrine cell derivation is demonstrated by the presence of *(left)* cytokeratin and *(right)* synaptophysin immunoreactivity. This tumor was immunoreactive with insulin.

- As a group, PEN are slightly more common in women than in men. They may occur at any age but are most common in adults, with the median age of occurrence in the sixth decade of life (the age at presentation may depend on whether the tumor is or is not associated with multiple endocrine neoplasia syndrome).
- Classification of PEN is based on the functional status of the tumor (production of pancreatic peptide hormone with an associated clinical syndrome) and includes nonfunctioning and functioning PEN. Functional capacity is not predicated on tumor size.

a. Nonfunctioning Pancreatic Endocrine Neoplasms

- Represent from 15% to 41% of all PEN.
- Not associated with a clinical syndrome, yet pancreatic hormone peptides can still be identified in tissue. The reasons for the lack of an associated syndrome may include (1) insufficient amount of hormone secretion into the bloodstream, (2) sufficient amount of hormone secretion

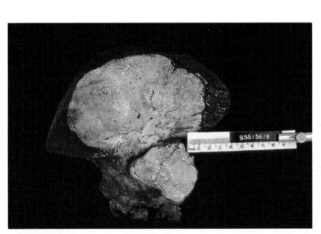

Figure 12–142. Pancreatic endocrine neoplasms are malignant neoplasms. In this example, the tumor invades the spleen.

but hormonal degradation occurs soon after secretion, and (3) functionally abnormal hormone secretion that is incapable of producing a clinical syndrome.

■ Clinical presentation includes an abdominal mass, pain in the abdomen and back, and/or jaundice due to pancreatic ductal obstruction.
■ Other findings may include ascites, weight loss, steatorrhea, fatigue, malaise, and mental confusion.

b. Functioning or Hormonally Active Pancreatic Endocrine Neoplasms
(Table 12–7)

■ Represent from 60% to 85% of all PEN.
■ Clinical presentation (signs and symptoms) depend on hormonal secretion by the tumor.

■ Insulin-producing tumors (insulinomas) are the most common, followed by gastrin-producing tumors (gastrinomas).

c. Insulinomas (Beta Cell Tumors)

■ Most common of the functioning PEN, representing from 30% to 70% of all functioning PEN.
■ The great majority are intrapancreatic or attached to the pancreas. Extrapancreatic neuroendocrine tumors associated with insulin production and symptoms related to hypoglycemia are extraordinarily rare.
■ Slightly more common in women than in men. Average age at presentation is in the middle of the fifth decade of life; rarely, it occurs in adolescence.
■ Clinical manifestations are due to hypoglycemia, with more than 80% of patients showing transient symptoms of

Table 12–7
COMPARISON OF FUNCTIONING PANCREATIC ENDOCRINE NEOPLASMS

Feature	Insulinoma	Gastrinoma	VIPoma	Glucagonoma	Somatostatinoma
Incidence	30%–70%	20%–25%	Approximately 3%	Rare (1%)	Very rare
Gender/age	F slightly > M; occurs in mid-5th decade, rarely in adolescence	M slightly > F; 5th–6th decades; rarely in adolescence	F > M; adults	F > M; adults	F > M; adults
Clinical	Solitary tumor; hypoglycemia, >80% of patients have transient symptoms of CNS dysfunction	ZES with symptoms related to gastric acid hypersecretion, including abdominal pain, diarrhea	VIPoma syndrome: watery diarrhea, hypokalemia, and achlorhydria (WDHA or Verner-Morrison syndrome)	Glucagonoma syndrome: necrolytic migratory erythema, impaired glucose intolerance, anemia (normochromic, normocytic), depression, constipation, venous thrombosis	Somatostatinoma syndrome: triad of diabetes, cholelithiasis, steatorrhea
Location	IP, any site	Majority located in "gastrinoma triangle"*; IP (head > tail and body) in patients without MEN 1; EP (duodenal wall) in patients with MEN 1	Vast majority (80%) are IP (body and tail); EP, including RP, adrenal gland, lung	IP (body and tail) or attached to pancreas	IP: head > tail, body; infiltrates into duodenum
Benign vs. malignant	>90% benign; <10% malignant	10%–40% benign; 60%–90% malignant	20%–30% benign; 70%–80% malignant	<30% benign; >70% malignant	10% benign; 90% malignant
Treatment	Surgery (simple excision or subtotal pancreatectomy)	Surgery for ZES in patients without MEN 1 is simple excision; for ZES in patients with MEN 1 possibly surgery; omeprazole is used to control gastric acid hypersecretion	Surgery (usually Whipple procedure)	Surgery (usually Whipple procedure)	Surgery (usually Whipple procedure
Prognosis	Excellent; 70%–90% have relief of symptoms or are cured	5-yr survival 62%–75%; 10-yr survival 47%–53%	Insufficient data	Insufficient data	Insufficient data
Metastases	5%–10%	Up to 60%; nodal metastasis early; liver metastasis late	40%	70%	70%
MEN 1	10%	Up to approximately 25%	Infrequent	Infrequent	Infrequent
MEN 1-related tumors (%)	30%	50%	12%	5%	Insufficient data

*The "gastrinoma triangle" is the triangle centered around the pancreatic head, including the duodenum.
IP, Intrapancreatic; EP, extrapancreatic; RP, retroperitoneum; ZES, Zollinger-Ellison syndrome; WDHA, watery diarrhea, hypokalemia, and achlorhydria syndrome.

CNS dysfunction ranging from drowsiness to loss of consciousness or coma. Most patients seek medical attention because of neuroglycopenia, and because of this the clinical differential diagnosis may include psychiatric or neurologic diseases.

- Laboratory tests include positive results for hyperinsulinemic hypoglycemia; the reactive or functional hypoglycemia that occurs following food or glucose ingestion is usually not a feature of insulinoma, but if present, it does not exclude an insulinoma.
- Diagnostic test results include an elevated insulin level in the presence of hypoglycemia. **Insulin suppression tests** in patients with insulinoma fail to show a decrease in circulating plasma immunoreactive insulin that parallels the decrease in glucose, thereby documenting the "inappropriate" insulin release characteristic of insulinomas. The monitored fast is the most reliable and sensitive of the insulin suppression tests. Other tests include the measurement of C peptide levels following the failure to suppress endogenous insulin release by insulinomas (this test is also used in recurrence of metastatic insulinoma after resection), and secretagogue tests based on the exaggerated release of insulin by insulinomas in response to secretagogues of insulin release (except plasma glucose), including tolbutamide, calcium, glucagon, and leucine.
- Insulinomas are generally solitary tumors that usually measure less than 3 cm in diameter and weigh less than 10 g. However, they may vary in size and may reach 15 cm in diameter and weigh up to 400 g. Multiple tumors can occur and may be found metachronously or at intervals years after the initial diagnosis. Multiple and multifocal (intrapancreatic) insulinomas also occur in patients with multiple endocrine neoplasia type 1 syndrome (MEN 1 or Wermer's syndrome), in which one tumor dominates both in size and hormonal status (see Chapter 15).
- Nonhypoglycemic presentations are rare and include mass effects or association with MEN 1.

d. Gastrinoma (G-Cell Tumors)

- This is the second most common of the functioning PEN, representing from 20% to 25% of all functioning PEN.
- Excessive gastrin secretion from gastrinomas results in **Zollinger-Ellison syndrome (ZES).**
- ZES is slightly more common in men than in women. Mean age at presentation is in the fifth to sixth decades of life; rarely it occurs in adolescence.
- In the majority of cases (60% to 75%) the tumor occurs as an isolated disease called **sporadic ZES,** unassociated with an inherited disease. In the remaining patients, ZES is a component of MEN 1 syndrome (**MEN 1–associated gastrinoma).**
- Rarely, hyperplasia and hyperfunction of gastric antral G cells may cause ZES-like symptoms, which have been referred to as pseudo-ZES.
- Islet cell hyperplasia is not a cause of ZES because pancreatic islets do not include gastrin cells.
- Except for patients with advanced (metastatic) disease, all symptoms in ZES patients result from gastric acid hypersecretion, including peptic ulceration and diarrhea.

- The most common associated complaint is abdominal pain due to gastric mucosal ulceration, which occurs in more than 75% of cases. The pain is indistinguishable from that of patients with peptic ulcer disease or peptic esophagitis, except that in ZES no relief is experienced following administration of antisecretory medication.
- Diarrhea is the second most common symptom in ZES after abdominal pain. It may occur independent of or associated with abdominal pain. Diarrhea results from direct mucosal contact by the increased volume of acid which causes structural alterations, including blunting of intestinal villi, superficial erosions, inflammation, edema, and hemorrhage.
- Additional clinical manifestations may include dysphagia, pyrosis, upper gastrointestinal bleeding, nausea, vomiting, and intestinal perforation.
- Endoscopic evaluation shows the presence of multiple ulcers in unusual locations, including the distal duodenum and jejunum. However, typical peptic ulcers occur in most patients, and up to one-quarter of patients have no ulcers.
- The majority of gastrinomas (approximately 80%) are located in a triangle centered around the pancreatic head and including the duodenum; this is referred to as the gastrinoma triangle.
- The majority of gastrinomas not associated with MEN 1 originate in the pancreas (in the head more often than the body and tail), but a small percentage of cases are extrapancreatic, arising in the duodenal wall (the most common extrapancreatic site). Unusual sites of occurrence include the stomach, jejunum, liver, biliary tract, kidney, and mesentery; these tumors tend to be small and multifocal.
- The majority (more than 90%) of gastrinomas associated with MEN 1 originate in the duodenum and are solitary and large.
- The single best screening test for ZES is the elevated fasting serum gastrin concentrations. In addition, patients with ZES have hypersecretion of acid (hyperchlorhydria). However, elevated fasting serum gastrin levels or hyperchlorhydria are not restricted to ZES and occur in a wide variety of diseases, including achlorhydria associated with pernicious anemia or atrophic gastritis, renal failure, following small bowel resection, retained gastric antrum syndrome, antral G-cell hyperplasia, and chronic gastric outlet obstruction.
- Given the number of diseases that can simulate ZES with fasting hypergastrinemia and hyperchlorhydria, **provocative tests** are required, including the secretin provocative test, calcium provocative test, and meal provocative test. In patients with ZES, **secretin provocative testing** results in a 200 pg/ml (or more) increase in gastrin levels following administration of a secretin bolus. Secretin provocative tests are negative in the other diseases associated with elevated fasting serum gastrin levels.
- In patients with MEN 1, hypercalcemia secondary to primary hyperparathyroidism is the most common clinical abnormality, followed by symptomatology related to the presence of a functional PEN. Patients with MEN 1 and ZES almost always have hyperparathyroidism at the time of diagnosis.

e. Other Functioning PEN

- The other types of functioning PEN are uncommon; they originate predominantly within the pancreas and include:

  1. **VIPoma** due to excess production of vasoactive intestinal polypeptide (VIP) causing **VIPoma syndrome,** characterized by watery diarrhea, hypokalemia, and achlorhydria (WDHA syndrome or Verner-Morrison syndrome). The great majority of VIPomas are of pancreatic origin. VIPomas also secrete peptide histidine methionine (PHM), flanking peptide of VIP, pancreatic polypeptide, and neurotensin. PHM may contribute to the VIPoma syndrome, but there is no evidence that PHM or neurotensin do.

  2. **Glucagonoma (alpha cell tumors)** due to excess production of glucagon causing **glucagonoma syndrome,** characterized by skin rash (necrolytic migratory erythema), impaired glucose intolerance sometimes with mild diabetes, anemia (normochromic, normocytic), severe depression or other psychiatric disturbances, constipation and other altered bowel habits, and severe life-threatening venous thrombosis.

  3. **Somatostatinoma (delta cell tumors)** due to excess production of somatostatin causing **somatostatinoma syndrome,** characterized by the triad of diabetes due to inhibition of insulin secretion, cholelithiasis caused by inhibition of gallbladder contraction, and steatorrhea (in 90% of cases) caused by inhibition of pancreatic and gallbladder secretion.

  4. No syndrome is associated with pure **pancreatic polypeptide producing tumors (PPoma).** However, there is a high incidence of PPomas in MEN 1-associated PEN, and pancreatic polypeptide hormone levels have been suggested as a screening tool in patients who either have MEN 1 syndrome or are thought to have it.

- Other syndromes that may infrequently occur with PEN include those with ectopic hormone production, including Cushing's syndrome due to production of ACTH; acromegaly due to production of growth hormone or growth hormone-releasing factor; carcinoid syndrome (flushing and diarrhea) due to production of serotonin; and paraneoplastic hypercalcemia due to production of parathyroid hormone or parathyroid hormone-related protein (PTHrP).

- PEN may produce multiple hormones, but the occurrence of an associated combined hormonal syndrome is rare. In general, clinical hormonal syndromes correlate with hypersecretion of only one hormone. Transitions from one syndrome to another may occur over time or following treatment.

Radiology

- Large tumors and hepatic metastases are readily identified by ultrasound or CT scan.
- Small tumors may be difficult to detect and require a combination of ultrasound, CT scan with contrast, and arteriography. This combination has resulted in a 70% specificity and 100% sensitivity.

- The appearance of nonfunctioning PEN on CT scans may be indistinguishable from that of adenocarcinoma. However, compared to adenocarcinoma, PEN tend to be larger (4 to 6 cm with some over 10 cm), and following contrast enhancement parts of the PEN are hypervascular (other parts are hypovascular); metastatic PEN are also hypervascular. There is absence of thickening of the celiac axis, a common finding in adenocarcinoma, and PEN may show evidence of calcifications, which are not a feature of adenocarcinoma.
- In contrast to nonfunctioning PEN, functioning PEN, particularly insulinomas, are small, measuring less than 2 cm, and rarely alter the contour of the pancreas.
- The appearance of insulinoma on CT scans includes the presence of a small, round to oval, well-delineated or marginated solid mass that enhances following intravenous contrast enhancement; this enhancement is transient, necessitating the use of rapid scanning.
- Gastrinomas also tend to be small and extrahepatic and are often difficult to identify radiographically. Pancreatic gastrinomas may present as a hypodense mass often with associated necrosis.

Pathology

Fine Needle Aspiration

- Extremely cellular aspirates are seen; smear background may have granular green tint on Diff-Quik stain.
- Cellular clusters (aggregates) and single-cell pattern are evident. Vascularized tissue fragments, including branching capillaries encased by neoplastic cells, may be seen.
- Cells are generally small and uniform with small, round, and often eccentrically located nuclei, inconspicuous nucleoli, and a limited amount of eosinophilic cytoplasm. The cytologic appearance may resemble that of plasma cells.
- Occasionally, large atypical cells may be present.

Gross

- Most neoplasms are fairly well defined; a capsule may or may not be evident.
- PEN tend to be firm, especially if considerable fibrosis is present; they are tan-gray to pink to red, or yellowish in color. Cystic changes may occur in larger tumors.
- Nonfunctioning tumors are large, measuring on average 4 to 6 cm, but larger sizes can be attained.
- Functioning tumors tend to be small, measuring less than 2 cm in diameter but larger than 0.5 cm in diameter (0.5 cm is the minimum size at which a PEN can be detected).

Histology

- The light microscopic features are the same for all PEN. Purely by light microscopy, it is not possible to determine whether a PEN is nonfunctional or functional, and if functional, what its hormone production might be. Two possible exceptions to this statement include (1) PEN with an amyloid stroma, which typically occurs in insulinomas, and (2) PEN found in the ampullary region with a glandular growth and calcifications, which are most suggestive of somatostatinomas.

- PEN may show many different growth patterns in any one tumor, but one type of growth predominates, including solid (diffuse or medullary), trabecular, ribbon-like, gyriform, or cerebriform patterns. Other patterns include glandular structures, acini, and strands of cells in dense fibrous tissue. Rarely, sarcomatoid growth, including fascicular or storiform patterns, can be seen.
- The neoplastic cells are usually small to medium-sized, usually round but occasionally elongated; they have fairly regular round to ovoid nuclei, abundant finely granular, eosinophilic cytoplasm, distinct nucleoli, and a stippled chromatin pattern. The nuclei are relatively isomorphic but occasionally are large, even giant sized. Variations in the usual cytoplasmic appearance include the presence of clear cytoplasm or, rarely, oxyphilic (oncocytic) changes.
- The stroma components also vary from hyalinized or fibrotic to vascular to fibrovascular. Stromal amyloid deposition, characterized by acellular, eosinophilic extracellular material, may be present.
- Calcifications, appearing as irregular stromal masses or psammomatoid bodies, are infrequently seen. The presence of calcifications or psammomatoid bodies may suggest the diagnosis of a somatostatin-secreting tumor.
- In general, limited changes are seen in the non-neoplastic exocrine pancreas; however, strategically situated PEN may cause pancreatic ductal obstruction, resulting in changes characteristic of chronic pancreatitis.
- In the presence of a solitary PEN or a PEN not associated with MEN 1, or in gastrinomas, the non-neoplastic pancreatic endocrine components show limited alterations. In the presence of MEN 1 or a gastrinoma (without MEN 1), islet cell hyperplasia or changes of nesidioblastosis may be present. In the case of a gastrinoma, these alterations are probably the result of the trophic effects of hypergastrinemia.
- Microscopic foci of PEN, measuring less than 0.5 cm in diameter, occur, often as an incidental finding in pancreata removed for other reasons or at autopsy. In contrast to hyperplastic islets, microscopic foci show associated intratumoral fibrosis or sclerosis or may have an amyloid stroma. Hyperplastic islets do not show associated fibrosis; however, this differentiation may be difficult or impossible to make.
- On the basis of histology alone it is difficult to predict the biologic behavior of a given PEN (i.e., benignancy versus malignancy). **Histologic criteria that may suggest malignant behavior** include invasion into adjacent pancreatic parenchyma, vascular invasion, and invasion into peripancreatic soft tissue; however, the only definitive criteria for malignancy in PEN is the presence of invasion into adjacent organs or the presence of metastatic disease.
- Histochemistry: Epithelial mucin stains (mucicarmine, PAS with diastase) are generally negative, but mucus droplets may be identified in glandular or ductal structures, or when goblet cells are present. Little or no glycogen, as identified by PAS stain, is apparent. Intracytoplasmic or extracellular PAS-positive globules (possibly containing α_1-antitrypsin) can be seen. Argyrophilic stains, including Grimelius' or Churukian-Schenk's stains, are often positive. Congo red stains are positive in PEN with stromal amyloid.

- *Immunohistochemistry*
  - For all PEN, immunoreactivity is seen with cytokeratin, chromogranin, synaptophysin, and neuron-specific enolase.
  - Most PEN react with one or more peptide hormone markers, including insulin, gastrin, glucagon, somatostatin, VIP, and pancreatic polypeptide; some will react with serotonin.
  - PEN are nonreactive with trypsin, amylase, lipase, and vimentin.
- *Electron microscopy:* Membrane-bound neurosecretory granules, characteristic of all neuroendocrine tumors, are present and resemble those of the islet cells from which the tumor arises. Neurosecretory granules may vary in size and shape depending on the specific hormone that is stored. Even in functionally active tumors, neurosecretory granules may not be recognizable.
- Morphometric studies, DNA ploidy studies, proliferation indices, and nucleolar organizer region-associated protein studies have yielded conflicting data about their efficacy in determining the biologic potential of PEN.
- Oncogenic studies of PEN, including analyses for mutations, activations, chromosomal deletions, gene amplifications, and promoter insertions, have produced conflicting data about the genetic alterations leading to tumorigenesis as well as about the biologic behavior of PEN.

Differential Diagnosis

- Solid and papillary epithelial carcinoma (Chapter 12D, #3).
- Acinar cell carcinoma (Chapter 12E, #9).
- Localized hyperplasia of pancreatic endocrine islets (in the presence of microscopic foci of PEN).
- Chronic pancreatitis with prominent islets due to loss of exocrine pancreatic parenchymal elements (Chapter 11G, #2).

Treatment and Prognosis

- Surgery is the treatment of choice for all PEN; however, the goal of surgical therapy and the outcome following surgery are affected by many variables related to the clinical situation, including the specific tumor type (i.e., insulinoma, gastrinoma, or other), presence or absence of metastatic disease, presence or absence of a clinical syndrome, and association with (i.e., MEN 1-associated PEN) or independent of (i.e., sporadic PEN) a familial setting.
- Surgical intervention may include simple excision (enucleation) or resection. The type of surgery depends on the type of tumor and its expected malignancy rate, its location, the medical status of the patient, and the expected quality of life for the patient after resection compared with that without resection.
  - Simple excision can be performed for small tumors that are not locally invasive or do not involve the pancreatic duct or vessels, but it is of critical importance to determine the relationship of the tumor to the pancreatic duct prior to surgical excision. Simple excision can be per-

formed for tumors in the tail and body of the pancreas and even for select tumors in the head of the pancreas (see discussion below under gastrinomas). Simple excision allows preservation of the pancreas and spleen.

- Pancreatic resection is commonly performed for gastrinomas, somatostatinomas, and glucagonomas because these tumors are often malignant.

■ Intraoperative ultrasound facilitates the precise operative detection and localization of the tumor, especially tumors lying deep within the pancreatic parenchyma that are difficult to detect by palpation.

■ For **insulinomas,** which are usually solitary intrapancreatic tumors, localization followed by simple excision is the treatment of choice.

- Medical therapy, used for insulinomas that cannot be localized but that can be symptomatically controlled, is primarily directed at control of symptoms referable to hypoglycemia by dietary management or by drug therapy, including diazoxide, which suppresses insulin secretion.

■ For **gastrinomas,** treatment is directed at controlling gastric acid hypersecretion as well as at the tumor itself.

- Gastric acid hypersecretion associated with ZES is managed by medical therapy rather than surgery. Omeprazole, a potent, long-acting inhibitor of gastric acid secretion, is the drug used. Surgical management depends on the location of the tumor and the clinical setting.

- Intrapancreatic nonmetastatic sporadic gastrinomas occur more often in the head than in the tail and body of the pancreas. In the tail and body, a subtotal or distal pancreatectomy can be performed. For gastrinomas of the head of the pancreas, simple excision rather than a Whipple procedure is advocated because this decreases postoperative morbidity and mortality; despite the higher rates of malignancy seen with gastrinomas, long-term survival (at least 10 years) occurs in the great majority of these patients (80% to 90%) with simple excision. Further, there is no increase in the survival of patients undergoing a Whipple procedure.

- The role of surgery in the treatment of gastrinomas in patients with ZES with MEN 1 is uncertain. In these patients, many gastrinomas are not in the pancreas but in the duodenum, where they are multiple and small. In these patients, extensive localization studies are indicated; patients with unequivocally positive imaging studies undergo surgical exploration and resection with palpation of the remainder of the duodenum from inside the lumen. One goal of surgical resection of duodenal gastrinomas is to reduce the risk of metastatic disease.

- Surgical management of gastric acid hypersecretion, including vagotomy and total gastrectomy, has largely been replaced by the availability of effective medical therapy. However, surgical management is still used for patients who do not respond to medical therapy or in whom the gastrinoma is unresectable owing to multicentricity, metastatic disease, or inability to localize the tumor.

■ For other, less common, types of PEN such as glucagonoma, somatostatinoma, and VIPoma and for nonfunctional PEN, surgical resection is indicated if the tumor can be completely removed and the patient is medically capable of undergoing surgery.

- Because these tumors tend to have a higher malignancy rate, resection rather than simple excision is often indicated. Tumors in the pancreatic head require the Whipple procedure, and tumors in the tail and body require partial pancreatectomy with splenectomy.

- Medical management for the less common functional PEN is only partially effective; therefore, debulking surgery may assist in ameliorating symptoms and in increasing the efficacy of medical management.

■ The role of surgery in the management of patients with MEN 1-associated PEN is controversial because these tumors are characteristically multiple, and removal of any one tumor may not result in cure or amelioration of symptoms. Further, these tumors may have a lower malignant potential than sporadic PEN, thereby calling into question the need for surgical removal. Effective medical management of the symptoms of hormonal excess may obviate the need for surgery in these patients.

- In patients with MEN 1, primary hyperparathyroidism, and ZES, initial surgery should include removal of the abnormal parathyroid glands; following this, if a dominant PEN is found, it should be surgically excised (type of surgery depends on location). Because these patients may also have duodenal tumors, the duodenum should be explored for the presence of tumor; if found, it should be treated accordingly (by surgery), which often reduces symptoms.

- In the rare examples of patients with MEN 2 and a PEN, simple resection of the tumor is indicated.

■ Surgery in the presence of metastatic PEN often is beneficial to the patient.

- Complete resection of metastatic foci may be curative and may result in long-term survival.

- Partial resection and/or debulking may be beneficial in relieving symptoms (e.g., pain) or in enhancing the efficacy of either medical management (of symptoms related to hormonal excess) or adjuvant therapy (e.g., chemotherapy).

■ Chemotherapy is a valuable adjunct in the treatment of patients with metastatic disease, but the role of radiotherapy is limited and of questionable efficacy.

Prognosis

Insulinoma

- More than 90% of insulinomas are benign and are cured by complete surgical resection. If a tumor cannot be imaged in the pancreas or liver by radiographic studies in a patient with an insulinoma, it is assumed to be benign.

- Less than 10% of insulinomas are malignant. Metastases may occur years following the diagnosis. Up to one-third of patients have metastasis at the time of diagnosis. Tumors that prove to be malignant usually measure more than 3 cm in diameter.

- Five-year and 10-year survival rates are excellent.

Gastrinoma

- Five-year survival rates for all patients with ZES range from 62% to 75%.

- Ten-year survival rates for all patients with ZES range from 47% to 53%.
- Tumor extent is an important prognostic factor. In patients with no tumor at laparotomy or in whom tumor is completely excised, 5- and 10-year survival rates reach 90% to 100%; in patients with incomplete resection of tumor or unresectable disease, 5-year survival is 43% and 10-year survival is 25%.
- Patients with ZES and MEN 1 frequently present at an earlier age and possibly at an earlier stage of disease than patients with ZES only and therefore may have a better prognosis.
- The majority (60% to 90%) of gastrinomas are malignant and 10% to 40% are benign.

Other Functional PEN
- Greater than 70% of glucagonomas are malignant.
- Ninety percent of somatostatinomas are malignant.
- Fifty percent of VIPomas are malignant.
- The majority of PPomas are benign.
- Surgically removed nonfunctioning tumors are frequently malignant.
- Metastatic disease from PEN occurs most frequently to regional lymph nodes and liver. Delayed metastases may occur years (a decade or more) after the initial diagnosis. Therefore, close and continuous follow-up of all patients with PEN is indicated because even the most innocuous-appearing PEN may ultimately prove to be malignant, further indicating that the pathologic parameters are not predictive of the biologic behavior of this tumor. Hence, the diagnostic designation of these tumors as pancreatic endocrine neoplasms appended by its hormonal secretion (e.g., insulin-producing, gastrin-producing, etc.) is preferable to such designations as islet cell tumor, insulinoma, gastrinoma, and so on because any type of PEN is potentially malignant.

2. Nesidioblastosis

Definition: Diffuse or focal islet cell hyperplasia resulting in symptoms related to hyperinsulinemic hypoglycemia. Nesidioblastosis is derived from the Greek word *nesos,* meaning island. Nesidioblastosis is a physiologic process for the budding-off of endocrine cells from the duct epithelium (islet neogenesis). However, the term is used to indicate an absolute increase in mass of insulin-producing cells. This term is used for all types of islet cell hyperplasia.

Synonyms: Islet adenomatosis; pancreatic endocrine microadenomatosis.

Clinical

- Hyperinsulinemic hypoglycemia in adults is primarily caused by a pancreatic endocrine tumor (insulinoma) and rarely due to islet cell hyperplasia.
- Hyperinsulinemic hypoglycemia in neonates, children, and adolescents is primarily caused by islet cell hyperplasia and rarely by a pancreatic endocrine tumor (insulinoma).

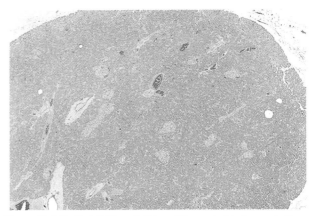

Figure 12–145. Nesidioblastosis (islet cell hyperplasia). An area in the resected pancreas shows multiple variably sized islets; the islets have an irregular contour and vary in size and shape. By conventional light microscopic staining (hematoxylin and eosin), it is difficult to identify individually scattered or dispersed pancreatic endocrine cells within the exocrine pancreas.

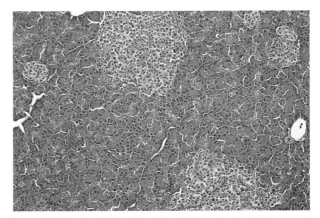

Figure 12–146. Nesidioblastosis (islet cell hyperplasia). Higher magnification shows variably sized islets. Even at this magnification, it is difficult to identify individually scattered pancreatic endocrine cells within the exocrine pancreas.

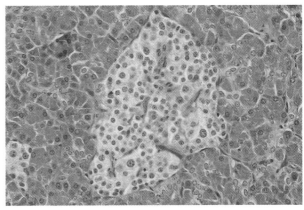

Figure 12–147. Additional features seen in nesidioblastosis (islet cell hyperplasia) include the presence of nesidiodysplasia (nuclear pleomorphism) with nucleomegaly.

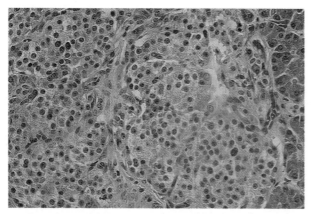

Figure 12–148. Another feature that can be seen in nesidioblastosis (islet cell hyperplasia) is the presence of ductuloinsular complexes, including the merging of endocrine cells with pancreatic exocrine ducts.

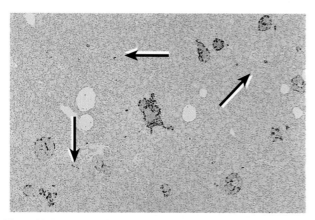

Figure 12–149. Nesidioblastosis. Chromogranin immunoreactivity delineates the islet cell nests as well as the scattered or dispersed endocrine cells *(arrows)* that lie admixed within the exocrine pancreas. The latter are virtually impossible to identify definitively by conventional stains.

■ In approximately 75% of patients, symptoms become manifest during the first 3 months of life; 90% of patients show symptoms within the first 12 months of life.

■ Nesidioblastosis in infants is often severe, with clinical manifestations that include somnolence, ataxia, seizures, and loss of consciousness. Patients may become hypoglycemic after only a few hours of fasting, and other patients become hypoglycemic even when receiving intravenous glucose therapy. Some infants develop hypoglycemia when given leucine or a high protein meal (leucine-sensitive hypoglycemia).

■ Neonates with hyperinsulinemic hypoglycemia tend to be large for gestational age, appearing obese and plethoric.

■ The symptoms of nesidioblastosis in older children may not be as severe as those in infants.

■ **Laboratory findings:** Abnormally high serum insulin concentrations and coexistent hypoglycemia.

■ Nesidioblastosis may be acquired or inherited.

　• Acquired causes of hyperinsulinemic hypoglycemia (other than islet cell hyperplasia) include ketotic hypoglycemia (which accounts for 90% of children with hypoglycemia beyond infancy), pituitary failure, and malicious insulin administration.

　• Inherited or genetic causes of hyperinsulinemic hypoglycemia include glycogen storage diseases or disorders of gluconeogenesis, Beckwith-Wiedemann syndrome characterized by neonatal hypoglycemia, omphalocele, macroglossia, gigantism, invariant visceromegaly, and susceptibility to abdominal malignancies (e.g., neuroblastoma), cerebrohepatorenal syndrome (Bowen-Zellweger syndrome).

■ The pathogenesis and etiology remain obscure.

Pathology

Gross

■ In focal nesidioblastosis the pancreas most often appears normal, but a small nodule or area of increased consistency, measuring less than 1 cm, may be found.

■ In diffuse nesidioblastosis the pancreas appears normal.

Histology

■ In focal nesidioblastosis there is a single focus or multiple foci in which a confluence of islets or dispersion of individual islet cells is seen within the exocrine pancreas. Ductuloinsular complexes, including a merging of endocrine cells with pancreatic exocrine ducts, are also seen.

■ In diffuse nesidioblastosis variably sized islets are seen throughout the pancreas. The islets have an irregular contour and vary in size and shape. Dispersed individual islet cells within the exocrine pancreas and ductuloinsular complexes are seen.

■ The cytomorphologic features, regardless of extent of disease, include the presence of nesidiodysplasia with islet cell hypertrophy and nuclear pleomorphism, including nucleomegaly.

■ The exocrine pancreas shows minimal alterations.

■ Histochemistry: Not of much assistance in diagnosis.

■ *Immunohistochemistry:* Chromogranin, synaptophysin, and neuron-specific enolase are useful for demonstrating the distribution of islet cells, including individually scattered endocrine cells within the exocrine pancreatic elements.

　• In focal nesidioblastosis, islets react with insulin, glucagon, somatostatin, and pancreatic polypeptide. Distribution is near normal, but insulin cells are more numerous. The presence of multiple pancreatic peptide immunoreactivity with near-normal distribution contrasts with the immunoreactive profile seen in PEN.

　• In diffuse nesidioblastosis, a reactive pattern similar to that seen in focal disease is found, but there appears to be no increase in the number of insulin cells.

■ *Electron microscopy:* Neurosecretory granules, predominantly beta and alpha granules are seen.

Differential Diagnosis

■ Factitious hypoglycemia (clinical differential diagnosis).

■ Pancreatic endocrine neoplasm (Chapter 12F, #1).

■ Prominent islets in chronic pancreatitis due to acinar and ductal atrophy (Chapter 11G, #2).

Treatment and Prognosis

- The goal of therapy is to avoid hypoglycemia.
  - In infants and younger children with hyperinsulinemia, more often caused by islet cell hyperplasia, medical therapy is used, including a combination of diazoxide and subcutaneous injections of somatostatin (inhibitors of insulin secretion) and, for short-term control, glucagon infusions. In addition, frequent feedings (low protein and high carbohydrate), avoidance of fasting, and glucose infusions, are administered.
  - If normoglycemia cannot be attained by medical therapy, surgical exploration is indicated. In these patients, the choice of surgery depends on whether or not a focal lesion can be identified.
  - If a focal lesion is found, partial pancreatectomy is performed. Patients with severe hypoglycemia continue on medical therapy, but a total pancreatectomy to control hypoglycemia may be necessary.
  - If a neoplasm is not found or if nesidioblastosis is diffuse, near-total (95%) pancreatectomy is indicated.
  - Patients with focal head of pancreas involvement may also require near-total or total pancreatectomy.
  - In older children and adults with hyperinsulinemia, more often caused by a tumor, localization and surgical removal is the treatment of choice.
- Prognosis is generally good.
  - For patients with focal disease, surgical resection often proves curative.
  - Patients with diffuse or multifocal disease are more problematic because recurrent hypoglycemia may follow subtotal pancreatectomy (in 75% to 80%); in these patients, near-total (95%) or total pancreatectomy resolves the hypoglycemic state.
- Early recognition and diagnosis are essential to avoid complications of persistent hypoglycemia, including permanent neurologic damage and severe mental retardation.

Additional Facts

- Hyperinsulinemic hypoglycemia in adults not due to a PEN is rare (**adult nesidioblastosis**). The histologic features seen in adults differ from those seen in infants and children; often nesidiodysplasia and ductuloinsular complexes are absent.

3. Neuroendocrine Tumor of the Pancreas: Carcinoid and Small Cell Neuroendocrine Carcinoma

- These types of neuroendocrine tumors are rare in the pancreas.

a. Carcinoid Tumors of the Pancreas

- Uncommon.
- All are considered malignant.
- Tumors are morphologically identical to those more commonly identified in other sites, such as the gastrointestinal tract.

- Carcinoid tumors characterized by carcinoid syndrome, including flushing, diarrhea, right-sided valvular heart disease, and bronchial asthma (wheezing), are uncommon but may be associated with a pancreatic-based tumor if the tumor secretes serotonin or metastasizes to the liver and produces sufficient serotonin.
- True carcinoids of the pancreas should include only those tumors that produce serotonin or its precursor 5-hydroxytryptophan.
- The cell of origin is probably a serotonin-secreting cell of pancreatic ducts.
- Pancreatic carcinoids are derived from the foregut and therefore stain with argyrophilic stains (e.g., Grimelius', Churukian-Schenk) but typically do not stain with argentaffin stains (e.g., Fontana-Masson stain).

b. Small Cell Neuroendocrine Carcinoma of the Pancreas

- Probably does not exist as a primary pancreatic tumor.
- If found in the pancreas, metastasis from another site, such as the lung, should be excluded.
- May be associated with hypercalcemia or ectopic ACTH production.

Additional Facts

- Neuroendocrine tumors of the pancreas or ampulla must be differentiated from the so-called **gangliocytic paraganglioma,** which is characterized by the following features:
  - Occur almost exclusively in the second portion of the duodenum near the ampulla of Vater; a small percentage may occur in the jejunum.
  - Occur in men more than women; most common in the fifth decade of life.
  - Present with gastrointestinal bleeding, nausea, or vomiting; there are no endocrinopathic clinical manifestations.
  - Can occur in association with neurofibromatosis or carcinoid tumor.

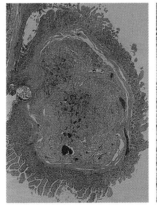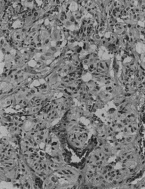

Figure 12–150. Gangliocytic paraganglioma. *Left,* Submucosal cellular proliferation with a nested and organoid growth, and fibrovascular stroma. *Right,* Higher magnification shows that the cell nests are composed of cells with a carcinoid-like appearance, including small, round uniform nuclei, stippled chromatin, and granular cytoplasm.

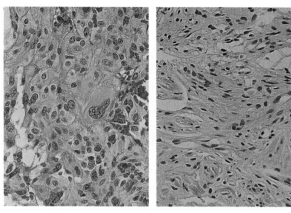

Figure 12–151. Gangliocytic paraganglioma. *Left,* Isolated ganglion cells include large polygonal cells with prominent round nuclei and eosinophilic nucleoli. *Right,* Other areas of the same tumor show the presence of spindle cells with features of a neurofibroma.

- Usually solitary, small, polypoid or pedunculated submucosal mass with associated surface ulceration or villous atrophy; it may be multiple and usually measures less than 2 cm in diameter.
- Histology: Composed of nested, organoid, and trabecular growth with fibrovascular stroma with an admixture of cell types, including (1) endocrine cells with a carcinoid-like appearance (small, round uniform nuclei, stippled chromatin, granular cytoplasm); (2) isolated ganglion cells (large polygonal cells with prominent round nuclei and eosinophilic nucleoli); (3) spindle cells with typical features of neurofibroma, including Schwann's cells and neurites.
- Insinuating growth within the lamina propria of the duodenal mucosa, extending into the submucosa or even to the serosa.
- *Immunohistochemistry:* Endocrine cells—immunoreactivity with neuroendocrine cell markers (chromogranin, synaptophysin), neuron-specific enolase, cytokeratin, CAM 5.2, somatostatin, pancreatic polypeptide, and rarely gastrin; ganglion cells—immunoreactivity with neuron-specific enolase, neurofilament, somatostatin, neuroendocrine cell markers (weakly positive); spindle cells—immunoreactivity with S-100 protein, neuron-specific enolase, neurofilament.
- Benign clinical course, even in the presence of nodal metastasis.
- May represent a hamartomatous process (related to the ventral primordium of the pancreas) rather than a neoplastic process.

4. Mixed Exocrine-Endocrine Pancreatic Tumors

- The existence of this mixed tumor is debatable; if it exists, it is extraordinarily rare.
- Acceptance is predicated on the presence of both exocrine cell and endocrine cell differentiation in a single tumor and also in any metastatic foci.
- Admixture of normal exocrine (non-neoplastic) elements in a PEN or admixture of normal (non-neoplastic) endocrine cells in a pancreatic exocrine tumor (e.g., adenocarcinoma) must be excluded.

5. Mixed Acinar-Endocrine Pancreatic Tumors

- Another rare tumor type.
- Occurs in adults.
- Presentation may include abdominal pain, nausea, backache, hematemesis; may also be found incidentally in a work-up for unrelated problems. It is not associated with systemic problems related to excess endocrine hormone secretion nor with the subcutaneous fat necrosis or polyarthralgia seen in acinar cell carcinomas.
- Occurs in all pancreatic sites.

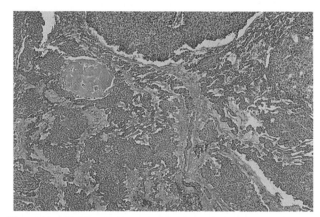

Figure 12–152. Mixed acinar-endocrine pancreatic tumor. On light microscopy, this tumor shows the presence of solid and acinar cell *(to the right of center)* growth patterns.

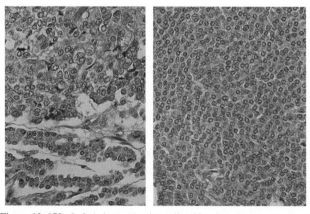

Figure 12–153. *Left,* Acinar appearing cells with acinar growth, prominent nucleoli, and cytoplasmic eosinophilic granularity. Less differentiated larger cells appear in the upper portion of this illustration. *Right,* Endocrine-appearing cells composed of small, round uniform nuclei, stippled chromatin, and granular cytoplasm are seen. The light microscopic appearance suggesting acinar and endocrine differentiation was confirmed by immunohistochemical studies that showed reaction by the acinar component with trypsin and lipase, and reaction by the endocrine component with neuroendocrine markers (chromogranin and synaptophysin). *Left,* The larger cell population seen in the upper portion of this illustration, which is the same solid large cell population seen in the upper portion of Figure 12–152, also showed acinar differentiation by immunohistochemical studies.

- Cellular tumor characterized by various combinations of growth patterns, including solid, trabecular, acinar, and glandular.
- Acinar and endocrine differentiation can be made cytomorphologically and confirmed with histochemical, immunohistochemical, and electron microscopic studies.
  - Histochemistry: Acinar differentiation—diastase-resistant, PAS-positive cytoplasmic granularity, butyrate esterase-positive; endocrine differentiation—argyrophilia.
  - *Immunohistochemistry:* Acinar differentiation—trypsin, lipase, chymotrypsin, and keratin reactivity; endocrine differentiation—chromogranin, synaptophysin, focal endocrine peptide hormones, including somatostatin, glucagon, gastrin, pancreatic polypeptide, and VIP, and keratin (absent serotonin).
  - *Electron microscopy:* Acinar differentiation—zymogen granules; endocrine differentiation—neurosecretory granules.
- Apparently aggressive tumors with associated metastasis either at presentation or subsequently (lymph nodes, liver, lung) and recurrence. May be lethal.

G. PANCREATIC MESENCHYMAL AND LYMPHOPROLIFERATIVE NEOPLASMS

- Rare primary pancreatic neoplasms.
- More often, these neoplasms occur as primary retroperitoneal tumors (mesenchymal) or primary peripancreatic or retroperitoneal lymph node tumors (lymphomas) with secondary involvement of the pancreas. An extrapancreatic retroperitoneal primary tumor should be excluded before a mesenchymal or lymphoproliferative neoplasm is considered as originating in the pancreas.

1. Mesenchymal Neoplasms

- Among the primary pancreatic benign mesenchymal tumors that may occur are vascular tumors (lymphangioma, hemangioma), and neurilemmoma.

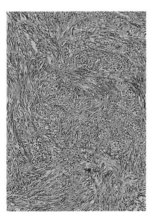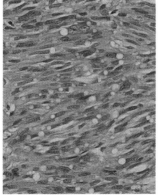

Figure 12–154. Leiomyosarcoma involving the tail of the pancreas. *Left,* Cellular tumor with a storiform growth composed of short intersecting fascicles. *Right,* Elongated, cigar-shaped, hyperchromatic nuclei with prominent perinuclear vacuolization. Immunoreactivity *(not shown)* was present with muscle markers. The tumor originated in the retroperitoneum and invaded the pancreatic tail directly.

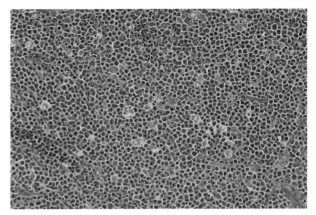

Figure 12–155. Malignant lymphoma involving the pancreas with a diffuse growth pattern, entirely composed of a large cell population. Immunohistochemistry *(not shown)* included reactivity with leukocyte common antigen (CD45RO) and B-cell lineage markers (CD20, L26). This malignant lymphoma also originated in the retroperitoneum with secondary involvement of the pancreas.

- Among the primary pancreatic malignant mesenchymal tumors that may occur are leiomyosarcoma, liposarcoma, malignant fibrous histiocytoma, fibrosarcoma, rhabdomyosarcoma, malignant peripheral nerve sheath tumor, and osteosarcoma.
- No gender predilection for these tumors; may occur in all ages.
- Clinical presentation may include abdominal pain and evidence of obstruction, including jaundice.
- For the above malignant tumors to be considered primary pancreatic mesenchymal tumors, the following criteria must be excluded:
  - Origin from an extrapancreatic retroperitoneal neoplasm with secondary involvement (by direct extension) of the pancreas.
  - Metastatic disease to the pancreas from a distant primary site.
  - Differentiation from an epithelial malignancy such as an anaplastic carcinoma with sarcomatoid features or metaplastic mesenchymal components.
  - Differentiation from a pseudoneoplastic or pseudosarcomatous pancreatic lesion such as inflammatory pseudotumor or inflammatory myofibroblastic tumor.

2. Lymphoproliferative Neoplasms

- Non-Hodgkin's malignant lymphomas (all types), Hodgkin's lymphomas, and plasma cell neoplasms (plasmacytomas) may occur in the pancreas.
- Like mesenchymal neoplasms, most lymphoproliferative tumors originate from outside the pancreas and involve the pancreas secondarily.
- No gender predilection for these tumors; may occur in all ages.
- Clinical presentation may include abdominal pain and evidence of obstruction, including jaundice.
- For a lymphoproliferative tumor to be considered primary in the pancreas, the following criteria must be excluded:
  - Origin from an extrapancreatic retroperitoneal or peripancreatic lymph node with secondary involvement of the pancreas.

- Systemic disease (lymphoma or multiple myeloma) that includes pancreatic involvement.
- Differentiation from a non-neoplastic lymphoproliferative lesion such as plasma cell granuloma or lymphoid hyperplasia.

H. SECONDARY TUMORS

- May occur via hematogenous and or lymphatic spread or by direct extension from a nearby primary tumor of the gastrointestinal tract (e.g., stomach, intestines) or retroperitoneum.
- The various tumors that metastasize to the pancreas are listed in Table 12–8; among the more common ones are lung carcinoma, malignant melanoma, renal cell carcinoma, and breast carcinoma.
- Virtually any type of tumor can metastasize to the pancreas.
- Metastatic disease to the pancreas is almost invariably associated with multiple metastases in other organs.
- Metastatic disease to the pancreas:
  - Seldom produces clinical symptoms or disturbances of pancreatic function.
  - More often than not results in multiple intrapancreatic metastatic nodules rather than a single mass.
  - Usually produce well-defined foci but seldom enlarge to the point of being palpable clinically.
  - Produce little disturbance of the pancreatic architectural pattern that is discernible by radiographic analysis.

I. AMPULLA OF VATER NEOPLASMS

Definition: Tumors originating from the duodenal mucosa of the ampulla or from around the ampulla.

- Tumors of the ampulla include benign and malignant epithelial and mesenchymal neoplasms (Table 12–9).
- Unlike periampullary tumors, ampullary tumors originate from the duodenal (intestinal) epithelium, whereas periampullary tumors may include neoplasms of pancreatic or common bile duct origin. This is not an academic distinction, however, because ampullary adenocarcinoma carries a decidedly better prognosis than carcinomas of the pancreas and common bile duct.
- Ampullary adenomas and adenocarcinomas are the most common tumors of this anatomic location.
- This section will only address ampullary adenoma and adenocarcinoma.

Table 12–8
SECONDARY PANCREATIC TUMORS

Gastrointestinal (colon, stomach) carcinoma
Lung carcinoma
Malignant melanoma
Renal cell carcinoma
Breast carcinoma
Prostatic carcinoma
Sarcomas
Malignant lymphomas

Table 12–9
AMPULLARY AND PERIAMPULLARY NEOPLASMS

Benign
Adenoma
Adenomyoma
Leiomyoma
Granular cell tumor
Neurofibroma
Malignant
Adenocarcinoma
Neuroendocrine carcinomas
Others

1. Ampullary Adenoma

Definition: Benign neoplasm of surface (duodenal) epithelial origin.

Clinical

- Uncommon, but represents the most common site of occurrence for small intestinal adenomatous neoplasms (least common site is the ileum).
- Strategically situated ampullary adenomas may obstruct biliary and pancreatic ducts, resulting in abdominal pain, jaundice, weight loss, and, rarely, pancreatitis. Intestinal obstruction, bleeding, and intussusception may also occur.
- Appear endoscopically as polypoid, papillary, or plaque-like growths with a soft consistency.
- May be associated with familial adenomatous polyposis.

Radiology

- Small tumors may be undetectable by radiologic assessment.
- Upper gastrointestinal studies reveal a "soap-bubble" appearance.

Pathology

Gross

- Majority of lesions are papillary or polypoid, multilobulated and soft; a small percent is sessile.

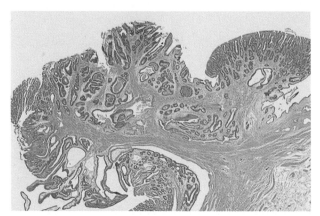

Figure 12–156. Ampulla of Vater adenoma. The tumor is exophytic and predominantly tubular in growth.

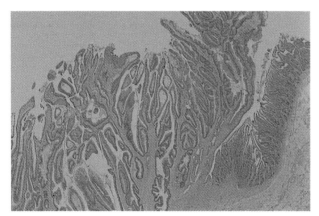

Figure 12–157. Ampulla of Vater adenoma. The tumor is exophytic and tubulovillous in growth.

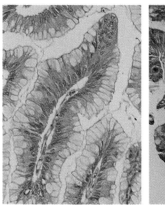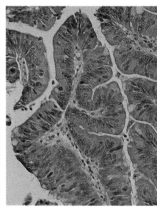

Figure 12–160. Comparison of the cytomorphologic features seen in the benign epithelium of an ampullary villous adenoma *(left)* versus those of the malignant epithelium in an ampullary adenocarcinoma *(right)*. In the adenoma, cellular maturation is retained with minimal cytologic atypia and basilar location of the nuclei; in the adenocarcinoma, the cytologic changes of malignancy include the presence of large pleomorphic nuclei, prominent nucleoli, irregular nuclear stratification, mitotic figures, and loss of cellular maturation (mucin production and brush border).

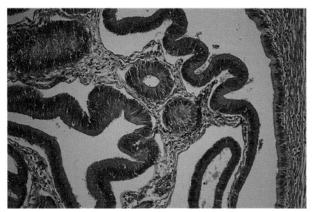

Figure 12–158. Ampullary adenoma. The proliferating cells grow within crypts and villi; the nuclei are stratified and show mild pleomorphic changes, inconspicuous nucleoli, and no mitoses. Normal cellular maturation is retained, including mucin production and surface brush border.

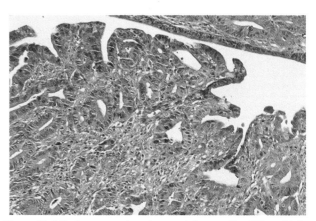

Figure 12–161. Intramucosal carcinoma of the ampulla of Vater. Malignant glandular epithelium did not extend beyond the mucosa and is composed of cells with marked nuclear pleomorphism, hyperchromasia, prominent nucleoli, increased nuclear-to-cytoplasmic ratio, and increased mitotic activity.

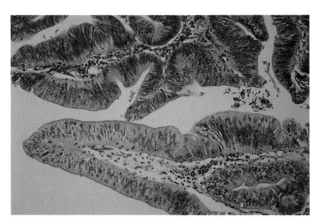

Figure 12–159. Ampullary adenoma with concomitant carcinoma in situ, characterized by cellular dysplasia, including pleomorphic and hyperchromatic nuclei, mitosis, and loss of cellular maturation.

- May attain large size, in particular, polypoid (villous) tumors, which may measure up to 8 cm in diameter.

Histology

- Growth patterns include villous (papillary) and villoglandular with fibrovascular cores; pure tubular growth (without villous features) can occur but is found in a minority of cases.
- Mucosal architecture is intact; proliferating cells replace normal cells and grow within crypts and villi. Nuclei show mild pleomorphic changes, inconspicuous nucleoli, and few, if any, mitoses. Normal cellular maturation is retained, including mucin-production and surface brush border.
- Goblet cells, columnar (absorptive) cells, Paneth's cells, and endocrine cells may also be seen in the neoplastic proliferation.

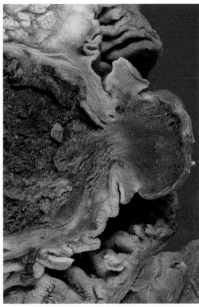

Figure 12–162. Ampullary adenocarcinoma. Large polypoid and indurated mass protrudes from the ampullary region into the duodenum. The duodenal surface mucosa overlying the tumor is focally ulcerated, and the tumor constricts the duodenal luminal diameter.

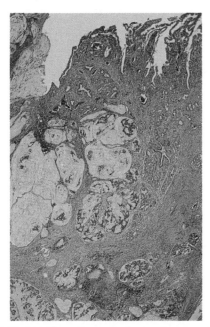

Figure 12–163. Ampullary adenocarcinoma, moderately well differentiated, invades through the submucosa. The invasive cancer includes malignant glandular epithelium with or without mucin pools.

■ Dysplastic foci may indicate the presence of concomitant carcinoma and should prompt detailed histologic evaluation of all resected tumor to exclude adenocarcinoma.

Differential Diagnosis

■ Ampullary adenocarcinoma (Chapter 12I, #2).
■ Ampullary adenomyoma.

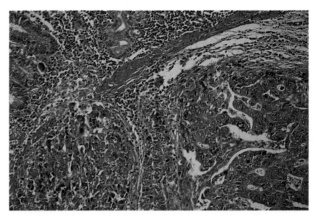

Figure 12–164. Ampullary adenocarcinoma. Invasive carcinoma with invasion through the submucosa. The neoplasm is moderately to poorly differentiated.

Treatment and Prognosis

■ Complete surgical resection is curative.
■ Like colonic lesions, there appears to be an adenoma-carcinoma sequence for ampullary adenomas representing the precursor lesion for ampullary adenocarcinoma.

Additional Facts

■ Villous adenomas, unlike tubular adenomas, are more likely to be symptomatic owing to their larger size and their tendency to cause bleeding.
■ Peroral biopsies may include only superficial components of the tumor, precluding full histologic evaluation of the neoplasm, in particular the depth of the lesion. Foci of adenocarcinoma may be missed due to sampling.

2. Ampullary Adenocarcinoma

Definition: Malignant neoplasm of surface (duodenal) epithelial origin.

Clinical

■ Represents the most common site of occurrence for small intestinal adenocarcinomas.
■ Equal gender predilection; occurs most commonly in the sixth to seventh decades of life.
■ Clinical presentation includes weight loss, anorexia, jaundice, abdominal pain, nausea, vomiting, fever, and hepatosplenomegaly. Jaundice may be intermittent owing to necrosis of tumor allowing for bile drainage through the biliary duct.
■ Appear endoscopically as ulcerated, fungating, or exophytic friable masses with a firm consistency.
■ May be associated with familial adenomatous polyposis; rarely occur in patients with Crohn's disease or gluten-sensitive enteropathy.

Radiology

■ Radiographic and endoscopic appearance of small tumors confined to the ampulla may not be abnormal.

- Barium studies may show an enlarged papilla with an irregular filling defect and irregular borders, sometimes with spiculation and ulceration.
- ERCP may reveal abrupt termination of the dilated common bile duct near the level of the ampulla.
- Ultrasound and CT scan may show dilatation of the common bile duct or pancreatic duct.

Pathology

Fine Needle Aspiration

- Duodenal or ampullary brushings may show dysplastic epithelial cells.

Gross

- May be polypoid, fungating, sessile, and ulcerative with an indurated consistency.
- An annular napkin-ring type of lesion constricting the lumen can be seen.
- With increasing use of endoscopy, smaller tumors measuring 1 cm in size can be detected.

Histology

- Similar to colonic adenocarcinomas, including the full spectrum of intestinal adenocarcinomas (well to moderately to poorly differentiated). The majority are moderately differentiated and mucin-producing; poorly differentiated ampullary adenocarcinomas occur but are uncommon.
- Growth patterns include villous (papillary) and villoglandular with fibrovascular cores.
- Cytologic changes characteristic of malignancy include the presence of large pleomorphic nuclei, prominent nucleoli, irregular nuclear stratification, increased mitotic activity with atypical forms, and necrosis (individual cell). Loss of cellular maturation (mucin production, brush border) may occur.
- Remnants of adenomas often are present. Adenomatous foci retain their cellular differentiation and have no dysplastic or anaplastic cytologic features.
- Invasive growth, including invasion through the muscularis propria, neurotropism, and vascular space invasion, may be seen.
- Malignant cytologic change may be confined to the mucosa without invasive growth; such a tumor is termed intramucosal carcinoma.
- Invasive carcinoma (extension into the submucosa) must be present in endoscopic biopsy material for a diagnosis of an ampullary neoplasm as malignant. Invasion may include obvious invasive glands in the submucosa with associated desmoplasia, incomplete epithelial-lined glandular lumina, or mucin pools with or without neoplastic cells.
- Glands situated in smooth muscle fascicles unaccompanied by stromal tissue are a feature of malignancy that can be detected on frozen section or in permanent sections. This feature assists in differentiating an adenocarcinoma from non-neoplastic or benign glands in the periampullary region.
- Poorly differentiated and anaplastic carcinomas can also occur. Some tumors may have a predominance of signet

ring cells. Unusual subtypes may include adenosquamous carcinoma.
- Generally, given the higher percentage of tumors that are better differentiated, neither histochemical or immunohistochemical studies are needed. For less differentiated tumors, epithelial mucin stains and cytokeratin stains may be helpful.
- Neuroendocrine cells (and Paneth's cells) can be seen in the neoplastic cell proliferation and confirmed by immunoreactivity with neuroendocrine cell markers such as chromogranin and synaptophysin; (neuro)endocrine functional activity is rare.
- Molecular biology: p53 mutations are found in ampullary carcinomas.

Differential Diagnosis

- Adenocarcinoma of the common bile duct.
- Adenocarcinoma of the pancreatic head (Chapter 12D, #1).
- Malignant lymphoma.

Treatment and Prognosis

- Pancreatoduodenectomy (Whipple procedure) is the treatment of choice.
- In situ adenocarcinoma found within an adenoma and with no evidence of invasion can be treated by local (transduodenal) resection. These tumors usually do not metastasize; ulcerating or napkin-ring type lesions tend to be higher stage tumors and associated with a worse prognosis than polypoid intramural tumors.
- Prognosis is better than that for pancreatic or common bile duct adenocarcinoma.
- Five-year survival rate is approximately 50% and rises to 80% in the absence of lymph node metastasis.
- Factors affecting prognosis include:
  - Presence or absence of nodal metastasis.
  - Tumor invasion limited to within the muscle of Oddi (stage I); this has a 5-year survival of 85%.
  - Tumor invasion beyond the muscle coat (stage II); 5-year survival is 25%.
- TNM classification and staging of ampullary adenocarcinomas are detailed in Table 12–10A and B.

Table 12–10A
TNM CLASSIFICATION OF AMPULLARY ADENOCARCINOMA (AMERICAN JOINT COMMITTEE ON CANCER STAGING)

T1	Tumor confined to ampulla
T2	Extension of tumor into the duodenal wall
T3	Tumor invades 2 cm or less into the pancreas
T4	Tumor invades more than 2 cm into the pancreas
N0	Regional lymph nodes not involved
N1	Regional lymph nodes involved
NX	Regional lymph nodes not assessed
M0	No distant metastasis
M1	Distant metastasis present
MX	Distant metastasis not assessed

Table 12–10B
STAGING OF AMPULLARY ADENOCARCINOMA
(AMERICAN JOINT COMMITTEE ON CANCER STAGING)

Stage I	T1, N0, M0
Stage II	T2–T3, N0, M0
Stage III	T1–T3, N1, M0
Stage IV	T4, any N, M0; any T, any N, M1

Additional Facts

■ Because of the difference in prognosis, it is important to distinguish ampullary from pancreatic or biliary tract adenocarcinoma.

■ Because of the anatomic complexity of the ampullary region, including the presence of the common bile duct and the pancreatic duct emptying into the duodenum, numerous small tortuous glands are normally seen extending into the adjacent muscularis. The pathologist must take this into account when viewing this anatomic region and try not to misinterpret the presence of normal glandular components as invasive carcinoma. Noncrowded glands with smooth, rounded contours composed of a single row of cuboidal to columnar epithelial cells with uniform, basally situated nuclei and without cytologic atypia are features of these small normally situated glands. It should be noted that adenomatous changes can occur in these deeply situated glands and should also not be interpreted as malignant unless architectural and cytomorphologic features of malignancy are present.

Bibliography

General Considerations

Ahlgren JD. Epidemiology and risk factors in pancreatic cancer. Semin Oncol 1996; 23:241–250.

Alter CL. Palliative and supportive care of patients with pancreatic cancer. Semin Oncol 1996; 23:229–240.

Beretta E, Malesci A, Zerbi A, et al. Serum CA 19-9 in the post-surgical follow-up of patients with pancreatic cancer. Cancer 1987; 60:2428–2431.

DelMaschio A, Vanzulli A, Sironi S, et al. Pancreatic cancer versus chronic pancreatitis: Diagnosis with CA 19-9 assessment, US, CT, and CT-guided fine needle aspiration. Radiology 1991; 178:95–100.

Devesa SS, Blot WJ, Stone BJ, et al. Recent cancer trends in the United States. J Natl Cancer Inst 1995; 87:175–182.

Edoute Y, Lemberg S, Malberger E. Preoperative and intraoperative fine needle aspiration cytology of pancreatic lesions. Am J Gastroenterol 1991; 86:1015–1019.

Fortner JG, Klimstra DS, Senie RT, Maclean BJ. Tumor size is the primary prognosticator for pancreatic cancer after regional pancreatectomy. Ann Surg 1996; 223:147–153.

Gordis L, Gold EB. Epidemiology and etiology of pancreatic cancer. In: Go VLW, DiMagno EP, Gardner JD, Lebenthal E, Reber HA, Scheele GA, eds. The Pancreas: Biology, Pathobiology and Disease. 2nd edition. New York: Raven Press, 1993, pp. 837–855.

Itzkowitz SH, Kim YS. New carbohydrate tumor markers. Gastroenterology 1986; 90:491–494.

Kojcan G, Rode J, Lees WR. Percutaneous fine needle aspiration cytology of the pancreas: Advantage and pitfalls. J Clin Pathol 1989; 42:341–347.

Lynch HY, Smyrk T, Kern SE, et al. Familial pancreatic cancer: A review. Semin Oncol 1996; 23:251–275.

McGrath PC, Sloan DA, Kenady DE. Surgical management of pancreatic carcinoma. Semin Oncol 1996; 23:200–212.

Parkin DM, Pisani P, Ferlay J. Estimates of the worldwide incidence of eighteen major cancers in 1985. Int J Cancer 1993; 54:594–606.

Safi F, Roscher R, Beger HG. Tumor markers in pancreatic cancer. Sensitivity and specificity of CA 19-9. Hepatogastroenterology 1989; 36:419–423.

Savarino V, Ceppa P, Biggi E, et al. Comparative study of percutaneous and preoperative fine-needle aspirations in the diagnosis of pancreatic cancer. Hepatogastroenterology 1986; 33:75–78.

Schnal SF, Macdonald JS. Chemotherapy of adenocarcinoma of the pancreas. Semin Oncol 1996; 23:220–228.

Scudera PL, Koizumi J, Jacobson IM. Brush cytology evaluation of lesions encountered during ERCP. Gastrointest Endosc 1990; 36:281–284.

Shemesh E, Czerniak A, Nass S, Klein E. Role of endoscopic retrograde cholangiopancreatectomy in differentiating pancreatic cancer coexisting with chronic pancreatitis. Cancer 1990; 65:893–896.

Thomas PRM. Radiotherapy for carcinoma of the pancreas. Semin Oncol 1996; 23:213–219.

Warshaw AL. Implications of peritoneal cytology for staging of early pancreatic cancer. Am J Surg 1991; 161:26–30.

Warshaw AL, Gu Z, Wittenberg J, Waxman AC. Preoperative staging and assessment of pancreatic cancer. Arch Surg 1990; 125:230–233.

Whipple AO. Surgical treatment of carcinoma of the ampullary region and head of pancreas. Am J Surg 1938; 40:260–263.

Whipple AO, Parsons WB, Mullins CR. Treatment of carcinoma of the ampulla of Vater. Ann Surg 1935; 102:763–779.

Benign Exocrine Neoplasms

Microcystic Adenomas

Albores-Saavedra J, Gould EW, Angeles-Angeles A, Henson DE. Cystic tumors of the pancreas. Pathol Annu 1990; 25(part 2):19–50.

Alpert LC, Truong LD, Bossart MI, et al. Microcystic adenoma (serous cystadenoma) of the pancreas. A study of 14 cases with immunohistochemical and electron-microscope correlation. Am J Surg Pathol 1988; 12:251–263.

Bogomoletz WV, Adnet JJ, Widgren S, et al. Cystadenoma of the pancreas: A histological, histochemical and ultrastructural study of seven cases. Histopathology 1980; 4:309–320.

Compagno J, Oertel JE. Microcystic adenomas of the pancreas (glycogen rich cystadenomas). A clinicopathologic study of 34 cases. Am J Clin Pathol 1978; 69:289–298.

Corbally MT, McAnena OJ, Urmacher C, et al. Pancreatic cystadenoma: A clinicopathologic study. Arch Surg 1989; 124:1271–1274.

Friedman AC, Lichtenstein JE, Dachman AH. Cystic neoplasms of the pancreas. Radiology 1983; 149:45–50.

Friedman H. Nonmucinous glycogen-poor cystadenoma of the pancreas. Arch Pathol Lab Med 1990; 114:888–891.

George DH, Murphy F, Michalski R, Ulmer BH. Serous cystadenocarcinoma of the pancreas: A new entity? Am J Surg Pathol 1989; 13:61–66.

Helpap B, Vogel J. Immunohistochemical studies on cystic pancreatic neoplasms. Path Res Pract 1989; 184:39–45.

Johnson CD, Stephens DH, Charboneau JW, et al. Cystic pancreatic tumors: CT and sonographic assessment. AJR 1988; 151:1133–1178.

Kamei K, Funabiki T, Ochiai M, et al. Some considerations on the biology of pancreatic serous cystadenoma. Int J Pancreatol 1991; 11:97–104.

Lauciricia R, Schwartz MR, Ramzy I. Fine-needle aspiration of pancreatic cystic epithelial neoplasms. Acta Cytol 1992; 36:881–886.

Lewandrowski KB, Warshaw AL, Compton CC. Macrocystic serous cystadenoma of the pancreas: A morphologic variant differing from microcystic adenoma. Hum Pathol 1992; 23:871–875.

Lo JW, Fung CHK, Yonan TN, Martinez N. Cystadenoma of the pancreas. An ultrastructural study. Cancer 1977; 39:2470–2474.

Minami M, Itai Y, Ohtomo K, Yoshida H, Yoshikawa K, Lio M. Cystic neoplasms of the pancreas: Comparison of MR imaging with CT. Radiology 1989; 171:53–56.

Montag AG, Fossati N, Michelassi F. Pancreatic microcystic adenoma coexistent with pancreatic ductal carcinoma. Am J Surg Pathol 1990; 14:352–355.

Mori K, Takeyama S, Hirosawa H, et al. A case of macrocystic serous cystadenoma of the pancreas. Int J Pancreatol 1995; 17:91–93.

Nguyen G-K, Vogelsang PJ. Microcystic adenoma of the pancreas. A report of two cases with fine needle aspiration cytology and differential diagnosis. Acta Cytol 1993; 37:908–912.

Nyongo A, Huntrakoon M, Taylor J, Ediger S, Parsa C. Microcystic adenoma of the pancreas with myoepithelial cells. A hitherto undescribed morphologic feature. Am J Clin Pathol 1985; 84:114–120.

Perez-Ordonez B, Naseem A, Lieberman PH, Klimstra DS. Solid serous adenoma of the pancreas: The solid variant of serous cystadenoma. Am J Surg Pathol 1996; 20:1401–1405.

Seizinger BR, Smith DI, Filling-Katz MR, et al. Genetic flanking markers refine diagnostic criteria and provide insights into the genetics of von Hippel-Lindau disease. Proc Natl Acad Sci U S A 1991; 88:2864–2868.

Shorten SD, Hart WR, Petras RE. Microcystic adenomas (serous cystadenoma) of the pancreas. A clinicopathologic investigation of eight cases with immunohistochemical and ultrastructural studies. Am J Surg Pathol 1986; 10:365–372.

Unger PD, Danque PO, Fuchs A, Kaneko M. DNA flow cytometric evaluation of serous and mucinous cystic neoplasms of the pancreas. Arch Pathol Lab Med 1991; 115:563–565.

Wenig BM, Heffner DK. Endolymphatic sac papillary tumor. Fact or fiction? Adv Anat Pathol 1996; 3:378–387.

Yoshimi N, Sugie S, Tanaka T, et al. A rare case of serous cystadenocarcinoma of the pancreas. Cancer 1992; 69:2449–2453.

Young NA, Villani MA, Khoury P, Naryshkin S. Differential diagnosis of cystic neoplasms of the pancreas by fine-needle aspiration. Arch Pathol Lab Med 1991; 115:571–577.

Cystic Teratomas

Assawamatiyanont S, King AD Jr. Dermoid cyst of the pancreas. Am Surgeon 1977; 43:503–504.

Iacono C, Zamboni G, Di Marcello R, et al. Dermoid cyst of the head of the pancreas area. Int J Pancreatol 1993; 14:269–273.

Jacobs JE, Dinsmore BJ. Mature cystic teratoma of the pancreas: Sonographic and CT findings. AJR 1993; 160:523–524.

Mester M, Trajber HJ, Compton CC, et al. Cystic teratomas of the pancreas. Arch Surg 1990; 125:1215–1218.

Pancreatic Neoplasms of Intermediate Biologic Potential
Ductal Alterations of Low-Malignant Potential

Adsay NV, Adair CF, Heffess CS, Klimstra DS. Oncocytic papillary mucinous cystic neoplasm of the pancreas. Am J Surg Pathol 1996; 20:980–994.

Bastid C, Bernard JP, Sarles H, Payan MJ, Sahel J. Mucinous ductal ectasia of the pancreas: A premalignant disease and a cause of obstructive pancreatitis. Pancreas 1991; 6:15–22.

DiGiuseppe JA, Hruban RH, Offerhaus GJA, et al. Detection of K-ras mutations in mucinous pancreatic duct hyperplasia from a patient with a family history of pancreatic carcinoma. Am J Pathol 1994; 144:889–895.

Fearon ER, Vogelstein B. A genetic model for colorectal tumorigenesis. Cell 1990; 61:759–767.

Fitzgerald PJ, Cubilla AL. Pancreas. In: Henson DE, Albores-Saavedra J, eds. The Pathology of Incipient Neoplasia. Philadelphia: W.B. Saunders, 1986, pp. 217–231.

Furukawa T, Takahashi T, Kobari M, Matsuno S. The mucus-hypersecreting tumor of the pancreas. Development and extension visualized by three-dimensional computerized mapping. Cancer 1992; 70:505–513.

Hruban RH, van Mansfield ADM, Offerhaus GJA, et al. K-ras oncogene activation in adenocarcinoma of the human pancreas. A study of 82 carcinomas using a combination of mutant-enriched polymerase chain reaction analysis and allele-specific oligonucleotide hybridization. Am J Pathol 1993; 143:545–554.

Itai Y, Ohhashi K, Nagai H, et al. "Ductectatic" mucinous cystadenoma and cystadenocarcinoma of the pancreas. Radiology 1986; 161:697–700.

Kawarada Y, Yano T, Yamamoto T, et al. Intraductal mucin-producing tumors of the pancreas. Am J Gastroenterol 1992; 87:634–638.

Kobayashi H, Itoh H, Konishi H. Duct ectasia due to mucus-producing cancers with intraductal extension: histopathologic correlation with radiologic imagings. Abdom Imaging 1995; 20:341–347.

Kodama T, Mori W. Morphological lesions of the pancreatic ducts. Significance of pyloric gland metaplasia in carcinogenesis of exocrine and endocrine pancreas. Acta Pathol Jpn 1983; 33:645–660.

Lemoine NR, Jain S, Hughes CM, et al. Ki-ras oncogene activation in preinvasive pancreatic cancer. Gastroenterology 1992; 102:230–236.

Longnecker DS. Intraductal papillary-mucinous tumors of the pancreas (editorial). Arch Pathol Lab Med 1995; 119:197–198.

Lynch HY, Smyrk T, Kern SE, et al. Familial pancreatic cancer: A review. Semin Oncol 1996; 23:251–275.

Milchgrub S, Campuzano M, Casillas J, Albores-Saavedra J. Intraductal carcinoma of the pancreas. Cancer 1992; 69:651–656.

Morohoshi T, Kanda M, Asanuma K, Klöppel G. Intraductal papillary neoplasms of the pancreas. A clinicopathologic study of six patients. Cancer 1989; 64:1329–1335.

Nagai E, Ueki T, Chijiiwa K, Tanaka M, Tsuneyoshi M. Intraductal papillary mucinous neoplasms of the pancreas associated with so-called "mucinous ductal ectasia." Histochemical and immunohistochemical analysis of 29 cases. Am J Surg Pathol 1995; 19:576–589.

Nickl NJ, Lawson JM, Cotton PB. Mucinous pancreatic tumors: ERCP findings. Gastrointest Endosc 1991; 37:133–138.

Nishihara K, Fukuda T, Tsuneyoshi M, et al. Intraductal papillary neoplasm of the pancreas. Cancer 1993; 72:689–696.

Obara T, Maguchi H, Saitoh Y, et al. Mucin-producing tumor of the pancreas. Natural history and serial pancreatogram changes. Am J Gastroenterol 1993; 88:564–569.

Obara T, Saitoh Y, Maguchi H, et al. Multicentric development of a pancreatic intraductal carcinoma through atypical papillary hyperplasia. Hum Pathol 1992; 23:82–85.

Oertel JE. The pancreas. Nonneoplastic alterations. Am J Surg Pathol 1989; 13(Suppl 1):50–65.

Oertel JE, Oertel YC, Heffess CS. Pancreas. In: Sternberg SS, ed. Diagnostic Surgical Pathology, 2nd ed. New York: Raven Press, 1994, pp. 1419–1457.

Ohta T, Nagakawa T, Akiyama T, et al. The "duct-ectatic" variant of mucinous cystic neoplasm of the pancreas. Clinical and radiologic studies of seven cases. Am J Gastroenterol 1992; 87:300–304.

Pour PM, Sayed S, Sayed G. Hyperplastic, preneoplastic and neoplastic lesions found in 83 human pancreases. Am J Clin Pathol 1982; 77:137–152.

Rickaert F, Cremer M, Devìre J, et al. Intraductal mucin-hypersecreting neoplasms of the pancreas. A clinicopathologic study of eight patients. Gastroenterology 1991; 101:512–519.

Santini D, Campione O, Salerno A, et al. Intraductal papillary-mucinous neoplasm of the pancreas. A clinicopathologic entity. Arch Pathol Lab Med 1995; 119:209–213.

Satoh K, Sasano H, Shimosegawa T, et al. An immunohistochemical study of the c-erb-2 oncogene product in intraductal mucin-hypersecreting neoplasms and in ductal cell carcinomas of the pancreas. Cancer 1993; 72:51–56.

Sessa F, Solcia E, Capella C, et al. Intraductal papillary-mucinous tumours represent a distinct group of pancreatic neoplasms. An investigation of tumour cell differentiation and K-ras, p53, and c-erb-2 abnormalities in 26 patients. Virchows Arch 1994; 425:357–367.

Shyr YM, Su CH, Tsay SH, Lui WY. Mucin-producing neoplasms of the pancreas. Intraductal papillary and mucinous cystic neoplasms. Ann Surg 1996; 223:141–146.

Tada M, Omata M, Ohto M. Ras gene mutations in intraductal papillary neoplasms of the pancreas. Cancer 1991; 67:634–663.

Tian F, Myles J, Howard JM. Mucinous pancreatic ductal ectasia of latent malignancy. An emerging clinicopathologic entity. Surgery 1992; 111:109–113.

Yamada M, Kozuka S, Yamao K, et al. Mucin-producing tumor of the pancreas. Cancer 1991; 68:159–168.

Yamguchi K, Ogawa Y, Chijiiwa K, Tanaka M. Mucin-hypersecreting tumors of the pancreas: assessing the grade of malignancy preoperatively. Am J Surg 1996; 171:427–431.

Mucinous Cystic Neoplasm

Albores-Saavedra J, Angeles-Angeles A, Nadji M, et al. Mucinous cystadenocarcinoma of the pancreas. Morphologic and immunocytochemical observations. Am J Surg Pathol 1987; 11:11–20.

Albores-Saavedra J, Gould EW, Angeles-Angeles A, Henson DE. Cystic tumors of the pancreas. Pathol Annu 1990; 25(part 2):19–50.

Alles AJ, Warshaw AL, Southern AF, et al. Expression of CA 72-4 (TAG 72) in the fluid contents of pancreatic cysts: A new marker to distinguish malignant cystic tumors from benign pancreatic neoplasms and pseudocysts. Ann Surg 1994; 219:131–134.

Bergman S, Medeiros JL, Radr T, et al. Giant cell tumor of the pancreas arising in the ovarian-like stroma of a mucinous cystadenocarcinoma. Int J Pancreatol 1995; 18:71–75.

Compagno J, Oertel JE. Mucinous cystic neoplasms of the pancreas with overt and latent malignancy (cystadenocarcinoma and cystadenoma). A clinicopathologic study of 41 cases. Am J Clin Pathol 1978; 69:573–580.

Dodd LG, Farrell TA, Layfield LJ. Mucinous cystic tumor of the pancreas: an analysis of FNA characteristics with an emphasis on the spectrum of malignancy associated features. Diagn Cytopathol 1995; 12:113–139.

Friedman AC, Lichtenstein JE, Dachman AH. Cystic neoplasms of the pancreas. Radiological-pathological correlation. Radiology 1983;149:45–50.

Gupta RK, Scally J, Steward RJ. Mucinous cystadenocarcinoma of the pancreas: diagnosis of fine needle aspiration cytology. Diagn Cytopathol 1989; 5:408–411.

Helpap B, Vogel J. Immunohistochemical studies on cystic pancreatic neoplasms. Path Res Pract 1989; 184:39–45.

Lewandrowski KB, Southern JF, Pins MR, et al. Cyst fluid analysis in the differential diagnosis of pancreatic cysts. A comparison of pseudocysts, serous cystadenomas, mucinous cystic neoplasms and mucinous cystadenocarcinoma. Ann Surg 1993; 217:4–7.

Lewandrowski KB, Warshaw AL, Compton CC, et al. Variability of cyst fluid carcinoembryonic antigen level, fluid viscosity, amylase content, and cytology among multiple loculi of a pancreatic mucinous cystic neoplasm. Am J Clin Pathol 1993; 100:425–427.

Logan SE, Voet RL, Tompkins RK. The malignant potential of mucinous cysts of the pancreas. West J Med 1982; 136:157.

Posen JA. Giant cell tumor of the pancreas of the osteoclastic type associated with a mucous secreting cystadenocarcinoma. Hum Pathol 1981; 12:944–947.

Rego JAG, Ruvira LV, Garcia AA, et al. Pancreatic mucinous cystadenocarcinoma with pseudosarcomatous mural nodules. A report of a case with immunohistochemical study. Cancer 1991; 67:494–498.

Talamini MA, Pitt HA, Hruban RH, et al. Spectrum of cystic tumors of the pancreas. Am J Surg Pathol 1992; 163:117–124.

Warshaw AL, Compton CC, Lewandrowski K, et al. Cystic tumors of the pancreas. New clinical, radiologic, and pathologic observations in 67 patients. Ann Surg 1990; 212:432–445.

Wenig BM, Albores-Saavedra J, Buetow PC, Heffess CS. Pancreatic mucinous cystic neoplasm with sarcomatous stroma: A report of three cases. Am J Surg Pathol 1997; 21:70–80.

Zamboni G, Castelli P, Pea M, et al. Mucinous cystic tumor of the pancreas recurring after 11 years as cystadenocarcinoma with foci of choriocarcinoma and osteoclastic-like giant cell tumor. Surg Pathol 1994; 5:253–262.

Solid and Papillary Epithelial Carcinoma

Adair CF, Wenig BM, Thompson LDR, Heffess CS. Solid and papillary epithelial carcinoma of the pancreas. Int J Surg Pathol 1995; 2:326.

Buetow PC, Buck JL, Pantongrag-Brown L, et al. Solid and papillary epithelial neoplasm of the pancreas: Imaging-pathologic correlation in 56 cases. Radiology 1996; 199:707–711.

Cappellari JO, Geisinger KR, Albertson DA, et al. Malignant papillary cystic tumor of the pancreas. Cancer 1990; 66:193–198.

Friedman AC, Lichtenstein JE, Fishman EK, et al. Solid and papillary epithelial neoplasm of the pancreas. Radiology 1985; 154:333–337.

Hamoudi AB, Misugi K, Grosfeld JL, Reiner CB. Papillary epithelial neoplasm of pancreas in a child. Report of a case with electron microscopy. Cancer 1970; 26:1126–1134.

Kissane JM. Pancreatoblastoma and solid and cystic papillary tumor: Two tumors related to pancreatic ontogeny. Semin Diag Pathol 1994; 11:152–164.

Klöppel G, Maurer R, Hofmann E, et al. Solid-cystic (papillary-cystic) tumours within and outside the pancreas in men: Report of two patients. Case report. Virchows Arch [A] 1991; 418:179–183.

Lee WY, Tzeng CC, Jin YT, et al. Papillary cystic tumor of the pancreas: A case indistinguishable from oncocytic carcinoma. Pancreas 1993; 8:127–132.

Matsunou H, Konishi F. Papillary-cystic neoplasm of the pancreas: A clinicopathologic study concerning the tumor aging and malignancy in nine cases. Cancer 1990; 65:283–291.

Miettinen M, Partanen S, Fraki O, Kivilaakso E. Papillary cystic tumor of the pancreas: An analysis of cellular differentiation by electron microscopy and immunohistochemistry. Am J Surg Pathol 1987; 11:885–895.

Nishihara K, Nagoshi M, Tsuneyoshi M, et al. Papillary cystic tumor of the pancreas. Assessment of their malignant potential. Cancer 1993; 71:82–94.

Pettinato G, Manivel JC, Rovetto C, et al. Papillary cystic tumor of the pancreas. A clinicopathologic study of 20 cases with cytologic, immunohistochemical, ultrastructural, and flow cytometric observations, and a review of the literature. Am J Clin Pathol 1992; 98:478–488.

Silverman JF, Geisinger KR. Pancreas. In: Silverman JF, Geisinger KR, eds. Fine Needle Aspiration Cytology of the Thorax and Abdomen. New York: Churchill Livingstone, 1996, pp. 135–170.

Stömmer P, Kraus J, Stolte M, Giedl J. Solid and cystic pancreatic tumors. Clinical, histochemical and electron microscopic features in ten cases. Cancer 1991; 67:1635–1641.

Yamaguchi K, Hirakata R, Kitamura K. Papillary cystic neoplasm of the pancreas: Radiological and pathological characteristics in 11 cases. Br J Surg 1990; 77:1000–1003.

Malignant Exocrine Neoplasms

Pancreatic Ductal Adenocarcinoma (also see references following General Considerations)

Alanen KA, Joensuu H, Klemi PJ, Nevalainen TJ. Clinical significance of nuclear DNA content in pancreatic carcinoma. J Pathol 1990; 160:313–320.

Allema JH, Reinders ME, van Gulik TM, et al. Prognostic factors for survival after pancreaticoduodenectomy for patients with carcinoma of the pancreatic head region. Cancer 1995; 75:2069–2076.

Allison DC, Bose KK, Hruban RH, Piantadosi S, et al. Pancreatic cancer cell DNA content correlates with long term survival following pancreaticoduodenectomy. Ann Surg 1991; 214:648–656.

Almoguera C, Shibata D, Forrester K, et al. Most human carcinomas of the exocrine pancreas contain mutant c-K-ras genes. Cell 1988; 53:549–554.

Barton CM, Staddon SL, Hughes CM, et al. Abnormalities of the p53 tumour suppressor gene in human pancreatic cancer. Br J Cancer 1991; 64:1076–1082.

Bätge B, Bosslet K, Sedlacek HH, et al. Monoclonal antibodies against CEA-related components discriminate between pancreatic duct type carcinomas and nonneoplastic duct lesions as well as nonduct type neoplasias. Virchows Arch [A] 1986; 408:361–374.

Borowitz MJ, Tuck FL, Sindelar WF, et al. Monoclonal antibodies against human pancreatic adenocarcinoma: Distribution of DU-PAN-2 antigen on glandular epithelia and adenocarcinomas. J Natl Cancer Inst 1984; 72:999–1005.

Chen J, Baithun SI. Morphological study of 391 cases of exocrine pancreatic tumors with special reference to the classification of exocrine pancreatic carcinoma. J Pathol 1985; 146:17–29.

Duff GL. The clinical and pathological features of carcinoma of the body and tail of the pancreas. Johns Hopkins Hosp Bull 1939; 65:69–100.

Eskelinen M, Lipponen P, Collan Y, et al. Relationship between DNA ploidy and survival in patients with exocrine pancreatic cancer. Pancreas 1991; 6:90–95.

Fortner JG, Klimstra DS, Senie RT, Maclean BJ. Tumor size is the primary prognosticator for pancreatic cancer after regional pancreatectomy. Ann Surg 1996; 223:147–153.

Gordis L, Gold EB. Epidemiology and etiology of pancreatic cancer. In: Go VLW, DiMagno EP, Gardner JD, et al, eds. The Pancreas: Biology, Pathobiology and Disease. 2nd edition. New York: Raven Press, 1993, pp. 837–855.

Grünewald K, Lyons J, Fröhlich A, et al. High frequency of Ki-ras codon 12 mutations in pancreatic adenocarcinoma. Int J Cancer 1989; 43:1037–1041.

Hyland C, Kheir SM, Kashlan MB. Frozen sections diagnosis of pancreatic carcinoma. A prospective study of 64 biopsies. Am J Surg Pathol 1981; 5:179–191.

Lemoine NR, Jain S, Hughes VM, et al. Ki-ras oncogene activation in preinvasive pancreatic cancer. Gastroenterology 1992; 102:230–236.

Metzgar RS, Hollingsworth MA, Kaufman B. Pancreatic mucins. In: Go VLW, DiMagno EP, Gardner JD, et al., eds. The Pancreas: Biology, Pathobiology and Disease. 2nd edition. New York: Raven Press, 1993, pp. 351–367.

Oertel JE, Oertel YC, Heffess CS. Pancreas. In: Sternberg SS, ed. Diagnostic Surgical Pathology. 2nd edition. New York: Raven Press, 1994, pp. 1419–1457.

Ohshio G, Manabe T, Watanabe Y, et al. Comparative studies of DU-PAN-2, carcino-embryonic antigen, and CA 19-9 in the serum and bile of patients with pancreatic and biliary tract diseases: Evaluation of the influence of obstructive jaundice. Am J Gastroenterol 1990; 85:1370–1376.

Klöppel G, Lingenthal G, Von Bulow M, Kern HF. Histological and fine structural features of pancreatic ductal adenocarcinomas in relation to growth and prognosis: studies in xenografted tumours and clinicohistopathological correlation in a series of 75 cases. Histopathology 1985; 9:841–856.

Raijman I, Levin B. Exocrine tumors of the pancreas. In: Go VLW, Di-Magno EP, Gardner JD, et al., eds. The Pancreas: Biology, Pathobiology and Disease. 2nd edition. New York: Raven Press, 1993, pp. 899–912.

Safi F, Roscher R, Beger HG. Tumor markers in pancreatic cancer. Sensitivity and specificity of CA 19-9. Hepatogastroenterology 1989; 36:419–423.

Sheer DG, Schlom J, Cooper HL. Purification and composition of the human tumor associated glycoprotein (TAG-72) defined by monoclonal antibodies CC49 and B72.3. Cancer Res 1988; 48:6811–6818.

Weger AR, Falkmer UG, Schwab G, et al. Nuclear DNA distribution pattern of parenchymal cells in adenocarcinomas of the pancreas and in chronic pancreatitis. Gastroenterology 1990; 99:237–242.

Histologic Variants of Ductal Adenocarcinoma

Aziz TZ, Bradfield JWB. Benign mucous squirts can mimic invasive carcinoma in villous adenomas. J Pathol 1985; 146:266A.

Berho M, Blaustein A, Willis I, et al. Microglandular carcinoma of the pancreas. Immunohistochemical and ultrastructural study of an unusual variant of pancreatic carcinoma that may closely resemble a neuroendocrine carcinoma. Am J Clin Pathol 1996; 105:727–732.

Bryko CM, Doll DC. Squamous cell carcinoma of the pancreas associated with hypercalcemia. Gastroenterology 1982; 83:1297–1299.

Cubilla AL, Fitzgerald PJ. Adenosquamous carcinoma. In: Hartmann WH, Sobin LH, eds. Atlas of Tumor Pathology. Tumors of the Exocrine Pancreas, Fascicle 19, Second series. Washington, D.C.: Armed Forces Institute of Pathology, 1984, pp. 168–173.

Huntrakoon M. Oncocytic carcinoma of the pancreas. Cancer 1983; 51:332–336.

Ishikawa O, Matsui Y, Aoki I, et al. Adenosquamous carcinoma of the pancreas: A clinicopathologic study and report of three cases. Cancer 1980; 46:1192–1196.

Lee WY, Tzeng CC, Jin YT, et al. Papillary cystic tumor of the pancreas: A case indistinguishable from oncocytic carcinoma. Pancreas 1993; 8: 127–132.

Morohoshi T, Held G, Klöppel G. Exocrine pancreatic tumours and their histological classification: A study based on 167 autopsy and 97 surgical cases. Histopathology 1983; 7:645–661.

Oertel JE, Heffess CS, Oertel YC. Pancreas. In: Sternberg SS, ed. Diagnostic Surgical Pathology. 2nd edition. New York: Raven Press, 1994, pp. 1419–1457.

Sommers SC, Meissner WA. Unusual carcinomas of the pancreas. Arch Pathol Lab Med 1954; 58:101–111.

Stömmer P, Kraus J, Langer E. Mikroglanduläre pankreaskarzinoma. Histologische, immunozytochemische und elektronenoptische befunde. Pathologe 1989; 10:354–358.

Zerbi A, De Nardi P, Braga M, et al. An oncocytic carcinoma of the pancreas with pulmonary and subcutaneous metastases. Pancreas 1993; 8:116–119.

Anaplastic Carcinoma

Alguacil-Garcia A, Weiland LH. The histologic spectrum, prognosis, and histogenesis of the sarcomatoid carcinoma of the pancreas. Cancer 1977; 39:1181–1189.

Berendt RC, Shnitka TK, Wiens E, et al. The osteoclast-type giant cell tumor of the pancreas. Arch Pathol Lab Med 1987; 111:43–48.

Bergman S, Medeiros JL, Radr T, et al. Giant cell tumor of the pancreas arising in the ovarian-like stroma of a mucinous cystadenocarcinoma. Int J Pancreatol 1995; 18:71–75.

Chen J, Baithun SI. Morphological study of 391 cases of exocrine pancreatic tumors with special reference to the classification of exocrine pancreatic carcinoma. J Pathol 1985; 146:17–29.

Dworak O, Wittekind C, Koerfgen HP, Gall FP. Osteoclastic giant cell tumor of the pancreas: An immuno-histochemical study and review of the literature. Pathol Res Pract 1993; 189:228–231.

Goldberg RD, Michelassi F, Montag AG. Osteoclast-like giant cell tumor of the pancreas: Immunophenotypic similarity to giant cell tumor. Hum Pathol 1991; 22:618–622.

Lewandrowski KB, Weston L, Dickersin GR, et al. Giant cell tumor of the pancreas of mixed osteoclastic and pleomorphic cell type. Evidence for a histogenetic relationship and mesenchymal differentiation. Hum Pathol 1990; 21:1184–1187.

Martin A, Texier P, Bahnini JM, Diebold J. An unusual epithelial pleomorphic giant-cell tumour of the pancreas with osteoclast-type cells. J Clin Pathol 1994; 47:372–374.

Posen JA. Giant cell tumor of the pancreas of the osteoclastic type associated with a mucous secreting cystadenocarcinoma. Hum Pathol 1981; 12:944–947.

Reyes CV, Wang T. Undifferentiated small cell carcinoma of the pancreas: a report of five cases. Cancer 1981; 47:2500–2502.

Rosai J. Carcinoma of the pancreas simulating giant cell tumor of bone. Electron microscopic evidence of its acinar origin. Cancer 1968; 22:333–344.

Silverman JF, Geisinger KR. Pancreas. In: Silverman JF, Geisinger KR, eds. Fine Needle Aspiration Cytology of the Thorax and Abdomen. New York: Churchill Livingstone, 1996, pp. 135–170.

Tschang TP, Garza-Garza R, Kissane JM. Pleomorphic carcinoma of the pancreas. An analysis of 15 cases. Cancer 1977; 39:2114–2126.

Wolfman NT, Karstaedt N, Kawamoto EH. Pleomorphic carcinoma of the pancreas: computed-tomographic, sonographic, and pathologic findings. Radiology 1985; 154:329–332.

Zamboni G, Castelli P, Pea M, et al. Mucinous cystic tumor of the pancreas recurring after 11 years as cystadenocarcinoma with foci of choriocarcinoma and osteoclastic-like giant cell tumor. Surg Pathol 1994; 5: 253–262.

Acinar Cell Carcinoma

Chen J, Baithun SI. Morphological study of 391 cases of exocrine pancreatic tumors with special reference to the classification of exocrine pancreatic carcinoma. J Pathol 1985; 146:17–29.

Cubilla AL, Fitzgerald PJ. Acinar cell cystadenocarcinoma. In: Hartmann WH, Sobin LH, eds. Atlas of Tumor Pathology. Tumors of the Exocrine Pancreas, Fascicle 19, Second series. Washington, D.C.: Armed Forces Institute of Pathology, 1984, pp. 213–219.

Klimstra DS, Heffess CS, Oertel JE, Rosai J. Acinar cell carcinoma of the pancreas. A clinicopathologic study of 28 cases. Am J Surg Pathol 1992; 16:815–837.

Lonardo F, Cubilla AL, Klimstra DS. Microadenocarcinoma of the pancreas—morphologic pattern or pathologic entity? A reevaluation of the original series. Am J Surg Pathol 1996; 20:1385–1393.

Morohoshi T, Kanda M, Horie A, et al. Immunocytochemical markers of uncommon pancreatic tumors. Acinar cell carcinoma, pancreatoblastoma, and solid cystic (papillary-cystic) tumor. Cancer 1987; 59:739–747.

Silverman JF, Geisinger KR. Pancreas. In: Silverman JF, Geisinger KR, eds. Fine Needle Aspiration Cytology of the Thorax and Abdomen. New York: Churchill Livingstone, 1996, pp. 135–170.

Webb JN. Acinar cell neoplasms of the exocrine pancreas. J Clin Pathol 1977; 30:103–112.

Pancreatoblastoma

Becker WF. Pancreatectoduodenectomy for carcinoma of the pancreas in an infant: Report of a case. Ann Surg 1957; 145:864–872.

Geisinger KR, Silverman JF. Fine-needle aspiration cytology of uncommon pancreatic neoplasms: A personal experience and review of the literature. Cytopathol Annu 1992; 23–48.

Kissane JM. Pancreatoblastoma and solid and cystic papillary tumor: two tumors related to pancreatic ontogeny. Semin Diag Pathol 1994; 11:152–164.

Klimstra DS, Wenig BM, Adair CF, Heffess CS. Pancreatoblastoma. A clinicopathologic study and review of the literature. Am J Surg Pathol 1995; 19:1371–1389.

Silverman JF, Holbrook CT, Pories WJ, et al. Fine-needle aspiration cytology of pancreatoblastoma with immunocytochemical and ultrastructural studies. Acta Cytol 1990; 34:632.

Pancreatic Endocrine Tumors

Bordi C, De Vita O, Pilato FP, et al. Multiple islet cell tumors with predominance of glucagon-producing cells and ulcer disease. Am J Clin Pathol 1987; 88:153–161.

Carrieaga MT, Henson DT. Liver, gallbladder, extrahepatic bile ducts, and pancreas. Cancer 1995; 75:171–190.

Clark ES, Carney JA. Pancreatic islet cell tumor associated with Cushing's syndrome. Am J Surg Pathol 1984; 8:917–924.

Comi RJ, Gorden P, Doppman JL. Insulinoma. In: Go VLW, DiMagno EP, Gardner JD, et al., eds. The Pancreas: Biology, Pathobiology and Disease. 2nd edition. New York: Raven Press, 1993, pp. 979–996.

Creutzfeldt W, Arnold R, Creutzfeldt C, Track NS. Pathomorphologic, biochemical, and diagnostic aspects of gastrinomas (Zollinger-Ellison syndrome). Hum Pathol 1975: 6:47–76.

Debas HT, Mulvihill SJ. Neuroendocrine gut neoplasms: important lessons from uncommon tumors. Arch Surg 1994; 129:965–971.

Galbut DL, Markowitz AM. Insulinoma: Diagnosis, surgical management and long-term follow-up. Review of 41 cases. Am J Surg 1980; 139:682–690.

Grimelius L, Hultquist G, Steinkvist B. Cytological differentiation of asymptomatic pancreatic islet cell tumours in autopsy material. Virchows Arch [A] 1975; 365:275–288.

Gunther RW, Klose KJ, Ruckert K, et al. Localization of small islet-cell tumours. Preoperative and intraoperative ultrasound, computed tomography, arteriography, digital subtraction angiography, and pancreatic venous sampling. Gastrointest Radiol 1985; 10:145–152.

Heitz PU, Kasper M, Polak JM, Klöppel G. Pancreatic endocrine tumors: immunocytochemical analysis of 125 tumors. Hum Pathol 1982; 13:263–271.

Klöppel G, Willemer S, Stamm B, et al. Pancreatic lesions and hormonal profile of pancreatic tumors in multiple endocrine neoplasia Type I. An immunocytochemical study of nine patients. Cancer 1986; 57:1824.

Liu T-H, Tseng H-C, Zhu Y, et al. Insulinoma. An immunocytochemical and morphologic analysis of 95 cases. Cancer 1985; 56:1420–1429.

Mukai K, Grotting JC, Greider MH, Rosai J. Retrospective study of 77 pancreatic endocrine tumors using the immunoperoxidase method. Am J Surg Pathol 1982; 6:387–399.

Norton JA, Doherty GM, Fraker DL. Surgery for endocrine tumors of the pancreas. In: Go VLW, DiMagno EP, Gardner JD, et al., eds. The Pancreas: Biology, Pathobiology and Disease. 2nd edition. New York: Raven Press, 1993, pp. 1009–1027.

Norton JA, Doppman JL, Jensen RT. Curative resection in Zollinger-Ellison syndrome: results of a 10 year prospective study. Ann Surg 1992; 215:8–12.

Norton JA. Neuroendocrine tumors of the pancreas and duodenum. Curr Probl Surg 1994; 31:77–156.

Rossi P, Allison DJ, Bezzi M, et al. Endocrine tumors of the pancreas. Radiol Clin North Am 1989; 27:129–161.

Ruttman E, Klöppel G, Bommer G, et al. Pancreatic glucagonoma with and without syndrome. Immunocytochemical study of 5 tumour cases and review of the literature. Virchows Arch [A] 1980; 388:51–67.

Shepherd JJ, Challis DR, Davies PF, et al. Multiple endocrine neoplasia, type 1. Gastrinomas, pancreatic neoplasms, microcarcinoids, the Zollinger-Ellison syndrome, lymph nodes, and hepatic metastases. Arch Surg 1993; 128:1133–1142.

Silverman JF, Geisinger KR. Pancreas. In: Silverman JF, Geisinger KR, eds. Fine Needle Aspiration Cytology of the Thorax and Abdomen. New York: Churchill Livingstone, 1996, pp. 135–170.

Islet Cell Hyperplasia (Nesidioblastosis)

Dobroschke J, Linder R, Otten A. Surgical treatment of nesidioblastosis in childhood. Prog Pediatr Surg 1991; 26:89–91.

Dohrmann P, Mengel W, Splieth J. Total pancreatectomy in a case of nesidioblastosis due to persisting hyperinsulinism following subtotal pancreatectomy. Prog Pediatr Surg 1991; 26:92–95.

Goudsward WB, Houthoff HJ, Koudstaal J, Zwierstra RP. Nesidioblastosis and endocrine hyperplasia of the pancreas: A secondary phenomenon. Hum Pathol 1986; 17:46.

Gould VE, Memoli VA, Dardi LE, Gould NS. Nesidiodysplasia and nesidioblastosis of infancy: Structural and functional correlations with the syndrome of hyperinsulinemic hypoglycemia. Pediatr Pathol 1983; 1:7–31.

Laidlaw GF. Nesidioblastoma, the islet tumor of the pancreas. Am J Pathol 1938; 14:125–134.

Resnick JM, Manivel JC. Immunohistochemical characterization of teratomatous and fetal neuroendocrine pancreas. Arch Pathol Lab Med 1994; 118:155–159.

Taguchi T, Suita S, Hirose R. Histological classification of nesidioblastosis: Efficacy of immunohistochemical study of neuron specific enolase. J Pediatr Surg 1991; 26:770–774.

Willberg B, Muller E. Surgery for nesidioblastosis—indications, treatment and results. Prog Pediatr Surg 1991; 26:76–83.

Pancreatic Carcinoid Tumor and Small Cell Neuroendocrine Carcinoma

Burke AP, Helwig EB. Gangliocytic paraganglioma. Am J Clin Pathol 1989; 92:1–9.

Collina G, Maiorana A, Trentini GP. Duodenal gangliocytic paraganglioma. Case report with immunohistochemical study on the expression of keratin polypeptides. Histopathology 1991; 19:476–478.

Corrin B, Gilby ED, Jones NF, Patrick J. Oat cell carcinoma of the pancreas with ectopic ACTH production. Cancer 1973; 31:1523–1527.

Dookhan DB, Miettinen M, Finkel G, Gibas Z. Recurrent duodenal gangliocytic paraganglioma with lymph node metastasis. Histopathology 1993; 22:399–401.

Hamid QA, Bishop AE, Rode J, et al. Duodenal gangliocytic paraganglioma. A study of 10 cases with immuno-cytochemcial neuroendocrine markers. Hum Pathol 1986; 17:1151–1157.

Hobbs RD, Stewart AF, Ravin ND, Carter D. Hypercalcemia in small cell carcinoma of the pancreas. Cancer 1984; 53:1552–1554.

Kepes JJ, Zacharias DL. Gangliocytic paragangliomas of the duodenum. Report of two cases with light and electron microscopic examination. Cancer 1971; 27:61–70.

Peart WS, Porter KA, Robertson JIS, Sandler M, Blalock E. Carcinoid syndrome due to pancreatic-duct neoplasm secreting 5-hydroxytryptophan and 5-hydroxytryptamine. Lancet 1963; 1:239–242.

Perrone T, Sibley RK, Rosai J. Duodenal gangliocytic paraganglioma. An immunohistochemical and ultrastructural study and a hypothesis concerning its origin. Am J Surg Pathol 1985; 9:31–41.

Reed RJ, Daroca PJ Jr, Harkin JC. Gangliocytic paraganglioma. Am J Surg Pathol 1977; 1:207–216.

Scheithauer BW, Nora FE, Lechago J, et al. Duodenal gangliocytic paraganglioma. Clinicopathologic and immunocytochemical study of 11 cases. Am J Clin Pathol 1986; 86:559–565.

van der Sluys Veer J, Choufoer JC, Querido A, et al. Metastasising islet-cell tumor of the pancreas associated with hypoglycemia and carcinoid syndrome. Lancet 1964; 1:1416–1419.

Mixed Exocrine-Endocrine Pancreatic Tumors

Eusebi V, Capella C, Bondi A, et al. Exocrine-paracrine cells in pancreatic exocrine carcinomas. Histopathology 1981; 5:599–613.

Reid JD, Song-Lim Y, Petrelli M, Jaffe R. Ductuloinsular carcinomas of the pancreas. A light, electron microscopic and immunohistochemical study. Cancer 1982; 49:908–915.

Mixed Acinar-Endocrine Pancreatic Tumors

Klimstra DS, Rosai J, Heffess CS. Mixed acinar-endocrine carcinomas of the pancreas. Am J Surg Pathol 1994; 18:765–778.

Pancreatic Mesenchymal and Lymphoproliferative Neoplasms

Abrebenal P, Sarfaty S, Gal R, et al. Plasma cell granuloma of the pancreas. Arch Pathol Lab Med 1984; 108:531–532.

Aranha GV, Simples PE, Veselik K. Leiomyosarcoma of the pancreas. Int J Pancreatol 1995; 17:95–97.

Borgia G, Ciampi R, Nappa S, et al. Pancreatic plasmacytoma. An unusual cause of obstructive jaundice. Arch Pathol Lab Med 1984; 108:773–774.

Cruikshank AH. Secondary tumours, lymphomas, and rare tumours. In: Pathology of the Pancreas. Berlin: Springer-Verlag, 1986, pp. 181–194.

Cubilla AL, Fitzgerald PJ. Sarcoma and malignant lymphoma. In: Hartmann WH, Sobin LH, eds. Atlas of Tumor Pathology. Tumors of the Exocrine Pancreas, Fascicle 19, Second series. Washington, D.C.: Armed Forces Institute of Pathology, 1984, pp. 220–221.

de Alava E, Torramade J, Vazquez JJ. Leiomyosarcoma of the pancreas. Virchows Arch [A] 1993; 422:419–422.

Elliott TE, Albertazzi VJ, Danto LA. Pancreatic liposarcoma. Case report with review of retroperitoneal liposarcomas. Cancer 1980; 45:1720–1723.

Ishikawa O, Matsui Y, Aoki Y, et al. Leiomyosarcoma of the pancreas. Report of a case and review of the literature. Am J Surg Pathol 1981; 5:597–602.

Nakashiro T, Tokunaga O, Watanabe T, et al. Localized lymphoid hyperplasia (pseudolymphoma) of the pancreas presenting with obstructive jaundice. Hum Pathol 1991; 22:724–726.

Pascal RR, Sullivan L, Hauser L, Ferzli G. Primary malignant fibrous histiocytoma of the pancreas. Hum Pathol 1989; 20:1215–1217.

Suster S, Phillips M, Robinson MJ. Malignant fibrous histiocytoma (giant cell type) of the pancreas. A distinctive variant of osteoclast-type giant cell tumor of the pancreas. Cancer 1989; 64:2303–2308.

Uzoaru I, Chou P, Reyes-Mugica M, et al. Inflammatory myofibroblastic tumor of the pancreas. Surg Pathol 1993; 5:181–188.

Secondary Tumors

Cruikshank AH. Secondary tumours, lymphomas, and rare tumours. In: Pathology of the Pancreas. Berlin: Springer-Verlag, 1986, pp. 181–194.

Ampulla of Vater Neoplasms

Asbun HJ, Rossi RL, Munson JL. Local resection for ampullary tumors. Is there a place for it? Arch Surg 1993; 128:515–520.

Baczako K, Büchler M, Beger HG, et al. Morphogenesis and possible precursor lesions of invasive carcinoma of the papilla of Vater: Epithelial dysplasia and adenoma. Hum Pathol 1985; 16:305–310.

Blackman E, Nash SV. Diagnosis of duodenal and ampullary epithelial neoplasms by endoscopic biopsy: a clinicopathologic and immunohistochemical study. Hum Pathol 1985; 16:901–920.

Buck JL, Elsayed AM. Ampullary tumors: Radiologic-pathologic correlation. Radiographics 1993; 13:193–212.

Fenoglio-Preiser CM, Pascal RR, Perzin KH. Tumors of the intestine. In: Hartmann WH, Sobin LH. Atlas of Tumor Pathology, Second series, Fascicle 27. Washington, D.C.: Armed Forces Institute of Pathology, 1990, pp. 175–250.

Ferrell LD, Beckstead JH. Paneth-like cells in an adenoma and adenocarcinoma in the ampulla of vater. Arch Pathol Lab Med 1991; 115:956–958.

Hyland C, Kheir SM, Kashlan MB. Frozen sections diagnosis of pancreatic carcinoma. A prospective study of 64 biopsies. Am J Surg Pathol 1981; 5:179–191.

Iwafuchi M, Watanabe H, Ishihara N, et al. Neoplastic endocrine cells in carcinomas of the small intestine. Hum Pathol 1987; 18:185–194.

Javier J, Lukie B. Duodenal adenocarcinoma complicating celiac sprue. Dig Dis Sci 1983; 25:150–153.

Komorowski RA, Beggs BK, Greenan JE, Venu RP. Assessment of ampulla of Vater pathology. An endoscopic approach. Am J Surg Pathol 1991; 15:1188–1196.

Komorowski RA, Cohen EB. Villous tumors of the duodenum. Cancer 1981; 47:1377–1386.

Kozuka S, Tsubone M, Yamaguchi A, Hachisuka K. Adenomatous residue in cancerous papilla of Vater. Gut 1981; 22:1031–1034.

Lashner BA. Risk factors for small bowel cancer in Crohn's disease. Dig Dis Sci 1992; 37:1179–1184.

Mingazzini PL, Malchiodi Albedi F, Blandamura V. Villous adenoma of the duodenum: Cellular composition and histochemical findings. Histopathology 1982; 6:235–244.

Newman DH, Doerhoff CR, Bunt TJ. Villous adenoma of the duodenum. Am Surgeon 1984; 50:26–28.

Noda Y, Watanabe H, Iida M, et al. Histologic follow-up of ampullary adenomas in patients with familial polyposis coli. Cancer 1992; 70:1847–1856.

Perzin KH, Bridge MF. Adenomas of the small intestine: A clinicopathologic review of 51 cases and a study of their relationship to carcinoma. Cancer 1981; 48:799–819.

Ribeiro MB, Greenstein AJ, Heimann TM, et al. Adenocarcinoma of the small intestine in Crohn's disease. Surg Gynecol Obstet 1991; 173: 343–349.

Scarpa A, Capelli P, Zamboni G, et al. Neoplasia of the ampulla of Vater. Ki-ras and p53 mutations. Am J Pathol 1993; 142:1163–1172.

Seifert E, Schulte F, Stolte M. Adenoma and carcinoma of the duodenum and papilla of Vater: A clinicopathologic study. Am J Gastroenterol 1992; 87:37–42.

Talbot IC, Neoptolemos JP, Shaw DE, Carr-Locke D. The histopathology and staging of carcinoma of the ampulla of Vater. Histopathology 1988; 12:155–165.

Willett CG, Warshaw AL, Convery K, Compton CC. Patterns of failure after pancreaticoduodenectomy for ampullary carcinoma. Surg Gynecol Obstet 1993; 176:33–38.

Witteman BJ, Janssens AR, Terpstra JL, et al. Villous tumors of the duodenum. Presentation of five cases. Hepatogastroenterology 1991; 38:550–553.

Yamaguchi K, Enjoji M. Carcinoma of the ampulla of Vater. A clinicopathologic study and pathologic staging of 109 cases of carcinoma and 5 cases of adenoma. Cancer 1987; 59:506–515.

CHAPTER 13

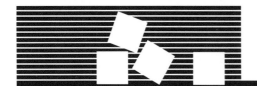

Non-Neoplastic Lesions of the Adrenal Gland

A. CLASSIFICATION OF NON-NEOPLASTIC LESIONS OF THE ADRENAL GLAND

Table 13–1
CLASSIFICATION OF NON-NEOPLASTIC LESIONS
OF THE ADRENAL GLAND

1. Adrenal heterotopia and accessory adrenal tissue
2. Congenital adrenal hypoplasia
3. Adrenal cytomegaly
4. Congenital adrenal hyperplasia
5. Addison's disease
6. Infectious diseases affecting the adrenal gland
7. Amyloidosis
8. Waterhouse-Friderichsen syndrome
9. Adrenal cysts
10. Adrenocortical nodules (nonhyperfunctioning)
11. Adrenocortical hyperplasia with hypercortisolism
12. Adrenocortical hyperplasia with hyperaldosteronism

B. ADRENAL HETEROTOPIA AND ACCESSORY ADRENAL TISSUE

Definition: True heterotopia refers to abnormal location of the entire adrenal gland, whereas accessory adrenal tissue usually consists of small rests of cortical cells.

Clinical

- Patients with adrenal heterotopia or adrenal rests rarely have any symptoms related to the abnormality. Most are incidental findings at surgery for unrelated problems.
- Heterotopia usually involves adrenal placement on the upper pole of the kidney, beneath the renal capsule. Rare examples have been located in the capsule of the liver.
- Accessory adrenal tissue, or adrenal rests, are most often seen along the migration path of the gonads. The most common site is in the area of the celiac axis, with rests

also frequently found around the kidney, in the broad ligament, in and around the spermatic cord, and in hernia sacs. Rarely they have been seen in the ovary and gallbladder wall, and one has been described in the cranial cavity.
- Accessory adrenal tissue is a very common finding, present in almost one third of individuals in an autopsy study.

Pathology

Gross

- Heterotopia is usually bilateral. The adrenal may be flattened and atrophic in appearance, although functionally it seems to be adequate to maintain normal cortisol levels.
- Accessory tissue appears as small, rounded, yellow, encapsulated nodules, a few millimeters in diameter.

Histology

- The adrenal rests are composed of lipid-rich cortical cells, usually without a medullary component. Some degree of zonal differentiation is present.
- In complete adrenal heterotopia no medulla is present.

Treatment and Prognosis

- Adrenal heterotopia is not associated with any endocrine abnormality.
- Adrenocortical rests require no treatment except in the rare instance of a cortical neoplasm arising in them. The rests may also be affected by any hyperplastic phenomenon resulting from adrenocorticotropic hormone (ACTH) stimulation.

C. CONGENITAL ADRENAL HYPOPLASIA

Definition: A sporadic or familial disorder characterized by a reduced volume of adrenocortical tissue.

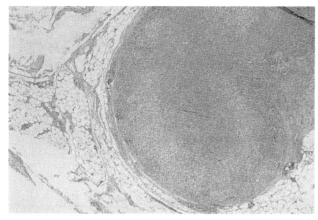

Figure 13–1. The soft tissue surrounding a hernia sac contains an encapsulated adrenocortical rest. As in most adrenal rests, no medullary tissue is present (see Fig. 13–2).

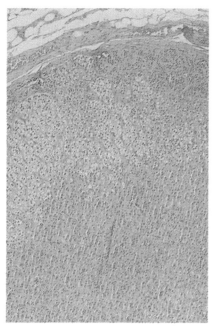

Figure 13–2. At a higher power the cellular composition is predominantly lipid-rich cells resembling those of the zona fasciculata. Zonation is readily observed in this example.

Clinical

- Congenital adrenal hypoplasia may be sporadic, or it may be an autosomal recessive or X-linked inherited disorder. Other cases are associated with glycerol kinase enzyme deficiency.
- The most common form, the cytomegalic type, is X-linked. More rare is the "miniature" type.
- Infants with congenital hypoplasia present with typical signs of adrenocortical insufficiency: vomiting, dehydration, weight loss, hyponatremia, and hyperkalemia.
- The onset of symptoms after birth is dependent on the amount of cortical tissue present.
- Males with X-linked cytomegalic type hypoplasia also manifest a hypothalamic form of hypogonadism due to gonadotropin-releasing hormone deficiency.

Pathology

Gross

- The miniature type of congenital adrenal hypoplasia is characterized by very small but normally formed adrenal glands. The size is variable and affects the clinical severity of disease.
- The cytomegalic type is characterized by small, dysmorphic glands.

Histology

- The histologic appearance of the miniature type of hypoplasia is similar to that of a normal gland for the patient's age, with normal zonation and cytologic features.
- The cytomegalic type is very abnormal histologically, with a distorted architectural pattern and strikingly atypical cytology. The cortical cells are large and vacuolated, with anisonucleosis, variable hyperchromasia, and frequent intranuclear cytoplasmic inclusions.

Treatment and Prognosis

- In the past congenital adrenal hypoplasia was uniformly fatal; however, with the availability of replacement glucocorticoid and mineralocorticoid therapy, the prognosis is very good.
- Important to successful therapy is early recognition of hypoadrenalism.

Additional Facts

- The cause of adrenocortical insufficiency is unknown but may be related to injury to the adrenal primordia in fetal life or lack of some key induction factor for the normal development of the cortex.
- Other causes of congenital adrenal insufficiency include anencephaly that results in agenesis or marked hypoplasia of the adrenals, familial glucocorticoid deficiency in which a selective deficiency of glucocorticoids due to an unknown cellular defect is found in the presence of high ACTH levels, glycerol kinase deficiency resulting in decreased glucocorticoid and mineralocorticoid levels, and adrenoleukodystrophy.
- Adrenoleukodystrophy is a demyelinating neurologic disorder that is associated with adrenocortical atrophy and hypoadrenalism. It is caused by a defect in oxidation of fatty acids, resulting in accumulation of cholesterol esters in tissues. The neonatal form is usually an autosomal recessive disorder, presenting with hypotonia, seizures, and rapid deterioration of sight and hearing at birth; mental and growth retardation are severe, and the children rarely live beyond 5 years of age. An X-linked childhood form becomes evident around 10 years of age, and an adult form may be seen in young adult men; these patients may present with adrenal insufficiency before neurologic disease is evident. The histology of adrenoleukodystrophy is characterized by large ballooned cortical cells containing lamellar inclusions. The lipid inclusions have a unique bilamellar and lamellar appearance ultrastructurally.

D. ADRENAL CYTOMEGALY

Definition: Cellular enlargement, both cytoplasmic and nuclear, with nuclear pleomorphism and hyperchromasia, involving the adrenocortical cells.

Clinical

■ Usually an incidental finding in a small percentage of neonates, cytomegaly is also seen in Beckwith-Wiedemann syndrome (symmetrical gigantism or hemihypertrophy, macroglossia, and exomphalos).

Pathology

Gross

■ The adrenals are enlarged in Beckwith-Wiedemann syndrome, with expansion of the cortex, and in some patients the medulla as well.
■ In incidental cytomegaly the adrenals are grossly normal in appearance.

Histology

■ The cytomegalic cells are located in the fetal cortex; they are variable in number in incidentally discovered cases in infants but are more numerous and diffusely distributed in Beckwith-Wiedemann syndrome.
■ The cells have increased cytoplasmic volume as well as enlarged nuclei. Nuclear pleomorphism, hyperchromasia and intranuclear cytoplasmic inclusions are often seen. Mitoses are exceptional.

Treatment and Prognosis

■ The cytomegaly is of little clinical significance; however, it is seen in x-linked congenital adrenal hypoplasia.
■ The association with Beckwith-Wiedemann syndrome has more serious implications, including hypoglycemia in the neonatal period and the later increased risk of malignant neoplasms, particularly Wilms' tumor and adreno-

cortical carcinoma, but also neuroblastoma and pancreatoblastoma.

E. CONGENITAL ADRENAL HYPERPLASIA

Synonym: Adrenogenital syndrome.

Definition: An autosomal recessive disorder resulting from defects in one of several enzymes necessary for the synthesis of cortisol and other steroid hormones from cholesterol, with the resultant increase in other steroid products, usually androgenic, leading to virilization in addition to deficiencies of various corticosteroids and mineralocorticoids.

Clinical

■ The enzyme defects in congenital adrenal hyperplasia (CAH) include 21-hydroxylase, 11-β-hydroxylase, 17-hydroxylase, 3β-hydroxysteroid dehydrogenase, and cholesterol desmolase. All these defects are associated with

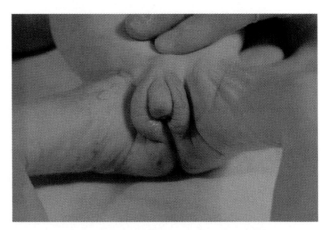

Figure 13–4. A female newborn with 21-hydroxylase deficiency has ambiguous external genitalia characterized by clitoromegaly and large rugated labioscrotal folds.

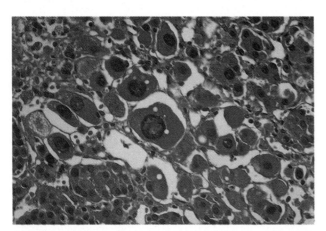

Figure 13–3. Adrenal cytomegaly, incidentally discovered at autopsy. The cells have increased cytoplasmic volume as well as nuclear enlargement. Nuclear pleomorphism, hyperchromasia, and intranuclear cytoplasmic inclusions are seen.

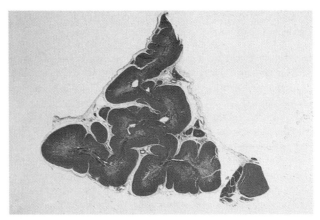

Figure 13–5. Congenital adrenal hyperplasia. The adrenal glands of a male infant, who died of adrenal insufficiency, are moderately enlarged with the typical "cerebriform" appearance.

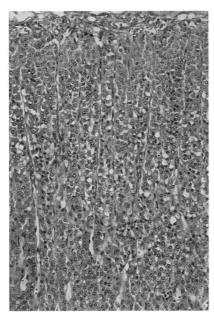

Figure 13–6. The same adrenal seen in Figure 13–5, with eosinophilic-compact (lipid-poor) cells.

deficiency of cortisol, but additional manifestations vary. Virilization affects both males and females.

- *21-Hydroxylase deficiency* is responsible for 95% of cases of CAH. The classic form is seen in between 1:5000 and 1:15,000 live births in the white population, with a much higher incidence in Alaskan Eskimos; it is characterized by deficient cortisol production, resulting in hypersecretion of ACTH, which in turn stimulates the adrenal cortex. The end result is the excessive production of cortisol precursors, particularly 17-hydroxyprogesterone. The virilization results from the accumulation of 17-hydroxypregnenolone, which is metabolized to androgenic steroids (dehydroepiandrosterone and androstenedione). Aldosterone production may also be reduced, in some cases producing a more acutely threatening clinical syndrome of hypotension and salt wasting. Aldosterone deficiency occurs in two thirds of patients. Males appear normal at birth, whereas females have ambiguous genitalia characterized by clitoromegaly with fusion of labioscrotal folds. Acne, development of genital hair, and bronzing of the skin are common. If treatment is delayed, the epiphyseal plates close prematurely. A nonclassic form of 21-hydroxylase deficiency presents later in childhood or at puberty with virilization. Rare patients with the enzyme defect may be asymptomatic.
- *11-β-hydroxylase deficiency* is the cause of approximately 5% of cases, and is the result of deficient metabolism of 11-deoxycortisol to cortisol, with secondary overproduction of androgens, as in the 21-hydroxylase defect. Accumulation of deoxycorticosterone in the pathway for mineralocorticoid production may lead to hypertension and hypokalemia in addition to the signs of hypocortisolism and virilization.
- *3-β-hydroxysteroid dehydrogenase deficiency* affects synthesis of glucocorticoids, mineralocorticoids, and sex steroids (both testosterone and estrogens). The androgen accumulated is weak and results in milder virilization of females and incomplete masculinization of male genitalia (hypospadias). Salt wasting is present in severe forms.
- *17-Hydroxylase deficiency* interrupts the synthesis of glucocorticoids and sex steroids, resulting in incomplete masculinization with hypospadias in males and amenorrhea in females and in manifestations of hypocortisolism.
- *Cholesterol desmolase deficiency* is usually fatal in childhood due to severe hypoadrenalism. Males have incomplete masculinization, whereas females lack virilization.

Pathology

Gross

- The adrenal glands in untreated CAH are two to several times the normal size, with weight dependent on age.
- The glands are brown, with a cerebriform surface, except in cholesterol desmolase deficiency, which is characterized by yellow areas and diffuse nodularity.

Histology

- The hyperplastic cerebriform appearance is noted microscopically as well as grossly. The proliferating cells are eosinophilic, compact lipid-poor cells, with a few lipid-rich cells in some cases. Cholesterol clefts, with foreign body reaction and calcifications, are seen in cholesterol desmolase–deficient cases.

Treatment and Prognosis

- Replacement therapy is directed toward the deficient steroid group(s). Cortisol is deficient in all of the enzyme defects. Mineralocorticoids and sex steroids are administered according to need.
- Surgical correction of ambiguous external genitalia or hypospadias is necessary in many instances.
- Prognosis is dependent on the severity of the steroid deficiency and on time of diagnosis. The diagnosis is usually more obvious in females due to the ambiguous genitalia; males are more likely to suffer longer effects of hypoadrenalism prior to recognition of CAH.
- Rare instances of benign and malignant adrenocortical neoplasms arising in patients with CAH have been reported.

Additional Facts

- Rarely, males with CAH have developed a peculiar form of testicular tumor in adolescence or young adulthood. These tumors are frequently bilateral, are responsive to ACTH stimulation, and produce cortisol. The tumors may be several centimeters in diameter, and they decrease in size with suppression of ACTH by dexamethasone. Although these lesions bear a striking histologic resemblance to Leydig cell tumors, the lack of crystalloids of Reinke and the ACTH dependence are more suggestive of an adrenocortical origin, possibly from adrenocortical rests. It is not clear whether these tumors represent true neoplasms or hyperplastic nodules. They have all pursued a benign course.

Table 13–2
CAUSES OF ADDISON'S DISEASE

Idiopathic, or Autoimmune

Infectious

Tuberculosis
Histoplasmosis
Coccidioidomycosis
North American blastomycosis
South American blastomycosis
Cryptococcosis
Cytomegalovirus
Herpes simplex virus
Varicella-zoster
Visceral leishmaniasis

Infiltrative Processes

Amyloidosis

Metastatic Carcinoma

Lung
Breast
Stomach
Colon

Malignant Lymphoma

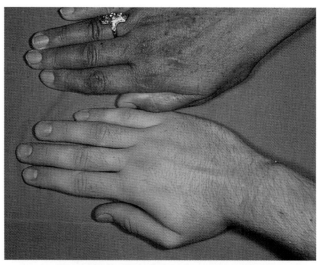

Figure 13–8. The hand in the upper portion of the field belongs to a patient with "bronzing" of the skin in Addison's disease. The lower hand is that of an individual without adrenal dysfunction.

F. ADDISON'S DISEASE (Table 13–2)

Synonym: Chronic adrenal insufficiency.

Definition: Chronic deficiency of glucocorticoids and mineralocorticoids due to a variety of causes, including autoimmune adrenalitis, infectious diseases, metastatic neoplasms, and accumulation of substances such as amyloid.

Clinical

■ Addison's disease affects individuals of any age.
■ The most common type of Addison's disease today is the idiopathic, or autoimmune, type; however, tuberculosis was the most common etiology until the past few decades.
■ Patients present with weakness, weight loss, and bronzing of the skin. Left untreated, dehydration, hypotension, and shock may develop, especially when the patient encounters other physiologic stresses, such as an infection.

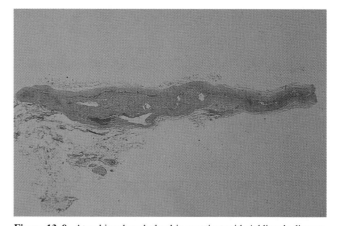

Figure 13–9. Atrophic adrenal gland in a patient with Addison's disease. Note the thinness of the cortical ribbon.

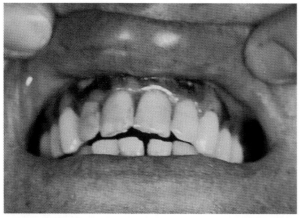

Figure 13–7. Mucosal hyperpigmentation in a patient with Addison's disease. The hyperpigmentation is due to the melanocyte-stimulating activity of adrenocorticotropic hormone.

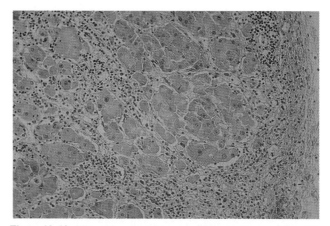

Figure 13–10. Idiopathic, or autoimmune, Addison's disease. Adrenalitis is present, with a moderate lymphoplasmacytic infiltrate interspersed among islands of residual cortex. The cortical cells are enlarged, with eosinophilic, lipid-poor cytoplasm and mild anisonucleosis.

- Bronzing of the skin in Addison's disease is due to high levels of ACTH resulting from the lack of feedback inhibition on the pituitary by the incompetent adrenal glands.
- The mechanism of autoimmune Addison's disease is not clear but is related to an autoimmune form of adrenalitis.
- Other endocrine associations are seen in two subsets of idiopathic Addison's disease, known as polyglandular autoimmune (PGA) syndromes. PGA I is defined as the presence of at least two of the following: Addison's disease, hypoparathyroidism, or chronic mucocutaneous candidiasis; a related disorder has additional associations of dental and nail dystrophy and a high incidence of juvenile diabetes, primary hypogonadism, and chronic active hepatitis. PGA II is an association of Addison's disease, autoimmune disease of the thyroid, and insulin-dependent diabetes.

Pathology

Gross

- The adrenal glands do not manifest hypofunction clinically until most of the cortical tissue is destroyed (as much as 90%). The glands, therefore, in clinically apparent Addison's disease are extremely small and may be difficult to identify.
- The gland is often only a wisp of fibrovascular tissue, brown to gray in color, without the usual orange rim of cortex.

Histology

- The cortex is thin and discontinuous, appearing as sparsely distributed patches of eosinophilic lipid-poor cells.
- A lymphoplasmacytic infiltrate is scattered through the remnant of the cortex. Lymphoid follicles may be present, similar to the pattern seen in lymphocytic thyroiditis. Unlike the infiltrate commonly seen as "nonspecific" adrenalitis, often an incidental autopsy or surgical observation, the inflammatory cells are centered on the residual islands of cortex. In nonspecific adrenalitis they are distributed around blood vessels and as aggregates in the cortex, unassociated with evidence of tissue damage.
- Cytomegaly is present in some cases.

Differential Diagnosis

- Nonspecific adrenalitis.

Treatment and Prognosis

- Therapy is directed at replacement of corticosteroid products and has dramatically altered the prognosis of Addison's disease.

Additional Facts

- Adrenal insufficiency may also be pituitary in origin, as in Sheehan's syndrome or lymphocytic hypophysitis. Such patients do not have the hyperpigmentation seen in Addison's disease.

G. INFECTIOUS DISEASES AFFECTING THE ADRENAL GLAND

Definition: Infections involving the adrenal gland are usually secondary to a systemic infection. Although many infections are capable of producing Addison's disease, destruction of most of the cortex is usually required before manifestations of hypoadrenalism are seen.

1. Tuberculosis

- Tuberculosis was the most common cause of Addison's disease during the first part of the twentieth century, causing about 70% of cases, while a minority of cases were considered idiopathic. With the advent of effective antituberculous drugs, the statistics have reversed.
- In contrast with idiopathic Addison's disease, computed tomographic (CT) or magnetic resonance imaging (MRI) scans show bilateral adrenal enlargement, often with calcification.
- The histologic pattern in adrenal tuberculosis is quite different from that of other organs: caseation necrosis with a diminished granulomatous reaction, in spite of well-developed granulomata in other sites.

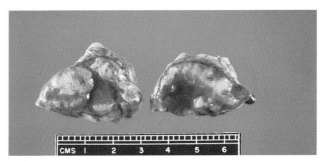

Figure 13–11. The adrenals from a patient who died of disseminated histoplasmosis. The glands are enlarged and contain large areas of caseation necrosis, a finding typical of tuberculosis and histoplasmosis in the adrenal. Well-formed granulomata are usually not prominent in the adrenal.

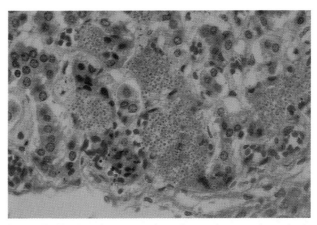

Figure 13–12. *Histoplasma capsulatum* is seen in macrophages in the adrenal gland of a patient with disseminated histoplasmosis (H & E). The organisms are tiny and ovoid; distinction from amastigotes of leishmania is readily accomplished with Gomori's methenamine silver (GMS) stain. ■

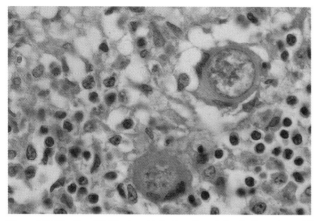

Figure 13–13. *Coccidioides immitis* in the adrenal gland of a patient with disseminated coccidioidomycosis. Sporangia in this field have been engulfed by giant cells, a common finding in this granulomatous fungal infection.

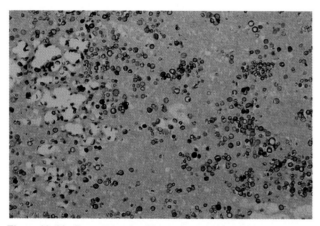

Figure 13–14. Cryptococcosis with massive necrosis of the adrenal gland in a patient with AIDS. The Gomori's methenamine silver (GMS) stain highlights the yeast forms, which are quite variable in size. Mucicarmine is also helpful in identifying the mucoid capsule of these organisms.

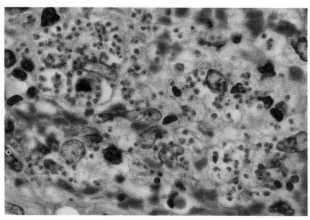

Figure 13–15. Visceral leishmaniasis in the adrenal gland of a woman from the Mediterranean area. The reaction is dominated by macrophages that are stuffed with the amastigote form of the organism (Gram's stain).

2. Histoplasmosis

- Adrenal involvement is present in most cases of disseminated histoplasmosis, although fewer than 10% develop Addison's disease.
- As in tuberculosis, necrosis is usually prominent, whereas well-formed granulomata are not seen. In some cases the necrosis is not extensive, and aggregates of histiocytes containing organisms are found in the gland.

3. Viral Infections

- Neonatal herpes simplex viral infection causes necrosis in the adrenal and in the liver that may be patchy or confluent but invokes little or no inflammatory reaction. Eosinophilic Cowdry A inclusions are easily found.
- Neonatal cytomegalovirus (CMV) infection is associated with multiorgan involvement. The adrenal lesions are similar to those in herpes simplex infection, with the exception of the characteristic intranuclear and cytoplasmic inclusions seen in CMV disease: large eosinophilic nuclear inclusions with a peripheral halo and small basophilic cytoplasmic inclusions.
- Acquired immunodeficiency syndrome–associated CMV infection has a predilection for adrenal involvement—it is the most commonly involved organ. In some patients confluent necrosis is severe enough to cause Addison's disease.

H. AMYLOIDOSIS

Definition: Abnormal accumulation of filamentous protein deposits in the interstitial tissue of the adrenal. Amyloidosis affecting the adrenal is most often the secondary type, related to chronic inflammatory disease, particularly granulomatous infections.

Clinical

- Amyloidosis is quite rare as a cause of Addison's disease. It is usually associated with chronic inflammatory dis-

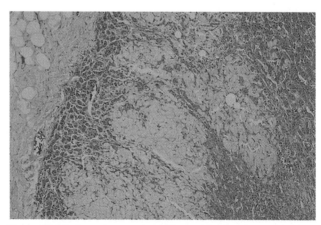

Figure 13–16. Amorphous eosinophilic amyloid deposits are present in the cortex of a patient with the secondary form of amyloidosis, which is more common than primary amyloidosis as a cause of Addison's disease. The adjacent cortical cells are compact and eosinophilic.

eases (secondary amyloidosis). Primary amyloidosis, associated with plasma cell dyscrasias and caused by abnormal immunoglobulins, usually affects the blood vessels but does not accumulate in the parenchyma; thus, it is not a significant cause of adrenal insufficiency.

- Accumulation of amyloid in the adrenal is silent until adequate replacement of cortex has occurred to cause adrenal insufficiency.

Pathology

Gross

- The accumulation of amyloid may greatly enlarge the gland. In such cases the cut surface is yellow-white, smooth, and waxy.
- The loss of adrenal function is dependent on the distribution of the amyloid. If the deposits are concentrated in the inner cortex, adrenal insufficiency may occur before the glands are noticeably enlarged.

Histology

- Amorphous smudgy-appearing pink deposits are seen in hematoxylin and eosin–stained sections, largely in the zona fasciculata and zona reticularis, crowding out the cortical tissue.
- The deposits are positive for Congo red, with apple-green birefringence, as well as for Crystal violet and amyloid-specific immunohistochemistry.
- Electron microscopy shows deposits consist of fine, non-branching filaments.

Treatment and Prognosis

- If amyloid deposition is extensive enough to cause Addison's disease, glucocorticoid and mineralocorticoid replacement is required.

I. WATERHOUSE-FRIDERICHSEN SYNDROME

Definition: A form of septicemic shock associated with sudden vascular collapse, disseminated intravascular coagulation, and adrenal hemorrhage.

Clinical

- A variety of organisms has been associated with the syndrome, although it has historically been linked to meningococcemia. Other causes include *Streptococcus pneumoniae, Haemophilus influenzae,* and neonatal echovirus infections.
- Rapid onset characterizes Waterhouse-Friderichsen syndrome, which is almost uniformly fatal.
- The disseminated intravascular coagulation is usually accompanied by a petechial rash.
- It is unlikely that the cause of shock in this syndrome is acute adrenal insufficiency; the adrenal hemorrhage is probably secondary.

Pathology

Gross

- The adrenals are acutely congested and may be nearly effaced by hemorrhage, but they are normal in size.

Histology

- The adrenal is massively hemorrhagic, with necrosis centered along the corticomedullary junction, which is most sensitive to hypoxemia.
- Fibrin thrombi in the sinusoids reflect the disseminated intravascular coagulation.

Treatment and Prognosis

- Although treatment with appropriate antibiotics may be aggressively instituted, the mortality rate from Waterhouse-Friderichsen syndrome is extremely high.

Additional Facts

- Neonatal hemorrhage due to delivery trauma, hypoxemia, and less fulminant episodes of septicemia may occur in the absence of Waterhouse-Friderichsen syndrome. In such cases the adrenal hemorrhage is most often unilateral. Although many are asymptomatic, some patients may develop a large hematoma or may experience rupture of the gland with hemorrhage into the retroperitoneum. Surgery may be required to control bleeding or to treat secondary abscess formation. Resolution of adrenal hematomas may be associated with calcification and cyst formation.
- Adrenal hemorrhage in adults is often caused by anticoagulant therapy. Vascular manipulation and surgical trauma to the gland are other causative factors.

J. ADRENAL CYSTS (Table 13–3)

Definition: Rare lesions characterized by cystic alteration of the adrenal. The chief non-neoplastic cysts include retention and embryonal cysts and endothelial cysts, as well as the pseudocyst.

- Adrenal cysts are rare, with an autopsy incidence of 0.06%. Most are incidental findings.
- Cysts occur over a wide age range but are most common in the fifth and sixth decades and are very rare in children.
- Male:female ratio is 1:3.

Table 13–3
ADRENAL CYSTS

Parasitic cysts
   Echinococcus granulosus
True epithelial cysts
   Glandular (retention) cyst
   Embryonal cyst
Endothelial cysts
   Lymphangiomatous
   Hemangiomatous
Pseudocysts (hemorrhagic cysts)

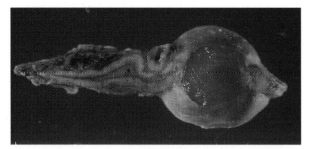

Figure 13–17. A serous, or lymphangiomatous, cyst of the adrenal gland. These translucent cysts are lined by a flattened layer of endothelium.

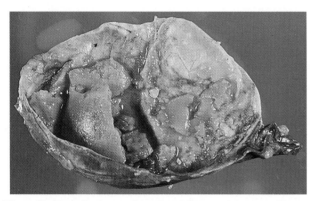

Figure 13–18. A simple cyst of the adrenal discovered at autopsy. The cyst wall is formed of fibrous tissue. No cyst lining is present. The large fibrin clots with organization within the cyst suggest that it may be an old hemorrhagic cyst.

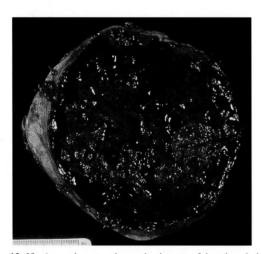

Figure 13–19. A pseudocyst, or hemorrhagic cyst, of the adrenal gland, is filled with organizing blood clot. The adrenal gland is tensely stretched over the cyst wall.

- Adrenal cysts are frequently asymptomatic; when symptoms occur, they are usually related to the mass effect of the lesion.
- Endothelial cysts and pseudocysts are the most common adrenal cysts, comprising more than 85% of this group of lesions.
- Epithelial cysts of the adrenal include true glandular (retention) cysts and embryonal cysts, which are very rare.

The classification of adrenal cysts is detailed in Table 13–3. These lesions should be distinguished from adrenocortical or medullary neoplasms with marked cystic degeneration.

1. Parasitic Cysts

- Most parasitic cysts are associated with *Echinococcus granulosus* infection, although adrenal involvement is very rare in echinococcosis and is generally associated with widely disseminated disease.
- The cyst may be several centimeters in diameter and usually has a smooth fibrous wall with internal loculations.
- The cyst fluid contains sandlike grains that represent scoleces of the parasite.

2. True Epithelial Cysts

- Usually small and incidental, these lesions are believed to be developmental accidents, possibly formed from rests of tissue of urogenital origin or from mesothelial inclusions.
- The cysts are lined by cuboidal or ciliated columnar epithelium and are filled with clear fluid.

3. Endothelial Cysts

- These multiloculated cysts are lined by flat endothelium and are believed to be related to hemangiomas and lymphangiomas.
- Lymphangiomatous cysts are the more common of the two types, and are also known as "serous" cysts. Although they are usually incidental, some cases attain a size adequate to become symptomatic surgical lesions.

4. Pseudocysts

- The pseudocyst has received more attention in recent years. Although they were frequently incidental autopsy findings in the past, radiographic advances and more widespread use of advanced diagnostic imaging techniques have increased the relative incidence in younger individuals and recognition of cysts as symptomatic lesions, usually causing abdominal pain.
- Pseudocysts appear radiographically as cysts with variable internal densities and peripheral calcification.
- Sizes range from 2 to 10 cm, except for very rare examples that attained a massive volume of 12 L.
- The pseudocyst wall is well-formed and fibrous and is filled with hemorrhagic material, organizing blood clot, and brown fluid. In some cases smooth muscle has been seen in the wall.
- Histologically, the cyst wall has no epithelial lining. There are descriptions of some cysts with a partial endothelial lining, suggesting that some of these may be the result of secondary hemorrhage in a vascular neoplasm or malformation. Adrenal cortex may form a partial rim around the pseudocyst wall. Foci of adrenocortical tissue have been described within the cavity of some lesions; the possibility of a hemorrhagic adrenocortical adenoma must be considered in such cases. The material in the cavity in-

cludes organizing clot, fibrous tissue, granulation tissue, and coagulated blood.

- Possible etiologies proposed for pseudocysts include resolving adrenal hemorrhage for any of a variety of reasons or hemorrhage into a hemangiomatous or lymphangiomatous lesion.
- Adrenal hemorrhage occurs in a variety of situations, including trauma, sepsis, therapeutic anticoagulation, clotting disorders, steroid therapy or administration of ACTH, neoplasia, adrenal vein thrombosis, traumatic delivery, and pregnancy. No etiology is discovered in many instances.

K. ADRENOCORTICAL NODULES (NONHYPERFUNCTIONING)

Definition: Multinodular adrenocortical proliferation, almost always bilateral, without clinical, biochemical, or histologic evidence of hyperfunction; nonfunctional nodules are the most common cause of adrenal enlargement.

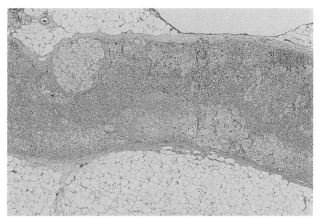

Figure 13–20. Incidental, nonhyperfunctioning adrenal cortical nodules are seen in this gland. The small nodules are composed of lipid-rich cells resembling the zona fasciculata. These nodules, which are almost always multiple and bilateral, are seen with increased frequency in the elderly and in patients with diabetes mellitus, vascular disease, and hypertension.

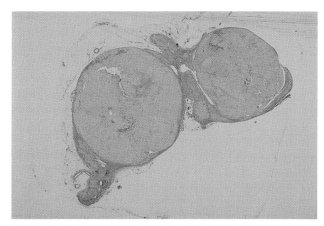

Figure 13–21. Large nonhyperfunctional cortical nodules were present bilaterally in this elderly man. The etiology is believed to be a regenerative response to zonal ischemia in patients with arteriopathy due to hypertension. Note the areas of normal intervening cortical tissue between nodules.

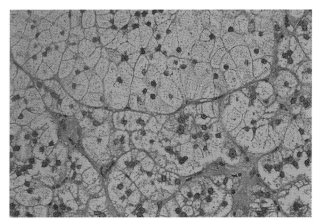

Figure 13–22. The cortical nodules seen in Figure 13–21 are composed of lipid-rich cells of the zona fasciculata type.

Clinical

- Very common incidental finding at surgery or during radiographic procedures for other problems.
- These lesions have been classified in the past as "nonfunctional adenomas"; however, the evidence supports a non-neoplastic origin.
- Nonhyperfunctional nodules are found over a wide age range, with incidence increasing with age.
- An increased incidence is seen in diabetes mellitus, hypertension, and cardiovascular or peripheral vascular disease.
- Incidental nodules larger than 1.5 cm in diameter are found in 20% of hypertensive patients at autopsy.
- The high incidence of incidental nodules with age, and apparent close association with vascular disease, is good evidence to support the theory that these lesions are secondary to arteriopathy associated with hypertension and represent a regenerative hyperplasia in response to localized ischemic injury.
- No clinical significance has been assigned to these lesions.

Radiology

- Advances in radiologic imaging techniques have led to an apparent increase in nonhyperfunctioning nodules during life.
- CT scan and MRI demonstrate adrenal enlargement, usually bilateral, but sometimes quite asymmetrical. A dominant nodule may have the appearance of a neoplasm, either primary or metastatic.

Pathology

Cytology

- Fine needle aspiration is an effective method for exclusion of metastatic disease in cases of adrenal enlargement due to nonfunctional nodules.
- The cytologic appearance is not distinguishable from normal cortex, or from a benign cortical neoplasm. Accurate localization is essential to assure sampling of the lesion.
- The cells are fragile, and the smears contain many naked nuclei in a background of foamy cytoplasmic material. The nuclei are round, with relatively dense chromatin.

Gross

- Nodules are usually multiple and bilateral; however, there may be significant disparity between glands regarding weight. In some cases one nodule is large enough to overshadow the smaller ones around it, but additional small nodules can almost always be found on close inspection.
- Size of individual nodules ranges from 1 mm to 3 cm in diameter, with most smaller than 1 cm.
- Larger nodules may contain foci of cystic degeneration or areas of calcification.

Microscopic

- The cells have abundant pale-staining finely vacuolated cytoplasm, resembling the cells of the zona fasciculata. Nodularity is quite obvious microscopically.
- The nodules are circumscribed but not encapsulated.
- Myelolipomatous foci may be present.

Differential Diagnosis

- Adrenocortical adenoma (Chapter 14B, #1).
- Nodular adrenocortical hyperplasia with Cushing's syndrome (Chapter 13L).

Treatment and Prognosis

- No therapy is required; however, these lesions may be clinically mistaken for neoplasms and be resected.
- Nuclear atypia and mitotic activity are not present.

L. ADRENOCORTICAL HYPERPLASIA WITH HYPERCORTISOLISM

Definition: Hypercortisolism with adrenal enlargement, usually bilateral, due to pituitary-based excess ACTH production, autonomous bilateral adrenal hyperplasia, or ectopic ACTH production.

Clinical

- 80% of cases of hypercortisolism are caused by overproduction of ACTH by the pituitary, usually due to an adenoma (Cushing's disease); 5% to 10%, by an adrenocortical adenoma; 10% to 15%, by ectopic ACTH production by an extra-adrenal tumor; 4%, by adrenocortical carcinoma; and a small number, by autonomous adrenocortical hyperplasia unrelated to ACTH.
- Hypercortisolism is associated with the following characteristic group of physical findings and related metabolic alterations known as Cushing's syndrome:
  - Truncal obesity.
  - Hirsutism.
  - Purple abdominal striae.
  - Osteoporosis.
  - Glucose intolerance.
  - Weakness and fatigue.
  - Amenorrhea.
  - Hypertension.
- Laboratory findings include elevated plasma cortisol levels without diurnal fluctuation, increased glucocorticoid

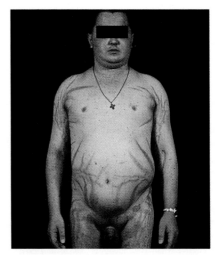

Figure 13–23. Large dark-purple striae are present on the trunk of a man with Cushing's syndrome. Truncal obesity and the characteristic "moon facies" are typical findings in patients with long-standing hypercortisolism.

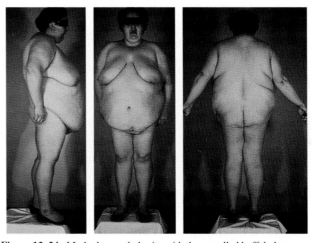

Figure 13–24. Marked truncal obesity with the so-called buffalo hump accumulation of fat along the dorsum of the neck and shoulders.

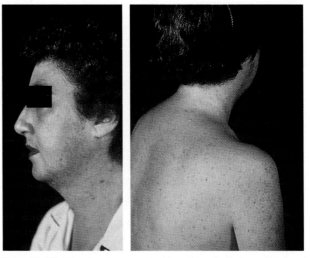

Figure 13–25. Hirsutism is present in this patient who had an adrenocorticotropic hormone–producing pituitary adenoma with hypercortisolism: Cushing's disease. Cushing's syndrome describes the manifestations of hypercortisolism without a pituitary tumor.

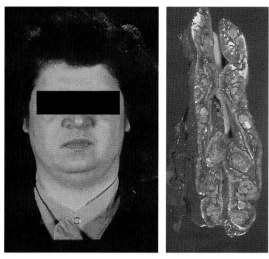

Figure 13–26. Diffuse cortical hyperplasia in a patient with Cushing's disease. The cortex is diffusely widened. There are scattered small nodules, which may be seen in adrenocorticotropic hormone-based hypercortisolism. The nodules are distinctly different from the macronodular and microadenomatous patterns of nodular cortical hyperplasia, which are usually seen in adrenal-dependent hypercortisolism, an uncommon cause of hypercortisolism.

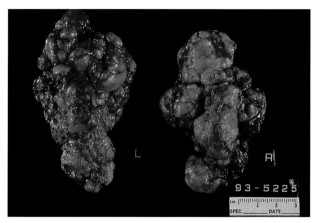

Figure 13–28. Bilateral macronodular hyperplasia in a patient with Cushing's syndrome (no pituitary adenoma was present). The large, variably sized nodules essentially replace the entire gland. No normal cortex is seen. This is an uncommon form of hypercortisolism.

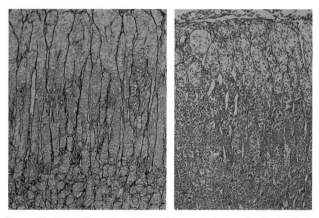

Figure 13–27. Diffuse adrenal cortical hyperplasia associated with Cushing's disease. Compact cells make up more than half the thickness of the cortical ribbon, while an outer zone of lipid-rich cells is present. The expanded zone of compact (zona reticularis) cells is an important histologic feature of diffuse hyperplasia with hypercortisolism. The reticulin stain *(left)*, demonstrates the zona fasciculata in which the normally lipid-rich cells have been converted into lipid-poor eosinophilic cells, seen in the hematoxylin-and-eosin stain *(right)*.

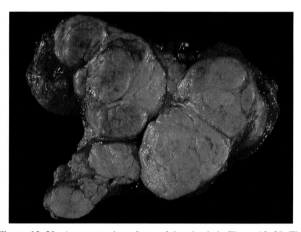

Figure 13–29. A cross section of one of the glands in Figure 13–28. The homogeneous orange-yellow nodules distort the gland. No residual uninvolved gland is seen.

excretion manifested by elevated urinary 17-ketosteroids without diurnal fluctuation, and failure of low-dose dexamethasone to suppress cortisol levels. Further distinction among causes of hypercortisolism is achieved by the high-dose dexamethasone suppression test: cortisol levels are suppressed in pituitary-dependent Cushing's syndrome, whereas tumors producing ectopic ACTH and adrenocortical hyperplasia rarely are suppressible, and adrenocortical adenomas that produce cortisol are essentially never suppressible. Another distinguishing test is administration of metyrapone, which blocks the final step in cortisol production, stimulating ACTH secretion with an adrenal response of increase in 11-deoxycortisol: adrenocortical hyperplasia is associated with a normal to

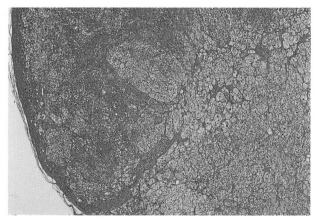

Figure 13–30. Bilateral macronodular cortical hyperplasia with Cushing's syndrome. Although the lipid-rich cells predominate, there are foci of eosinophilic compact cells within the nodules as well.

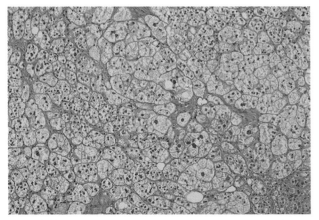

Figure 13–31. A nodule from an adrenal with macronodular cortical hyperplasia composed predominantly of lipid-rich cells.

exaggerated response, whereas adrenocortical adenomas are not affected (Table 13–4).

■ Whereas Cushing's syndrome in adults, usually in the third and fourth decades, is most often due to a pituitary adenoma, children younger than 8 years of age are much more likely to have an adrenocortical adenoma.

■ For pituitary-based hypercortisolism, the female:male ratio is 3:1.

■ Most patients with pituitary-dependent hypercortisolism have a pituitary adenoma that secretes ACTH; however, in a small number of patients no pituitary tumor can be identified; a pituitary hyperplasia or hypothalamic dysfunction is believed to be responsible for the small group without a demonstrable adenoma.

Pathology

a. Diffuse Hyperplasia, Pituitary-Dependent Hypercortisolism

■ Diffuse, symmetrical hyperplasia due to an oversecretion of ACTH by the pituitary is the most common cause of hypercortisolism.

■ Adrenal glands are usually no more than twice the normal weight.

■ The cortex is diffusely, but usually mildly, thickened, with a yellow outer zone and a brownish inner zone. Scattered small nodules may be present.

■ Larger nodules may be seen in patients with long-standing disease; they may achieve diameters of approximately 5 cm.

■ The microscopic appearance reveals a widened inner zone of compact cells of the zona reticularis type (corresponding to the grossly brown zone), which comprises half of the volume of cortex. The outer zone is composed of lipid-rich cells; similar cells are seen in nodules that may be present. The relative thickening of the zona reticularis is important in recognizing subtle cases of diffuse hyperplasia. The expansion of the lipid-poor zona reticularis zone is accomplished at the expense of the lipid-rich clear cells of the zona fasciculata, which are transformed into eosinophilic lipid-poor cells.

■ The changes in mild cases of diffuse hyperplasia closely resemble those seen in patients who have experienced chronic illness or prolonged hospitalization. Demonstration of hypercortisolism with lack of diurnal rhythm is necessary for confirming cortical hyperplasia in such cases.

b. Diffuse Hyperplasia due to Ectopic ACTH Syndrome

■ Adrenal enlargement due to an ACTH-producing tumor, excluding pituitary adenoma, is characterized by cortical thickening that is greater than that seen in pituitary-based hypercortisolism, with gland weights commonly exceeding 12 g each. Adrenals usually do not exceed 30 g in this disorder.

• The cortex is diffusely brown, and usually 4 mm in thickness.

■ The expanded cortex is composed of long fascicles of compact, lipid-poor cells. Nodules are not seen in most cases. The cortex lacks the distinct outer zone of clear cells seen in pituitary-based hypercortisolism.

■ Metastases from the ACTH-producing tumor may be present in the glands. Nuclear pleomorphism is common in cortical cells adjacent to metastatic lesions.

c. Macronodular Adrenal Hyperplasia with Hypercortisolism

■ This small subset of patients, when distinguished from pituitary-based hypercortisolism with nodule formation by laboratory studies, is composed of those in whom the adrenal hyperplasia appears to be at least partially autonomous, similar to that seen in cortical neoplasms.

Table 13–4
ETIOLOGY OF HYPERCORTISOLISM: LABORATORY DIFFERENTIAL DIAGNOSIS

	Pituitary Based	Cortical Neoplasm	Ectopic ACTH	Primary Adrenal Hyperplasia
Plasma cortisol	High, no diurnal variation	High, no diurnal variation	High, no diurnal variation	High, no diurnal variation
Plasma ACTH	High	Low	High	Low
Response to ACTH with glucocorticoid production	Rise	None	Usually none	Variable, may rise
Dexamethasone suppression	Suppresses with high dose only	No suppression	No suppression	No suppression
Response to metyrapone	Rise in 12-deoxycortisol	No response	No response, usually	Variable, often rise in 12-deoxycortisol

ACTH, adrenocorticotropic hormone.

- Both micronodular ("microadenomatous") and macronodular forms occur: the micronodular pattern is more consistently associated with clear-cut autonomous behavior (discussed later).
- This group of patients is resistant to high-dose dexamethasone suppression but usually responsive to ACTH and metyrapone. Plasma ACTH levels are variable and are often somewhat elevated. The mechanism for this hyperplasia has not been defined, although there may be some relationship to the pituitary gland in its origin. Pituitary adenomas have not been described in this group.
- Adrenal glands usually weigh from 30 to 50 g but may approach 100 g.
- Multinodular adrenal hyperplasia is characterized grossly by nodularity that completely replaces the gland, unlike pituitary-based hyperplasia with nodules, in which there are areas of diffuse hyperplasia between scattered nodules. The nodules vary greatly in size, from 2 to 3 mm to 3 cm. They are variegated and yellowish brown.
- The cells in multinodular hyperplasia are an admixture of groups of compact cells and lipid-rich cells. This admixture contrasts with simple diffuse hyperplasia associated with a pituitary adenoma, in which the nodules, when present, are composed of clear cells. In macronodular hyperplasia the cortex between distinct nodules is also hyperplastic, with subtle microscopic nodularity.

d. Microadenomatous Adrenal with Hypercortisolism

- Synonyms for this lesion include primary pigmented nodular adrenocortical disease, micronodular adrenal disease, and primary adrenocortical nodular disease.
- A very rare form of autonomous adrenal hyperplasia, both sporadic and familial cases, has been reported.
- Unlike macronodular cortical hyperplasia as described earlier, microadenomatous adrenal disease is clearly pituitary independent. Plasma ACTH levels are extremely low, and the adrenals do not respond to administration of ACTH. Neither is there any response to metyrapone or dexamethasone.
- The adrenals are normal to slightly enlarged and are dotted with 1- to 3-mm cortical nodules, which are usually darkly pigmented (brown to black). An occasional nodule may be larger than 3 mm; nodules as large as 1.8 cm have been described. Small nodules may protrude from the surface of the gland.
- The cortex between nodules appears atrophic, in contrast with that seen in macronodular hyperplasia.
- The cellular composition of the nodules is largely compact, lipid-poor cells, although scattered groups of lipid-rich cells are common. Slight nuclear pleomorphism may be seen. The pigment in the cytoplasm of the cells is believed to be lipofuscin, although neuromelanin has also been postulated to contribute to the color of these lesions.
- The etiology of this disorder is unknown; however, an autoimmune process with antibodies to ACTH receptors has been suggested.
- Bilateral adrenalectomy is the treatment of choice.

M. ADRENOCORTICAL HYPERPLASIA WITH HYPERALDOSTERONISM

Definition: A diffuse non-neoplastic proliferation of the zona glomerulosa of the adrenal cortex associated with excessive secretion of aldosterone.

Clinical

- In contrast with hypercortisolism, hyperaldosteronism is more often caused by an adrenocortical adenoma than by hyperplasia of the adrenal cortex. Approximately 80% of patients with hyperaldosteronism have an adrenal adenoma. The remaining patients have bilateral hyperplasia of the zona glomerulosa.
- Age of presentation is usually in the fourth through sixth decades.
- The female:male ratio is 3:1.
- The clinical presentation is hypertension with hypokalemia. Plasma renin levels are low.

Pathology

Gross

- The adrenals are not enlarged, although nonfunctional cortical nodules may be present as a result of the hypertension.

Histology

- The histologic changes in diffuse hyperplasia with hyperaldosteronism are often very subtle. In the normal adrenal gland the zona glomerulosa is extremely thin, discontinuous, and often difficult to see.
- Hyperplasia of the zona glomerulosa is recognized by the presence of V-shaped proliferations of glomerulosa cells extending in a wedgelike fashion toward the center of the gland. The proliferation may be accompanied by an increase in delicate fibrous tissue within the zona glomerulosa. The zona glomerulosa may extend as a thin continuous band between the wedges of proliferating cells.

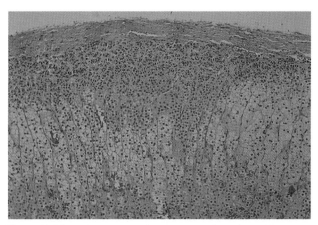

Figure 13–32. Diffuse hyperplasia of the zona glomerulosa in a patient with hyperaldosteronism. The wedge-shaped proliferation angled toward the center of the gland is an essential feature of this disease. Continuity of the zona glomerulosa is also a helpful indicator of hyperplasia.

■ Spironolactone bodies, small laminated spherical inclusions that are positive with periodic acid–Schiff–diastase and Luxol fast blue, may be identified in patients who have recently been treated with spironolactone.

■ Hyperplasia of the zona glomerulosa may accompany an aldosterone-producing cortical adenoma, which should be excluded before making a diagnosis of diffuse zona glomerulosa hyperplasia as the etiology for hyperaldosteronism.

■ Small nonfunctional nodules composed of lipid-rich cells resembling the zona fasciculata frequently accompany both diffuse hyperplasia of the zona glomerulosa and aldosterone-producing adrenocortical adenomas. These probably are secondary to the patient's hypertension.

Differential Diagnosis

■ Aldosterone-producing adrenocortical adenoma (Chapter 14B, #1a).

Treatment and Prognosis

■ Response to bilateral adrenalectomy is somewhat unpredictable in patients with hyperaldosteronism. In many instances there appear to be other factors influencing the aldosterone levels, independent of the adrenal. In such cases hypertension is not cured by a rather radical surgical approach of resecting all of the patient's adrenal tissue. Patients in whom no cortical adenoma is found are generally treated conservatively with antihypertensives.

Bibliography

Adrenal Heterotopia and Accessory Adrenal Tissue

Busuttil A. Ectopic adrenal within the gallbladder wall. J Pathol 1974; 113:231–233.
Dolan MF, Janovski N. Adrenohepatic union. Arch Pathol 1968; 86:22–24.
Falls JL. Accessory adrenal cortex in the broad ligament: Incidence and functional significance. Cancer 1955; 8:143–150.
Graham LS. Celiac accessory adrenal glands. Cancer 1953; 114:149–152.
Lack EE, Kozakewich HPW. Embryology, developmental anatomy, and selected aspects of non-neoplastic pathology. In: Lack EE, ed. Pathology of the Adrenal Glands. Vol. 14. New York: Churchill Livingstone, 1990, pp. 19–24.
Schechter DC. Aberrant adrenal tissue. Ann Surg 1968; 167:421–426.
Symonds DA, Driscoll SG. An adrenal cortical rest within the fetal ovary. Am J Clin Pathol 1973; 60:562–564.
Wiener MF, Dallgard SA. Intracranial adrenal gland. Arch Pathol 1959; 67:228–233.

Congenital Hypoplasia

Hay ID, Smail PJ, Forsyth CC. Familial cytomegalic adrenocortical hypoplasia: An X-linked syndrome of pubertal failure. Arch Dis Child 1981; 56:715–721.
Kruse K, Sippell WG, Schnakenburg KV. Hypogonadism in congenital adrenal hypoplasia: Evidence for a hypothalamic origin. J Clin Endocrinol Metab 1984; 58:12–17.
Lack EE, Kozakewich HPW. Embryology, developmental anatomy, and selected aspects of non-neoplastic pathology. In: Lack EE, ed. Pathology of the Adrenal Glands. Vol. 14. New York: Churchill Livingstone, 1990, pp. 36–38.
Silla IN, Voorhess ML, MacGillivray MH, et al. Prolonged survival without therapy in congenital adrenal hypoplasia. Am J Dis Child 1983; 137:1186–1188.
Wise JE, Matalon R, Morgan AM, McCabe ERB. Phenotypic features of patients with congenital adrenal hypoplasia and glycerol kinase deficiency. Am J Dis Child 1987; 141:744–747.

Adrenal Cytomegaly

Borit A, Kosek J. Cytomegaly of the adrenal cortex. Arch Pathol 1969; 88:58–64.
Lack EE, Kozakewich HPW. Embryology, developmental anatomy, and selected aspects of non-neoplastic pathology. In: Lack EE, ed. Pathology of the Adrenal Glands. Vol. 14. New York: Churchill Livingstone, 1990, pp. 30–32.
Oppenheimer EH. Adrenal cytomegaly: Studies by light and electron microscopy. Arch Pathol 1970; 90:57–64.
Pettinati MJ, Haines JL, Higgins RR, et al. Wiedemann-Beckwith syndrome: Presentation of clinical and cytogenetic data on 22 new cases and review of the literature. Hum Genet 1986; 74:143–148.
Sotelo-Avila C, Gooch WM. Neoplasms associated with the Beckwith-Wiedemann syndrome. Perspect Pediatr Pathol 1976; 3:255–262.
Wiedemann HR. Tumors and hemihypertrophy associated with Wiedemann-Beckwith syndrome. Eur J Pediatr 1983; 141:129–132.

Congenital Adrenal Hyperplasia

Brook CGC, Zachmann M, Prader A, Murset G. Experience with long-term therapy in congenital adrenal hyperplasia. J Pediatr 1974; 85:12–19.
Lack EE, Kozakewich HPW. Embryology, developmental anatomy, and selected aspects of non-neoplastic pathology. In: Lack EE, ed. Pathology of the Adrenal Glands. Vol. 14. New York: Churchill Livingstone, 1990, 38–47.
Mininberg DT, Levine LS, New MI. Current concepts in congenital adrenal hyperplasia. Pathol Annu 1982; 2:179–195.
New MI, Levine LS. Congenital adrenal hyperplasia. Adv Hum Genet 1973; 4:251–326.
Page DL, DeLellis RA, Hough AJ. Congenital adrenal hyperplasia. In: Page DL, DeLellis RA, Hough AJ, eds. Tumors of the Adrenal. Fascicle 23, second series. Washington, DC: Armed Forces Institute of Pathology, 1986, pp. 56–58.
Rutgers JL, Young RH, Scully RE. The testicular "tumor" of the adrenogenital syndrome: A report of six cases and review of the literature on testicular masses in patients with adrenocortical disorders. Am J Surg Pathol 1988; 12:503–513.
Van Seters AP, Van Aalderen, Moolenaar AJ, et al. Adrenocortical tumour in untreated congenital adrenal hyperplasia associated with inadequate ACTH suppressibility. Clin Endocrinol 1981; 14:325–334.
White PC, New MI, Dupont B. Congenital adrenal hyperplasia. Part I. N Engl J Med 1987; 316:1519–1524.

Addison's Disease

Dunlop D. Eighty-six cases of Addison's disease. Br Med J 1963; Oct 12:887–896.
Griffel B. Focal adrenalitis: Its frequency and correlation with similar lesions in the thyroid and kidney. Virchows Arch [Pathol Anat] 1974; 364:191–198.
Lack EE. Lymphoid "hypophysitis" with end-organ insufficiency. Arch Pathol 1975; 99:215–219.
Lack EE, Kozakewich HPW. Embryology, developmental anatomy, and selected aspects of non-neoplastic pathology. In: Lack EE, ed. Pathology of the Adrenal Glands. Vol. 14. New York: Churchill Livingstone, 1990, pp. 47–52.
Nerup J. Addison's disease—clinical studies: A report of 108 cases. Acta Endocrinol 1974; 76:127–141.
Neufeld M, Maclaren NK, Blizzard RM. Two types of autoimmune Addison's disease associated with different polyglandular autoimmune (PGA) syndromes. Medicine 1981; 60:355–362.
Vita JA, Silverberg SJ, Goland RS, et al. Clinical clues to the cause of Addison's disease. Am J Med 1985; 78:461–466.

Infectious Diseases Affecting the Adrenal Gland

Dunlop D. Eighty-six cases of Addison's disease. Br Med J 1963; Oct 12:887–896.
Goodwin RA Jr, Shapiro JL, Thurman GH, et al. Disseminated histoplasmosis: Clinical and pathologic correlations. Medicine 1980; 59:1–33.
Greene LW, Cole W, Greene JB, et al. Adrenal insufficiency as a complication of the acquired immunodeficiency syndrome. Ann Intern Med 1984; 101:497–499.
Guttman PH. Addison's disease: A statistical analysis of five hundred and sixty-six cases and a study of the pathology. Arch Pathol 1930; 10:742–785.

Klatt EC, Shibata D. Cytomegalovirus infection in the acquired immuno-deficiency syndrome: Clinical and autopsy findings. Arch Pathol Lab Med 1988; 112:540–544.

Lack EE, Kozakewich HPW. Embryology, developmental anatomy, and selected aspects of non-neoplastic pathology. In: Lack EE, ed. Pathology of the Adrenal Glands. Vol. 14. New York: Churchill Livingstone, 1990, pp. 52–56.

Nerup J. Addison's disease—clinical studies: A report of 108 cases. Acta Endocrinol 1974; 76:127–141.

Singer DB. Pathology of neonatal herpes simplex virus infection. In: Rosenberg S, Bernstein J, eds. Perspectives in Pediatric Pathology. Vol 6. New York: Masson Publishing, 1981, pp. 243– 262.

Amyloidosis

Heller EL, Camarata SJ. Addison's disease from amyloidosis of the adrenal glands. Arch Pathol 1950; 49:601–604.

Lack EE, Kozakewich HPW. Embryology, developmental anatomy, and selected aspects of non-neoplastic pathology. In: Lack EE, ed. Pathology of the Adrenal Glands. Vol. 14. New York: Churchill Livingstone, 1990, p. 57.

Waterhouse-Friderichsen Syndrome

Khuri FJ, Alton DJ, Hardy BE, et al. Adrenal hemorrhage in neonates: Report of 5 cases and review of the literature. J Urol 1980; 124:684–687.

Kuhajda F, Hutchins GM. Adrenal corticomedullary junction necrosis: A morphologic marker for hypotension. Am Heart J 1979; 98:294–297.

Mostoufizadeh M, Lack EE, Gang DL, et al. Postmortem manifestations of echovirus 11 sepsis in five newborn infants. Hum Pathol 1983; 14:818–823.

Adrenal Cysts

Cerny JC, Warshawsky A, Hall J, et al. The preoperative diagnosis of adrenal cysts. J Urol 1970; 104:787–790.

Cheema P, Cartagena R, Stanbitz W. Adrenal cysts: Diagnosis and treatment. J Urol 1981; 126:393–399.

Foster DG. Adrenal cysts: Review of the literature and report of a case. Arch Surg 1966; 92:131–143.

Gaffey MJ, Mills SE, Fechner RE, et al. Vascular adrenal cysts: A clinico-pathologic and immunohistochemical study of endothelial and hemorrhagic (pseudocystic) variants. Am J Surg Pathol 1989; 13:740–747.

Incze JS, Lui PS, Merriam JC, et al. Morphology and pathogenesis of adrenal cysts. Am J Pathol 1979; 95:423–432.

Medeiros LJ, Lewandrowski KB, Vickery AL. Adrenal pseudocyst: A clinical and pathologic study of eight cases. Hum Pathol 1989; 20:660–665.

Medeiros LJ, Weiss LM, Vickery AL. Epithelial-lined (true) cyst of the adrenal gland: A case report. Hum Pathol 1989; 20:491– 492.

Page DL, DeLellis RA, Hough AJ. Cysts. In: Page DL, DeLellis RA, Hough AJ, eds. Tumors of the Adrenal. Fascicle 23, second series. Washington, DC: Armed Forces Institute of Pathology, 1986, pp. 175–178.

Adrenocortical Nodules (Nonhyperfunctioning)

Cohen RB. Observations on cortical nodules in human adrenal glands. Cancer 1966; 19:552–556.

Copeland PM. The incidentally discovered adrenal mass. Ann Surg 1984; 199:116–122.

Dobbie JW. Adrenocortical nodular hyperplasia: The aging adrenal. J Pathol 1969; 99:1–18.

Geelhoed GW, Druy EM. Management of the adrenal "incidentaloma." Surgery 1982; 92:866–874.

Lack EE, Kozakewich HPW. Adrenal cortical nodules, hyperplasia, and hyperfunction. In: Lack EE, ed. Pathology of the Adrenal Glands. Vol. 14. New York: Churchill Livingstone, 1990, pp. 78–83.

Neville AM. The nodular adrenal. Invest Cell Pathol 1978; 1:99–111.

Neville AM, O'Hare MJ. Aspects of structure, function, and pathology. In: James VHT, ed. The Adrenal Gland. New York: Raven Press, 1979, pp. 1–65.

Page DL, DeLellis RA, Hough AJ. The multinodular adrenal. In: Page DL, DeLellis RA, Hough AJ, eds. Tumors of the Adrenal. Fascicle 23, second series. Washington, DC: Armed Forces Institute of Pathology, 1986, pp. 73–78.

Adrenocortical Hyperplasia with Hypercortisolism

Arce B, Licea M, Hung S, Padron R. Familial Cushing's syndrome. Acta Endocrinol 1978; 87:139–147.

Burke CW. Disorders of cortisol production: Diagnostic and therapeutic progress. Recent Adv Endocr Metab 1978; 1:61–90.

Choi Y, Werk EE Jr, Sholiton LJ. Cushing's syndrome with dual pituitary-adrenal control. Arch Intern Med 1970; 125:1045–1049.

Cohen RB, Chapma WB, Castleman B. Hyperadrenocorticism (Cushing's disease): A study of surgically resected adrenal glands. Am J Pathol 1959; 35:537–561.

Hidai H, Fujii H, Otsuka K, et al. Cushing's syndrome due to huge adrenocortical multinodular hyperplasia. Endocrinol Jpn 1975; 22:555–560.

Jex RK, van Herden JA, Carpenter PC, Grant CS. Ectopic ACTH syndrome. Am J Surg 1985; 149:276–282.

Lack EE, Kozakewich HPW. Adrenal cortical nodules, hyperplasia, and hyperfunction. In: Lack EE, ed. Pathology of the Adrenal Glands. Vol. 14. New York: Churchill Livingstone, 1990, pp. 83–104.

Neville AM, O'Hare MJ. Aspects of structure, function, and pathology. In: James VHT, ed. The Adrenal Gland. New York: Raven Press, 1979, pp. 1–65.

Neville AM, Symington T. Bilateral adrenocortical hyperplasia in children with Cushing's syndrome. J Pathol 1972; 107:65–106.

Orth DN. The old and the new in Cushing's syndrome. N Eng J Med 1984; 310:649–651.

Page DL, DeLellis RA, Hough AJ. Hyperplasia. In: Page DL, DeLellis RA, Hough AJ, eds. Tumors of the Adrenal. Fascicle 23, second series. Washington, DC: Armed Forces Institute of Pathology, 1986, pp. 56–78.

Plotz CM, Knowlton AI, Ragan C. The natural history of Cushing's syndrome. Am J Med 1952; 13:597–614.

Prinz RA, Brooks MH, Lawrence AM, Paloyan E. The continued importance of adrenalectomy in the treatment of Cushing's disease. Arch Surg 1979; 114:481–484.

Ruder HJ, Loriaux DL, Lipsett MB. Severe osteopenia in young adults associated with Cushing's syndrome due to micronodular adrenal disease. J Clin Endocrinol Metab 1974; 39:1138–1147.

Schweitzer-Cagianut M, Froesch ER, Hedinger E. Familial Cushing's syndrome with primary adrenocortical microadenomatosis (primary adrenocortical nodular dysplasia). Acta Endocrinol 1980; 94:529–535.

Shenoy BV, Carpenter PB, Carney JA. Bilateral primary pigmented nodular adrenocortical disease. Am J Surg Pathol 1984; 8:335–344.

Singer W, Kovacs K, Ryan N, Horvath E. Ectopic ACTH syndrome: Clinicopathological correlations. J Clin Pathol 1978; 31:591–598.

Smals AGH, Pieters GFFM, van Haelst UJG, Kloppenborg PWC. Macronodular adrenocortical hyperplasia in long-standing Cushing's disease. J Clin Endocrinol Metab 1984; 58:25–31.

Adrenocortical Hyperplasia with Hyperaldosteronism

Ferris JB, Brown JJ, Fraser R, et al. Hypertension with aldosterone excess and low plasma-renin: Preoperative distinction between patients with and without adrenocortical tumor. Lancet 1970; 2:995–1000.

Grant CS, Carpenter P, van Heerden JA, et al. Primary aldosteronism: Clinical management. Arch Surg 1984; 119:585–590.

Lack EE, Kozakewich HPW. Adrenal cortical nodules, hyperplasia, and hyperfunction. In: Lack EE, ed. Pathology of the Adrenal Glands. Vol. 14. New York: Churchill Livingstone, 1990, pp. 105–108.

Page DL, DeLellis RA, Hough AJ. Hyperplasia. In: Page DL, DeLellis RA, Hough AJ, eds. Tumors of the Adrenal. Fascicle 23, second series. Washington, DC: Armed Forces Institute of Pathology, 1986, pp. 62–63.

Weinberger MH, Grim CE, Hollifield JW, et al. Primary aldosteronism: Diagnosis, localization, and treatment. Ann Intern Med 1979; 90:386–395.

CHAPTER 14

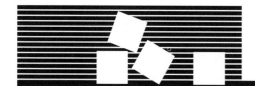

Neoplasms of the Adrenal Gland

A. CLASSIFICATION OF NEOPLASMS OF THE ADRENAL GLAND

Table 14–1
CLASSIFICATION OF NEOPLASMS OF THE ADRENAL GLAND

A. Neoplasms of the Adrenal Cortex

1. Adrenocortical adenoma
2. Adrenocortical carcinoma

B. Neoplasms of the Adrenal Medulla

1. Adrenomedullary hyperplasia
2. Pheochromocytoma
3. Neuroblastoma and ganglioneuroblastoma
4. Ganglioneuroma
5. Composite tumors of the adrenal medulla
6. Primary malignant melanoma

C. Miscellaneous Neoplasms and Tumor-Like Lesions

1. Malignant lymphoma
2. Myelolipoma
3. Adenomatoid tumor
4. Hemangioma
5. Angiosarcoma
6. Nerve sheath tumors
7. Metastatic neoplasms
8. Other rare neoplasms (smooth muscle, gonadal stromal type)

B. NEOPLASMS OF THE ADRENAL CORTEX

1. Adrenocortical Adenoma

Definition: A benign neoplastic proliferation of adrenocortical cells, almost always associated with endocrine hyperfunction discernible by clinical, biochemical, or histological evidence.

Synonyms: Adrenocortical adenoma, adrenal adenoma.

Clinical

- Most adrenocortical adenomas exhibit some evidence of hyperfunction. It is this feature that defines the separation of adenomas from the dominant nonhyperfunctioning adrenocortical nodule. Although many adenomas are associated with clinical endocrine abnormalities, in others the secretory product may be so limited that it is detectable only by biochemical studies. Some adenomas may produce too little steroid hormone to effect biochemically diagnostic elevations; the only evidence of hyperfunction in such cases may be histologic evidence of atrophy in the adjacent cortex.

- Endocrine syndromes associated with adenomas include, in order of frequency, hyperaldosteronism (Conn's syndrome), hyperadrenocorticism (Cushing's syndrome), virilization, and, very rarely, feminization. Most patients present either with pure hyperaldosteronism or Cushing's syndrome. The presence of virilization, feminization, or mixed syndromes increases the probability of malignancy in adrenocortical neoplasms.

- Cortical adenomas are responsible for 80% of cases of hyperaldosteronism. The clinical findings are weakness, with hypertension and hypokalemia. The prevalence of Conn's syndrome (hyperaldosteronism associated with adrenocortical adenoma) in the hypertensive population is approximately 0.5% to 8.0%. Most tumors are diagnosed in the fourth through sixth decades, with a predilection for females.

- Adenomas are responsible for only 5% to 10% of cases of Cushing's syndrome compared with 80% of cases associated with pituitary adenoma and most of the remainder related to ectopic adrenocorticotropic hormone (ACTH) secretion by other neoplasms. Hypercortisolism due to adrenocortical adenoma is usually seen in children. In children younger than 8 years of age, Cushing's syndrome is more often due to an adrenocortical neoplasm; however, pituitary adenoma is more commonly the cause of hypercortisolism in children older than 8 years of age. In adults, hypercortisolism is usually caused by pituitary adenomas in females (usually premenopausal) and by ectopic ACTH in men (increasing with age).

- Virilizing tumors are seen over a wide age range and encompassing prepubertal children and in adult females. They usually secrete dehydroepiandrosterone or dehydroepiandrosterone sulfate, and, less commonly, testosterone. The majority of virilizing adrenocortical tumors in adults are malignant, but they are often benign in children.

- Feminizing adrenocortical neoplasms are usually seen in men between 25 and 45 years of age. The clinical findings

288

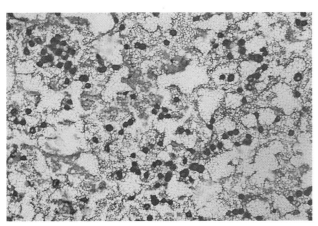

Figure 14–1. Fine needle aspirate of an adrenocortical adenoma contains mainly naked nuclei, in a background of vacuolated cytoplasm. The distinction from normal or hyperplastic adrenal cortex cannot be reliably made (Diff-Quik).

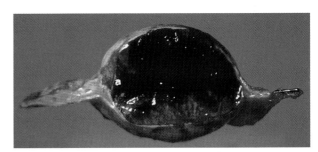

Figure 14–4. A "black adenoma." The pigment responsible for the dark color is believed to be lipofuscin. This tumor was associated with Cushing's syndrome. The adjacent cortex is thin.

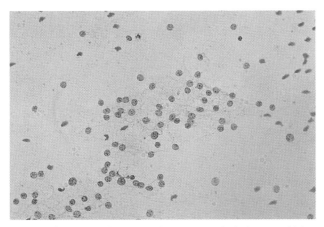

Figure 14–2. Fine needle aspirate of an adrenocortical adenoma with better preserved cells demonstrates vesicular chromatin and wisps of finely vacuolated cytoplasm (Papanicolaou).

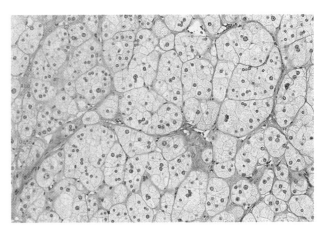

Figure 14–5. Lipid-rich clear cells in a cortical adenoma with hypercortisolism. The cells resemble those of the normal zona fasciculata.

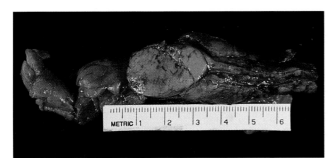

Figure 14–3. A circumscribed yellow-orange cortical adenoma from a patient with Cushing's disease. The lesion is solitary and is associated with thinning of the adjacent cortex.

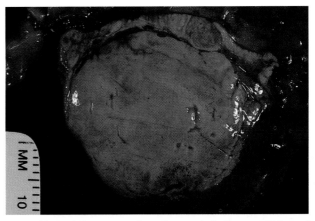

Figure 14–6. "Aldosteronoma," an adrenocortical adenoma with hyperaldosteronism. The poor circumscription reflects the lack of encapsulation in most aldosteronomas. The irregular thickening with vague nodularity of the adjacent cortex is a common finding, in contrast with the atrophic residual gland associated with adenomas producing Cushing's syndrome.

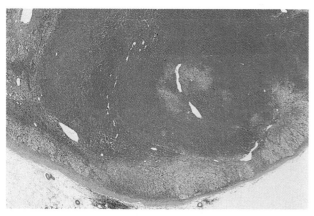

Figure 14–7. This aldosterone-producing cortical adenoma is unencapsulated and "merges" with the surrounding non-neoplastic cortex.

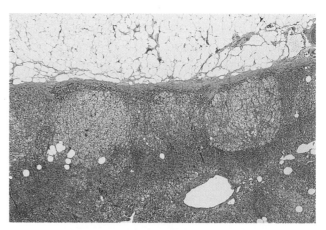

Figure 14–10. The adrenal cortex adjacent to an aldosterone-producing cortical adenoma frequently contains nodules of clear cells that are cytologically distinct from those of the tumor. These additional nodules are believed to represent nonhyperfunctional nodules related to the patient's hypertension.

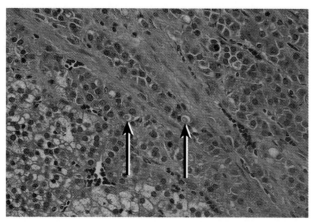

Figure 14–8. Although compact, or lipid-poor, cells predominate in this aldosterone-producing adenoma, these neoplasms frequently have an admixture of clear and compact cells. Spironolactone bodies are present *(arrows)*.

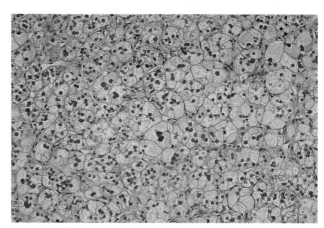

Figure 14–11. Adrenocortical adenomas may exhibit focal nuclear pleomorphism and hyperchromasia, as does this aldosterone-producing adenoma. These cells are not indicative of malignancy.

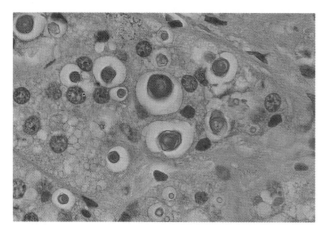

Figure 14–9. Spironolactone bodies in an adrenocortical adenoma associated with hyperaldosteronism. The patient had been treated with spironolactone for 3 to 4 weeks.

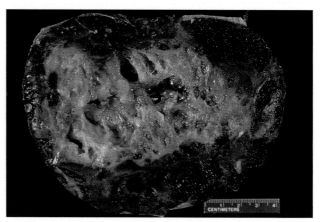

Figure 14–12. A cortical adenoma with massive hemorrhage that has resulted in a neoplasm with fibrosis, vascular proliferation, and cystic degeneration. Such tumors may resemble vascular neoplasms or pseudocysts. A search for a rim of neoplastic cortex and islands of tumor trapped deep within the cyst is helpful in arriving at a diagnosis of cortical neoplasia.

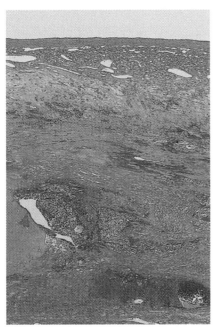

Figure 14–13. An adrenocortical adenoma with marked cystic degeneration due to hemorrhage. The central hemorrhage and necrosis are not the same as the patchy tumor cell necrosis and hemorrhagic areas in adrenocortical carcinoma and should not be misinterpreted.

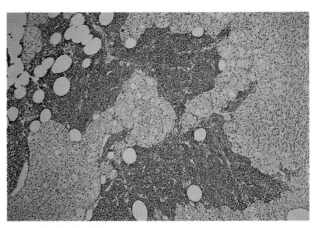

Figure 14–15. Myelolipomatous changes are common in adrenocortical adenomas, as in other proliferations of the adrenal cortex.

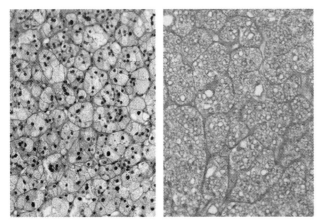

Figure 14–14. Adrenocortical adenoma with associated degenerative changes. *Left,* Viable tumor is seen composed of benign neoplastic cortical cells with tumor nests separated by fibrovascular stroma. *Right,* Adjacent to the viable tumor were foci showing degenerative changes, including tumor necrosis, but with retention of the architectural pattern. Trichrome stains (not shown) would assist in highlighting the architectural pattern of the remaining tumor islands.

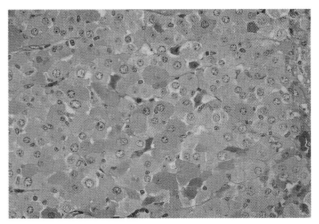

Figure 14–16. Adrenal oncocytic adenoma with large cells with abundant eosinophilic granular cytoplasm. The nuclei are relatively uniform, with prominent nucleoli.

include gynecomastia, decreased libido, feminized hair pattern, and testicular atrophy. The findings are due to increased estrogen levels. Most feminizing adrenal neoplasms are malignant.

■ "Mixed" endocrine syndromes usually include Cushing's syndrome with virilization or feminization and are usually associated with malignant cortical neoplasms.

■ Adrenocortical adenoma with hyperaldosteronism is diagnosed biochemically by documenting low serum potassium levels (usually <4.0 mEq per liter, although some individuals may be normokalemic), suppressed plasma renin levels, and elevated plasma aldosterone levels, although these studies are not entirely specific.

■ Adrenocortical adenoma with Cushing's syndrome must be distinguished biochemically from pituitary-dependent Cushing's disease. Both diseases are associated with elevated plasma cortisol and 17-hydroxycorticoid levels, which are not suppressed by low-dose dexamethasone. High-dose dexamethasone almost always suppresses pituitary-based hypercortisolism, but not that due to an adrenocortical adenoma. Plasma ACTH level is elevated in pituitary adenomas with hypercortisolism but is usually undetectable in patients with adrenocortical adenomas that produce Cushing's syndrome.

■ Nonfunctional adrenocortical adenomas are probably rare, whereas the nonfunctional and non-neoplastic adrenocortical nodule described in Chapter 13K is quite common. The distinction between these two entities rests on subtle differences in the cortex adjacent to the nodule. The few true nonhyperfunctioning adenomas are most often incidental findings, although large examples may be associated with flank or abdominal pain.

Radiology

- Computed tomographic (CT) scan is useful in localizing adrenal adenomas, particularly the larger lesions as typically seen in Cushing's syndrome. Adenomas associated with hyperaldosteronism, however, may be quite small and difficult to identify. The frequent use of the CT scan for evaluation of a variety of abdominal complaints has also increased the incidence of detection of adrenal masses during life; most incidentally discovered lesions are nonhyperfunctioning and represent cortical nodules rather than adenomas.
- Magnetic resonance imaging (MRI) is also useful in localization and has the added advantage of helping categorize lesions by the signal intensity of the T2-weighted image: pheochromocytomas have a high intensity signal; metastases have an intermediate signal, and nonhyperfunctioning cortical nodules or adenomas have a low intensity signal. Distinctions between hyperfunctioning and nonfunctioning adenomas cannot be made.
- Radionuclide scanning using radioactive iodine–labeled cholesterol is an indicator of steroid hormone secretion that demonstrates differential uptake between hyperfunctioning adenomas and the remaining cortex. The technique appears to be helpful in characterizing the nonhyperfunctional cortical nodules, which fail to exhibit differential uptake as compared with the rest of the cortex.
- Radiographic images of adrenocortical adenomas with extensive degenerative changes such as hemorrhage and cystic alterations may be misleading, suggesting the possibility of pheochromocytoma or adrenocortical carcinoma.

Pathology

Cytology

- The typical smear contains predominantly naked nuclei scattered rather evenly in a background of foamy to slightly granular cytoplasm. Distinct borders are difficult to discern, but occasional intact cells with small, round nuclei with homogeneous chromatin, inconspicuous nucleoli, and vacuolated cytoplasm are seen. Focal enlarged and irregular nuclei may be present. Mitotic figures are not noted. Necrosis is not usually present. Some cases may be characterized by better preservation of the cortical cells, which are usually arranged in acinar groupings; the cytologic features are otherwise similar.
- The chief utility of fine needle aspiration of adrenal masses is the exclusion of metastatic disease involving the adrenal. Distinction between benign and malignant adrenocortical neoplasms may by very difficult based solely on cytologic criteria. The clinical and radiographic features, combined with such cytologic findings as necrosis and widespread marked nuclear atypia, may lend support to a malignant diagnosis.
- The close cytologic resemblance of most adenomas to normal cortex makes distinction between lesional and nonlesional samples difficult; reliance on careful radiologic localization for verification of the source of a sample is important.

Gross

- The gross appearance of adrenocortical adenomas varies to some degree with the steroid hormone produced; however, overlap in size and appearance occurs between groups.
- *Adenoma with hyperaldosteronism:* unilateral and solitary, with an average size of 1.5 cm and yellow color, they are frequently unencapsulated or incompletely encapsulated. The tumor may be accompanied by mild nodularity of remaining cortex.
- *Adenoma with hypercortisolism:* unilateral and solitary, with an average size of 4 cm, and mottled yellow-brown color, they are usually encapsulated. The remaining cortex usually appears atrophic.
- *Adenoma with virilization:* unilateral and solitary, with an average size of 5 cm (some much larger) and reddish-brown color, they are encapsulated.
- Adenomas associated with feminization are rare (most such neoplasms are malignant); they resemble tumors associated with virilization.
- Pigmented, or "black," adenomas are rare adrenocortical neoplasms that are distinguished from typical adenomas only by their diffusely brown to black gross appearance. Cushing's syndrome is the most commonly associated endocrine disorder, but hyperaldosteronism has also been reported in a few patients. The pigment responsible for the gross appearance is visible as brown intracytoplasmic granular material by light microscopy. It is believed to represent primarily lipofuscin, although some may be neuromelanin.

Histology

- Although there are some associations of cell type with secretory product in cortical neoplasms, tumors frequently exhibit a mixture of patterns that make specific classification of endocrine function based on histology difficult at best. There are some generalizations and some specific findings of interest related to type of endocrine function.
- Necrosis, although considered a criterion for malignancy, must be judged cautiously. Adenomas, particularly when large or following venographic studies, may undergo central necrosis. This finding is not indicative of malignancy. The necrosis observed in cortical carcinomas is usually patchy and is not localized to the center of the tumor. Other criteria of malignancy should be found to reinforce the significance of necrosis in a neoplasm.
- Central degenerative changes, when long-standing, may include resolving hemorrhage and necrosis with vascular proliferation and cystic alteration. These changes must be distinguished from a vascular neoplasm; the presence of residual viable cortical cells or ghost cells within the area of concern indicates an underlying adrenocortical neoplasm.
- Hemorrhage in an adrenocortical adenoma may be massive, greatly increasing the size and weight of adenomas and sometimes masking the true neoplastic process involved.
- Myelolipomatous foci are common in cortical adenomas.

a. Adenoma with Hyperaldosteronism

- The tumor is circumscribed, but a distinct fibrous capsule is usually lacking; the tumor cells usually appear different from the normal cortex by virtue of size and cytoplasmic staining features.
- The normal cortex may contain small cortical nodules that are probably secondary to the patient's hypertension. These nodules may confuse the issue of distinguishing between an adenoma and a nodular cortical hyperplasia. However, hyperaldosteronism due to hyperplasia is a diffuse process involving the zona glomerulosa rather than a multinodular process.
- There may be considerable variation in the cytologic features: large, pale vacuolated cells with abundant lipid and vesicular nuclei predominate; these cells resemble the cells of the zona fasciculata. In addition, a range of cells with less cytoplasm but rich in lipid to small cells with a rim of eosinophilic cytoplasm and more condensed chromatin (similar to the zona glomerulosa and zona reticularis) may be seen.
- In addition to nonhyperfunctional cortical nodules, there may be hyperplasia of the zona glomerulosa in the adjacent or contralateral cortex. This expansion of the zona glomerulosa may be diffuse or regional.
- A unique feature of "aldosteronomas" is the presence of "spironolactone bodies," eosinophilic laminated cytoplasmic inclusions surrounded by a clear space. They measure 2 to 12 mm in diameter, and they are periodic acid–Schiff (PAS) positive, diastase resistant, and medium to dark blue with Luxol fast blue. The inclusions are found after treatment with spironolactone and may be seen for a few months after cessation of therapy. Spironolactone bodies contain phospholipids and may be derived from endoplasmic reticulum. The effect of spironolactone in controlling blood pressure lasts only 5 to 6 weeks; the number of spironolactone bodies diminishes as the efficacy of the medication wanes.

b. Adenoma with Hypercortisolism

- More distinctly circumscribed than aldosteronomas, these adenomas are contained within a pseudocapsule of compressed cortex and connective tissue, or, if large, within the adrenal capsule.
- The tumor cells are most often quite large, with abundant finely vacuolated pale cytoplasm and vesicular nuclei (fasciculata-like), arranged in nests or cords. There are also smaller, more eosinophilic, lipid-poor cells resembling the zona reticularis. Lipofuscin may be prominent in some tumors.
- Enlarged atypical nuclei may be seen, but they are usually quite focal. Mitoses are rarely seen.
- The non-neoplastic adrenal cortex is usually atrophic, although there may be intervening nonfunctioning cortical nodules, which should be distinguished from nodular cortical hyperplasia. The cytologic features of the adenoma are usually different from the nonfunctional nodules in a given case.

c. Adenomas with Virilization

- The distinction between benign and malignant virilizing cortical neoplasms may be difficult. Half of these neoplasms occur in children; the criteria for malignancy in childhood adrenocortical neoplasms are not well-defined, and the criteria used for adult tumors cannot be reliably applied. Many tumors with mitoses, marked nuclear atypia, and other features associated with malignancy in adults may be seen in childhood tumors that pursue a benign course.
- In adults, these tumors are more likely to behave aggressively, even if all of the histologic criteria of malignancy are not present.
- The usual histologic pattern is one in which small eosinophilic cells resembling the zona reticularis predominate; however, areas of lipid-rich cells may be seen as well.
- An unusual variant of virilizing adrenocortical adenoma is associated with production of testosterone in some cases. The tumor cells are large and eosinophilic and resemble ovarian theca-lutein cells.

d. Adenomas with Feminization

- Feminizing adrenocortical neoplasms are rare. In adults, most of these tumors have the histologic features of malignancy and are classified as adrenocortical carcinomas, although there are reports of "adenomas" with benign behavior in children.
- The histologic features are similar to those of virilizing tumors.

Differential Diagnosis

- Adrenocortical carcinoma (Chapter 14B, #2).
- Adrenocortical nodule (nonfunctional) (Chapter 13K).
- Nodular adrenocortical hyperplasia (Chapter 13L).
- Metastatic carcinoma, especially renal cell carcinoma.
- Pheochromocytoma with lipid degeneration (Chapter 14C, #2).

Treatment and Prognosis

- Surgical therapy for adrenocortical adenoma associated with Cushing's syndrome is usually effective in reversing the clinical effects of hypercortisolism within 1 year of resection. There is a risk of adrenocortical insufficiency due to long-standing suppression of the contralateral cortex by the tumor; supportive administration of mineralocorticoids and glucocorticoids as well as ACTH may be required for a year or longer.
- Hyperaldosteronism due to an adenoma usually responds quickly to resection of the involved gland; however, some patients may have persistent hypertension due to hyperplastic changes in the zona glomerulosa of the contralateral gland.
- Complete surgical resection (adrenalectomy) is the desired therapy for virilizing and feminizing cortical tumors; evaluation for evidence of metastases is essential

owing to the high incidence of malignancy, particularly in adults. Failure of the clinical syndrome to resolve is evidence of extra-adrenal spread.

Additional Facts

■ *Oncocytic adrenocortical neoplasms* are uncommon, with only a few cases documented in the literature. Most cases have been clinically nonfunctional, usually discovered incidentally. One virilizing tumor with benign histologic and clinical features has been reported. Initially these lesions were all believed to be benign; however, one 10-cm oncocytic tumor exhibited locally aggressive behavior (invasion of the inferior vena cava, kidney, and liver) but no metastatic disease. This aggressive lesion lacked definitive histologic features of malignancy. Patient ages have been in the fifth through seventh decades, with no apparent gender predilection. Oncocytic adrenocortical neoplasms are characterized grossly by a homogeneous tan to yellow-brown color; they have been as large as 10 cm and weighed as much as 865 g. The histologic pattern is usually a diffuse proliferation of large polygonal cells with abundant granular eosinophilic cytoplasm, somewhat eccentrically placed and variably sized round vesicular nuclei, and one or more prominent nucleoli. Mitoses and necrosis are not usually seen. Electron microscopy has documented the presence of a vast number of mitochondria filling the cytoplasm. Of importance is the obligatory finding of three of Weiss' criteria for malignancy in all oncocytic adrenal tumors: diffuse growth pattern, high nuclear grade, and predominance of eosinophilic cells; it is not clear, owing to the small number of cases, whether a modification of these criteria would be predictive of behavior in these tumors.

2. Adrenocortical Carcinoma (Tables 14–2 through 14–5)

Definition: A malignant neoplasm arising from cells of the adrenal cortex, which may manifest syndromes of pure or mixed endocrine syndromes (Cushing's syndrome, virilization, feminization) or which may be clinically nonfunctional.

Clinical

■ Adrenocortical carcinomas are rare, accounting for 0.02% of cancers.
■ A broad age distribution is seen, with cases concentrated in the first two decades and in the fifth through seventh decades.
■ No definite gender or racial predilections are seen, although some series suggest a slight female predominance.
■ Common presenting symptoms include a palpable abdominal mass, abdominal pain, weight loss, or evidence of endocrine hyperfunction.
■ Cushing's syndrome is the most commonly encountered endocrine syndrome, usually as a mixed hypercortisolism/virilization syndrome. Pure virilizing or feminiz-

Table 14–2

CRITERIA FOR MALIGNANCY IN ADRENOCORTICAL NEOPLASMS: WEISS

Histologic Feature	Definition
High nuclear grade	Fuhrman's nuclear grade III or IV
Mitotically active*	>5/50 HPF
Atypical mitotic figures*	Abnormal spindles or chromosome distribution
Eosinophilic tumor cell cytoplasm	≥75% of tumor, rather than clear cells
Diffuse growth pattern	>⅓ of tumor area
Necrosis	Involving confluent nests of cells or larger areas
Venous invasion*	Vessel with smooth muscle in wall
Sinusoidal invasion	Vascular space without smooth muscle
Capsular invasion	Into or through capsule, with stromal reaction

*Found only in tumors with malignant clinical behavior.
Malignancy = 3 or more criteria.
Adapted from Weiss LM. Comparative histologic study of 43 metastasizing and nonmetastasizing adrenocortical tumors. Am J Surg Pathol 1984; 8:163–169.

Table 14–3

NONHISTOLOGIC CRITERIA FOR MALIGNANCY IN ADRENOCORTICAL NEOPLASMS: HOUGH AND ASSOCIATES

Tumor weight >100 g
Urinary 17-ketosteroids >100 mg/g creatinine/24 hr
Nonresponsive to ACTH administration
Cushing's syndrome with virilization ("mixed" endocrine syndrome)
Virilization
No endocrine syndrome
Weight loss of >10 lb in 3 mo

Table 14–4

HISTOLOGIC CRITERIA FOR MALIGNANCY IN ADRENOCORTICAL NEOPLASMS: HOUGH AND ASSOCIATES

Diffuse growth pattern predominates
Vascular invasion
Tumor cell necrosis (>2 HPF in diameter)
Broad fibrous bands (>1 HPF in diameter)
Capsular invasion
Mitotic rate >1/10 HPF
Moderate to marked cellular pleomorphism

Table 14–5

HISTOLOGIC CRITERIA FOR MALIGNANCY IN ADRENOCORTICAL NEOPLASMS: VAN SLOOTEN AND ASSOCIATES

Extensive regressive changes, including necrosis, hemorrhage, fibrosis, or calcification
Loss of normal architecture
Moderate to marked nuclear atypia
Moderate to marked nuclear hyperchromasia
Abnormal nucleoli
Mitotic rate >2/10 HPF
Vascular or capsular invasion

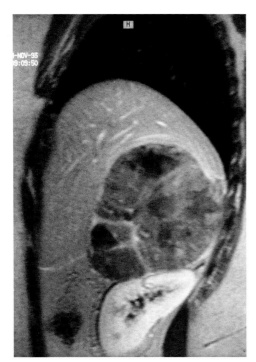

Figure 14–17. A sagittal view by magnetic resonance imaging showing a very large suprarenal mass with coarse fibrous septations and variable internal densities. The histologic diagnosis is adrenocortical carcinoma.

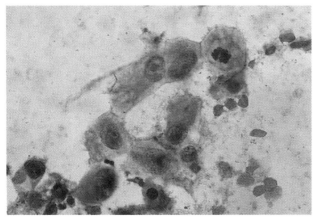

Figure 14–18. Fine needle aspirate of adrenocortical carcinoma. Highly pleomorphic cortical carcinomas such as this one are common and may be impossible to distinguish from a metastatic carcinoma.

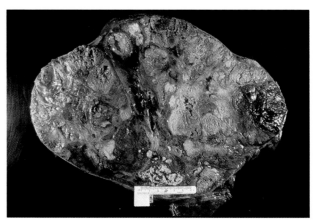

Figure 14–19. This tumor has gross features commonly seen in adrenocortical carcinoma: hemorrhage, coarse nodularity, necrosis, and large size.

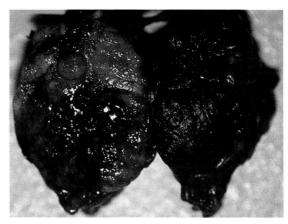

Figure 14–20. Size is not a reliable criterion for malignancy in adrenocortical neoplasms. This small, pigmented aldosterone-producing tumor proved to be a cortical carcinoma by histologic features as well as by its behavior. Metastatic disease was present at the time of surgery.

ing tumors are infrequently seen, and hyperaldosteronism as an isolated syndrome is exceedingly rare. The overall incidence of endocrine manifestations in adrenocortical carcinoma varies greatly in series of cases—from 24% to 96%.

■ Laboratory findings depend on the endocrine function of the tumor. Cushing's syndrome is manifested by high levels of corticosteroids that are not suppressed by high-dose dexamethasone, and, unlike Cushing's syndrome seen in adenomas, carcinomas fail to increase cortisol levels in response to ACTH. The frequent mixture of Cushing's syndrome with virilization or hyperaldosteronism is also different from the pure Cushing's syndrome of adenomas. Marked elevation of urinary 17-ketosteroids due to the more frequent production of excess androgens is seen more often in carcinomas than in adenomas.

■ In the past many patients have had metastatic disease involving liver, lung, or bone at the time of presentation (24% to 50%), although the earlier discovery of these neoplasms with more advanced imaging in recent years may alter the epidemiology of cortical carcinoma.

Radiology

■ CT and MRI scans are the most widely used methods of localization. Cortical carcinomas are usually much larger than adenomas and are more often partially necrotic or hemorrhagic.

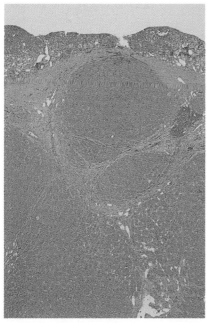

Figure 14–21. Adrenocortical carcinoma. Features suggestive of malignancy in this field include dissection of the tumor into nodules by broad fibrous bands and predominance of cells with eosinophilic cytoplasm.

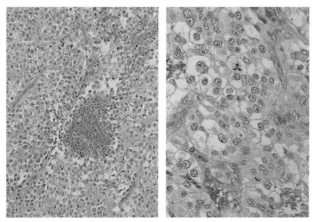

Figure 14–22. Adrenocortical carcinoma with areas of confluent tumor cell necrosis *(left)* and a high mitotic rate, including atypical mitotic figures *(right)*.

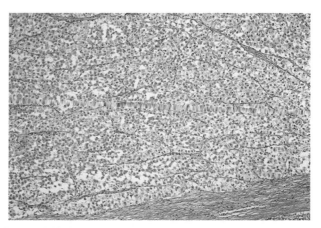

Figure 14–23. The presence of a trabecular growth pattern, as seen here, is suggestive of malignancy in cortical neoplasms.

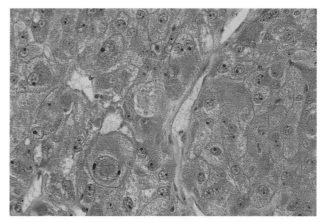

Figure 14–24. Adrenocortical carcinomas may contain a variety of cellular patterns. The predominance of cells with eosinophilic cytoplasm and high nuclear grade are among the criteria for malignancy in adrenocortical neoplasms. An intranuclear cytoplasmic pseudoinclusion is seen in this field.

Pathology

Cytology

- The cytologic features depend on the degree of differentiation, characterized by resemblance to normal cortical cells. More well-differentiated tumors may be difficult to distinguish from cortical adenomas, whereas more pleomorphic carcinomas may be difficult to distinguish from metastatic carcinomas.
- Smears are usually very cellular, and unlike normal cortex and adenomas, the cytoplasm is usually intact. There is loss of cohesiveness, with many single cells admixed with loose groups of cells.

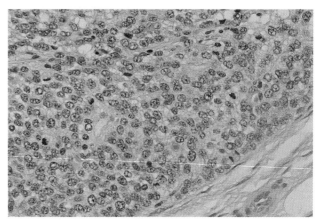

Figure 14–25. Small cells with an increased nuclear:cytoplasmic ratio are cause for concern in adrenocortical neoplasms. Such areas are often a fertile spot to search for mitoses, as in this cortical carcinoma.

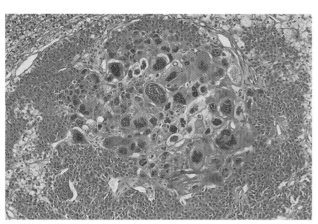

Figure 14–26. Marked nuclear pleomorphism with bizarre cells is seen in this area of an adrenocortical carcinoma. Focal nuclear pleomorphism may be seen in adenomas, but it is not of this degree. Other features of malignancy were present in this neoplasm, including predominance of eosinophilic cells, which are seen in this field.

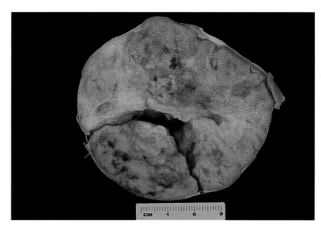

Figure 14–29. An oncocytic adrenocortical neoplasm is brownish yellow and contains large fibrous septae. The histologic criteria in this tumor and its behavior indicate malignancy.

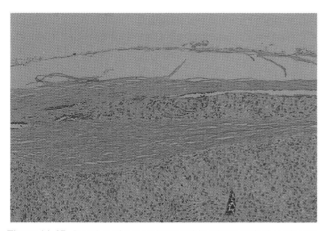

Figure 14–27. Invasion of a capsular vessel in adrenocortical carcinoma. Frequent mitotic figures, confluent necrosis, high nuclear grade, and predominance of eosinophilic cells were additional criteria for malignancy identified in this case.

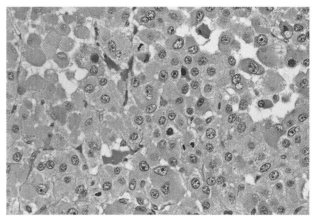

Figure 14–30. Few cases of oncocytic adrenocortical carcinoma are documented; although this neoplasm has not metastasized in a brief follow-up period, the mitotic rate and other features suggest that it is best classified as a carcinoma. The abundant eosinophilic cytoplasm and nuclear morphology are "oncocytic."

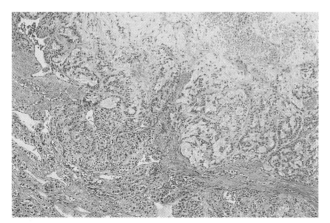

Figure 14–28. Myxoid change and a pseudoglandular pattern are unusual features that might suggest an extra-adrenal origin in this carcinoma; however, other areas were typical of adrenocortical carcinoma, and there was no evidence of disease in any other location.

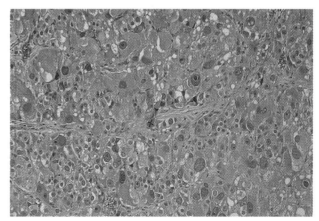

Figure 14–31. This adrenal neoplasm in an 8-month-old girl was associated with striking virilization. In spite of the "malignant" appearance of many adrenocortical neoplasms in children, they usually exhibit benign behavior. Size appears to be the best predictor of behavior in children: tumors weighing more than 500 g are almost always malignant.

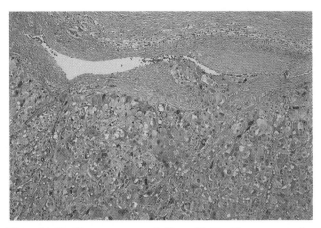

Figure 14–32. The same case seen in Figure 14–31, with tumor protruding into a capsular vein. Vascular invasion does not appear to predict aggressive behavior in childhood cortical tumors.

- Although loss of cytoplasmic lipid vacuoles is common in carcinomas, some more "well-differentiated" carcinomas may contain vacuolated cells, which are helpful in recognizing the neoplasm as being of cortical origin. The lipid-rich cells differ from those in adenomas in their nuclear features: the nuclei are enlarged and hyperchromatic and contain nucleoli. Mitoses, if present, are highly suggestive of malignancy.
- Carcinomas in which the cells have little or no lipid are more difficult to distinguish from metastatic lesions. The cytoplasm is eosinophilic and granular and varies greatly in amount; some tumor cells may have an abundance of cytoplasm, whereas others have a high nuclear:cytoplasmic ratio. The nuclei tend to be quite atypical, with hyperchromasia and pleomorphism that may become extremely bizarre. Nucleoli are usually prominent and large. Necrosis of tumor cells is helpful in supporting a malignant diagnosis.
- Immunohistochemistry and electron microscopy may be helpful in the differential diagnosis between adrenocortical carcinoma and metastatic carcinoma, as discussed later.

Gross

- Reported average weights of cortical carcinomas vary greatly, from 705 to more than 1210 g; however, the weight ranges are quite large—from less than 40 to more than 3000 g. The range of recorded weights overlaps significantly with the weight range of cortical adenomas. Although weight has been used as a predictor of behavior in cortical neoplasms, it has become clear that weight is not, by itself, a reliable criterion for malignancy. This is particularly true with the increasing use of advanced radiologic imaging techniques, which are capable of detecting these neoplasms when they are much smaller and sometimes incidental.
- Tumors as small as 38 g have metastasized, whereas others weighing as much as 1800 g have behaved in a benign fashion.
- Nonhyperfunctioning tumors tend to be larger at the time of diagnosis than those associated with clinical endocrine dysfunction.

- Cortical carcinomas may be grossly encapsulated or, especially if large, infiltrative; adjacent organs may be involved. Large tumors often completely efface the adrenal gland.
- The contour of the neoplasm is usually multinodular. The cut surface is yellow to brown and is usually mottled by patches of hemorrhage and necrosis, which may be extensive. Degenerative changes lead to cystic areas occasionally.

Histology

- Although a variety of histologic patterns may be observed, including the typical nesting configuration of adrenocortical adenomas, the presence of diffuse or solid and broad trabecular areas is common in carcinomas and should alert one to the possibility of malignancy. Occasionally pseudoglandular or myxoid patterns may seen.
- Broad bands of fibrous tissue often dissect the tumor into coarse irregular nodules.
- Necrosis may be absent in smaller tumors but is a common finding overall; it may be focal and involving only small clusters of tumor cells, or it may be extensive, with confluent "geographic" patches.
- Eosinophilic, lipid-poor tumor cells tend to predominate, although aggregates of cells with pale, vacuolated cytoplasm may be present as well. The amount of cytoplasm is quite variable. Pleomorphic cells with very atypical nuclei and abundant cytoplasm may be impressive, but these cells are not restricted to carcinomas. A more disturbing cell type is the rather monotonous cell with a high nuclear:cytoplasmic ratio; these cells populate areas of intense cellularity and are usually fruitful areas for counting mitotic figures. The small cells have relatively large rounded hyperchromatic nuclei, with coarse chromatin and prominent nucleoli.
- Hyaline globules may be present in the cytoplasm of some carcinomas.
- The presence of readily identified mitotic figures is usually indicative of malignancy and is usually accompanied by other criteria for carcinoma. A rate of 6 or more mitoses per 50 HPF has been suggested as an indicator of malignancy, although not all carcinomas will have such a high mitotic rate.
- Vascular invasion and extensive local capsular invasion are highly suspicious for malignancy; involvement of true venous structures (in contrast with sinusoids) appears to be conclusive evidence of malignancy.
- The distinction between cortical adenoma and carcinoma is usually relatively simple; however, there are cases in which an unequivocal classification cannot be made. Several sets of criteria for malignancy have been compiled in conjunction with review of series of clinically benign and malignant adrenocortical neoplasms. The criteria of Hough and associates use both clinical and pathologic parameters, whereas Weiss and van Slooten and colleagues included only pathologic findings. These parameters are summarized in Tables 14–2 through 14–5. Numerical values are assigned to each criterion in the methods of Hough and van Slooten, with a minimum score required for the diagnosis of malignancy.
- *Immunohistochemistry:* Immunohistochemistry is not helpful in distinguishing between adrenocortical adenoma

and adrenocortical carcinoma; however, it is useful in the differential diagnosis between cortical carcinoma and a variety of metastatic lesions. Cortical carcinomas are positive for vimentin but are usually negative for cytokeratin, epithelial membrane antigen, carcinoembryonic antigen, S100, HMB-45, and blood group isoantigens. Use of some low-molecular-weight cytokeratins may yield scattered positive cells in some cases. The immunostaining pattern is helpful in distinguishing between adrenocortical carcinoma and hepatocellular or renal cell carcinoma, which may be a histologic differential diagnostic problem.

- *Electron microscopy:* Few cytoplasmic lipid vacuoles are seen. Mitochondria are variably shaped but usually elongated, and they often have tubular cristae. Stacks of rough endoplasmic reticulum and myelin figures are usually present.
- *Flow cytometric DNA analysis:* Although aneuploidy tends to favor malignancy in cortical neoplasms, there is some overlap with adenomas, particularly larger ones.

Differential Diagnosis

- Adrenocortical adenoma.
- Metastatic carcinoma, especially hepatocellular or renal cell carcinoma.
- Pheochromocytoma.

Treatment and Prognosis

- Adrenocortical carcinomas are extremely aggressive—more than 60% of patients have metastatic disease at the time of diagnosis. Patients who develop metastatic disease rarely live longer than 1 year.
- The treatment includes resection of the primary lesion, followed by chemotherapy using mitotane.
- Tumor stage is useful in predicting survival: *Stage I,* tumor is 5 cm or smaller and confined to the adrenal; *Stage II,* tumor is larger than 5 cm and confined to the adrenal; *Stage III,* tumor, any size, is confined to the adrenal with regional lymph node involvement or locally invasive without lymph node metastases; *Stage IV,* tumor is locally invasive with regional lymph node involvement, or tumor with involvement of adjacent organ, or any tumor with distant metastases. Approximately one third of patients with stage I or II tumors survive 5 years.

Additional Facts

- *Adrenocortical neoplasms in children* cannot be categorized reliably using the systems established for adult cortical neoplasms. Although childhood cortical tumors have been assigned a poor prognosis in the past, current detection methods, surgical technique, and endocrine replacement therapy appear to have altered the outcome significantly. Reevaluation of criteria has shown that pediatric tumors may exhibit increased mitotic rate, atypical mitoses, necrosis, vascular and capsular invasion, fibrous bands, and marked nuclear pleomorphism, without aggressive clinical behavior. Tumor size may have prognostic significance, with a weight greater than 500 g usually associated with malignant behavior; however, as in adult

tumors, there is overlap in the weights of benign and malignant tumors in different studies.

C. NEOPLASMS OF THE ADRENAL MEDULLA

1. Adrenomedullary Hyperplasia

Definition: Diffuse or nodular increases in medullary tissue and associated hypersecretion of catecholamines, most often as a precursor to pheochromocytoma in multiple endocrine neoplasia syndrome (MEN).

Clinical

- Although most instances of adrenomedullary hyperplasia (AMH) are reported in patients with MEN, there are occasional patients who appear to have a sporadic form of hyperplasia, with similar clinical manifestations.
- *Sporadic* cases of AMH are characterized by signs and symptoms of pheochromocytoma, including hypertension (paroxysmal or sustained), headaches, palpitations, and

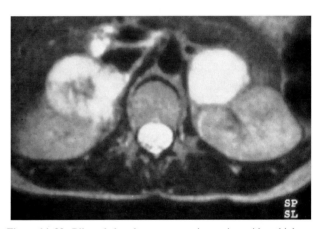

Figure 14–33. Bilateral pheochromocytomas in a patient with multiple endocrine neoplasia, type 2A. The large tumors are bright on the T2-weighted image by magnetic resonance imaging.

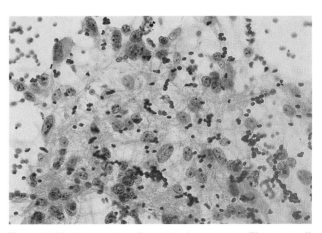

Figure 14–34. Fine needle aspirate, pheochromocytoma. The tumor cells cluster in a loose acinar arrangement. Fibrillar cytoplasmic processes create a meshlike background. Mild nuclear pleomorphism is seen. Bizarre nuclei may be present in some cases and does not signify malignancy.

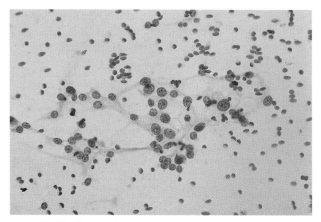

Figure 14–35. Fine needle aspirate, pheochromocytoma. A tumor with smaller cells, aggregating in acinar clusters. The salt-and-pepper chromatin pattern reflects the neuroendocrine origin. Wisplike processes of granular cytoplasm are present.

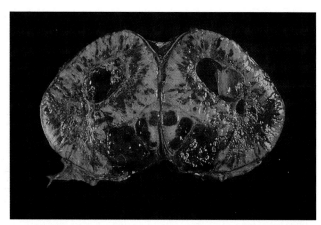

Figure 14–38. Pheochromocytoma with variegated red-tan color and central area of cystic degeneration, a common finding in pheochromocytomas.

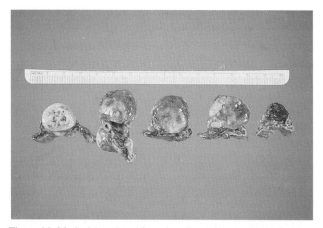

Figure 14–36. Serial sections of an adrenal containing multiple pheochromocytomas in a patient with multiple endocrine neoplasia, type 2A. A compound tumor of the medulla was found in the opposite adrenal.

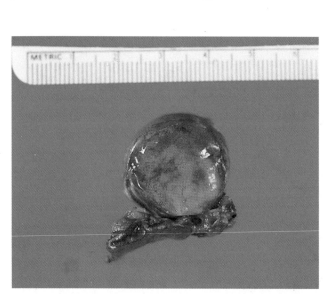

Figure 14–37. Cross section of the adrenal seen in Figure 14–36. The tiny nodules, measuring a few millimeters in diameter, represent part of the spectrum of adrenal medullary hyperplasia, which is typically seen in cases of familial pheochromocytoma.

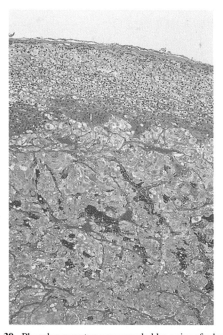

Figure 14–39. Pheochromocytoma surrounded by a rim of adrenal cortex. The capsule of a pheochromocytoma is often composed of the adrenal remnant and its capsule.

diaphoresis in the absence of a detectable tumor. These patients have no family history of MEN syndromes. Urinary catecholamine or metanephrine levels are elevated.

■ *Familial* AMH is usually associated with MEN 2 and is believed to be the precursor of pheochromocytomas in this setting. Unlike patients with sporadic AMH, familial AMH may be detected before it is symptomatic due to laboratory screening in families at risk. The earliest indication of AMH is elevation of the epinephrine:norepinephrine ratio in the urine. When symptoms become evident, they are generally those seen in pheochromocytoma.

■ AMH has been reported in Beckwith-Wiedemann syndrome, which may be sporadic or familial.

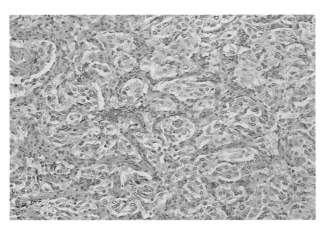

Figure 14–40. The classic "zellballen" pattern in pheochromocytoma: rounded nests of chief cells circumscribed by an intricate fibrovascular network. The vascular proliferation is particularly prominent in this example. The chief cells in this tumor display slight nuclear pleomorphism, which can be striking in some cases.

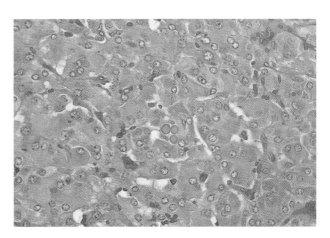

Figure 14–43. Hyaline globules are periodic acid-Schiff–positive, diastase resistant. There is some evidence that their presence is a feature that favors a benign outcome. These globules are not specific. They may be found in a variety of vascular neoplasms.

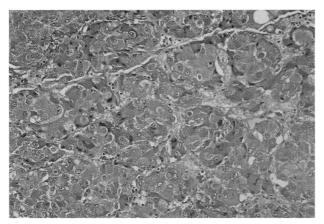

Figure 14–41. Large polygonal tumor cells in this pheochromocytoma have prominent cytoplasmic amphophilic granularity and mild nuclear pleomorphism.

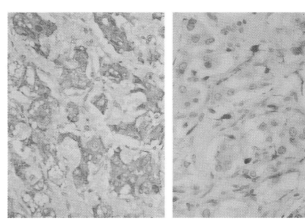

Figure 14–44. Immunohistochemical pattern of pheochromocytoma. Chief cells are positive for chromogranin *(left);* sustentacular cells are S100 positive *(right).*

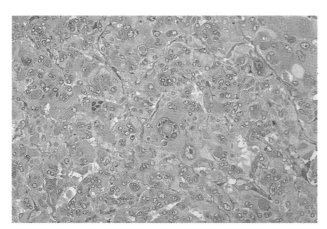

Figure 14–42. Nuclear pleomorphism is more prominent in this pheochromocytoma with eosinophilic granular cytoplasm. Intranuclear cytoplasmic pseudoinclusions are common.

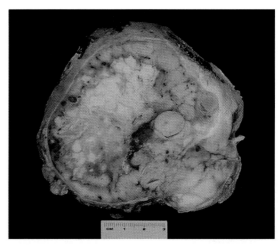

Figure 14–45. This malignant pheochromocytoma demonstrates the gross nodular pattern that is helpful in distinguishing between benign and malignant sympathoadrenal paragangliomas.

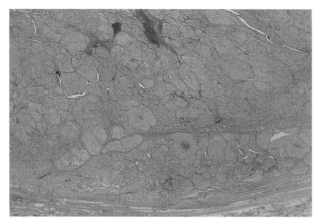

Figure 14–46. A malignant pheochromocytoma, with large, irregularly sized cell nests (zellballen).

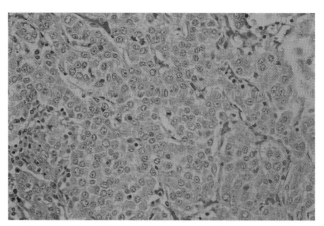

Figure 14–49. Malignant pheochromocytoma seen in Figure 14–48, demonstrating a very high mitotic rate.

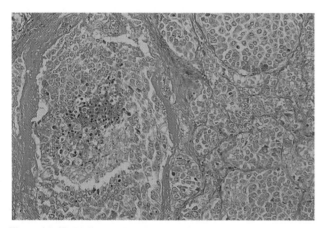

Figure 14–47. Malignant pheochromocytoma, large cell nests with central necrosis. The mitotic rate is also very high in this lesion.

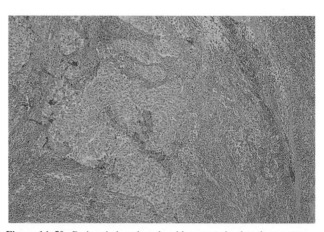

Figure 14–50. Periaortic lymph node with metastatic pheochromocytoma from the primary tumor illustrated in Figure 14–48. Metastatic disease is the ultimate proof of malignancy in pheochromocytoma. Some pheochromocytomas with a benign histologic appearance metastasize, supporting the unpredictable reputation of these neoplasms.

Radiology

■ CT scans may show no abnormality or, in more advanced diffuse or nodular AMH, may demonstrate adrenal enlargement (bilateral in most cases).

Pathology

Gross

■ Changes of AMH are usually bilateral but may be asymmetrical.
■ Adrenal enlargement may not be evident grossly. In such cases morphometric demonstration of an increased volume and weight of medullary tissue or direct dissection of the medullary tissue from the gland is necessary to document AMH. The normal medullary weights range from 0.37 to 0.48 g per gland. A decrease in the overall cortical to medullary ratio, which is normally 4:1, is also helpful.
■ In more advanced cases of AMH the medulla may be diffusely expanded or multinodular, extending into the tail of

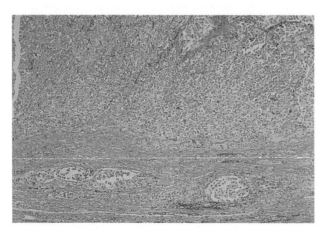

Figure 14–48. Malignant pheochromocytoma with extensive regional vascular invasion. This patient developed regional lymph node metastases several months after resection of the adrenal tumor.

the gland, where medullary tissue is not normally seen. In such cases the overall adrenal weight is increased. The distinction of nodular AMH from multiple pheochromocytomas in MEN-associated medullary disease is somewhat arbitrary; nodules smaller than 1 cm are classified as "hyperplastic," whereas those 1 cm or larger in diameter are considered pheochromocytomas.

- The hyperplastic medullary tissue may be gray to tan to dark red; the nodular areas tend to blend indistinctly with the surrounding medulla.

Histology

- The microscopic proliferation of medullary cells may be diffuse or variably nodular. The adjacent cortex may be compressed. As the hyperplasia advances, nodules become larger and more distinct.
- Various patterns may be seen, as in pheochromocytoma, including solid, trabecular, or the typical zellballen nesting pattern.
- The cells may exhibit significant nuclear pleomorphism and hyperchromasia; the cytoplasm may be vacuolated or very granular. These changes are believed to reflect the hypersecretory activity of the hyperplastic medullary cells.
- Mitotic figures may be seen, although they are usually few in number.

Differential Diagnosis

- Pheochromocytoma (Chapter 14C, #2).

Treatment and Prognosis

- Resection of one or both adrenal glands has resulted in resolution or improvement of symptoms in a large proportion of patients with sporadic AMH; bilateral adrenalectomy has been used in many patients with MEN 2 with favorable results.
- AMH is considered a benign, preneoplastic disease by most; however, the clinical risks of hypersecretion of catecholamines and the potential for malignancy in pheochromocytoma are key concerns in clinical management decisions.

2. Pheochromocytoma

Definition: A neoplastic proliferation of the neuroendocrine cells of the adrenal medulla and of their supporting, or "sustentacular," cells. This term has specifically referred to paragangliomas of the adrenal medulla but has also been used to designate all paragangliomas of the sympathoadrenal neuroendocrine system (including the "extra-adrenal" pheochromocytomas). Signs and symptoms are related to release of catecholamines, chiefly epinephrine and norepinephrine.

Synonyms: Adrenal paraganglioma, sympathoadrenal paraganglioma, chromaffinoma, chromaffin cell tumor, chromophile tumor, medullary adenoma, adrenergic tumor.

Clinical

- Pheochromocytomas are uncommon, with an autopsy incidence of 0.005% to 0.1%. In the past as many as 76% of pheochromocytomas were not diagnosed during life; however, these do not appear to have been nonfunctional or "silent" tumors, since most of those patients died of sudden cardiac or cerebrovascular events, often related to a surgical procedure for an unrelated problem.
- 90% of cases are sporadic, whereas 10% are familial.
- Familial cases of pheochromocytoma may occur in the absence of other familial disease syndromes or may be seen in association with MEN 2A (most common), MEN 2B, von Recklinghausen's disease, and von Hippel-Lindau disease.
- Tumors occur over a very broad age range from infancy to old age, but the incidence peaks in the fifth decade. Familial cases are usually diagnosed at an earlier age, usually within the first 2 decades.
- No definite gender predilection has been noted; however, some studies suggest a slight preponderance of females.
- Only approximately 10% of pheochromocytomas occur in children.
- Common presenting symptoms include headache (>90%), palpitations, diaphoresis, flushing of the skin, anxiety, nausea, and constipation. Dyspnea, chest pain, visual disturbances, abdominal pain, fatigue, and paresthesias are less frequent complaints. The triad of headache, palpitations, and sweating are particularly predictive of a diagnosis of pheochromocytoma.
- Hypertension, with or without tachycardia, is the key physical finding, with half of patients experiencing sustained hypertension with episodes of marked hypertension, whereas the remaining have paroxysmal hypertensive episodes. A few patients with pheochromocytomas are normotensive.
- 10% to 15% of patients have a palpable abdominal mass.
- Laboratory biochemical evaluation is the cornerstone of diagnosis: 24-hour urine samples are assayed for elevations of epinephrine, norepinephrine, total catecholamines, and for their metabolites, metanephrine, normetanephrine, and vanillylmandelic acid. Plasma catechol amines (epinephrine and norepinephrine) may also be determined; they have a higher sensitivity for diagnosing pheochromocytoma than do urine assays. Urine metanephrine and vanillylmandelic acid levels, the most widely used assays, detect 80% to 90% of tumors.
- Clinical presentation reflects the pattern of catecholamine secretion: Norepinephrine-secreting tumors produce sustained hypertension; tumors with significant epinephrine secretion in addition to norepinephrine produce episodic hypertension; and pure epinephrine-secreting tumors may produce hypotension. Dopamine is the dominant product of a small number of pheochromocytomas; these patients are usually normotensive and may present a diagnostic dilemma.

Radiology

- CT scan, m-iodobenzylguanidine (I-MIBG) scan, MRI, ultrasonography, and venous cannulation with sampling for catecholamine levels all are useful in localization of pheochromocytomas.
- CT scan is the most widely used imaging method for localization. The adrenal glands and sites of extra-adrenal

paragangliomas are readily visualized. Pheochromocytomas are nonhomogeneous, well-circumscribed tumors. The lack of homogeneity is the result of areas of hemorrhage, necrosis, or cystic degeneration. MRI is similarly useful, with the added advantage of improved differential distinction among pheochromocytoma, metastases to the adrenal, and many adrenocortical neoplasms.

- The ^{131}I-MIBG scan uses a radioactive material that is taken up by neuroendocrine tumors, including pheochromocytomas, neuroblastomas, parathyroid proliferative diseases, paragangliomas, and some carcinoids and medullary thyroid carcinomas. Almost all benign pheochromocytomas, but only half of malignant cases, are detectable with this procedure. I-MIBG is also useful in identifying metastatic disease in tumors with uptake of the radioisotope.

Pathology

Cytology

- Fine needle aspiration of adrenal masses, as well as retroperitoneal extra-adrenal lesions, is a common method of preoperative diagnosis, which is helpful in distinguishing between metastatic and primary lesions. Biochemical and clinical evidence for the diagnosis of pheochromocytoma are usually adequate to make a preoperative diagnosis without resorting to fine needle aspiration; indeed, aspiration of pheochromocytoma may result in life-threatening hemorrhage or in a hypertensive crisis. Most of the cytologic diagnoses of pheochromocytoma are made in patients with atypical clinical presentation or equivocal biochemical evidence.
- Smears are usually cellular, with loose clusters of polygonal to somewhat elongated cells with poorly defined cytoplasmic borders. Delicate wisplike processes may extend from some of the cells; the cytoplasm is finely granular.
- The nuclei are quite variable, with some marked anisonucleosis in some cases. Hyperchromasia is usually evident, with a coarse chromatin pattern. Nucleoli vary from cell to cell in terms of being inconspicuous to very prominent. Intranuclear cytoplasmic pseudoinclusions may be present and are numerous in some cases. Naked nuclei are common.
- An unfortunate but helpful clue in the diagnosis may be noted during the procedure: hypertension, with palpitations, diaphoresis, or other manifestations.

Gross

- Sporadic pheochromocytomas are usually single unilateral tumors 3 to 5 cm in diameter. Multiple and bilateral tumors are common in a familial setting, particularly in MEN 2. The multiple neoplasms in MEN 2 may be accompanied by a diffuse increase in the medullary tissue due to adrenomedullary hyperplasia.
- Pheochromocytomas are circumscribed, with larger tumors possessing a definite capsule. Compressed adrenal cortex may be splayed over the capsule of large tumors.
- The cut surface is gray to pink-tan or red, with areas of hyperemia or recent hemorrhage. Areas of remote hemorrhage, fibrosis, cystic degeneration, and necrosis are more common in large tumors. The tumor may darken to a brown or mahogany color after exposure to air due to oxidation of catecholamines.
- The *chromaffin reaction* is a gross method of demonstrating the presence of catecholamines. After immersion in a dichromate fixative, the tumor becomes deep brown in color as a result of oxidation of epinephrine and norepinephrine. The pigments are visible microscopically but are water soluble and are thus largely removed in routine processing of tissue.

Histology

- Architectural patterns most frequently encountered are trabecular (most common), alveolar or nesting, and diffuse. Less often, pseudoacinar structures may be superimposed on an alveolar pattern. Focal spindling of cells is also reported; extensive spindling is believed by some to be more common in malignant pheochromocytomas, although not all studies support this impression.
- Vascularity is prominent, with capillaries in a delicate fibrovascular meshwork surrounding groups of tumor cells arranged in nest or cords. The vascularity in some cases is so prominent as to give the tumor an angiomatous appearance.
- Although most tumors are surrounded by at least a thin capsule of fibrovascular tissue, extension of tumor into the adrenal cortex may be seen; this does not imply invasion and malignancy.
- The cytologic features of pheochromocytomas vary greatly from case to case. Polygonal cells with finely granular eosinophilic to somewhat basophilic cytoplasm are most often seen; the nuclear:cytoplasmic ratio is approximately 1:2. The nuclei are central to eccentric in position; they are ovoid, with stippled "salt-and-pepper" chromatin and small nucleoli. From this typical cell, numerous variations emerge. Some tumors may contain small cells with a higher nuclear:cytoplasmic ratio, whereas others have abundant granular cytoplasm that varies from pink to purple. Some tumor cells resemble ganglion cells, with prominent nucleoli and basophilic Nissl-like material. The cytoplasm may contain eosinophilic, PAS-positive globules, which appear to be related to high level of secretory activity. Nuclear pleomorphism may be striking with groups of cells with bizarre hyperchromatic nuclei many times the size of most surrounding pheochromocytes. Intranuclear cytoplasmic pseudoinclusions are common and may be especially striking in pleomorphic nuclei.
- Degenerative changes are seen more often in large tumors; they include areas of sclerosis, hemosiderin accumulation, resolving hemorrhage, and cystic changes.
- Stromal amyloid has been reported in as many as 70% of pheochromocytomas and should be considered in the differential diagnosis of medullary thyroid carcinoma.
- *Histochemistry:* Argyrophilic granules can be demonstrated using a number of techniques, including the Grimelius, Pascual, and Churukian-Schenk stains.
- *Immunohistochemistry:* The most useful immunostains are for chromogranin, which stains the chief cells, and S100, which stains the sustentacular cells found at the periphery of clusters of chief cells. Other markers that are positive in the chief cells include synaptophysin, neuron-specific enolase, and neurofilament proteins as well as serotonin, leu- and met-enkephalins, pancreatic polypep-

tide, and vasoactive intestinal peptide. Previous reports suggested that a decrease in the number of sustentacular cells, as demonstrated by S100 staining, is associated with likelihood of malignant behavior in head and neck paragangliomas and in sympathoadrenal paragangliomas. However, some recent reevaluations conclude that density of sustentacular cells is not a reliable predictor of behavior in either group of paragangliomas.

■ *Flow cytometric/DNA measurement:* Although studies of normal medulla and adrenomedullary hyperplasia reveal a diploid or euploid DNA distribution, nondiploid and aneuploid DNA patterns were found in most benign and all malignant pheochromocytomas.

■ *Electron microscopy:* The diagnostic feature is the presence of membrane-bound dense-core neurosecretory granules. The granules range in size from 150 to 250 nm. In most pheochromocytomas norepinephrine granules are most abundant; they differ from epinephrine granules by the presence of a large eccentric electron-lucent zone between the dense core and the granule membrane. In predominantly epinephrine-secreting tumors and in normal medullary cells neurosecretory granules have only a uniform narrow halo surrounding the electron-dense core. Tumor cells may have poorly formed intercellular junctions, as well as variable basal lamina.

Malignancy in Pheochromocytoma

■ The reported incidence of malignancy in adrenal pheochromocytomas varies by series; however, the traditional 10% figure is near the average of most studies. Extra-adrenal pheochromocytomas have a significantly higher rate of malignancy, from 14% to 50%.

■ The distinction between benign and malignant pheochromocytomas has long been problematic, with the only widely accepted and definitive proof of malignancy being metastasis to other organs. Sites of metastasis are usually liver, lymph nodes, bone, and lungs.

■ Tumors with benign histologic features may metastasize, whereas tumors with bizarre pleomorphism may behave in a benign fashion. Metastatic deposits may likewise appear very atypical or may be histologically indistinguishable from benign paraganglioma. This unpredictability has frustrated pathologists and surgeons in spite of many attempts to define criteria for malignancy.

■ The conclusions from several studies of pheochromocytoma have conflicted in many areas concerning malignant criteria. The following features have been associated with an increased incidence of malignant behavior, although there are some exceptions to each and no single criterion has proved entirely reliable:

Tumor size: Malignant tumors averaged 383 and 759 g versus 73 and 156 g, respectively, for benign tumors in two large series. One malignant tumor, however, weighed only 35 g.

Coarsely nodular or multinodular gross appearance: Benign tumors are more often unicentric and uniform, whereas gross nodularity is more common in malignant tumors. There is, however, overlap between benign and malignant categories.

Confluent tumor necrosis: Necrosis involving contiguous groups of tumor cells is seen in one third of malignant tumors.

Mitotic rate: A mitotic rate of greater than 3/30 HPF favors malignancy; benign tumors usually have less than 1/30 HPF. Some malignant tumors, however, have very low mitotic rates. Atypical mitoses are uncommon, but are a strong indicator of malignancy.

Extensive local invasion and or vascular invasion: Invasion is a helpful feature if extensive; however, tumors that do not behave aggressively may have some evidence of capsular invasion (or poor encapsulation) and may protrude into vessels in the area of the capsule.

Large zellballen with central degeneration: The nests seen in an alveolar pattern are usually small and compact; larger nests or nodules, when present, suggest malignancy. Central necrosis within these large zellballen is also an ominous finding.

Lack of hyaline globules: The presence of numerous eosinophilic intracytoplasmic globules is very suggestive of benignity; however, globules are not readily apparent in all benign pheochromocytomas. Their absence, therefore, is not definitive evidence of malignancy.

Dopamine secretion: Tumors that secrete predominantly or exclusively dopamine are more often malignant. This group of tumors is also difficult to diagnose due to lack of typical symptoms of pheochromocytoma.

Small cells with high nuclear:cytoplasmic ratio: Malignant tumors have been noted in some studies to be composed predominantly of small cells; however, there is some overlap with benign tumors in this respect.

Monotony of cytologic pattern: Nuclear pleomorphism is more often a feature of benign tumors; a monotonous cellular pattern is common in malignant pheochromocytomas.

Spindle cell pattern: Although some have reported an association of spindling of tumor cells with malignancy, others have noted a predominantly spindle cell pattern in rare clinically benign tumors. The presence of spindle cells should be evaluated in conjunction with other criteria of malignancy.

Differential Diagnosis

■ Adrenocortical adenoma (Chapter 14B, #1).
■ Adrenocortical carcinoma (Chapter 14B, #2).
■ Metastatic carcinoma, particularly renal cell carcinoma (Chapter 14D, #7).
■ Metastatic neuroendocrine neoplasms, including pancreatic islet cell tumors, medullary thyroid carcinoma, and gastrointestinal and pulmonary carcinoid tumors.
■ Alveolar soft part sarcoma.

Treatment and Prognosis

■ Preoperative management of hypertension is essential and has contributed to a dramatic decrease in operative mortality.

■ Surgical resection is the treatment of choice—adrenalectomy or, for extra-adrenal tumors, resection of the lesion. The possibility of multiple lesions or metastatic disease requires intraoperative evaluation of both adrenal glands, as well as the paracaval and para-aortic areas and regional lymph nodes.

■ Because a diagnosis of malignancy may rely on subsequent clinical behavior in the absence of definitive histologic evidence, close follow-up of patients with pheochromocytomas is needed.

■ Treatment for malignant pheochromocytomas depends on extent of disease. Locally aggressive tumors with invasion of adjacent tissues or regional lymph node metastases may be adequately treated by radical surgery. If resection is incomplete or if distant metastases are present, radiation therapy and chemotherapy have been used; however, the limited number of cases makes results difficult to interpret.

■ 5-year survival of patients with malignant pheochromocytoma is reported as 43%, with approximately half of the patients dead after a rapidly progressive course, whereas the remainder may survive for many years with more indolent disease.

■ Follow-up of serum and urinary catecholamines and their metabolites is an extremely useful method of monitoring patients for recurrent disease.

■ Recurrent elevation of catecholamines in children or in patients with familial history of pheochromocytoma may indicate development of multifocal lesions rather than metastatic or recurrent disease.

Additional Facts

■ Several studies have reported an association of brown adipose tissue in the periadrenal area, and elsewhere in the abdomen, with pheochromocytoma. Although explanations implicating activation of this fatty tissue by catecholamines have been proposed, a recent examination of periadrenal adipose tissue associated with pheochromocytoma and in control patients found no difference in incidence or amount of brown fat between the groups.

■ Carney's triad is an unusual nonfamilial association of functioning paragangliomas (usually extra-adrenal), gastric epithelioid leiomyosarcoma, and pulmonary chondro-

mas. Young females are usually affected. Adrenal pheochromocytomas have been seen in a few cases.

■ Other disorders that may manifest the clinical signs and symptoms of pheochromocytoma include coarctation of the abdominal aorta, adrenal myelolipoma, renal cysts, and acute mercury poisoning. "Pseudopheochromocytoma" has been used to describe this clinical situation. Rare patients appear to have a hyperactive adrenergic system. Psychological disorders must also be considered in the clinical differential of pheochromocytoma.

■ Paragangliomas of the head and neck region are more closely affiliated with the parasympathetic autonomic system than with the sympathetic system, as are the adrenal and extra-adrenal abdominal paragangliomas. Paragangliomas of the head and neck are found in the intercarotid, jugulotympanic, aorticopulmonary, vagal, orbital, laryngeal, and pulmonary distribution. Head and neck paragangliomas are usually clinically nonfunctional, although they do frequently contain catecholamines. The histology, immunohistochemistry, and ultrastructure are similar to sympathoadrenal paragangliomas. Although only approximately 2% of the head and neck paragangliomas metastasize, they may by virtue of their location and extension to vital structures cause significant morbidity and mortality.

3. Neuroblastoma and Ganglioneuroblastoma (Tables 14–6 and 14–7)

Definition: Malignant neoplasm derived from the undifferentiated cells of the sympathetic nervous system. These lesions represent a spectrum from the primitive neuroblastoma to tumors in which differentiation into ganglion cells and schwannian stroma may be focal or nearly complete (ganglioneuroblastomas). The distinction between neuroblastoma and ganglioneuroblastoma has not been well-defined. Clinically, the term "neuroblastoma" is used in therapeutic protocols and staging to refer to the spectrum of pathologic entities that encompass neuroblastoma and ganglioneuroblastoma. A combination of histopathologic, molecular-genetic, and clinical features separates the lesions into prognostic groups that sometimes overlap strict histologic nomenclature.

Table 14–6
INTERNATIONAL STAGING SYSTEM FOR NEUROBLASTOMA AND GANGLIONEUROBLASTOMA

Stage	Criteria
I	Localized tumor confined to the area of the origin; complete gross excision, with or without microscopic residual disease; identifiable ipsilateral and contralateral lymph nodes negative microscopically
IIa	Unilateral tumor with incomplete gross excision; identifiable ipsilateral and contralateral lymph nodes negative microscopically
IIb	Unilateral tumor with complete or incomplete gross excision; positive ipsilateral regional lymph nodes; identifiable contralateral lymph nodes negative microscopically
III	Tumor infiltrating across the midline with or without regional lymph node involvement; or unilateral tumor with contralateral regional lymph node involvement; or midline tumor with bilateral regional lymph node involvement
IV	Dissemination of tumor to distant lymph nodes, bone, bone marrow, liver, and/or other organs (exclusive of cases defined as stage IV-S)
IV-S	Localized primary tumor as defined for stage I or II with dissemination limited to the liver, skin, and/or bone marrow

Adapted from Brodeur GM, Seeger RC, Barrett A, et al. International criteria for diagnosis, staging, and response to treatment in patients with neuroblastoma. J Clin Oncol 1988; 6:1874–1881.

Table 14–7
NEUROBLASTOMA AND GANGLIONEUROBLASTOMA:
CLINICAL AND LABORATORY PROGNOSTIC FACTORS

	Favorable	Unfavorable
Age at diagnosis	<1 yr	>1 yr
Stage	I, II, IV-S	III, IV
Location	Thoracic	
Symptoms and signs	Opsoclonus-myoclonus	
Serum ferritin		>142 ng/ml
Serum neuron-specific enolase		>100 ng/ml
Urinary catecholamines	Elevated VMA/HVA	Low VMA/HMA; VLA positive
N-*myc* amplification	1 diploid copy	≥3 copies
Quantitative DNA analysis	Hyperdiploid or aneuploid	Diploid (linked to N-*myc* amplification)

VMA, vanillylmandelic acid; HVA, homovanillic acid; VLA, vanillacetic acid.

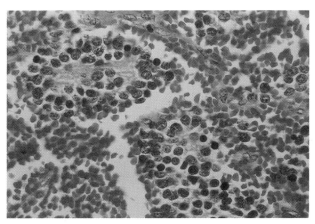

Figure 14–53. Fine needle aspirate, adrenal neuroblastoma. The tumor fragments in this cell block are characteristic of neuroblastoma, with Homer Wright rosettes.

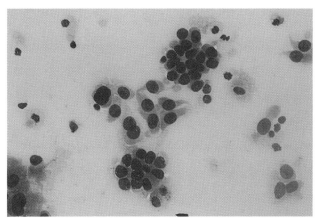

Figure 14–51. Fine needle aspirate, adrenal neuroblastoma in a 1-year-old child. The small cells resemble those of many other small blue cell tumors of childhood, although the cytoplasmic processes in this example are helpful in suggesting the diagnosis (Diff-Quik).

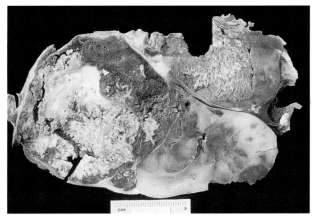

Figure 14–54. A large adrenal neuroblastoma with the typical variegated appearance with areas of necrosis and hemorrhage. The chalky-appearing flecks represent foci of calcification.

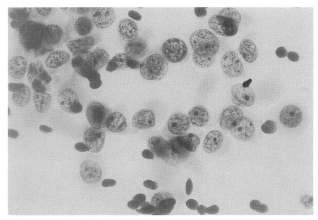

Figure 14–52. Fine needle aspirate, adrenal neuroblastoma, demonstrating the "salt-and-pepper" chromatin characteristic of many neuroendocrine tumors (Papanicolaou).

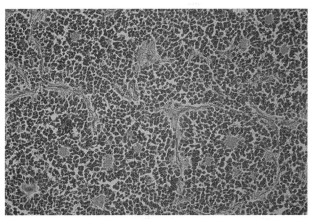

Figure 14–55. The classic pattern of neuroblastoma with well-developed Homer Wright rosettes in a background of small cells with a very high nuclear:cytoplasmic ratio.

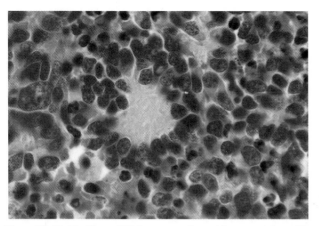

Figure 14–56. The Homer Wright rosettes of neuroblastoma are formed by a cluster of tumor cells arranged around a central core of neurofibrillary material.

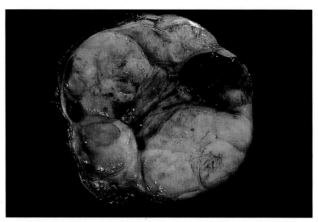

Figure 14–59. Ganglioneuroblastoma with a lobulated gray-white cut surface. The texture is firmer than neuroblastoma. This case had few immature neuroblastic areas; no necrosis is seen grossly.

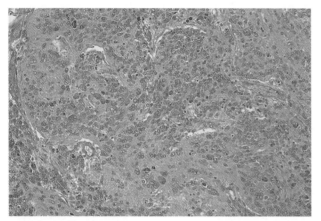

Figure 14–57. Neuroblastoma with areas of more prominent stroma and neuronal differentiation. Other areas of this neoplasm had higher cellularity, with little fibrillar stroma.

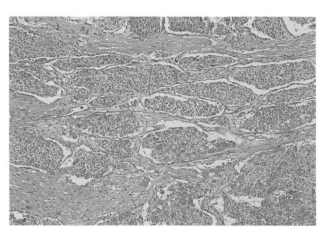

Figure 14–60. Ganglioneuroblastoma with islands of neuroblasts scattered among differentiated ganglioneuromatous areas. This adrenal tumor occurred in an adult woman.

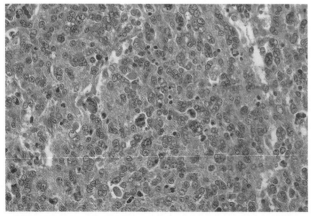

Figure 14–58. Neuronal differentiation in neuroblastoma is characterized by nuclear enlargement with a more vesicular chromatin pattern and more prominent nucleolus. The eosinophilic cytoplasm becomes more obvious and cell borders are visible. Karyorrhexis is seen in this field.

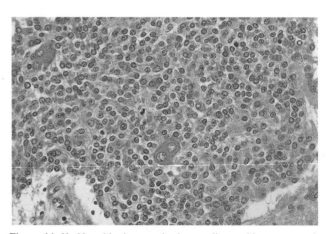

Figure 14–61. Neuroblastic areas in the ganglioneuroblastoma seen in Figure 14–60 contain cells with distinct neuronal differentiation.

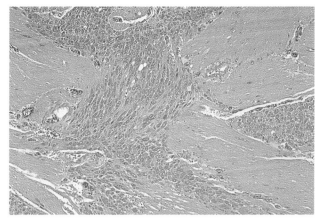

Figure 14–62. Ganglioneuromatous areas in the tumor seen in Figure 14–60, with bands of schwannian stroma admixed with ganglion cells in various stages of maturation.

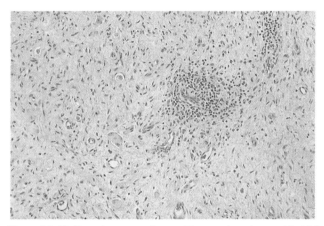

Figure 14–63. Paraspinous ganglioneuroblastoma in a 1-year-old child with a predominantly ganglioneuromatous pattern contains aggregates of small lymphocytes, which should not be confused with neuroblasts.

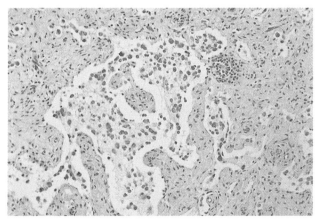

Figure 14–64. The ganglioneuroblastoma that was illustrated in Figure 14–63 contained rare microscopic islands of neuroblastic cells with fibrillar stroma.

Clinical

- Most common adrenal neoplasm in children, neuroblastoma/ganglioneuroblastoma is the fourth most common malignant tumor in children. The incidence of neuroblastoma is 8.7 per million and the incidence of ganglioneuroblastoma is approximately 1.8 per million. The detection rate for neuroblastoma/ganglioneuroblastoma in infants is higher in Japan due to a mass screening program.
- No gender predilection; slightly less common in black population.
- Familial cases are rare but reported; also rare are the associations with von Recklinghausen's disease, Beckwith-Wiedemann syndrome, and Hirschsprung's disease.
- 85% of cases are diagnosed before 5 years of age; however, rare cases are reported in adults over a wide age range.
- Slightly more than half of cases are intra-abdominal, with 36% to 38% arising in the adrenal. Other sites include the thorax (14% to 20%), neck (3.4% to 5%), pelvis (3.4% to 5%), and head (2%), basically any location along the sympathetic chain or in the adrenal medulla.
- The most common presentation is an abdominal mass; however, paraspinal neuroblastomas, particularly those with a "dumbbell" configuration that extend through a vertebral foramen, may cause loss of neurologic function due to spinal cord impingement. Neuroblastomas or ganglioneuroblastomas may cause other "location-dependent" symptoms related to their size. Children with metastatic disease at presentation may manifest more generalized symptoms and findings such as fever, weight loss, irritability, bone pain, proptosis and periorbital ecchymosis due to orbital involvement, cutaneous metastatic nodules ("blueberry muffin baby"), anemia, or thrombocytopenia.
- A number of paraneoplastic phenomena may be seen: hypertension out of proportion to measured catecholamine levels (in as many as 20% of patients), watery diarrhea syndrome due to vasoactive intestinal polypeptide, opsoclonus myoclonus ("dancing eyes, dancing feet"), ectopic ACTH syndrome, Horner's syndrome and heterochromia iridis.
- Mass screening for neuroblastoma in children at age 6 months using a qualitative vanillylmandelic acid spot test has increased the incidence of neuroblastoma in the more favorable age group (<1 year); however, the most recent consensus is that mass screening is not efficacious in reducing the population mortality due to neuroblastoma.
- Laboratory evaluation for suspected neuroblastoma includes quantitative urine levels of 3-methoxy-4-hydroxymandelic acid (vanillylmandelic acid), a metabolite of norepinephrine, and 3-methoxy-4-hydroxyphenylacetic acid (homovanillic acid), a metabolite of dopamine. Vanillylmandelic acid is elevated in 75% of patients at the time of diagnosis and homovanillic acid is elevated in 80%. An elevated ratio of vanillylmandelic acid to homovanillic acid is associated with a more aggressive course, as is the presence of vanillacetic acid.
- Clinical evaluation of patients with neuroblastoma routinely includes CT scan with contrast or MRI, chest radiograph, and radionuclide bone scan. Bone marrow aspirate and biopsy are also essential owing to the high incidence of bone marrow metastasis.

Radiology

- CT scan and MRI are useful in the preoperative evaluation of neuroblastoma. The tumors usually have well-defined margins that can be effectively visualized by MRI, providing information on extent of disease (vascular structures and adjacent organs involved and laterality of the neoplasm). Neuroblastomas usually have a relatively uniform intensity, with low-density areas corresponding to necrosis. Calcifications may be seen by CT scan. By MRI the tumors have a high signal intensity with T2-weighted images and low signal intensity with T1-weighted images.

Pathology

Cytology

■ Neuroblastic areas of neuroblastoma/ganglioneuroblastoma yield a monotonous population of small round nuclei with stippled chromatin. Individual cell borders are not distinct; the fibrillar cytoplasm of the cells forms a cobweb-like background.

■ Ganglioneuromatous areas yield ganglion cells of variable maturity, some binucleated or multinucleated. Ganglion cell differentiation is associated with an increase in cytoplasmic volume; elongated cytoplasmic processes may be seen. Fragments of eosinophilic stroma containing scattered spindle cells may be present; however, the cellularity of tumors with a predominance of mature ganglioneuromatous components is generally much lower than the cellular yield of those with abundant neuroblastic areas.

Gross

■ Usually circumscribed, neuroblastoma/ganglioneuroblastoma usually range in size from 5 to 10 cm but may be larger.

■ The appearance is quite variable: a single circumscribed mass or multinodular lesion may be seen. Encapsulation is variably present and may simply reflect the adrenal investiture.

■ Since neuroblastomas and ganglioneuroblastomas represent a spectrum of tumors with variable proportions of primitive neuroblastic tissue and maturing stroma-rich ganglioneuromatous areas, the gross appearance may range from extremely soft gray tissue with extensive hemorrhage and necrosis, sometimes with chalky punctate calcifications, to more rubbery yellow-gray neoplasms that are similar to typical ganglioneuromas. An important gross feature is the presence of distinct nodule(s) of neuroblastoma in a tumor otherwise characteristic for ganglioneuroma; this "nodular stroma-rich" pattern of ganglioneuroblastoma is associated with an unfavorable prognosis.

Histology

■ The microscopic appearance ranges from pure neuroblastomas to ganglioneuroblastomas in which primitive neuroblastic elements are mixed with maturing ganglion cells and schwannian stroma.

■ *Neuroblastoma:* Small, round nuclei with stippled (salt-and-pepper) chromatin and indistinct nucleoli appear to be embedded in a meshlike eosinophilic fibrillary matrix. Cell borders are not discernible. The nuclei may be randomly distributed in this neurofibrillary matrix or may be arranged in palisades or in rosettes around a center of fibrillary material, forming "pseudorosettes" (or Homer Wright rosettes).

■ *Maturation: Ganglioneuroblastoma (differentiation into ganglion and Schwann's cells):* Ganglion cell differentiation is characterized by nuclear enlargement, an increase in eosinophilic cytoplasm with discernible cells borders, and, as maturation progresses, eccentric placement of the nucleus, a vesicular chromatin pattern, a prominent nucleolus, and the appearance of granular basophilic Nissl substance in the cytoplasm. In most tumors ganglionic maturation is associated with the appearance of a schwannian stroma with abundant fasciculated eosinophilic fibrillar material containing scattered spindle cells. The proportion of ganglioneuromatous tissue required to merit classification of a neuroblastic tumor as "ganglioneuroblastoma" is not uniformly agreed on; conventional terminology indicates that tumors with more than 5% ganglion cells should be considered ganglioneuroblastoma, whereas some prefer reserving the term for tumors in which the preponderant component is ganglioneuromatous tissue (tumors with minor components of ganglionic differentiation would be termed "differentiating neuroblastoma"). Nomenclature is somewhat superseded by the Shimada age-linked histologic grading system discussed later.

■ Neuroblastic and ganglioneuromatous areas may contain aggregates of small lymphocytes that may resemble neuroblasts. The distinction becomes important in ganglioneuromas and more differentiated ganglioneuroblastomas. Leukocyte common antigen immunohistochemistry is helpful in this regard.

■ Several histologic grading systems have been developed for neuroblastoma/ganglioneuroblastoma. The most widely used system, developed by Shimada, is the following:

• *Stroma-rich tumors:* With abundant schwannian stroma, these encompass the spectrum of ganglioneuroblastomas. Three subgroups include the following:

  • *Well differentiated:* Lacks gross nodules of neuroblastic cells. Largely ganglioneuromatous, with only occasional scattered groups of primitive neuroblasts that do not form microscopic nodules that disrupt the stroma. Favorable histology—100% survival.

  • *Intermixed:* Lacks gross nodules of neuroblastic cells; however, there are microscopic aggregates of primitive neuroblasts displacing the stroma. Favorable histology—92% survival.

  • *Nodular:* Grossly visible nodules distinguish between the primitive neuroblastic and mature ganglioneuromatous components of the neoplasm. Unfavorable histology—18% survival.

• *Stroma-poor tumors:* Grade based on age at diagnosis, correlated with mitosis-karyorrhexis index (MKI), and quantity of differentiating elements. Undifferentiated: less than 5% of neuroblasts with ganglionic maturation.

  • *Favorable prognosis groups* (84% survival):

    • Less than 1.5 years old with MKI less than 200.

    • 1.5–4 years old, differentiating tumor, with MKI less than 100.

- *Unfavorable prognosis groups* (4.5% survival):
  - Less than 1.5 years old with MKI higher than 200.
  - 1.5–4 years old differentiating tumor with MKI higher than 100.
  - More than 1.5 years old with undifferentiated tumor.
  - More than 5 years old.
- *Immunohistochemistry:* Although not reliable as specific markers of neural differentiation, neuron-specific enolase and synaptophysin are usually positive; Leu-7 and chromogranin are variably positive; broad-spectrum screening panels of "cocktails" of antibodies against the range of subunits of neurofilament proteins are usually positive.
- Neuroblastomas are also cytokeratin negative and negative or minimally reactive for vimentin. Two antibodies that are reactive in neuroblastoma, although only in frozen sections or flow cytometric material, are HSAN 1.2 (very specific for neuroblastoma) and HLA epitope W6/32.
- *Electron microscopy:* Dense-core granules are most readily identified; neural tubules, neurofilaments, and neural processes may be seen, more abundantly in more differentiated tumors.
- *Molecular genetics:* N-*myc* oncogene amplification is associated with likelihood of disease progression. Amplification is rare in stages I and II but is found in approximately half of the cases of stages III and IV neuroblastoma. Amplification of N-*myc* is not usually seen in stage IV-S neuroblastoma or in patients with opsoclonus-myoclonus, two settings associated with a very favorable prognosis. Proto-oncogenes *ras, ret,* and c-*src* have been linked with neuroblastoma as well; however, the prognostic implications are not as strong as with N-*myc*. The N-*myc* oncogene in neuroblastoma is translocated from its normal position on chromosome 2 to 1p.
- *Flow cytometric DNA analysis:* Aneuploidy and low percentage of cells in the S, G2, and M phases of the cell cycle are associated with a favorable prognosis and correlate with favorable histologic patterns and stages.

Differential Diagnosis

- Pheochromocytoma (Chapter 14C, #2).
- Wilms' tumor.
- Lymphoma/leukemia (Chapter 14D, #1).
- Rhabdomyosarcoma.
- Ewing's sarcoma (see the following "Additional Facts").
- Primitive neuroectodermal tumors (see the following "Additional Facts").

Treatment and Prognosis

- Several systems for staging have been employed. The Evans Staging system and a recent modification, the International Staging System, are frequently used in the United States.
- Surgery alone may be adequate therapy for stages I and IIa; the addition of chemotherapy and/or radiation is required in higher-stage disease.
- 65% of patients have disseminated disease at the time of diagnosis; 60% of those are classified as stage IV; 5% are considered stage IV-S, which has a very favorable prognosis in spite of dissemination.
- Stage IV-S patients are usually infants, with a median age of 3 months. Although most have an adrenal primary, some have no identifiable primary tumor. If an adrenal primary tumor is present, it must be no higher than stage II. These patients commonly have massive hepatomegaly secondary to metastases. Bone marrow involvement (true bone metastases place the patient in stage IV), cutaneous metastatic nodules, and regional lymph node metastases are frequently present as well. The cutaneous nodules are often bluish purple, earning the clinical appellation "blueberry muffin baby." Infants younger than 1 year of age with stage IV-S neuroblastoma/ganglioneuroblastoma are typically long-term survivors. Because of the frequency of spontaneous regression in children younger than 1 year of age, surgical resection is often the sole initial treatment modality; chemotherapy and radiation may be withheld if there is no evidence of disease progression. The prognosis is poor in children older than 1 year of age.
- The most effective drugs in the treatment of neuroblastoma/ganglioneuroblastoma are cyclophosphamide, cisplatin, doxorubicin, teniposide, vincristine, peptichemio, and melphalan.
- High-dose chemotherapy with or without radiation, followed by allogeneic or autologous bone marrow transplantation, and immunotherapy are areas of research interest in stage IV neuroblastoma/ganglioneuroblastoma.
- Long-term survival is affected by several clinical, histologic, and genetic factors; however, overall long-term survival by stage of disease is a useful parameter: *Stage I,* more than 90%; *Stage II,* 70% to 80%; *Stage III,* 25%. Survival of stage IV patients is exquisitely age sensitive: more than 60% if younger than 1 year of age at diagnosis; 20% if between 1 and 2 years of age at diagnosis; and 10% if older than 2 years of age at diagnosis. *Stage IVS,* more than 80% (most of these patients are younger than 1 year of age).

Additional Facts

- "In situ neuroblastoma," a term coined to describe a small nodule of neuroblastic cells smaller than 1 cm in diameter in the adrenal with no other evidence of tumor, is found in 1 per 224 infants at autopsy. They appear to regress spontaneously, as the incidence of clinically evident neuroblastoma/ganglioneuroblastoma is 1 per 10,000. All of these lesions have been located within the adrenal gland. The relationship of these lesions to the neuroblastic nodules observed in the normal developing adrenal gland is not clear; neither has their possible role as a precursor to overt neuroblastoma been defined.
- Some neuroblastomas exhibit such prominent cystic change that they may be confused with adrenal cysts or hematomas. These lesions generally fall within the favorable prognostic group using the Shimada age-linked histologic classification.
- Spontaneous regression and maturation are common findings in neuroblastoma/ganglioneuroblastoma that have been observed clinically and histologically.

- Opsoclonus-myoclonus is believed to be a paraneoplastic cerebellar dysfunction, probably autoimmune in origin. Found in approximately 5% of patients, it is associated with a favorable prognosis.
- Although there is much evidence to suggest that neuroblastoma/ganglioneuroblastoma are congenital tumors, rare cases have been reported in adults over a broad age range. The distribution of adult neuroblastoma/ganglioneuroblastoma is similar to that in children. Although adult tumors may pursue a longer course as a result of slower growth, they appear to be less responsive to chemotherapy than are childhood neuroblastoma/ganglioneuroblastoma. Bone marrow disease in adults is particularly resistant, resulting in difficulty in achieving clinical remissions of disease.
- Primitive neuroectodermal tumors (PNETs) and Ewing's sarcoma are two small cell malignant neoplasms with evidence of neuroectodermal differentiation that may be difficult to distinguish from classic neuroblastoma histologically. Particularly PNET, which by definition contains at least occasional Homer Wright rosettes, may pose difficulties in the differential diagnosis. Immunohistochemistry may be quite helpful. Although PNET, like neuroblastoma, expresses neuron-specific enolase, neurofilament proteins, and S100, PNET also expresses vimentin, HNK-1, HBA-71, and sometimes cytokeratin, unlike neuroblastoma. Ewing's sarcoma is also positive for HBA-71 and vimentin but does not express neurofilaments or S100; it is variably positive for neuron-specific enolase. Most PNETs and Ewing's sarcoma are associated with the genetic translocation t(11; 22)(q24; q12), which has not been found in neuroblastoma.

4. Ganglioneuroma

Definition: A benign neoplasm composed of mature sympathetic ganglion cells and neurites (with variable myelination), with Schwann cells and collagen. These lesions represent the mature end of the histologic spectrum from neuroblastoma to ganglioneuroblastoma to ganglioneuroma.

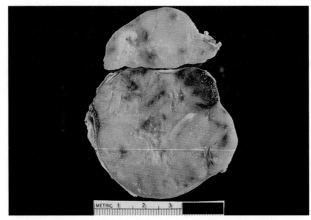

Figure 14–65. A ganglioneuroma with the typical gray and fairly homogeneous cut surface. The texture is rubbery, in contrast with the soft texture of neuroblastoma, which is reminiscent of fetal brain tissue.

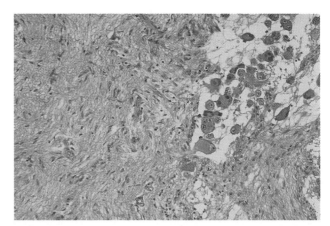

Figure 14–66. Ganglioneuroma is characterized by well-developed abundant schwannian stroma and patches of ganglion cells, which are often slightly dysmorphic.

Clinical

- Ganglioneuromas are uncommon neoplasms occurring in an older age group than neuroblastomas or ganglioneuroblastomas. Most are diagnosed in patients in the first three decades of life, although they occur over a broad age range. Adrenal ganglioneuromas are more common in the third through fifth decades.
- A gender predilection for females has been reported.
- Ganglioneuromas are associated with the sympathetic nervous system, occurring along the length of the sympathetic chains, often paravertebral, and in association with related structures. They are found in the posterior mediastinum > retroperitoneum > adrenal gland (30%) > pelvic cavity > neck > parapharyngeal area. Unusual reported locations include the gastrointestinal tract, kidney, skin, uterus, ovary, orbit, and upper respiratory tract mucosa.
- Adrenal ganglioneuromas are usually smaller than those found in the mediastinum or retroperitoneum and are usually asymptomatic; occasional patients express complaints of vague abdominal or flank pain. The larger masses of the mediastinum or retroperitoneum more often present with symptoms related to compression of adjacent structures. Rarely, hypertension, watery diarrhea syndrome (with elevated vasoactive intestinal peptide), virilization, or myasthenia gravis have been reported. Occasional patients have elevation of urinary catecholamines.

Radiology

- Ganglioneuromas are often incidentally discovered during routine radiographic studies. Calcifications present in 41% of tumors may be seen on plain radiographs.

Pathology

Cytology

- Limited material may be obtained due to the preponderance of stroma with collagen and Schwann cells.
- Ganglion cells of variable size, and somewhat dysmorphic, are usually present in a few scattered groups. They may be binucleated or multinucleated.

- Surrounding the ganglion cells is an eosinophilic fibrillar matrix containing spindled nuclei with somewhat corrugated nuclear contour. Collagen bundles are scattered through the matrix.
- Fine needle aspiration of these lesions is somewhat tenuous, since small immature neuroblastic areas may be missed in sampling.

Gross

- Usually circumscribed, ganglioneuromas often appear to be encapsulated, particularly the extra-adrenal examples; however, they usually are surrounded by a fibrous pseudo-capsule rather than a true capsule.
- The average size for all ganglioneuromas is 8 cm; however, adrenal tumors tend to be smaller than mediastinal and retroperitoneal tumors, which may become very large.
- The light gray to tan cut surface is rubbery to gelatinous; it may be homogeneous, fasciculated, or whorled.
- Degenerative alterations, often with cyst formation, hemorrhage, or myxoid change, may occur, particularly in larger tumors.
- Close attention to the gross features is extremely important. Note should be made of grossly distinctive areas or nodules of different color or texture, particularly if they appear darker or purplish, or if they are hemorrhagic. Such areas should be sampled to exclude neuroblastic foci, because stroma-rich ganglioneuroblastomas may be grossly quite similar to ganglioneuroma.

Histology

- Ganglion cells are present in variable numbers. They are round to polygonal, with eccentrically placed vesicular nuclei and a single prominent nucleolus. Binucleated forms and multinucleated forms are often seen and are helpful in distinguishing between entrapped non-neoplastic ganglion cells in a peripheral nerve sheath tumor and the neoplastic ganglion cells of ganglioneuroma. Nissl substance is often seen in larger ganglion cells; and brown, finely granular "neuromelanin" may be observed.
- Neuritic processes are readily demonstrated using a silver stain. Myelin may or may not be present.
- The more voluminous component of ganglioneuroma consists of proliferating Schwann with spindled nuclei, and a variable quantity of collagen fibers. The Schwann cells and collagen often form interlacing bundles. Ganglion cells are usually distributed in small groups within the schwannian stroma. Individual ganglion cells may be surrounded by a rim of satellite cells.
- Mature adipose tissue may be incorporated into the schwannian stroma at the advancing edge of the tumor. Blunt fingers of tumor may protrude into surrounding tissue from the periphery of a ganglioneuroma.
- *Immunohistochemistry:* Aggregates of mature lymphocytes are occasionally found within ganglioneuromas. These must be distinguished from immature neuroblastic cells of a ganglioneuroblastoma. Leukocyte common antigen may be helpful in problem cases. As expected, the ganglion cells express neural markers such as neurofilament proteins, synaptophysin, S100, and neuron-specific enolase. The schwannian component is also S100 positive.

- *Electron microscopy:* The bulky stromal component is represented by numerous nerve bundles, which are largely unmyelinated, and mature Schwann's cells, which are completely surrounded by basal lamina. Each Schwann's cell is associated with multiple axons. The collagen bundles are not long-spacing collagen.

Differential Diagnosis

- Ganglioneuroblastoma (Chapter 14C, #3).
- Neurilemmoma (Chaper 14D, #6).
- Neurofibroma (Chapter 14D, #6).

Treatment and Prognosis

- Surgical excision is the treatment of choice.
- Ganglioneuromas are benign and slow-growing tumors, although they may become quite large.
- Rare cases of malignant transformation of ganglioneuroblastoma into a neurofibrosarcoma (malignant schwannoma) or malignant peripheral nerve sheath tumor have been reported. In some cases there has been a previous history of radiation or chemotherapy, but others appear to represent spontaneous malignant transformation. Histologic features seen in malignant nerve sheath tumors include increased cellularity, mitotic activity, and tumor necrosis.

Additional Facts

- Rare examples of virilizing ganglioneuromas have been reported. The presence of Leydig cells with crystalloids of Reinke in one well-documented case suggest that cells of the adrenal gland may transform into gonadal stromal cells. More commonly, virilization is associated with adrenocortical neoplasms.
- Ganglioneuromas appear to occur either de novo or as the result of maturation of neuroblastoma or ganglioneuroblastoma. Patients who have been treated for confirmed neuroblastoma may be found to have residual mass lesions, either in the site of the primary or in metastatic sites; in many instances excision of such lesions revealed pure mature ganglioneuroma. In other cases consecutive biopsies have demonstrated a progressive pattern of maturation from neuroblastic neoplasms to ganglioneuroma. A similar maturation sequence may occur spontaneously, without chemotherapy or radiation. Although some support the theory that apparently de novo ganglioneuromas are actually the end point of maturation of an unrecognized congenital or childhood neuroblastoma/ganglioneuroblastoma, the differences in anatomic distribution and delay in presentation lend credence to the possibility of two mechanisms of origin for ganglioneuroblastoma.

5. Composite Tumors of the Adrenal Medulla

Synonyms: Composite pheochromocytoma, compound tumor of adrenal medulla.

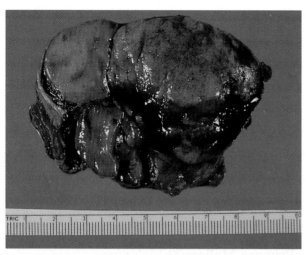

Figure 14–67. Compound tumor of the adrenal medulla: mixed pheochromocytoma and ganglioneuroblastoma surrounded by a rim of adrenal cortex. The patient had multiple pheochromocytomas in the other adrenal, as well as medullary thyroid carcinoma with liver metastases (multiple endocrine neoplasia, type 2A).

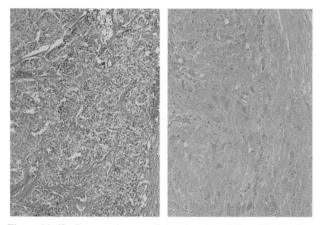

Figure 14–68. Compound tumor of the adrenal medulla, with pheochromocytoma *(left)* and ganglioneuroblastoma *(right)*.

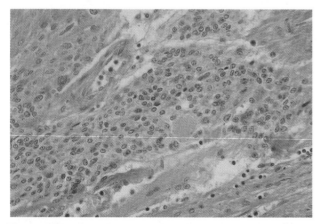

Figure 14–69. Neuroblastic areas in a compound tumor of the adrenal medulla (also shown in Figures 14–67 and 14–68).

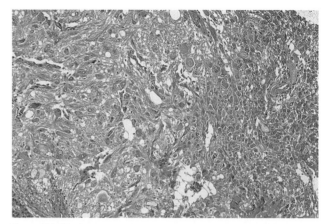

Figure 14–70. Compound tumor of the adrenal medulla with areas of pheochromocytoma merging with ganglioneuromatous areas (also shown in Figures 14–67 to 14–69).

Definition: A neoplasm in which there are components of pheochromocytoma and neuroblastoma, ganglioneuroblastoma, or ganglioneuroma.

Clinical

- These neoplasms represent approximately 3% of sympathoadrenal paragangliomas.
- Age and gender distribution reflects that of pheochromocytoma.
- Two cases have been associated with von Recklinghausen's disease; another occurred in a patient with bilateral, multiple pheochromocytomas associated with MEN 2A (Sipple's syndrome).
- Most occur in the adrenal gland; however, an extra-adrenal location is reported.
- Symptoms associated with catecholamine hypersecretion as seen in typical pheochromocytomas, such as hypertension, palpitations, diaphoresis, and headaches, are common. A few patients have presented with watery diarrhea syndrome due to secretion of excess vasoactive intestinal peptide. Symptoms related to the mass effect of the neoplasm may predominate.
- Laboratory evaluation reveals results similar to those in patients with pure pheochromocytoma, except in the instances of vasoactive intestinal peptide excess.

Pathology

Cytology

- Limited sampling may fail to illustrate the biphasic nature of this neoplasm. Since pheochromocytoma is usually the dominant component in composite tumor fine needle aspirates are more likely to yield pheochromocytes.
- The areas of pheochromocytoma are characterized by loose aggregates of polygonal cells with variably granular cytoplasm and poorly defined cell borders. Wispy projections of cytoplasm may be seen. The chromatin is clumped and rather coarse. Anisonucleosis and rare bizarre nuclei may be present; some cells have prominent nucleoli.

- The ganglioneuroma/ganglioneuroblastoma yield elongated spindled nuclei in an eosinophilic and somewhat fibrillar background. Scattered ganglion cells with abundant cytoplasm, vesicular nuclei, and a single prominent nucleolus are present. If an immature neuroblastic component is sampled, groups of small cells with a very high nuclear to cytoplasmic ratio are seen; the chromatin is somewhat stippled but evenly distributed; a fine fibrillar background may be noted. It is important to distinguish between small round lymphocytes, which are often present in ganglioneuromas, and neuroblastic cells.

Gross

- Diameters as large as 15 cm have been reported.
- Usually circumscribed, the gross appearance depends on the relative proportions of pheochromocytoma and neuroblastoma/ganglioneuroblastoma/ganglioneuroma. The color ranges from gray-white to tan to purple, often with areas of hemorrhage.
- The texture is usually firm to rubbery, but larger areas of immature neuroblastic tumor may be soft and sometimes necrotic.
- A thin rim of yellow adrenal cortex may be seen at the periphery of the tumor.

Histology

- Composite tumors show areas with any of the variety of patterns typically seen in pheochromocytomas. The pheochromocytoma is usually the predominant component.
- Admixed with the areas of pheochromocytoma are histologically distinct areas that may have features of neuroblastoma, ganglioneuroblastoma, or ganglioneuroma, as previously described.
- Transitional areas in which the features of pheochromocytes and ganglionic cells seem to blend may be difficult to categorize.
- *Immunohistochemistry:* Chromogranin staining is strong and diffuse in pheochromocytes; it is absent or weak in the perikarya of ganglion cells but concentrated in the distal neuronal processes. S100 is present in a sustentacular cell distribution in the pheochromocytoma component but is much more abundant in ganglioneuromatous areas with schwannian differentiation. S100 distribution may also be helpful in differentiating between areas of pheochromocytoma and neuroblastoma: neuroblastoma lacks the sustentacular cell pattern of S100 staining.

Differential Diagnosis

- Pheochromocytoma (Chapter 14C, #2).
- Ganglioneuroblastoma/ganglioneuroma (Chapter 14C, #3, 4).

Treatment and Prognosis

- The clinical course of composite tumors has not been well-delineated because of the tumor's rarity. Most have occurred in adults; therefore, it is not clear whether the histologic grading and stage have the same implications as in childhood neuroblastoma/ganglioneuroblastoma.

- Aggressive behavior with metastasis and poor clinical outcome has been reported in approximately half of the reported cases with a neuroblastic component, including one in which both a malignant pheochromocytomatous and a neuroblastic component metastasized.
- Complete surgical removal is desirable; radiation and chemotherapy have been used with inconclusive results.

Additional Facts

- The occurrence of "composite" tumors with both neuronal and neuroendocrine differentiation is logical in light of the neural crest origin of both cell lines.
- Occasionally pheochromocytomas exhibit focal neuronal differentiation.

6. Primary Malignant Melanoma

Definition: Malignant neoplasm composed of cells with light microscopic, immunohistochemical, or ultrastructural evidence of melanocytic differentiation. The diagnostic criteria for primary adrenal melanoma require, in

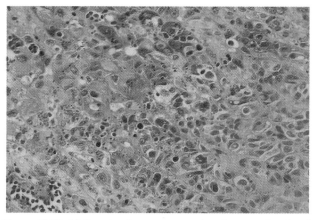

Figure 14–71. Malignant melanoma, apparently primary to the adrenal gland. The presence of melanin is helpful in suggesting the correct diagnosis. Amelanotic cases are less readily recognized.

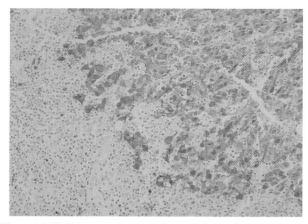

Figure 14–72. Primary malignant melanoma of the adrenal, with scant melanin, is diffusely positive by immunostaining for S100 protein.

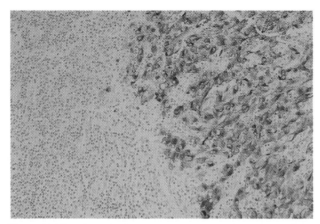

Figure 14–73. Primary malignant melanoma of the adrenal seen in Figure 14–72, with strong positive staining for HMB-45.

addition, unilateral adrenal involvement; no current or prior history of suspicious pigmented lesions of the skin, eye, or mucosal surfaces; and absence of extra-adrenal primary melanoma after a thorough autopsy.

Clinical

- The few reported case have occurred in adults, with no gender predilection.
- Common presenting symptoms include abdominal or flank pain, weight loss, malaise, or a palpable abdominal mass.
- Patients should be studied carefully to exclude other more common sites of primary melanoma, such as the skin, mucous membranes, and eye.

Radiology

- By CT scan, ultrasonography, or arteriography the lesions are hypovascular and may contain large necrotic or cystic areas.

Pathology

Gross

- Usually large (≤17 cm).
- The cut surface is usually brown to black and may be partially cystic hemorrhagic and necrotic.

Histology

- The tumor cells may vary in size from small and monotonous to large, bizarre cells.
- The presence of a nesting or a biphasic pattern with epithelioid cells alternating with spindle cells may provide helpful clues to the diagnosis.
- Brown to black pigment is usually present but varies in quantity. A Fontana-Masson stain may help highlight pigment.
- *Immunohistochemistry:* S100 and HMB-45 are positive.
- *Electron microscopy:* Premelanosomes in various stages of development are seen.

Differential Diagnosis

- Pigmented adrenocortical nodules (Chapter 13K).
- Bilateral pigmented micronodular hyperplasia (Chapter 13K).
- Pigmented ganglioneuroblastoma (Chapter 14C, #3).
- Black adenomas of the adrenal cortex (Chapter 14B, #1).
- Pigmented pheochromocytomas (Chapter 14C, #2).

Treatment and Prognosis

- Resection of tumors localized to the adrenal may be helpful in controlling symptoms.
- The prognosis is very poor, with death due to disseminated disease within a year of diagnosis.

Additional Facts

- The origin of primary adrenal melanomas is not clear; however, the common neural crest origin of the adrenal chromaffin cells that populate the medulla and of melanocytes lends credence to the concept of melanoma arising in the adrenal medulla.

D. MISCELLANEOUS NEOPLASMS AND TUMOR-LIKE LESIONS

1. Malignant Lymphoma

Definition: A malignant neoplastic proliferation of any of a variety of lymphoid cell lines. Primary lymphomas of the adrenal are rare.

Clinical

- Primary non-Hodgkin's lymphomas of the adrenal gland are reported almost exclusively in adults, in the fifth through ninth decades, with a mean age of 60 years.
- Male:female ratio is 3:1.

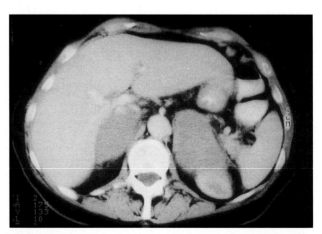

Figure 14–74. Computed tomographic scan demonstrating bulky suprarenal masses with homogeneous density, representing primary adrenal lymphoma. Bilaterality is a peculiar common attribute of adrenal lymphomas.

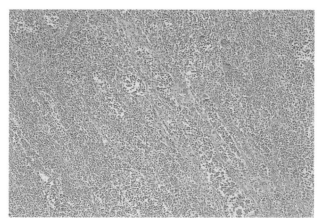

Figure 14–75. Diffuse effacement of the adrenal in a patient with primary adrenal lymphoma. The neoplasm was limited to both adrenal glands.

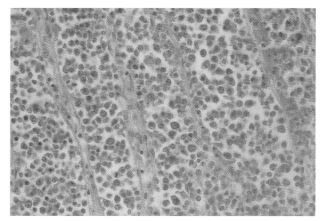

Figure 14–76. Primary adrenal lymphoma, large cell type, the most common pattern of primary lymphomas in this location. Most are of B-cell immunophenotype.

- Presenting symptoms include abdominal pain, fever, anemia, weight loss, and manifestations of adrenal insufficiency.
- Involvement is bilateral in approximately 50%.

Radiology

- CT scan and ultrasonography are useful in localization for percutaneous needle biopsy or fine needle aspiration but do not readily exclude adrenocortical neoplasms or metastases to the adrenal gland.

Pathology

Cytology

- Fine needle aspiration provides a useful diagnostic alternative to laparotomy, since resection is not the treatment of choice.
- The presence of a monotonous large cell lymphoid population is the most common finding and can be readily diagnosed as malignant lymphoma.
- Small cell and mixed small and large cell lymphomas may be more difficult to classify based solely on the cytomor-

phology. Cell suspensions for flow cytometric immunophenotyping or immunohistochemical phenotyping may provide definitive classification if adequate material is obtained.

Gross

- Adrenal lymphomas are frequently bilateral and range in size from 2 to 17 cm.
- The cut surface is white-gray and fleshy and may be partially necrotic.
- Extension of the adrenal tumor into surrounding soft tissue in many cases makes exclusion of a retroperitoneal lymphoma secondarily involving the adrenal difficult.

Histology

- The histologic pattern is dependent on the type of malignant lymphoma present. All cases of primary adrenal lymphoma have been non-Hodgkin's lymphoma. Large cell lymphoma is the most common pattern reported in this location.
- The malignant lymphoid cells infiltrate and replace the adrenomedullary and cortical tissue, resulting in adrenal insufficiency in advanced bilateral cases.
- *Immunohistochemistry:* Most adrenal lymphomas are of the B-cell phenotype and are positive for leukocyte common antigen and L26; rare T-cell lymphomas are reported (UCHL-1 positive; L26 negative).

Differential Diagnosis

- Poorly differentiated adrenocortical carcinoma (Chapter 14B, #2).
- Metastatic poorly differentiated carcinoma (Chapter 14D, #7).
- Malignant melanoma (either primary adrenal or metastatic) (Chapter 14C, #6).
- Malignant pheochromocytoma (Chapter 14C, #2).

Treatment and Prognosis

- Chemotherapeutic regimens and radiation therapy are selected based on the histologic classification of the lymphoma.
- Surgical resection does not improve survival.
- The prognosis of primary adrenal lymphoma is very poor, with death usually within several months of diagnosis in spite of aggressive therapy.

Additional Facts

- Primary adrenal lymphoma is rare; some of the reported cases must be viewed critically because it is difficult to exclude secondary involvement of the adrenal by the much more common lymphoma arising in retroperitoneal lymph nodes. The reports of pure bilateral adrenal involvement without regional lymph node involvement support the concept of a true primary adrenal malignant lymphoma.

2. Myelolipoma (Table 14–8)

Definition: A benign tumor-like lesion composed of both mature adipose tissue and hematopoietic elements.

Clinical

■ Most often discovered in the fifth to seventh decades of life.
■ No gender predilection.

Table 14–8
MYELOLIPOMATOUS LESIONS OF THE ADRENAL GLAND

As an Isolated Entity
Myelolipoma
Secondarily Associated with Other Lesions
Adrenocortical hyperplasia
Adrenocortical nodule
Adrenocortical adenoma

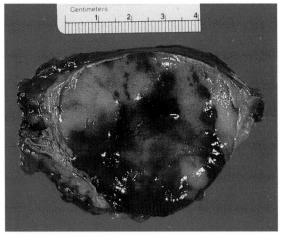

Figure 14–77. Myelolipoma surrounded by a rim of normal adrenal. The yellow cut surface resembles adipose tissue; the reddish areas are foci of concentration of hematopoietic elements.

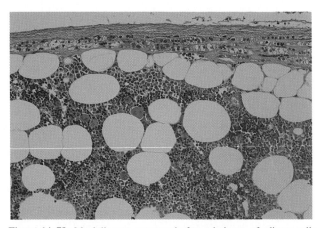

Figure 14–78. Myelolipoma, composed of an admixture of adipose cells and hematopoietic elements, including myeloid, erythroid, and megakaryocytic components. The thinned cortex surrounds this circumscribed mass.

■ Incidence in adults between 36 and 65 years of age and is 1 in 7600.
■ Most often found in the adrenal, but also reported in mediastinum, perirenal/peri-adrenal region, presacral area, liver, and gastrointestinal tract.
■ Most commonly an incidental finding in an asymptomatic patient; however, patients may complain of abdominal or flank pain, or rarely present with massive retroperitoneal hemorrhage. Other findings include hematuria, hypertension, or hormonal dysfunction.
■ Endocrine dysfunction reported in association with myelolipomas include Cushing's syndrome, Conn's syndrome, Addison's disease, virilization, diabetes mellitus, and congenital adrenal hyperplasia. Because secondary myelolipomatous foci are common (and may be quite extensive) in many adrenal neoplasms and hyperplastic lesions an underlying causative lesion other than myelolipoma must be excluded. It is likely that many reports of syndromes such as Cushing's and Conn's syndromes and virilization linked to myelolipomas actually represent myelolipomatous changes overshadowing an underlying cortical adenoma or hyperplastic process.

Radiology

■ The improved resolution and frequency of use of imaging techniques such as CT and MRI scans have increased the detection rate of myelolipomas, often as incidental findings.
■ The radiographic appearance does not distinguish between metastatic lesions and adrenal myelolipomas.
■ CT-directed fine needle aspiration cytology can be useful in distinguishing between metastases and myelolipoma of the adrenal.

Pathology

Cytology

■ An admixture of mature adipocytes and hematopoietic cells, including myeloid and erythroid precursors and megakaryocytes, is characteristic of myelolipoma.
■ The chief cytologic differential diagnosis in CT-directed fine needle aspiration of myelolipoma is inadvertent sampling of normal bone marrow from vertebral body or rib.

Gross

■ Sizes range from small incidental findings in autopsy or surgical specimens to masses measuring as large as 34 cm in diameter.
■ Circumscribed, but not usually encapsulated, the border of the myelolipoma often blends with a thin rim of compressed adrenal tissue.
■ The cut surface is yellow and fatty, with variably sized patches of mottled red to purple tissue.
■ Areas of hemorrhage and infarction are more common in larger examples.

Histology

■ Mature adipocytes are admixed with aggregates of hematopoietic cells representing myeloid, erythroid, and megakaryocytic elements.

- The relative proportions of adipose and hematopoietic tissue vary; the marrow elements may be inconspicuous in some cases.
- Metaplastic bone or areas of fibrosis or hyalinization may be present.

Differential Diagnosis

- Myelolipomatous foci in adrenocortical neoplasm or hyperplasia.
- Extramedullary hematopoiesis.

Treatment and Prognosis

- Surgical excision is the treatment of choice for symptomatic or large incidental lesions. Observation is acceptable for small, clinically silent lesions.
- Myelolipomas are benign and do not recur after complete excision.
- Large myelolipomas are at risk for rupture and massive retroperitoneal hemorrhage.

Additional Facts

- Although etiology and nature of myelolipoma is not well-defined, they do not appear to represent true neoplasms.
- Theories regarding the presence of myelolipomatous masses in the adrenal, either alone or associated with adrenocortical proliferations, suggest the following possibilities: metaplastic changes in adrenal stromal cells, metaplastic changes in adrenocortical cells, bone marrow emboli lodging in the adrenal gland, and embryonic rests of bone marrow in the adrenal gland. Metaplastic change in stromal cells is the favored origin of myelolipomatous proliferations in the adrenal.

3. Adenomatoid Tumor

Definition: Rare benign neoplasm of probable mesothelial origin characterized by vacuolated epithelioid cells that form glandlike structures.

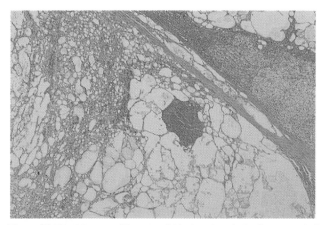

Figure 14–79. Adenomatoid tumor within the adrenal gland composed of variably sized glandlike structures.

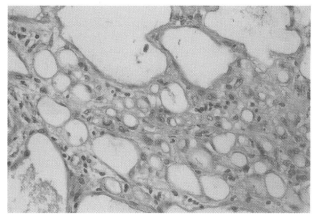

Figure 14–80. The glandlike structures of an adenomatoid tumor are lined by flattened epithelioid cells. Cords and nests of these cells are also seen; in these areas large intracytoplasmic vacuoles may be seen, giving some of the cells a signet-ring appearance.

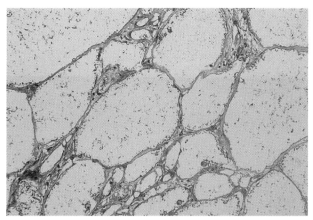

Figure 14–81. Cytokeratin immunostaining demonstrated by the epithelioid cells of an adenomatoid tumor of the adrenal. The tumors are believed to be mesothelial in origin.

Clinical

- Only a few examples of adenomatoid tumor of the adrenal gland are reported. They are characteristically found in the genital tract, particularly involving the epididymis, uterus, or fallopian tube.
- Most adenomatoid tumors are small and incidental.

Pathology

Gross

- Most measure only a few centimeters in diameter.
- Poorly circumscribed, the tumor may have an infiltrative border.
- The cut surface is white to gray; the lesion may appear solid or may contain punctate to slightly larger cystic spaces.
- Foci of calcification may be present.

Histology

- The border may appear infiltrative, with microscopic projections into the surrounding adrenal or periadrenal soft tissue.

- The tumor is composed of nests and cords of epithelioid cells with uniform round nuclei and frequent intracytoplasmic vacuoles. The vacuoles may be quite large and lend a signet ring appearance to the cells. Tubular or glandlike spaces are seen in many areas; the epithelioid cells may be flattened in these tubule-like areas.
- The stroma varies in quantity and consists of fibroblastic cells and collagen. Some areas may be hyalinized. Foci of calcification may be present in the stroma.
- *Histochemical stains:* Mucicarmine and PAS (with and without diastase) are negative.
- *Immunohistochemistry:* The tumor cells have the staining characteristics of mesothelial cells: positive for cytokeratin, epithelial membrane antigen, and vimentin. Chromogranin is negative.
- *Electron microscopy:* tumor cells with well-formed desmosomes, elongated thin microvilli typical of mesothelial cells, and tonofilaments.

Differential Diagnosis

- Lymphangioma (Chapter 14D, #4).
- Metastatic adenocarcinoma, especially signet ring cell type (Chapter 14D, #7).

Treatment and Prognosis

- Adenomatoid tumors are benign and do not recur after surgical excision.

4. Hemangioma

Definition: Rare benign neoplastic proliferation of blood vessels; the predominant pattern is cavernous, although capillary-type hemangiomas occur as well.

Clinical

- Most commonly an incidental autopsy finding, even surgical cases are usually asymptomatic and incidental.
- Found over a broad age range, from 25 to 79 years.

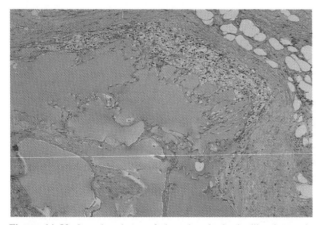

Figure 14–82. Lymphangioma of the adrenal gland: dilated vascular spaces filled with serous fluid adjacent to the adrenal cortex. The differential diagnosis includes adenomatoid tumor. The lining cells are positive for endothelial markers rather than cytokeratin.

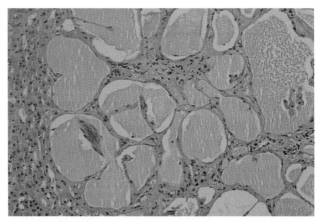

Figure 14–83. Lymphangioma of the adrenal gland: the endothelial cells are flat, without nuclear atypia.

- More common in females.
- The few symptomatic cases are related to large tumor size and local mass effect.

Radiology

- Radiography is a common means of incidental discovery of adrenal hemangiomas.
- CT scan reveals a hypodense lesion with contrast enhancement.
- Ultrasonographic images have variable echogenicity related to size of proliferating vessels and extent of thrombosis.
- The lesions may be identified on plain radiographs if calcification is present.

Pathology

Gross

- Sizes range from 2 (most incidental tumors) to 22 cm for symptomatic lesions.
- Most are solitary and unilateral, but bilateral examples occur.
- Tumors are encapsulated; smaller examples may be surrounded at least partially by a rim of residual adrenal gland.
- The cut surface is hemorrhagic, with variably sized blood-filled spaces. The color is red-purple, with yellow areas if necrosis is present. Calcification, phleboliths, and areas of fibrosis are common, especially in larger tumors.

Histology

- Proliferating well-formed vascular spaces of variable size are arranged in an orderly fashion, sometimes forming distinct lobules. The supportive stroma is predominantly fibrous but may appear more cellular in capillary-type hemangiomas. Large dilated vascular spaces are more common—the cavernous pattern of hemangioma.
- The endothelial cells may be plump, but they are uniform and lack nuclear pleomorphism and hyperchromasia. They form a complete, even lining within the vascular spaces.

Differential Diagnosis

- Adrenocortical adenoma with marked degenerative changes (Chapter 14B, #1).
- Angiosarcoma (Chapter 14D, #5).
- Pheochromocytoma with vascular ectasia (Chapter 14C, #2).

Treatment and Prognosis

- Hemangiomas are benign; if treatment is required for alleviation of symptoms, surgical resection is preferred.

Additional Facts

- Adrenocortical adenomas with marked degenerative changes and secondary vascular proliferation are often mistaken for hemangiomas or, occasionally, for angiosarcoma. Central hemorrhage or infarction in cortical adenomas resolves with loss of cortical cells, which are replaced by areas of variably dense fibrosis and vascular proliferation that may be quite pronounced. The vessels in such cases are usually variable in size, often resembling the components of a cavernous hemangioma; they are usually associated with hemosiderin deposits, fibrosis, and sometimes with cholesterol granulomas. Close observation of the remaining adrenocortical tissue may reveal an abnormally thickened rim of cortical cells surrounding the vascular proliferation; and often islands of preserved cortical cells or "ghosts" of necrotic cortical cells are found deep within the fibrovascular process, indicating the underlying cortical neoplasm, which represents the primary lesion. Degenerative change with neovascularization in cortical adenomas is much more common than adrenal hemangiomas.
- *Lymphangiomas* also occur rarely in the adrenal gland. They, like hemangiomas, are frequently incidental findings, although some may become quite large and replace much of the cortex. They are distinguished from hemangiomas by the presence of serous fluid within the vascular spaces and frequently by associated lymphoid tissue. Treatment and behavior are similar to hemangiomas.

5. Angiosarcoma

Definition: A rare malignant vasoformative neoplasm in which the neoplastic cellular component exhibits endothelial cell differentiation, usually with epithelioid feature when encountered in the adrenal.

Synonym: Epithelioid angiosarcoma.

Clinical

- Most commonly encountered in the sixth and seventh decades, angiosarcomas are seen over an age range from 45 to 85 years.
- No gender predilection.
- Presenting symptoms include a palpable abdominal mass, flank or abdominal pain, weight loss, fever, and weakness,

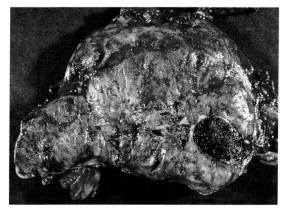

Figure 14–84. Primary adrenal angiosarcoma with a fleshy yellow cut surface that may not immediately suggest the vascular nature of this neoplasm. Areas of necrosis and hemorrhage are common.

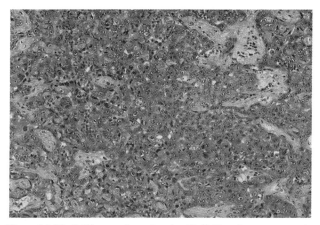

Figure 14–85. Solid areas of an adrenal epithelioid angiosarcoma may be difficult to distinguish from adrenal cortical carcinoma or metastatic carcinoma. The sheets of cells have eosinophilic cytoplasm with vesicular nuclei and prominent nucleoli. Mitoses are common.

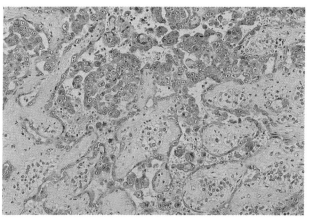

Figure 14–86. Vasoformative areas in adrenal epithelioid angiosarcoma are more diagnostic. The endothelial cells are large and very atypical, with crowded papillary tufts projecting into the vascular lumen.

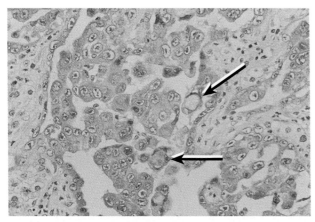

Figure 14–87. The epithelioid tumor cells have eosinophilic cytoplasm and marked nuclear atypia. Mitoses are frequent. Some of the tumor cells contain intracytoplasmic lumina *(arrows)*.

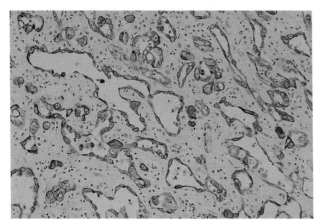

Figure 14–88. Strong immunostaining for cytokeratin in adrenal epithelioid angiosarcoma may cause confusion with adrenocortical carcinoma or metastatic carcinoma, particularly in areas of solid growth.

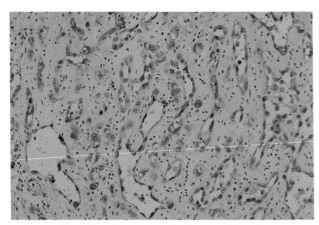

Figure 14–89. Factor VIII–associated antigen immunohistochemical stain in adrenal epithelioid angiosarcoma. The tumor cells are positive for a variety of endothelial-related stains, including CD34 (QBEND) and *Ulex europeus* lectin.

over a period of weeks to several months. The tumors may be asymptomatic and incidentally discovered.
- Rarely paraneoplastic endocrine abnormalities are reported.

Radiology

- CT scan or ultrasonography demonstrates retroperitoneal or suprarenal partially cystic to solid neoplasms with contrast enhancement.

Pathology

Gross

- Size ranges from 6 to 10 cm.
- The tumors may be circumscribed to grossly infiltrative.
- The cut surface is gray to yellow to red, variably cystic to solid, with hemorrhage and necrosis.

Histology

- An infiltrative border is usually evident in spite of gross circumscription. The residual adrenal cortex as well as periadrenal soft tissue are often invaded by tumor.
- Hemorrhage is usually extensive, as is necrosis.
- The tumor cells are arranged in solid sheets or nests that merge with vasoformative areas. The vascular spaces are lined by cells identical to those in the more solid areas; they form an endothelial lining that varies from single cells to tufts of tumor cells projecting into the vascular lumina.
- The tumor cells are epithelioid in appearance: polygonal cells with abundant eosinophilic cytoplasm, round-to-oval vesicular nuclei with hyperchromasia, and prominent central nucleoli. Nuclear pleomorphism and mitotic activity are common findings. Some cells contain intracytoplasmic lumina in which red blood cells may be seen.
- A background stroma is composed of fibrous tissue with areas of acute and chronic inflammation.
- *Histochemistry:* Mucicarmine and PAS with and without diastase are negative.
- *Immunohistochemistry:* Neoplastic cells are positive for Factor VIII–related antigen, CD-34 (QBEND), vimentin, cytokeratin (most cases), B72.3, and *Ulex europeus* lectin (only one third of cases); no staining is seen with smooth muscle actin, S-100, chromogranin, desmin, or epithelial membrane antigen.
- *Electron microscopy:* The epithelioid tumor cells are found in sheets, or they may line vascular lumina. Occasional cells contain intracytoplasmic lumina, in which red blood cells may be seen. Basal lamina surrounds the tumor cells; and pinocytotic vesicles may be identified. Weibel-Palade bodies, if found, are characteristic of endothelial differentiation: they appear as intracytoplasmic rod-shaped bodies with an internal parallel array of microtubules.

Differential Diagnosis

- Adrenocortical carcinoma (Chapter 14B, #2).
- Metastatic adenocarcinoma (Chapter 14D, #7).
- Pheochromocytoma (Chapter 14C, #2).
- Primary or metastatic melanoma (Chapter 14C, #6).

Treatment and Prognosis

■ Surgical resection is the preferred therapy.
■ Approximately one third of patients develop metastatic disease, usually involving the lungs, and die within 2 years; however, long-term survival is reported in an equal number of patients.

Additional Facts

■ The epithelioid appearance of the tumor cells in adrenal angiosarcoma, combined with the positive immunohistochemistry for cytokeratin, may cause confusion with the much more common epithelial malignancies of the adrenal gland (i.e., adrenocortical carcinoma and metastatic carcinoma.) Immunohistochemical markers of endothelial cell differentiation, Factor VIII–associated antigen, CD-34, and *Ulex europeus* lectin are helpful discriminators in this differential diagnosis.

6. Nerve Sheath Tumors

Definition: A spectrum of benign and malignant neoplasms, all uncommon in the adrenal gland, characterized by a proliferation of schwannian cells with or without a neu-

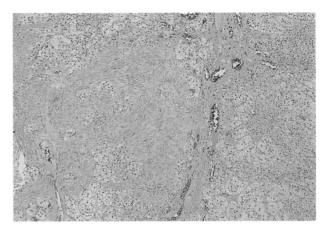

Figure 14–92. This incidental autopsy finding of a spindle cell proliferation histologically and immunohistochemically resembling the cells of a nerve sheath tumor. The significance of these lesions is unknown. They have been referred to as "tumefactive spindle cell proliferations."

ritic component. Included in this group are neurilemmoma, neurofibroma, and malignant peripheral nerve sheath tumors.

Clinical

■ Although all nerve sheath tumors are rare in the adrenal gland, cases are reported over a wide age range.
■ No gender predilection is evident.
■ Nerve sheath tumors, benign and malignant, may be seen in association with von Recklinghausen's disease.
■ Most malignant peripheral nerve sheath tumors have been associated with ganglioneuromas, either in patients with a history of irradiation for neuroblastoma/ ganglioneuroblastoma or as a *de novo* occurrence.
■ Both incidental and symptomatic cases are reported. Symptomatology is usually related to mass effect of the lesion, and includes abdominal or flank pain.

Pathology

■ *Neurofibroma:* Grossly unencapsulated, with a white to gray-yellow rubbery cut surface, with variable cystic or myxoid changes. The histologic pattern is one of a mixture of neurites, fibroblasts, and collagen fibers. Immunohistochemistry: Scattered spindle cells are S100 positive.
■ *Neurilemmoma, or schwannoma:* An encapsulated tumor, with a white to pink-yellow rubbery cut surface, with variable cystic changes and focal calcification. The spindle cell proliferation may be compact, orderly, and cellular in areas (Antoni A area), with foci of nuclear palisading; other areas are less cellular and orderly and have a myxoid background (Antoni B area). The cellular component is predominantly Schwann's cells, with few if any neurites. Occasional mitotic figures may be seen. Scattered pleomorphic nuclei may be seen, especially in degenerated or "ancient" neurilemmomas. "Cellular schwannomas" represent a more cellular variant in which the Antoni A areas predominate; mitotic activity (usually <4/10 HPF) is common; the cellularity and mitoses may cause confusion with malignant nerve sheath tumors, fibrosarcoma, or leiomyo-

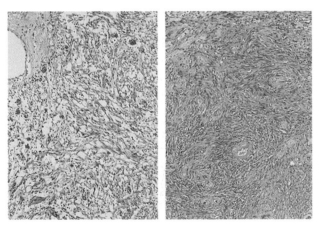

Figure 14–90. Neurilemmoma of the adrenal gland, with Antoni A *(right)* and Antoni B areas *(left)*.

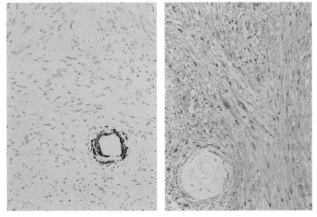

Figure 14–91. Immunohistochemical staining for S100 *(right)* and smooth muscle actin *(left)* in an adrenal neurilemmoma.

sarcoma. *Immunohistochemistry:* S100 is strongly and diffusely positive in neurilemmomas; this feature is particularly helpful in excluding malignant nerve sheath tumors (in which S100 staining is weaker and usually focal) and other soft tissue sarcomas.

■ *Malignant peripheral nerve sheath tumor:* Sometimes seen arising as a fusiform mass from a peripheral nerve, the cut surface is usually fleshy white-tan and may be somewhat hemorrhagic or necrotic. The very cellular spindle cell proliferation is characterized by wavy nuclei and indistinct cell borders; fascicular, whorled, or loose myxoid patterns may be seen. Nuclear palisading, as seen in neurilemmomas, is uncommon and focal. Pleomorphism and mitotic activity are commonly seen and are helpful in excluding neurofibroma. Neurilemmoma, also in the differential diagnosis, may exhibit atypical nuclei and mitoses; the distinction between malignant peripheral nerve sheath tumors may be made on the basis of lack of the Antoni A/Antoni B patterns and on the S100 staining pattern in that type of tumor. *Immunohistochemistry:* S100 stains only scattered cells or groups of cells and is present in 50% to 90% of cases.

Differential Diagnosis

■ Ganglioneuroma (Chapter 14C, #3).
■ Ganglioneuroblastoma (Chapter 14C, #2).
■ Smooth muscle neoplasms (Chapter 14D, #8).
■ Secondary adrenal involvement by a variety of primary soft tissue sarcomas of the retroperitoneum (Chapter 14D, #7).
■ Malignant melanoma, primary or metastatic, of adrenal (Chapter 14C, #6).

Treatment and Prognosis

■ Benign nerve sheath tumors may be treated, if symptomatic, by surgical excision, which is curative.
■ Malignant peripheral nerve sheath tumors frequently recur locally and metastasize in spite of aggressive surgical therapy.

Additional Facts

■ Incidental proliferations of neural tissue may be found at autopsy or in adrenal glands resected for another disease process. These lesions consist of a single nodule or multiple small nodules, which may be circumscribed or, occasionally, have an infiltrative border. The spindle cells have wavy nuclei and variable cellularity; they may resemble a neurofibroma, neurilemmoma, or even a traumatic neuroma. Most are centered in the medulla. Although the natural history of these lesions is a mystery, they may represent incipient neurofibromas or neurilemmomas.

7. Metastatic Neoplasms

Definition: Secondary deposits from a malignant neoplasm primary to another site, exclusive of contiguous infiltration of the adrenal by a neoplasm in an adjacent organ or

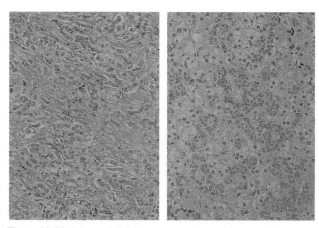

Figure 14–93. Metastatic lobular breast carcinoma involving both adrenal glands. Linear groups of tumor cells with sclerotic collagenous stroma are seen on the left; cords and clusters of tumor cells subtly infiltrate the cortex, seen on the right.

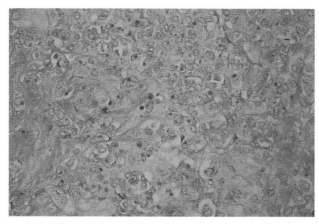

Figure 14–94. A periodic acid-Schiff–diastase stain demonstrates small mucin droplets in the cytoplasm of the tumor cells in the metastatic breast carcinoma seen in Figures 14–92 and 14–93.

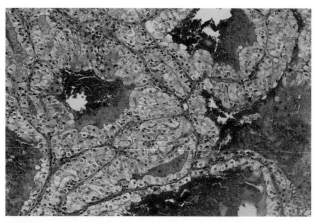

Figure 14–95. Metastatic renal cell carcinoma of the clear cell type is readily recognized. The pooling of blood within the glandular spaces is typical of renal cell carcinoma.

soft tissue. The adrenal is the fourth most common recipient of metastatic disease after lung, liver, and bone.

Clinical

- Adrenal metastases are present in 9% to 27% of patients with cancer; involvement is bilateral in 41%.
- Lung and breast carcinomas are the most common tumors to metastasize to the adrenal.
- Most metastatic lesions are clinically silent with regard to adrenal function; however, rare instances of Addison's disease have been reported as a result of metastases of a variety of primary malignancies, including carcinomas of the lung and breast, renal cell carcinoma, carcinomas of the gastrointestinal tract, seminoma, pancreatic carcinoma, transitional cell carcinoma, and melanoma. Rarely, adrenocortical carcinoma may also metastasize to the contralateral gland and cause adrenal insufficiency.
- Destruction of 90% of the cortex must occur before overt adrenal insufficiency occurs; however, the symptoms of Addison's disease may be subtle and may be overlooked in the patient who is chronically ill with cancer. Laboratory testing for hypoadrenalism is helpful in patients with bilateral metastatic lesions.
- Manifestations of adrenal insufficiency include weakness, wasting, intolerance of physical stress, and hyperpigmentation of skin and mucous membranes.

Radiology

- Metastatic disease, even relatively small lesions, are readily detected by CT scan; however, unilateral metastatic lesions cannot easily be distinguished from primary adrenal neoplasms.
- CT-directed fine needle aspiration is an effective method for preoperative exclusion of metastatic disease in the event of a unilateral adrenal lesion and may be helpful in identifying the source of metastases when the primary site is undetermined.

Pathology

Gross

- Lesions may be unilateral or bilateral; although frequently multiple, they may be solitary.
- Gross lesions are usually readily identified, and, if large, are often partially necrotic. Some lesions are subtle, replacing the medulla and causing enlargement of the gland without a distinct nodule.

Histology

- Although most metastatic lesions are readily recognized as secondary lesions, some neoplasms may be difficult to distinguish from primary adrenal neoplasms such as adrenocortical carcinoma and pheochromocytoma. The differential diagnosis between some poorly differentiated metastatic carcinomas and adrenocortical carcinoma can be especially problematic. Metastatic neuroendocrine malignancies may mimic pheochromocytoma (particularly malignant ones).

- *Immunohistochemistry:* Adrenocortical carcinomas are usually vimentin positive but negative or only weakly positive for cytokeratin and negative for epithelial membrane antigen. These stains may be helpful in the differential with metastatic carcinoma—if the carcinoma is strongly positive for cytokeratin and/or epithelial membrane antigen.

Treatment and Prognosis

- The outlook for patients with adrenal metastases is dismal. Treatment depends on the primary source and tumor type.

8. Other Rare Neoplasms

- *Smooth muscle tumors:* Leiomyomas and leiomyosarcomas of the adrenal are extremely rare; they are believed to arise from vascular smooth muscle.
- *Gonadal stromal-type tumors:* Tumefactive spindle-cell lesions resembling ovarian thecal metaplasia, granulosa-theca cell tumor, and Leydig cell tumor with crystalloids of Reinke have been described but are exceedingly rare.

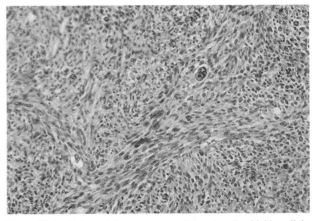

Figure 14–96. Primary leiomyosarcoma of the adrenal, a highly cellular spindle cell proliferation with hyperchromatic pleomorphic nuclei arranged in interweaving fascicles.

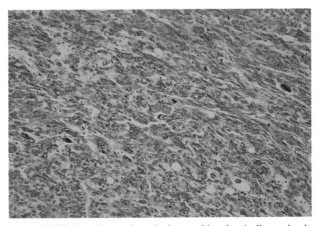

Figure 14–97. Smooth muscle actin immunohistochemically marks the primary adrenal leiomyosarcoma seen in Figure 14–96.

Bibliography

Neoplasms of the Adrenal Cortex

Adrenocortical Adenoma

Bhettay E, Bonnici F. Pure oestrogen-secreting feminizing adrenocortical adenoma. Arch Dis Child 1977; 52:241–243.

Caplan RH, Virata RL. Functional black adenoma of the adrenal cortex. Am J Clin Pathol 1974; 62:97–103.

Conn JW, Hinerman DL. Spironolactone-induced inhibition of aldosterone biosynthesis in primary aldosteronism: Morphological and functional studies. Metabolism 1977; 26:1293–1307.

Erlandson RA, Reuter VE. Oncocytic adrenal cortical adenoma. Ultrastruct Pathol 1991; 15:539–547.

Favre L, Jacot-des-Combes E, Morel P, et al. Primary aldosteronism with bilateral adrenal adenomas. Virchows Arch [Pathol Anat] 1980; 388:229–236.

Garret R, Ames RP. Black-pigmented adenoma of the adrenal gland. Arch Pathol 1973; 95:349–353.

Granger JK, Houn H-Y, Collins C. Massive hemorrhagic functional adrenal adenoma histologically mimicking angiosarcoma: Report of a case with immunohistochemical study. Am J Surg Pathol 1991; 15:699–704.

Hamwi GJ, Gwinup G, Mostow JH, Besch PK. Activation of testicular adrenal rest tissue by prolonged excessive ACTH production. J Clin Endocrinol Metab 1963; 23:861–869.

Hough AJ, Hollifield JW, Page DL, Hartmann WH. Prognostic factors in adrenal cortical tumors. Am J Clin Pathol 1979; 72:390–399.

Kable WT, Yussman MA. Testosterone-secreting adrenal adenoma. Fertil Steril 1979; 32:610–611.

Katz RL. Kidney, adrenal, and retroperitoneum. In: Bibbo M, ed. Comprehensive Cytopathology. Philadelphia: WB Saunders, 1991, pp. 771–805.

Kovacs K, Horvath E, Feldman PS. Pigmented adenoma of adrenal cortex associated with Cushing's syndrome. Urology 1979; 7:641–645.

Lack EE, Travis WD, Oertel JE. Adrenal cortical neoplasms. In: Lack EE, ed. Pathology of the Adrenal Glands. Vol. 14. New York: Churchill Livingstone, 1990, pp. 115–136.

Macadam RF. Black adenoma of the human adrenal cortex. Cancer 1971; 27:116–119.

Orth DN, Liddle GW. Results of treatment in 108 patients with Cushing's syndrome. N Engl J Med 1971; 285:243–247.

Page DL, DeLellis RA, Hough AJ. Adrenal cortical adenoma. In: Page DL, DeLellis RA, Hough AJ, eds. Tumors of the Adrenal. Fascicle 23, second series. Washington, DC: Armed Forces Institute of Pathology, 1986, pp. 81–114.

Reidbord H, Fisher ER. Aldosteronoma and nonfunctioning adrenal cortical adenoma. Arch Pathol 1969, 88.155–161.

Ross NS, Aron DC. Hormonal evaluation of the patient with an incidentally discovered adrenal mass. N Engl J Med 1990; 323:1401–1405.

Sasano H, Suzuki T, Sano O, et al. Adrenocortical oncocytoma: A true nonfunctioning adrenocortical tumor. Am J Surg Pathol 1991; 15: 949–956.

Sasano N, Ojima M, Masuda T. Endocrinologic pathology of functioning adrenocortical tumors. Pathol Ann 1980; 15:105–142.

Wadih GE, Nance KV, Silverman JF. Fine-needle aspiration cytology of the adrenal gland: Fifty biopsies in 48 patients. Arch Pathol Lab Med 1991; 116:841–846.

Young WF, Hogan MJ, Klee GG, et al. Primary aldosteronism: Diagnosis and treatment. Mayo Clin Proc 1990; 65:96–110.

Adrenocortical Carcinoma

Bugg MF, Ribeiro RC, Roberson PK, et al. Correlation of pathologic features with clinical outcome in pediatric adrenocortical neoplasia. Am J Clin Pathol 1994; 101:625–629.

Cagle PT, Hough AJ, Pysher TJ, et al. Comparison of adrenal cortical tumors in children and adults. Cancer 1986; 57:2235–2237.

Cibas ES, Medeiros LJ, Weinberg DS, et al. Cellular DNA profiles of benign and malignant adrenocortical tumors. Am J Surg Pathol 1990; 14:948–955.

El-Naggar AK, Evans DB, Mackay B. Oncocytic adrenal cortical carcinoma. Ultrastruct Pathol 1991; 15:549–556.

Evans HL, Vassilopoulou-Sellin R. Adrenal cortical neoplasms: A study of 56 cases. Am J Clin Pathol 1996; 105:76–86.

Fuhrman SA, Lasky LC, Limas C. Prognostic significance of morphologic parameters in renal cell carcinoma. Am J Surg Pathol 1982; 6:655–663.

Gandour MJ, Grizzle WE. A small adrenocortical carcinoma with aggressive behavior: An evaluation of criteria for malignancy. Arch Pathol Lab Med 1986; 110:1076–1079.

Hough AJ, Hollifield JW, Page DL, Hartmann WH. Prognostic factors in adrenal cortical tumors: A mathematical analysis of clinical and morphologic data. Am J Clin Pathol 1979; 72:390–399.

Katz RL. Kidney, adrenal, and retroperitoneum. In: Bibbo M, ed. Comprehensive Cytopathology. Philadelphia: WB Saunders, 1991, pp. 771–805.

King DR, Lack EE. Adrenal cortical carcinoma: A clinical and pathologic study of 49 cases. Cancer 1979; 44:239–244.

Komminoth P, Roth J, Schröder S, et al. Overlapping expression of immunohistochemical markers and synaptophysin mRNA in pheochromocytomas and adrenocortical carcinomas: Implications for the differential diagnosis of adrenal gland tumors. Lab Invest 1995; 72:424–431.

Lack EE, Mulvihill JJ, Travis WD, Kozakewich HPW. Adrenal cortical neoplasms in the pediatric and adolescent age group: Clinicopathologic study of 30 cases with emphasis on epidemiological and prognostic features. Pathol Annu 1992; 27:1–53.

Lack EE, Travis WD, Oertel J. Adrenal cortical neoplasms. In: Lack EE, ed. Pathology of the Adrenal Glands. Vol. 14. New York: Churchill Livingstone, 1990, pp. 136–163.

Luton J-P, Cerdas S, Billaud L, et al. Clinical features of adrenocortical carcinoma, prognostic factors, and the effect of mitotane therapy. N Engl J Med 1990; 322:1195–1201.

Medeiros LJ, Weiss LM. New developments in the pathologic diagnosis of adrenal cortical neoplasms: A review. Am J Clin Pathol 1992; 97:73–83.

Miettinen M. Neuroendocrine differentiation in adrenocortical carcinoma: New immunohistochemical findings supported by electron microscopy. Lab Invest 1992; 66:169–174.

Nader S, Hickey RC, Sellin RV, Samaan NA. Adrenal cortical carcinoma: A study of 77 cases. Cancer 1983; 552:707–711.

Ribeiro RC, Neto RS, Schell MJ, et al. Adrenocortical carcinoma in children: A study of 40 cases. J Clin Oncol 1990; 8:67–74.

Van Slooten H, Schberg A, Smeenk D, Moolenaar A. Morphologic characteristics of benign and malignant adrenocortical tumors. Cancer 1985; 55:766–773.

Wadih GE, Nance KV, Silverman JF. Fine-needle aspiration cytology of the adrenal gland: Fifty biopsies in 48 patients. Arch Pathol Lab Med 1991; 116:841–846.

Weiss LM. Comparative histologic study of 43 metastasizing and nonmetastasizing adrenocortical tumors. Am J Surg Pathol 1984; 8:163–169.

Weiss LM, Medeiros LJ, Vickery AL. Pathologic features of prognostic significance in adrenal cortical carcinoma. Am J Surg Pathol 1989; 13:202–206.

Wick MR, Cherwitz DL, McGlennen RC, Dehner LP. Adrenocortical carcinoma: An immunohistochemical comparison with renal cell carcinoma. Am J Pathol 1986; 122:343–352.

Neoplasms of the Adrenal Medulla

Adrenomedullary Hyperplasia

Carney JA, Sizemore GW, Tyce GM. Bilateral adrenal medullary hyperplasia in multiple endocrine neoplasia, type II: The precursor of bilateral pheochromocytoma. May Clin Proc 1975; 50:3–10.

DeLellis RA, Wolf HJ, Gagel RT, et al. Adrenal medullary hyperplasia: A morphometric analysis of patients with familial medullary thyroid carcinoma. Am J Pathol 1976; 83:177–190.

Lack EE. Adrenal medullary hyperplasia and pheochromocytoma. In: Pathology of Adrenal and Extra-adrenal Paraganglia: Major Problems in Pathology. Vol. 29. Philadelphia: WB Saunders, 1994, pp. 220–228.

Montalbano FP, Barnovsky ID, Ball H. Hyperplasia of the adrenal medulla: A clinical entity. JAMA 1962; 182:264–267.

Rudy FR, Bates RD, Cimorelli AJ, et al. Adrenal medullary hyperplasia: A clinicopathologic study of four cases. Hum Pathol 1980; 11:650–657.

Visser JW, Axt R. Bilateral adrenal medullary hyperplasia: A clinicopathologic entity. J Clin Pathol 1975; 28:298–304.

Pheochromocytoma

Bravo EL. Pheochromocytoma: New concepts and future trends. Kidney Int 1991; 40:544–556.

Bravo EL, Gifford RW Jr. Pheochromocytoma: Diagnosis, localization, and management. N Engl J Med 1984; 311:1298–1303.

Feldman JM, Blalock JA, Zern RT, et al. Deficiency of dopamine-beta-hydroxylase: A new mechanism for normotensive pheochromocytomas. Am J Clin Pathol 1979; 72:175–185.

Greene JP, Guay AT. New perspectives in pheochromocytomas. Urol Clin North Am 1989; 16:487–503.

Katz RL. Kidney, adrenal, and retroperitoneum. In: Bibbo M, ed. Comprehensive Cytopathology. Philadelphia: WB Saunders, 1991, pp. 771–805.

Lack EE. Adrenal medullary hyperplasia and pheochromocytoma. In: Pathology of Adrenal and Extra-adrenal Paraganglia: Major Problems in Pathology. Vol. 29. Philadelphia: WB Saunders, 1994, pp. 229–264.

Linnoila RI, Keiser HR, Steinberg SM, Lack EE. Histopathology of benign versus malignant sympathoadrenal paragangliomas: Clinicopathologic study of 120 cases including unusual histologic features. Hum Pathol 1990; 21:1168–1180.

Medeiros LJ, Katsas GG, Balogh K. Brown fat and adrenal pheochromocytoma: Association or coincidence? Hum Pathol 1985; 16:970–972.

Medeiros LJ, Wolf BC, Balogh K, Federman M. Adrenal pheochromocytoma: A clinicopathologic review of 60 cases. Hum Pathol 1985; 16:580–589.

Melicow MM. One hundred cases of pheochromocytoma (107 tumors) at the Columbia-Presbyterian Medical Center, 1926–1976: A clinicopathologic analysis. Cancer 1977; 40:1987–2004.

Modlin IM, Farndon JR, Shepherd A, et al. Phaeochromocytomas in 72 patients: Clinical and diagnostic features, treatment, and long-term results. Br J Surg 1979; 66:456–465.

Padberg B-C, Garbe E, Chilles E, et al. Adrenomedullary hyperplasia and phaeochromocytoma: DNA cytomorphometric findings in 47 cases. Virchows Arch A [Pathol Anat] 1990; 416:443–446.

Proye MAC, Fossati P, Fontaine P, et al. Dopamine-secreting pheochromocytoma: An unrecognized entity? Classification of pheochromocytomas according to their type of secretion. Surgery 1986; 100: 1154–1161.

Ramsay JA, Asa SL, van Nostrand AWP, et al. Lipid degeneration in pheochromocytomas mimicking adrenal cortical tumors. Am J Surg Pathol 1987; 11:480–486.

Samaan NA, Hickey RC, Shutts PE. Diagnosis, localization, and management of pheochromocytoma: Pitfalls and follow-up in 41 patients. Cancer 1988; 62:2451–2460.

Sheps SG, Jiang N-S, Klee GG, van Heerden JA. Recent developments in the diagnosis and treatment of pheochromocytomas. Mayo Clin Proc 1990; 65:88–95.

Steinhoff MM, Wells SA Jr, Deschryver-Kecskemeti K. Stromal amyloid in pheochromocytomas. Hum Pathol 1992; 23:33–36.

Stenstrom G, Svardsudd K. Pheochromocytoma in Sweden, 1958–1981: An analysis of the National Cancer Registry data. Acta Med Scand 1986; 220:225–232.

Sutton MGS, Sheps SG, Lie JT. Prevalence of clinically unsuspected pheochromocytoma: Review of a 50-year autopsy series. Mayo Clin Proc 1981; 56:354–360.

Swenson SJ, Brown ML, Sheps SG, et al. Use of I^{131}-MIGB scintigraphy in the evaluation of suspected pheochromocytoma. Mayo Clin Proc 1985; 60:299–304.

Van Heerden JA, Sheps SG, Hamberger B, et al. Pheochromocytoma: Current status and changing trends. Surgery 1982; 91:367–373.

Wadih GE, Nance KV, Silverman JF. Fine-needle aspiration cytology of the adrenal gland: Fifty biopsies in 48 patients. Arch Pathol Lab Med 1991; 116:841–846.

Webb TA, Sheps SG, Carney JA. Differences between sporadic pheochromocytoma and pheochromocytoma in multiple endocrine neoplasia, type 2. Am J Surg Pathol 1980; 4:121–126.

Welbourn RB. Early surgical history of phaeochromocytoma. Br J Surg 1987; 74:594–596.

Neuroblastoma and Ganglioneuroblastoma

Brodeur GM. Molecular pathology of human neuroblastomas. Semin Diagn Pathol 1994; 11:118–125.

Brodeur GM, Nakagawara A. Molecular basis of clinical heterogeneity in neuroblastoma. Am J Surg Pathol 1992; 14:111–116.

Brodeur GM, Seeger RC, Barrett A, et al. International criteria for diagnosis, staging, and response to treatment in patients with neuroblastoma. J Clin Oncol 1988; 6:1874–1881.

Carlsen NLT. Neuroblastoma—epidemiology and pattern of regression: Problems in interpreting results of mass screening. Am J Pediatr Hematol Oncol 1992; 14:103–110.

Davis S, Rogers MAM, Pendergrass TW. The incidence and epidemiologic characteristics of neuroblastoma in the United States. Am J Epidemiol 1987; 126:1063–1074.

Dehner LP. Primitive neuroectodermal tumor and Ewing's sarcoma. Am J Surg Pathol 1993; 17:1–13.

Evans AE, D'Angio GJ, Randolph J. A proposed staging for children with neuroblastoma. Cancer 1980; 27:374–378.

Gansler T, Chatten J, Varello M, et al. Flow cytometric DNA analysis of neuroblastoma: Correlation with histology and clinical outcome. Cancer 1986; 58:2453–2458.

Joshi VV, Chatten J, Sather HN, Shimada H. Evaluation of the Shimada classification in advanced neuroblastoma with a special reference to the mitosis-karyorrhexis index: A report from the Children's Cancer Study Group. Mod Pathol 1991; 4:139–148.

Joshi VV, Silverman JF. Pathology of neuroblastic tumors. Semin Diagn Pathol 1994; 11:107–117.

Kaye JA, Warhol MJ, Kretschmar C, et al. Neuroblastoma in adults: Three case reports and a review of the literature. Cancer 1986; 58:1149–1157.

Kretschmar CS. Childhood neuroblastoma: Clinical and prognostic features. In: Lack EE, ed. Pathology of the Adrenal Glands. Vol. 14. New York: Churchill Livingstone, 1990, pp. 257–275.

Lack EE. Neuroblastoma, ganglioneuroblastoma, and related tumors. In: Pathology of Adrenal and Extra-adrenal Paraganglia: Major Problems in Pathology. Vol. 29. Philadelphia: WB Saunders, 1994, pp. 315–351.

Look T, Hayes A, Shuster JJ, et al. Clinical relevance of tumor cell ploidy and N-*myc* gene amplification in childhood neuroblastoma: A Pediatric Oncology Group study. J Clin Oncol 1991; 9:581–591.

McGahey BE, Moriarty AT, Nelson WA, Hull MT. Fine-needle aspiration biopsy of small round blue cell tumors of childhood. Cancer 1992; 69:1067–1073.

Murphy SB, Cohn SL, Craft AW, et al. Do children benefit from mass screening for neuroblastoma? Consensus statement from the American Cancer Society workshop on neuroblastoma screening. Lancet 1991; 337:344–345.

Oppedal BR, Storm-Mathisen I, Lie S, Brandtzaeg P. Prognostic factors in neuroblastoma: Clinical, histopathologic, and immunohistochemical features and DNA ploidy in relation to prognosis. Cancer 1988; 62:772–780.

Philip T. Overview of current treatment of neuroblastoma. Am J Pediatr Hematol Oncol 1992; 14:97–102.

Rosen EM, Cassady JR, Frantz CN, et al. Neuroblastoma: The Joint Center for Radiation Therapy/Dana-Farber Cancer Institute/Children's Hospital experience. J Clin Oncol 1984; 2:719–732.

Shimada H, Chatten J, Newton WA, et al. Histopathologic prognostic factors in neuroblastic tumors: Definition of subtypes of ganglioneuroblastoma and an age-linked classification of neuroblastomas. J Natl Cancer Inst 1984; 73:405–416.

Shochat SJ, Corbelletta NL, Repman MA, Schengrund C-L. A biochemical analysis of thoracic neuroblastomas: A Pediatric Oncology Group study. J Pediatr Surg 1987; 22:660–667.

Silverman JF, Dabbs DJ, Ganick DJ, et al. Fine needle aspiration cytology of neuroblastoma, including peripheral neuroectodermal tumor, with immunocytochemical and ultrastructural confirmation. Acta Cytol 1988; 32:367–376.

Triche TJ. Differential diagnosis of neuroblastoma and related tumors. In: Lack EE, ed. Pathology of the Adrenal Glands. Vol. 14. New York: Churchill Livingstone, 1990, pp. 323–350.

Tsuda T, Obara M, Hirano H, et al. Analysis of N-*myc* amplification in relation to disease stage and histologic types in human neuroblastoma. Cancer 1987; 60:820–826.

Tsuda H, Shimosato Y, Upton MP, et al. Retrospective study on amplification of N-*myc* and c-*myc* genes in pediatric solid tumors and its association with prognosis and tumor differentiation. Lab Invest 1988; 59:321–327.

Ganglioneuroma

Aguirre P, Scully RE. Testosterone-secreting adrenal ganglioneuroma containing Leydig cells. Am J Surg Pathol 1983; 7:699–703.

Carpenter WB, Kernohan JW. Retroperitoneal ganglioneuromas and neurofibromas: A clinicopathological study. Cancer 1963; 16:788–797.

Fletcher CDM, Fernando IN, Braimbridge MV, et al. Malignant nerve sheath tumor arising in a ganglioneuroma. Histopathology 1988; 12:445–454.

Ghali VS, Gold JE, Vincent RA, Cosgrove JM. Malignant peripheral nerve sheath tumor arising spontaneously from retroperitoneal ganglioneuroma: A case report, review of the literature, and immunohistochemical study. Hum Pathol 1992; 23:72–75.

Hayes FA, Green AA, Rao BN. Clinical manifestations of ganglioneuroma. Cancer 1989; 63:1211–1214.

Keller SM, Papazoglou S, McKeever P, et al. Late occurrence of malignancy in a ganglioneuroma 19 years following radiation therapy to a neuroblastoma. J Surg Oncol 1984; 25:227–231.

Lack EE. Neuroblastoma, ganglioneuroblastoma, and related tumors. In: Pathology of Adrenal and Extra-adrenal Paraganglia: Major Problems in Pathology. Vol. 29. Philadelphia: WB Saunders, 1994, pp. 351–362.

Ricci A Jr, Parham DM, Woodruff JM, et al. Malignant peripheral nerve sheath tumors arising from ganglioneuromas. Am J Surg Pathol 1984; 8:19–29.

Composite Tumors of the Adrenal Medulla

Fernando PB, Cooray GH, Thanabalasundram RS. Adrenal pheochromocytoma with neuroblastomatous elements: Report of a case with autopsy. Arch Pathol 1951; 52:182–188.

Franquemont DW, Mills SE, Lack EE. Immunohistochemical detection of neuroblastomatous foci in composite adrenal pheochromocytoma-neuroblastoma. Am J Clin Pathol 1994; 102:163–170.

Layfield LJ, Glasgow BJ, Du Puis MH, Bhuta S. Aspiration cytology and immunohistochemistry of a pheochromocytoma-ganglioneuroma of the adrenal gland. Acta Cytol 1987; 31:33–39.

Lewis D, Geschickter CF. Tumors of the sympathetic nervous system. Arch Surg 1934; 28:16–58.

Nakagawara A, Ikeda K, Tsuneyoshi M, et al. Malignant pheochromocytoma with ganglioneuroblastomatous elements in a patient with von Recklinghausen's disease. Cancer 1985; 55:2794–2798.

Tischler AS, Dayal Y, Balogh K, et al. The distribution of immunoreactive chromogranins, S-100, and vasoactive intestinal peptide in compound tumors of the adrenal medulla. Hum Pathol 1987; 18:909–917.

Trump DL, Livingston JN, Baylin SB. Watery diarrhea syndrome in an adult with ganglioneuroma-pheochromocytoma: Identification of vasoactive intestinal peptide, calcitonin, and catecholamines in assessment of their biologic activity. Cancer 1977; 40:1526–1532.

Wahl HR, Robinson D. Neuroblastoma of the mediastinum with pheochromoblastomatous elements. Arch Pathol 1943; 35:571–578.

Primary Malignant Melanoma

Carstens PHB, Kuhns JG, Ghazi C. Primary malignant melanomas of the lung and adrenal. Hum Pathol 1984; 15:910–914.

Das Gupta T, Brasfield RD, Paglia MA. Primary melanomas in unusual sites. Surg Gynecol Obstet 1969; 128:841–844.

Sasidharan K, Babu AS, Pandey AP, et al. Primary melanoma of the adrenal gland: A case report. J Urol 1977; 117:663–665.

Travis WD, Oertel JE, Lack EE. Miscellaneous tumors and tumefactive lesions of the adrenal gland. In: Lack EE, ed. Pathology of the Adrenal Glands. Vol. 14. New York: Churchill Livingstone, 1990, pp. 360–362.

Miscellaneous Neoplasms and Tumor-Like Lesions

Malignant Lymphoma

Bauduer F, Delmer A, Le Tourneau, et al. Primary adrenal lymphoma. Acta Hematol 1992; 88:213–215.

Harris GJ, Tio FO, von Hoff DD. Primary adrenal lymphoma. Cancer 1989 63:799–803.

Hayes JA, Christensen OE. Primary adrenal lymphoma. J Pathol Bacteriol 1961; 82:193–219.

Ohsawa M, Tomita Y, Hashimoto M, et al. Malignant lymphoma of the adrenal gland: Its possible correlation with Epstein-Barr virus. Mod Pathol 1996; 9:534–543.

Schnitzer B, Smid D, Lloyd RV. Primary T-cell lymphoma of the adrenal glands with adrenal insufficiency. Hum Pathol 1986; 17:634–636.

Shea TC, Spark R, Kane B, Lange RF. Non-Hodgkin's lymphoma limited to the adrenal gland with adrenal insufficiency. Am J Med 1985; 78:711–714.

Sparagana M. Addison's disease due to reticulum cell sarcoma apparently confined to the adrenals. J Am Geriatr Soc 1970; 18:550–554.

Myelolipoma

Bennett BD, McKenna TJ, Hough AJ, et al. Adrenal myelolipoma associated with Cushing's disease. Am J Clin Pathol 1980; 73:443–447.

Gee WF, Chikos PM, Greaves JP, et al. Adrenal myelolipoma. Urology 1975; 5:562–566.

Olsson CA, Krane RJ, Klugo RC, Selikowitz SM. Adrenal myelolipoma. Surgery 1973; 73:665–670.

Page DL, DeLellis RA, Hough AJ. Myelolipoma and related lesions. In: Page DL, DeLellis RA, Hough AJ, eds. Tumors of the Adrenal Gland. Fascicle 23, second series. Washington, DC: Armed Forces Institute of Pathology, 1986, pp. 162–182.

Adenomatoid Tumor

Craig JR, Hart WR. Extragenital adenomatoid tumor: Evidence for the mesothelial theory of origin. Cancer 1979; 43:1678–1681.

Simpson PR. Adenomatoid tumor of the adrenal gland. Arch Pathol Lab Med 1990; 114:725–727.

Travis WD, Lack EE, Azumi N, et al. Adenomatoid tumor of the adrenal gland with ultrastructural and immunohistochemical demonstration of a mesothelial origin. Arch Pathol Lab Med 1990; 114:722–724.

Hemangioma

Orringer RD, Lynch JA, McDermott WV. Cavernous hemangioma of the adrenal gland. J Surg Oncol 1983; 22:106–108.

Rothberg M, Bastidas J, Mattey, Bernas E. Adrenal hemangiomas: Angiographic appearance of a rare tumor. Radiology 1978; 126:341–344.

Travis WD, Oertel JE, Lack EE. Miscellaneous tumors and tumefactive lesions of the adrenal gland. In: Lack EE, ed. Pathology of the Adrenal Glands. Vol. 14. New York: Churchill Livingstone, 1990, pp. 362–364.

Vargas AD. Adrenal hemangioma. Urology 1980; 16:389–390.

Angiosarcoma

Bosco PJ, Silverman ML, Zinman LM. Primary angiosarcoma of adrenal gland presenting as a paraneoplastic syndrome: Case report. J Urol 1991; 146:1101–1103.

Granger JK, Houn HY, Collins C. Massive hemorrhagic functional adrenal adenoma histologically mimicking angiosarcoma: Report of a case with immunohistochemical study. Am J Surg Pathol 1991; 15:699–704.

Kareti LR, Katlein S, Siew S, Blauvelt A. Angiosarcoma of the adrenal gland. Arch Pathol Lab Med 1988; 112:1163–1165.

Livaditou A, Alexiou G, Floros D, et al. Epithelioid angiosarcoma of the adrenal gland associated with chronic arsenical intoxication? Pathol Res Pract 1991; 187:284–289.

Wenig BM, Abbondanzo SL, Heffess CS. Epithelioid angiosarcoma of the adrenal glands: A clinicopathologic study of nine cases with a discussion of the implications of "epithelial-specific" markers. Am J Surg Pathol 1994; 18:62–73.

Nerve Sheath Tumors

Bedard YC, Horvath E, Kovacs K. Adrenal schwannoma with apparent uptake of immunoglobulin. Ultrastruct Pathol 1986; 10:505–509.

Oliver WR, Reddick RL, Gillespie GY, Siegel GP. Juxtaadenal schwannoma: Verification of the diagnosis by immunohistochemistry and ultrastructural studies. J Surg Oncol 1985; 30:259–261.

Ricci A Jr, Parham DM, Woodruff JM, et al. Malignant peripheral nerve sheath tumors arising from ganglioneuromas. Am J Surg Pathol 1984; 8:19–29.

Travis WD, Oertel JE, Lack EE. Miscellaneous tumors and tumefactive lesions of the adrenal gland. In: Lack EE, ed. Pathology of the Adrenal Glands. Vol. 14. New York: Churchill Livingstone, 1990, pp. 362–364.

Metastatic Neoplasms

Campbell CM, Middleton RG, Rigby OF. Adrenal metastasis in renal cell carcinoma. Urology 1983; 21:403–405.

Cedermark BJ, Blumenson LE, Pickren JW, Elias EG. The significance of metastases to the adrenal gland from carcinoma of the stomach and esophagus. Surg Gynecol Obstet 1977; 145:41–48.

Cedermark BJ, Blumenson LE, Pickren JW, et al. The significance of metastasis to the adrenal glands in adenocarcinoma of the colon and rectum. Surg Gynecol Obstet 1977; 144:537–546.

Foucar E, Dehner LP. Renal cell carcinoma occurring with contralateral adrenal metastasis. Arch Surg 1979; 114:959–963.

Seidenwurm DJ, Elmer EB, Kaplan LM, et al. Metastases to the adrenal glands and the development of Addison's disease. Cancer 1984; 54:552–557.

Travis WD, Oertel JE, Lack EE. Miscellaneous tumors and tumefactive lesions of the adrenal gland. In: Lack EE, ed. Pathology of the Adrenal Glands. Vol. 14. New York: Churchill Livingstone, 1990, pp. 365–368.

Vieweg WVR, Reitz RE, Weinstein RL. Addison's disease secondary to metastatic carcinoma: An example of adrenocortical and adrenomedullary insufficiency. Cancer 1973; 31:1240–1243.

Other Rare Neoplasms

Choi SH, Liu K. Leiomyosarcoma of the adrenal gland and its angiographic features: A case report. J Surg Oncol 1981; 16:145–148.

Lack EE, Graham CW, Azumi N, et al. Primary leiomyosarcoma of the adrenal gland: Case report with immunohistochemical and ultrastructural study. Am J Surg Pathol 1991; 15:899–905.

Pollock WJ, McConnell, Hilton C, Lavine RL. Virilizing Leydig cell adenoma of adrenal gland. Am J Surg Pathol 1986; 10:816–822.

CHAPTER 15

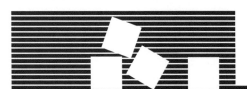

Classification of Multiple Endocrine Neoplasia Syndromes

Table 15–1

MULTIPLE ENDOCRINE NEOPLASIA SYNDROME, TYPE IA (WERMER'S SYNDROME)

Components	Frequency of Involvement
Parathyroid hyperplasia or adenoma	90%–100%
Pancreatic or gastrointestinal neuroendocrine hyperplasia or neoplasm	75%
Pituitary adenoma	66%

Table 15–2

MULTIPLE ENDOCRINE NEOPLASIA SYNDROME, TYPE II (SIPPLE'S SYNDROME OR TYPE IIA)

Components	Frequency of Involvement
C-cell hyperplasia or medullary thyroid carcinoma	~100%
Pheochromocytoma	50%
Parathyroid hyperplasia or adenoma	25%

Table 15–3

MULTIPLE ENDOCRINE NEOPLASIA, TYPE III (GORLIN'S SYNDROME OR TYPE IIB)

Components	Frequency of Involvement
C-cell hyperplasia or medullary thyroid carcinoma	~100%
Pheochromocytoma	34%
Parathyroid hyperplasia or adenoma	4%

Bibliography

DeLellis RA. Multiple endocrine neoplasia syndromes revisited. Clinical, morphologic and molecular features revisited. Lab Invest 1995;72:494–505.

CHAPTER 16

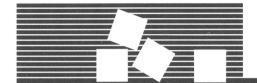

Endocrine Abnormalities Associated with Human Immunodeficiency Virus Infection and Acquired Immunodeficiency Syndrome

- Endocrine abnormalities may be an important component in the manifestations of human immunodeficiency virus (HIV) infection and acquired immunodeficiency syndrome (AIDS).
- Endocrine organ dysfunction may be the direct result of HIV infection or other opportunistic infections or may result from the development of malignancies associated with HIV infection or as a complication of medications used in the treatment of the HIV-infected or AIDS patient.
- Hormonal-related dysfunctions (in production, secretion, or metabolism) may represent a response to severe illness rather than a cytopathologic change in endocrine organs.
- The causes of AIDS-related endocrine disease include opportunistic infections, malignancies, and medication-induced endocrine toxicities (Table 16–1).
- HIV-associated endocrine dysfunctions may present early in the disease course with subtle clinical manifestations, or they may be part of the severe systemic disease occurring in the latter stages of AIDS and may be marked.
- Clinical manifestations vary and may include manifestations related to:
  - Adrenal gland: adrenal insufficiency.
  - Hypothalamic-pituitary axis: hyponatremia, growth failure (in pediatric AIDS).
  - Thyroid: primary hypothyroidism, "euthyroid sick syndrome," in which the thyroid gland is normal but due to severe systemic nonthyroidal illness alterations in thyroid physiology occur, including decreased circulating T_3 levels as a consequence of impaired conversion of T_4 to T_3, but T_4 levels vary and may be increased.
  - Pancreas: acute pancreatitis, chronic pancreatitis, pancreatic abscess, hyperamylasemia due to nephropathy,

glucose intolerance, diabetes mellitus, steatorrhea, and obstructive jaundice.
  - Parathyroid: hypercalcemia.
  - Gonads: decreased circulating sex steroids, including testosterone, estradiol, or progesterone; very high levels of pituitary gonadotropins, including luteinizing hormone and follicle-stimulating hormone. Chronic disease results in gonadal atrophy with disturbances in menstrual function and ovulation and reduced spermatogenesis.

Table 16–1
ETIOLOGY OF AIDS-RELATED ENDOCRINE DISEASE

Opportunistic Infections

1. Viruses
   Cytomegalovirus
   Herpetic
2. Mycobacteria
   Tuberculosis
   M. avium intracellulare
3. Fungi
   Cryptococcus neoformans
   Aspergillus
4. Protozoa
   Toxoplasma gondii
   Pneumocystis carinii
   Cryptosporidium
   Microsporidiosis

Malignancies

Kaposi's sarcoma
Malignant lymphomas

Medication-Induced Endocrine Toxicity

Pentamidine
Trimethoprim-sulfamethoxazole
Ocreatide

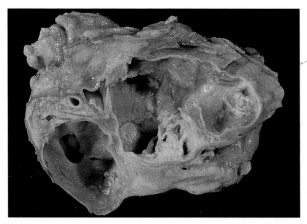

Figure 16–1. Cytomegalovirus pancreatitis. Autopsy specimen from a patient with AIDS showing cystic alteration and replacement of the pancreatic parenchyma.

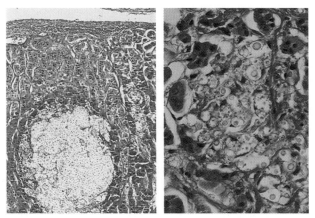

Figure 16–4. Adrenal cryptococcal infection. *Left,* Cystic lesion filled with microorganisms is seen within the adrenal cortex. *Right,* Higher magnification shows the spherical and encapsulated cryptococcal organisms.

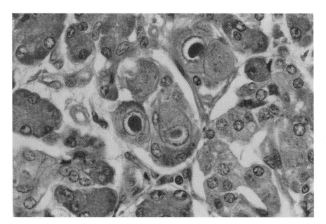

Figure 16–2. Cytomegalovirus pancreatitis. Classic intranuclear inclusions of cytomegalovirus in pancreatic exocrine tissue.

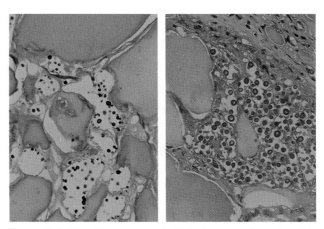

Figure 16–5. Thyroid cryptococcosis. *Left,* Grocott methenamine silver (GMS) and *right,* mucicarmine stains delineate the microorganisms.

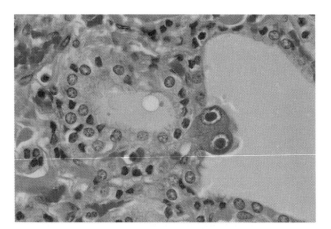

Figure 16–3. AIDS patient with cytomegalovirus thyroiditis showing classic intranuclear inclusions in thyroid follicular epithelial cells.

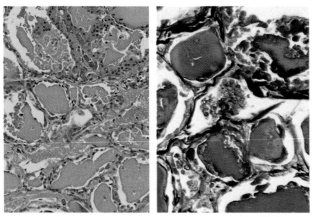

Figure 16–6. *Pneumocystis carinii* infection of the thyroid. *Left,* The classic eosinophilic "fluffy" exudate can be seen by light microscopy. *Right,* GMS stains the *Pneumocystis* organisms black, appearing as spherical, encapsulated organisms with irregular (convoluted) contours.

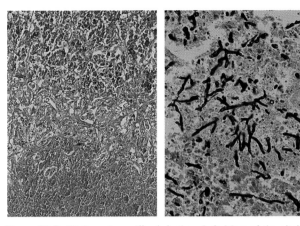

Figure 16–7. Pituitary *Aspergillus* infection. *Left,* Most of the pituitary gland is necrotic. Remnants of the gland are seen toward the top of this panel. *Right,* GMS stain shows the fungal forms, which demonstrate features consistent with *Aspergillus* species, including hyphae and acute angle branching.

Bibliography

Cappell MS. The pancreas in AIDS. In: Broder S, Merigan TC Jr, Bolognesi D, eds. Textbook of AIDS Medicine. Baltimore: Williams & Wilkins, 1994, pp. 555–565.

Cavalieri RR. The effects of nonthyroid disease and drugs on thyroid function tests. Med Clin North Am 1991; 75:27–39.

Dluhy RG. The growing spectrum of HIV-related endocrine abnormalities. J Clin Endocrinol Metab 1990; 70:563–564.

Hellerstein MK. Endocrine abnormalities. In: Cohen PT, Sande MA, Voberding PA, eds. The AIDS Knowledge Base: A Textbook on HIV Disease from the University of California, San Francisco and San Francisco General Hospital. Boston: Little, Brown, 1994, pp. 1–10.

Merenich JA, McDermott MT, Asp AA, Harrison SM, Kidd GS. Evidence of endocrine involvement early in the course of human immunodeficiency virus infection. J Clin Endocrinol Metab 1990; 70:566–571.

Schambelan M, Grunfeld C. Endocrine abnormalities associated with HIV infection and AIDS. In: Broder S, Merigan TC Jr, Bolognesi D, eds. Textbook of AIDS Medicine. Baltimore: Williams & Wilkins, 1994, pp. 629–636.

Wartofsky L, Burman KD. Alterations in thyroid function in patients with systemic illness: The "euthyroid sick syndrome." Endocrine Rev 1982; 3:164–217.

APPENDICES

EMBRYOLOGY, ANATOMY, AND HISTOLOGY

APPENDIX A

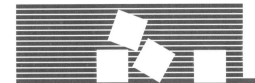

Pituitary Gland

Embryology

- The pituitary gland derives from two separate primordia:
  - Adenohypophysis, or anterior pituitary, is of ectodermal derivation and includes the pars distalis, pars intermedia, and pars tuberalis.
  - Neurohypophysis, or posterior pituitary, has no functional relationship with the anterior lobe. It derives as an evagination of the diencephalon and includes the posterior lobe, infundibulum, and neural stalk.
- The anterior pituitary develops from a diverticulum, the Rathke's pouch, around the 4th week of gestation and grows cranially between the developing sphenoid bone, becoming an elongated structure with a narrow proximal end around the 5th week of gestation.
- While obliteration of the proximal segment and separation from the oral epithelium occurs, the distal segment of Rathke's pouch connects with the infundibulum, a downgrowth from the diencephalon of neuroectodermal derivation; persistence of remnants of Rathke's pouch can give rise to a pharyngeal hypophysis.
- Extensive cellular proliferation of the anterior wall of Rathke's pouch gives rise to the pars distalis; a cephalic proliferation of the adenohypophysis or pars tuberalis envelops the infundibulum.
- The posterior wall of Rathke's pouch gives rise to a poorly defined pars intermedia or intermediate lobe, which is rudimentary in adults and in direct contact with the posterior pituitary; obliteration of the lumen of Rathke's pouch is recognizable only in the adult gland as colloid-filled cysts.
- The neurohypophysis gives rise to the median eminence, infundibular stem, and pars nervosa, retaining its connection with the brain through the infundibular stalk.
- Fusion of the thin walls of the upper portion of the infundibulum forms the pituitary stalk, and neuroepithelial cell proliferation in the distal end enlarges to form the posterior pituitary.
- The pituitary gland is grossly recognizable by the end of the 3rd month of gestation.
- The hormonal secretion of the adenohypophysis is under hypothalamic control, and the pars distalis is the main source of pituitary hormones secreting growth hormone (GH), or somatotropin, adrenocorticotropic hormone (ACTH), prolactin (PRL) or luteotropic hormone, thyrotropin (thyroid-stimulating hormone [TSH]), and gonadotropin (follicle-stimulating hormone [FSH] and luteinizing hormone [LH]).
- The pars intermedia is the source of melanocyte-stimulating hormone (MSH) in the lower mammals, but it is not secreted as such in the adults.
- The neurohypophysis, or pars nervosa, is composed of nerve fibers and axon terminals of the hypothalamohypophysial tract, pituicytes (which are modified glial cells), neurosecretory material, and fibrovascular connective tissue.
- Nerve tracts from the hypothalamus (via the hypophysial stalk) to the posterior lobe transport vasopressin and oxytocin in association with carrier proteins called "neurophysins."

Anatomy

- The adult pituitary gland is a reddish, ovoid body measuring approximately 13 mm in transverse diameter, 9 mm in anteroposterior diameter, and 6 mm in vertical diameter; the weight of the gland is about 500 mg, 80% of which constitutes the anterior lobe; the pituitary gland is slightly heavier in females and increases during pregnancy and in multiparous woman.
- The pituitary gland lies in the sella turcica and is enclosed by the dura mater; it is attached to the hypothalamus by the pituitary stalk, which penetrates the diaphragm sella (dural roof) through a small, 5-mm, central opening; it is separated from the sphenoid bone by a loose, richly vascularized connective tissue layer.
- The relationship of the pituitary gland to the adjacent structures is of clinical importance.
  - The sella is in close proximity with the internal carotid arteries, the optic nerves, and the cavernous sinuses; the latter is of particular importance in relation to pituitary tumors for its predisposition toward tumor invasion.
  - Anteriorly and below the sphenoid sinus, the pituitary gland is separated from the sella by thin connective tissue and bone.

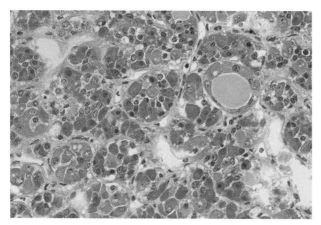

Figure A–1. Normal anterior pituitary gland section showing chromophobic, acidophilic, and basophilic cells and a pseudofollicle.

• Directly above the diaphragm sella lies the optic chiasm, clinically important because of the visual impairment associated with tumor growth.

Innervation

■ There is no nerve supply to the pars distalis.
■ The hormonal secretion of the pars distalis is controlled by synthesized hypothalamic-releasing hormones that are carried in the blood.
■ Some axons are found in the perisinusoidal connective tissue ending in close association with somatotrophs without regulation of hormonal secretion.

Arteries and Veins

■ The blood supply is involved in the secretory activity of the adenohypophysis.
■ The inferior hypophysial arteries branch of the internal carotid artery supplies primarily the posterior lobe.
■ The superior hypophysial arteries branch of the internal carotid artery and posterior communicating arteries supply primarily the median eminence and pituitary stalk.
■ Branches of the superior hypophysial arteries after penetrating the infundibulum give rise to the external capillary plexus.

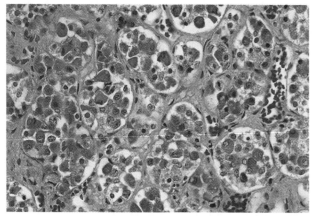

Figure A–2. Normal anterior pituitary gland. Cells are arranged in nests bounded by a capillary network.

■ The blood collected from the median eminence and pituitary stalk converge into veins forming the portal system. There are two portal systems:
  • The long portal system originates in the tuber cinereum, whereas the short portal system originates in the lower infundibulum and ends distally in the pars distalis; therefore, the pars distalis circulation is through the portal system, which carries hypothalamic-releasing and inhibiting factors to the target cells.
■ The veins of the hypophysis drain into the cavernous sinuses.

Histology

■ The anterior lobe is largely enclosed by a dense connective tissue capsule and is subdivided into three regions: the central wedge and the lateral wings.
■ Cells are arranged into small groups of cells or cell nests surrounded by a thin fibrovascular stroma containing a few reticular fibers that constitute the supporting framework of the gland; stroma is scanty.
■ On routine hematoxylin and eosin sections and based on their avidity for acid or basic dyes, three cell types can be identified:
  • **Acidophilic cells** in the lateral wings.
  • **Basophilic cells** in the median wedge.
  • **Chromophobes** scattered throughout the anterior lobe.
■ Histochemical stains do not identify specific hormone production by the cells and the periodic acid–Schiff (PAS) selectively stains the granules of the basophilic cells.
■ The significant variation in size and shape of the specific granules by electron microscopy are considered valuable criteria to distinguish cell types.
■ Immunohistochemical and immunoelectron microscopy demonstrate the presence of five types of cells:
  • **Growth hormone** cells, or **somatotrophs,** are the most numerous cells distributed in the lateral wings of the pituitary gland. They account for about 40% to 50% of the pituitary cell population. They stain with acid dyes and contain round secretory granules measuring from 300 to 600 nm in diameter, selectively stained by the antibody to growth hormone.
  • **Prolactin** cells, or **lactotrophs,** tend to be distributed throughout the gland but tend to be more numerous at the posterolateral edges. They account for 15% to 25% of the pituitary cell population. They also stain with acid dyes. By electron microscopy and immunohistochemistry two types of cells with variable size granules have been identified: one population of cells containing granules with a variable size from 500 to 700 nm in diameter stained diffusely strong with the antibody against prolactin, whereas a second type of cell have smaller granules measuring from 250 to 350 nm in diameter and showed juxtanuclear staining. During pregnancy the lactotrophs increase considerably in number and the greatest activity postpartum is initiation and maintenance of lactation.
  • **ACTH-producing** cells, or **corticotrophs,** represent 15% to 20% of the pituitary cell population. These cells are located in the median wedge, tend to penetrate the

posterior lobe (basophil invasion), and are more noticeable in advanced age. They are basophilic and the positive reaction of the cytoplasm with PAS is related to the glycoprotein content of the proopiomelanocortin precursor and the peptides. These cells have granules that may vary from 200 to 350 nm in diameter. Immunohistochemistry demonstrates the presence of ACTH and other derivatives of the proopiomelanocortin molecules such as β-lipotropin (β-LPH) and endorphins. The most common morphologic abnormality is the **Crooke's hyaline change,** which consists of perinuclear accumulation of a faintly eosinophilic, glassy, homogeneous substance displacing the granules to the cell periphery. Crooke's hyaline material is composed of type 1 microfilaments, contains no ACTH, and accumulates under conditions of exogenous or endogenous hypercortisolism.

- **Thyrotrophs (TSH)** are cells located in the anteromedial portion of the anterior pituitary, which represent about 5% of the pituitary cell population. These cells have elongated shapes, with granules ranging in size from 100 to 300 nm in diameter. The cells have a basophilic cytoplasm and are PAS positive. Immunohistochemistry demonstrates the presence of TSH. These cells hypertrophy following thyroidectomy and atrophy after thyroxine administration.
- **Gonadotrophs** account for 10% of the pituitary cell population. They are distributed in the anterior lobe and also have variably sized granules from 200 to 350 nm in diameter. Cytoplasmic PAS-positive reaction is due to glycoprotein content. Immunohistochemistry demonstrates the presence of LH and FSH.

■ The follicular cells or stellate cells are nonsecretory cells arranged in follicle-like structures containing colloid material. The cytoplasm contains glycogen, lipid droplets, and polyribosomes. They may also appear as stellate cells with branching process among the secretory cells. Although their function is not well known, they seem to be phagocytic. The filaments of the processes react with the antibody to gliofibrillar acid protein.

Congenital Abnormalities

Agenesis

■ Complete absence of the pituitary gland is rare and incompatible with life. It is associated with holoprosencephaly secondary to hypothalamic malformation and also with severe endocrine abnormalities of the gonads and thyroid, and hypoplasia of the adrenal glands.

Hypoplasia

■ Hypoplasia of the pituitary gland is associated with hypoplasia of the adrenal glands. It can be suspected in patients with small sella turcica with endocrine problems and growth manifestations. It may also occur in ectopic location of the pituitary gland with other dysfunctional abnormalities. It has been reported in holoprosencephaly and anencephaly. In the latter, the pituitary gland is flattened, the anterior lobe is always present and may appear enlarged owing to vascular congestion, whereas the neurohypophysis is hypoplastic or missing.

■ Hypoplasia has been also associated with a flattened or small sella turcica in which the absence of the opening of the diaphragm sella indicates failure of the development of the pituitary stalk. The hypoplastic pituitary gland has a decreased number of ACTH cells, whereas the other cells are identifiable and normal in number.

Pituitary Duplication

■ Extremely rare condition associated with cleft palate, oral malformations, and accessory anterior lobe masses in the roof of the pharynx.

Anomalous Craniopharyngeal Canal

■ Defined as a canal that appears along the course of the tract of Rathke's pouch during bone development. It is found in 0.9% of newborns and 0.4% of older patients. The contents of the canal vary from blood vessels, connective tissue, and accessory pituitary tissue.

Bibliography

Asa SL, Kovacs K. Functional morphology of the human fetal pituitary. Pathol Annu 1984; 19:275–315.
Fawcett DW. Hypophysis. In: Bloom and Fawcett, Textbook of Histology. 11th edition. Philadelphia: WB Saunders, 1986, pp. 479–499.
Kontogeorgos G. Pituitary tumors. In: Polak JM, ed. Diagnostic Histopathology of Neuroendocrine Tumors. Edinburgh: Churchill Livingstone, 1993, pp. 227–230.
Kovacs K, Horvath E. Tumors of the pituitary gland. In: Hartman WH, Sobin LH, eds. Atlas of Tumor Pathology. Second series, Fascicle 21. Washington, DC: Armed Forces Institute of Pathology, 1986, pp. 1–50.
Lloyd RV. Cytology and function of the pituitary gland. In: Surgical Pathology of the Pituitary Gland. Vol. 27. In: Major Problems in Pathology. Philadelphia: WB Saunders, 1993, pp. 5–17.
Lloyd RV. Embryology and anatomy of the pituitary gland. In: Surgical Pathology of the Pituitary Gland. Vol. 27. In: Major Problems in Pathology. Philadelphia: WB Saunders, 1993, pp. 1–4.
Moore KL, Persaud TVN. The pituitary gland. In: The Developing Human: Clinically Oriented Embryology. 5th edition. Philadelphia: WB Saunders, 1993, pp. 405–408.
Pernicone PJ, Scheithauer BW, Horvath E, Kovacs K. Pituitary and sellar region. In: Sternberg SS, ed. Histology for Pathologists. New York: Raven Press, 1992, pp. 279–299.
Tindall GT, Barrow DL. Anatomy. In: Disorders of the Pituitary. St. Louis: CV Mosby, 1986, pp. 1–22.
Treip CS. The hypothalamus and pituitary gland. In: Adams JH, Duchen LW, eds. Greenfield's Neuropathology. 5th edition. New York: Oxford University Press, 1992, pp. 1046–1082.

Congenital Anomalies of the Pituitary Gland

Adams JH, Duchen LW. The hypothalamus and pituitary gland. In: Greenfield's Neuropathology. New York: Oxford University Press, 1992, pp. 1067–1068.
Badawy SZ, Pisarska MD, Wasenko JJ, Buran JJ. Congenital hypopituitarism as part of suprasellar dysplasia: A case report. J Reprod Med 1994; 39:643–648.
Kim TS, Cho S, Dickson DW. A prosencephaly: Review of the literature and report of a case with cerebellar hypoplasia, pigmented epithelial cyst, and Rathke's cleft cyst. Acta Neuropathol (Berl) 1990; 79:424–431.
Kollias SS, Ball WS, Prenger EC. Review of the embryologic development of the pituitary gland and report of a case of hypophyseal duplication detected by MRI. Neuroradiology 1995; 37:3–12.
Lloyd RV. Non-neoplastic pituitary lesions. In: Surgical Pathology of the Pituitary Gland. Vol. 27. Philadelphia: WB Saunders, 1993, p. 25.

Maghnie M, Triulzi F, Larizza D, et al. Hypothalamic-pituitary dysfunction in growth-hormone–deficient patients with pituitary abnormalities. J Clin Endocrinol Metab 1991; 73:79–83.

Mosier HD. Hypoplasia of the pituitary and adrenal cortex. J Pediatr 1956; 48:633–639.

Reid JD. Congenital absence of the pituitary gland. J Pediatr 1960; 56:658–664.

Rimoin DL. Genetic disorders of the pituitary gland. In: Emery AEH, Rimoin DL, eds. Principles and Practice of Medical Genetics. Vol. 2. Edinburgh: Churchill Livingstone, 1983, pp. 1134–1151.

Shashi V, Clark P, Rogol AD, Wilson WG. Absent pituitary gland in brothers with an oral-facial-digital syndrome resembling OFDS II and VI: A new type of OFDS? Am J Med Genet 1995; 57:22–26.

APPENDIX B

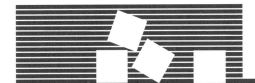

Thyroid Gland

Embryology

- The thyroid gland is the first endocrine gland to appear during embryonic development deriving from three primordia, the median anlage, and lateral anlages.
- The median anlage develops around the 24th day of gestation as a small, median endodermal thickening on the primitive pharynx. This thickening forms a diverticulum that attaches to the tongue by a narrow tube, the thyroglossal duct. Its opening in the base of the tongue constitutes the foramen cecum.
- As a result of further cellular proliferations, the hollow thyroid diverticulum obliterates and divides into the right and left lobes, connected by the isthmus, around the 7th week of gestation.
- During development the thyroid descends and assumes a definitive position in the anterior neck. By this time the thyroglossal duct degenerates. The proximal opening persists as the foramen cecum of the tongue. In approximately 50% of people the inferior end of the thyroglossal duct persists as the pyramidal lobe, which is attached to the hyoid bone by fibrous or muscular tissue.
- The endodermal cell mass, which constitutes the thyroid primordium, is separated into cords by invasion of vascular mesenchyme and divides into smaller groups around the 10th week of gestation. A single layer of cells becomes arranged around a lumen and the primitive follicles make their appearance around the 11th week of gestation. At this time storage of colloid, iodine concentrates, and hormone synthesis can be demonstrated.
- The lateral anlagen corresponds to the ultimobranchial body, which derives from the pharyngeal pouches.
- The ultimobranchial body from which the C cells originate fuses and incorporates into the thyroid, whose calcitonin production regulates normal calcium levels in the body. The C cells differentiate from the neural crest cells that migrate into the pharyngeal pouches from the branchial arches.

Anatomy

- The thyroid gland is a bilobed, reddish-tan organ located in the lower part of the neck, on either side of the larynx and trachea.

- The thyroid is connected by a narrow band of tissue, the isthmus, which overlies the three tracheal rings below the cricoid cartilage.
- The weight of the gland varies from 15 to 25 g in adults, is heavier in women than in men, and varies during pregnancy, iodine intake, and other pathologic conditions.
- The thyroid is enclosed by a connective tissue capsule that is firmly attached to the gland, and septa divide the gland into lobules.
- The lateral thyroid lobes have a conical shape measuring 5 cm long, 3 cm transversally, and 2 cm posteriorly, being the base of the lobe at the level of the fourth and fifth tracheal rings.
- Each lobe in the posterior lateral aspect is attached to the cricoid cartilage by the lateral ligament of the thyroid gland.
- The superficial surface of the gland is convex; the medial surface is adapted to the larynx and trachea and, inferiorly, is related to the side of the trachea in front of, and to the laryngeal nerve posteriorly, which runs in the tracheoesophageal space. The rounded posterior border below is related to the inferior thyroid artery.
- The isthmus connects both lobes and measures 1.2 cm transversely, and it extends anterior to the second and third tracheal rings. It is covered by the sternohyoid muscles, the anterior jugular veins, the fascia, and the skin.
- In almost 50% of the population, a segment of thyroid tissue, designated the "pyramidal lobe," projects upward from the isthmus ascending to the hyoid bone; the pyramidal lobe generally appears as a fibrous tract but in pathologic conditions may become prominent or cystic.

Innervation

- The nerves derived from the superior, middle, and inferior sympathetic cervical ganglia.
- In the thyroid gland through perivascular and interfollicular plexuses, nerves end near the follicular basement membrane, influencing thyroid secretion indirectly by action in the blood vessels.

Arteries and Veins

- The thyroid gland is a richly vascularized organ; the vascular supply is derived from the superior and inferior thyroid arteries.

341

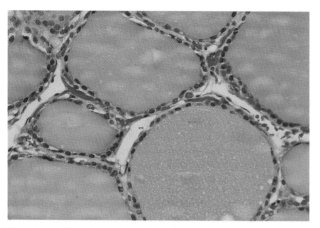

Figure B–1. Normal thyroid gland. Variably sized follicles are lined by cuboidal follicular epithelium and homogeneous eosinophilic colloid.

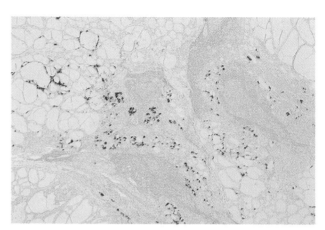

Figure B–4. Normal thyroid gland. Calcitonin immunoreactivity identifying dispersed C cells in the thyroid parenchyma and in the remnant of the ultimobranchial body (solid cell nests).

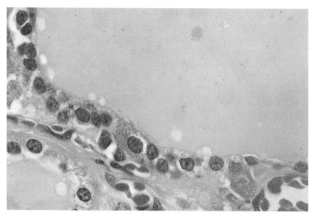

Figure B–2. Normal thyroid gland. Follicle shows C cells with granular basophilic cytoplasm.

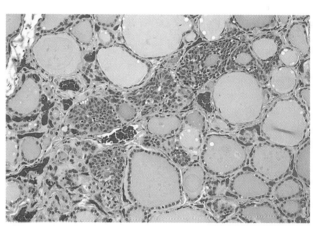

Figure B–5. Normal thyroid gland. Remnant of the ultimobranchial body (solid cell nests). Follicles within the solid cell nests are surrounded by C cells and lumina with eosinophilic material.

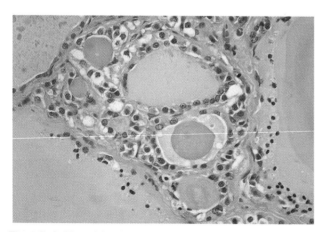

Figure B–3. Normal thyroid gland. Single parafollicular and small interstitial clusters of C cells with clear cytoplasm are shown.

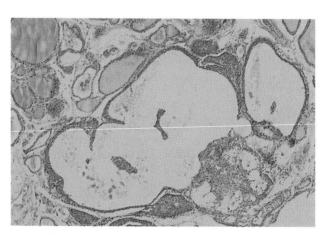

Figure B–6. Normal thyroid gland. Solid cell nests with prominent cystic configuration.

- The superior thyroid artery arises from the external carotid artery; it descends forward and downward to the superior pole of the thyroid gland, and it lies superficial to the external branch of the superior laryngeal nerve.
- The superior thyroid artery divides into (1) a large branch that runs down over the anterior surface of the gland to the isthmus and anastomoses with the superior thyroid artery of the contralateral side; and (2) a smaller posterior branch that courses the posterior lateral surface of the gland and through small ramus communicans anastomoses with the inferior thyroid artery from the same side.
- The inferior thyroid artery, larger than the superior thyroid artery, originates from the thyrocervical trunk, a branch of the subclavian artery, and passes behind and close to the carotid sheath and under the common carotid artery. It divides into anterior and posterior branches at the level of the junction of the inferior and middle thirds of the thyroid gland.
- The recurrent laryngeal nerve runs behind the inferior thyroid artery or main branches of the artery on the left side.
- Occasionally, an artery accessory to or replacing the inferior thyroid artery, is the vessel known as thyroid ima artery, a branch of the brachycephalic artery.
- In the thyroid gland the arteries penetrate the substance of the gland and divide into numerous branches throughout the parenchyma, giving origin to a rich capillary network that ends in capillaries around the follicles.
- Efferent vessels anastomose and accompany the arteries to the surface of the gland, forming a large venous plexus in the fascia covering the gland; from there, the veins follow closely the arteries and form three trunks, generally two superior veins that empty into the internal jugular vein; the inferior thyroid veins empty into the innominate veins or the internal jugular or subclavian vein.

Lymphatics

- The thyroid lymphatics originate in the interfollicular spaces of the gland and form two plexuses: intraglandular and extraglandular.
  - The intraglandular plexus runs in the interlobular connective tissue, accompanies the arteries, and connects with the extraglandular plexus in the outer surface of the gland, from where it connects with larger trunks, the superior and inferior lymphatics.
  - The superior group arises from the medial and lateral area draining into the deep cervical or internal jugular chain.
  - The lateral group arises from the anterolateral and posterolateral surfaces of the superior pole, ending in the deep cervical lymph nodes.
  - The inferior group channels drain the lower portions of the lobe and isthmus into the lower deep cervical lymph nodes, including the supraclavicular into the pretracheal, paratracheal, and mediastinal lymph nodes.

Histology

- The thyroid gland is divided by connective tissue septa into lobules, each one of these containing from 20 to 40 follicles; each follicle is considered a functional unit of the thyroid gland.

- The **thyroid follicles** consist of rounded structures of variable size lined by a single layer of cuboidal or flattened cells and a lumen containing a proteinaceous colloid material, the storage product of the secretory activity of the follicular cells.
- Colloid is eosinophilic, strongly positive with the periodic acid–Schiff stain and exhibits acidophilia in sections stained with Masson's trichrome stain; calcium oxalate crystals are visualized in the colloid in normal and pathologic conditions.
- The height of the cells varies according to the functional status of the gland. The follicles are surrounded by a basal membrane, and they remain in close relationship with lymphatics, a rich capillary network, and nerves present around the individual follicles.
- The cells have an eosinophilic or amphophilic cytoplasm, a central rounded or ovoid nucleus with delicate chromatin, and a single nucleolus.
- *Immunohistochemistry:* The follicular cells react with a number of keratins, with vimentin to a lesser degree, and specifically with the antibody to thyroglobulin.
- *Electron microscopy:* Numerous microvilli are seen in the luminal surface of the follicular cells. The cells are joined laterally by junctional complexes. The cytoplasm has abundant rough endoplasmic reticulum, a well-developed Golgi apparatus in a supranuclear or paranuclear position, and lysosomes in the apical cytoplasm.
- **Thyroid C cells:** The C cells, or parafollicular cells, represent a second population of distinct cells in the thyroid gland.
- C cells are encountered at the junction of the upper and middle thirds of the lateral lobes.
- In contrast with follicular cells, C cells are larger and are composed of round, polyhedral or spindle-shaped cells with larger nuclei and a lighter cytoplasm, ranging from clear or faintly basophilic to granular appearing; although considered difficult to identify in routine stain sections, they can be easily recognized because of their location in the follicles and the morphologic characteristics.
- The C-cell number varies from the neonatal period to adulthood; from numerous cells found at birth to single cells or smaller groups in the adult thyroid parenchyma.
- *Histochemistry:* C cells can be selectively stained by silver techniques, including Grimelius stain, Churukian-Schenk and the silver nitrate of Cajal, revealing brown to black cytoplasmic granules.
- *Immunohistochemistry:* C cells are specifically identified by immunoperoxidase techniques with antibodies to calcitonin; in addition to calcitonin, the cells contain calcitonin gene–related peptide (demonstrated by hybridization techniques), somatostatin, and serotonin. C cells also express keratins, and stained positive for neuron-specific enolase, chromogranin, synaptophysin and polyclonal carcinoembryonic antigen.
- *Electron microscopy:* C cells are enclosed in the basement membrane of the follicular cells without reaching the lumen of the follicles owing to interposition of the follicular cells; characteristic of these cells are the presence of round electron-dense membrane-bound granules that range from 100 to 300 nm in diameter.

■ **Solid cell nests:** consists of collection of cells with a squamoid appearance lacking intercellular bridges, most probably representing the remnant of the ultimobranchial body from which the C cells originate. These clusters of cells are found in the location of major concentration of C cells, and their visualization depends on the number of serial sections obtained from the lateral thyroid lobes. The cells have a polygonal or oval shape with elongated nuclei.

■ Occasionally, solid cell nests exhibit pseudofollicles with a luminal content that stains positive with the Alcian blue stain owing to the presence of acid mucopolysaccharides and less often have a cystic appearance.

■ The cells of solid cell nests show a positive reaction with low- and high-molecular-weight keratins, and some of the cells demonstrate calcitonin and polyclonal carcinoembryonic antigen reactivity.

Bibliography

Fawcett DW. The thyroid. In: Bloom and Fawcett: A Textbook of Histology. 11th edition. Philadelphia: WB Saunders, 1986, pp. 500–510.

Hollinshead WH. The neck. In: Anatomy for Surgeons. The Head and Neck. 3rd edition. Philadelphia: Harper and Row, 1982, pp. 499–515.

LiVolsi VA. Developmental biology and anatomy of the thyroid including the aberrant thyroid. In: Benington JL, ed. Surgical Pathology of the Thyroid: Series of Major Problems in Pathology. Philadelphia: WB Saunders, 1990, pp. 3–13.

LiVolsi VA. Thyroid. In: Sternberg SS, ed. Histology for Pathologists. New York: Raven Press, 1992, pp. 301–310.

Moore KL, Persaud TVN. Development of the thyroid gland. In: The Developing Human: Clinical Oriented Embryology. 5th edition. Philadelphia: WB Saunders, 1993, pp. 200–203.

Murray D. The thyroid gland. In: Kovacs K, Asa SL, eds. Functional Endocrine Pathology. Boston: Blackwell Scientific, 1991, pp. 293–301.

Pintar LJ, Toran-Allerand CD. Normal development of the hypothalamic-pituitary-thyroid axis. In: Braverman LE, Utiger RD, eds. Werner and Ingbar's The Thyroid: A Fundamental and Clinical Text. 6th edition. Philadelphia: JB Lippincott, 1991, pp. 7–21.

Rosai J, Carcangiu ML, De Lellis RA. Tumors of the thyroid. In: Rosai J, Sobin LH, eds. Atlas of Tumor Pathology. Fascicle 5. Third series. Washington, DC: Armed Forces Institute of Pathology, 1992, pp. 1–17.

Warwick R, Williams PL. The thyroid. In: Gray's Anatomy. 35th British edition. Philadelphia: WB Saunders, 1973, pp. 1373–1375.

APPENDIX C

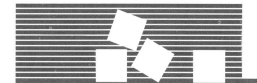

Parathyroid Glands

Embryology

- The parathyroid glands are of endodermal origin and originate as symmetrical nodular epithelial proliferations on the dorsal aspects of the third and fourth pharyngeal pouches around the 5th week of gestation.
- The superior gland develops from the fourth pharyngeal pouch, which is connected with the pharynx, from which it separates. The fourth pharyngeal pouch is a complex bilobed structure composed of a ventral component, the ultimobranchial body that fuses with the lateral aspect of the thyroid lobe, and a dorsal epithelial proliferation that separates to become the superior parathyroid gland, assuming the usual adult position along the posteromedial aspect of the thyroid gland. The superior parathyroid glands tend to be more constant in position than the inferior glands.
- The inferior parathyroid gland develops from the third pharyngeal pouch, also a complex bilobed structure, associated with the thymus, from which it separates after migrating caudally to a position near the lower pole of the thyroid gland.
- The most common "anomaly" of the parathyroid glands is ectopia, which usually represents a variation in embryologic migratory pattern.

Anatomy

- Most individuals have at least four parathyroid glands; and approximately 13% of the population has supernumerary glands, ranging in number from 1 additional gland to as many as 12 glands in rare instances.
- Rare individuals with fewer than four glands have been reported; however, there is doubt in at least some of the cases that all the glands were identified.
- Supernumerary glands may be well formed (about half of the cases) or may be less distinct aggregate of parathyroid tissue located near the normal glands.
- There is considerable variation in the location of the parathyroid glands in adults, although their distribution follows a predictable pattern based on their embryologic development.
- The superior glands are more constantly placed than the lower glands. The superior glands are located along the posterior edge of the thyroid superior to the intersection between the recurrent laryngeal nerve and the inferior thyroid artery (approximately 80%). Twenty percent are found posterior to the upper pole of the thyroid, where they may be intimately associated with the thyroid capsule. The superior glands may rarely be retroesophageal or retropharyngeal, or even intrathyroidal.
- The lower glands are more variably placed. Although the most common location is around the posterolateral or inferior aspects of the lower pole of the thyroid gland (approximately 60%), they may be found within the portion of the thymus that is adjacent to the lower pole of the thyroid. Since the inferior glands pursue a lengthy developmental migratory course, they may be found from the level of the hyoid bone to the mediastinum, where they may be situated in thymic tissue or in the pericardium.
- The parathyroid glands are soft yellow-brown to dark brown, circumscribed ovoid structures. Some parathyroids are bilobed or flattened.
- Each measures approximately 3 to 6 mm in length; and the combined weight increases from early infancy (mean, 5 to 9 mg) to the third or fourth decade (mean, for males, 120 mg; for females, 142 mg).
- The actual parenchymal cell mass represents about 74% of the weight of adult parathyroid glands.

Innervation

- Innervation is derived from the sympathetic ganglia (superior or middle cervical ganglia) either directly or indirectly through a plexus in the fascia of the posterior surface of the thyroid lobes. The nerves are probably vasomotor rather than secretomotor.

Arteries and Veins

- The parathyroid glands receive their blood supply from the abundant anastomosis between the thyroid arteries and arteries from the other neck organs. The arterial supply is derived from branches of the superior and inferior thyroid arteries. If ectopic in location, the arterial supply may be from the esophageal or pharyngeal arteries.

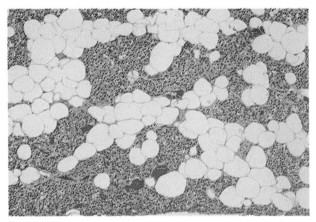

Figure C–1. Normal parathyroid gland. Strands and nests of cells with prominent adipose tissue component.

■ Venous drainage is through the superior or inferior lateral veins.

Lymphatics

■ Rich lymphatic drainage is associated with that of the thyroid and thymus.

Histology

■ The capsule of the parathyroid glands consists of delicate fibrous tissue.
■ Within the glands is an arborizing meshwork of arterioles and venules and a myriad of capillaries that give the glands an extremely rich blood supply.
■ The glands of children are very cellular, with little stromal collagen and very few stromal fat cells. The number of stromal fat cells begins to increase around puberty and continues to increase until the third to fifth decades.
■ Stromal fat is quite variable in its distribution among individuals as well as within a single gland, making the relative percentage of stromal fat a tenuous feature in evalua-

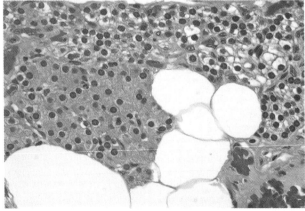

Figure C–2. Normal parathyroid gland. Principal or chief cells (upper and right portion of illustration), oxyphilic cells (to the left of center), and adipose tissue.

tion of parathyroid proliferations. Women generally have a higher percentage than men. Generally, stromal fat represents about 50% of total stromal volume.
■ Stromal fat content is affected by several variables, including nutrition, body habitus, general state of health, and heredity.
■ In infants and children the chief cells are arranged in solid sheets, with minimal intervening stroma. Oxyphilic and transitional oxyphilic cells are not normally observed. The chief cells are small and have faintly eosinophilic cytoplasm with less intracellular fat than the cells of adult parathyroid glands. More variable architectural features appear beginning in puberty with the accumulation of more stromal tissue.
■ The parenchymal cells of adult parathyroid glands are arranged in solid groups, cords, nests, and follicle-like structures, with intervening stromal tissue. The follicle-like structures often contain eosinophilic periodic acid–Schiff-positive material that resembles colloid. This material is not immunoreactive for thyroglobulin. A resemblance of this colloid-like substance to amyloid at a light microscopic and ultrastructural level has been noted.
■ The adult parathyroid contains predominantly chief cells, although they are larger and contain more intracytoplasmic fat than the chief cells in children. The cytoplasm is amphophilic or slightly eosinophilic to somewhat clear. Prominent lipid droplets are present in 70% to 80% of the chief cells. Chief cells that are "active" in the secretory process contain little or no cytoplasmic lipid. They also contain more secretory granules as evidenced by silver stains or by chromogranin staining. The nuclei of chief cells are round and tend to be rather hyperchromatic owing to a coarse chromatin pattern typical of neuroendocrine cells.
■ Oxyphilic cells and transitional oxyphilic cells are also found in the adult parathyroid. Transitional oxyphilic cells appear to represent an intermediate phase in the transition from chief cells to oxyphilic cells. The oxyphilic cells may be interspersed in small groups among the chief cells, or they may form nodules. The relative number of oxyphilic cells and the tendency to form oxyphilic cell nodules increase with age. The oxyphilic cells are larger than chief cells and have striking eosinophilic granular cytoplasm. Ultrastructural studies indicate that the cytoplasmic granularity results from the enormous number of mitochondria in these cells. Although the oxyphilic cells in normal glands do not seem to be actively secreting parathormone, hyperfunctioning oxyphilic neoplasms have been reported. The nuclei of oxyphilic cells are usually pyknotic.

Congenital Abnormalities

■ Parathyroid agenesis is rare.
■ DiGeorge syndrome includes complete or partial absence of the third and fourth pharyngeal pouches and their derivatives: the thymus, the parathyroid glands, and the C cells. The disease is manifested by multiple facial malformations, hypoplasia of the thyroid, hypoparathyroidism, and cardiac abnormalities.

Bibliography

Abu-Jawdeh GM, Roth SI. Parathyroid glands. In: Sternberg SS, ed. Histology for Pathologists. New York: Raven Press, 1992, pp. 311–318.

Åkerström G, Malmaeus J, Bergström R. Surgical pathology of human parathyroid glands. Surgery 1984; 95:14–21.

DeLellis RA. The normal parathyroid gland. In: Rosai J, Sobin LH, eds. Tumors of the Parathyroid Gland. Fascicle 6. Third series. Washington, D.C.: Armed Forces Institute of Pathology, 1991, pp. 1–14.

Grimelius L, Åkerström G, Johansson H, Bergström R. Anatomy and histopathology of human parathyroid glands. Pathol Annu 1981; 16:1–24.

Grimelius L, Åkerström G, Johansson H, et al. The parathyroid glands. In: Kovacs K, Asa SL, eds. Functional Endocrine Pathology. Boston: Blackwell Scientific, 1991, pp. 375–395.

Moore KL, Persaud TVN: The branchial or pharyngeal apparatus. In: The Developing Human: Clinically Oriented Embryology. 5th edition. Philadelphia: WB Saunders, 1993, pp. 195–200.

Wang C-A. The anatomic basis of parathyroid surgery. Ann Surg 1976; 183:271–275.

APPENDIX D

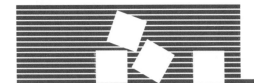

Pancreas

Embryology

- The pancreas arises from outgrowths of endodermal cells of the caudal segment of the foregut, between the layers of the ventral mesentery (between the 5th and 6th week).
- The bilobed pancreatic evagination develops in the angle formed by the hepatic duct and the duodenum in the ventral mesentery.
- The ventral bud consists of two parts: the left part that later atrophies and the right part that gives origin to the uncinate process and caudal half of the head of the pancreas.
- The rotation of the duodenum and the common bile duct carries the ventral pancreas to the right posteriorly.
- The larger dorsal pancreatic bud arises between the stomach and the common bile duct in the dorsal mesentery and ultimately becomes the tail, body, isthmus, and cephalad part of the pancreas.
- The ventral bud that lies behind the dorsal pancreatic bud fuses intimately with the dorsal pancreas, forming a single glandular structure that remains in the concave space of the retroperitoneal duodenum.
- The fusion of the ductal system of both anlagen give rise to the main pancreatic duct (Wirsung), which empties into the second portion of the duodenum either alone or together with the common bile duct through the ampulla of Vater, around the 7th week.
- The duct of the dorsal bud (Santorini), proximal to the usual site of fusion, persists as an accessory pancreatic duct that opens in the duodenal lumen through the minor papilla or becomes a tributary of the main duct.
- Around the 15th week the pancreas consists of a network of branching solid epithelial, actively mitotic tubules (primitive ducts) from which acini and islets develop from cell clusters at the end of these tubules.
- The pancreatic parenchyma becomes organized into lobes and lobules.
- Many of the ductular cells assume an acinar arrangement along the wall of the ducts.
- The acini tend to be at the periphery of the lobules, while the islets that remain associated with the ductal system are localized in the center of the lobule.
- Mesodermal cells differentiating into fibroblasts form the primitive pancreatic stroma that decreases after the 4th month.

- Shortly thereafter, pancreatic islets develop from the outer surface of the primitive tubules and begin to organize into a cordlike cluster of cells penetrated by capillaries and encroached by connective tissue. These are known as "primary islands"; they are few in number, and they reach maturation around the 5th month. Most of these islands degenerate (this process is accompanied by infiltration of lymphocytes in the connective tissue) and become scarce at birth.
- Secondary islands appear around the 3rd month of gestation and become more numerous and discrete about the 5th month, increasing in size and number through fetal development. These islets constitute the permanent islets.
- Specific granules are demonstrable in the islets cells around the 16th week of gestation. The first identifiable cell is the A cell at 9 weeks, followed by D cells and B cells around the 11th week of gestation; PP cells are the last to appear; of note is that B cells tend to be scattered as isolated cells or cell clusters in the pancreatic parenchyma or along the ductular epithelium.

Anatomy

- The pancreas is a lobulated, retroperitoneal pinkish-gray, poorly encapsulated organ, 12 to 15 cm long, with a weight range of 65 to 150 g (slightly heavier in males); in the newborn the pancreas weighs 2 to 3 g, and its weight increases to 40 g at the time of adolescence.
- It extends along the posterior abdominal wall, behind the stomach, from the duodenum to the spleen, and consists of a head, a body connected by a narrow neck to the head, and the tail.
  - The head lies within the duodenal curvature with the uncinate process projecting upward and to the left behind the superior mesenteric vessels.
  - The neck merges with the body.
  - The body is anteriorly and inferiorly covered by peritoneum, and it is in direct contact with the aorta and the origin of the superior mesenteric artery, posteriorly.
  - The tail, which extends into the hilum of the spleen, in close relation with the splenic vessels, lies in contact with the inferior part of the gastric surface of the spleen.

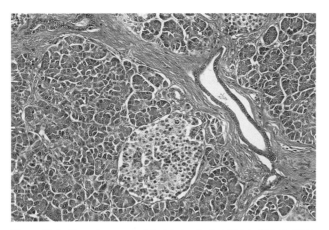

Figure D–1. Normal pancreas. Interlobular duct and islet of Langerhans.

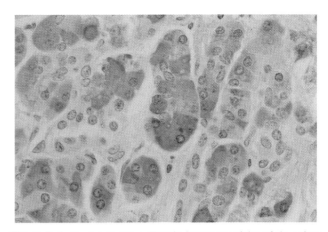

Figure D–4. Normal pancreas. Trypsin immunoreactivity of the acinar cells.

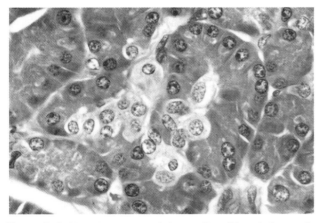

Figure D–2. Normal pancreas. Acinar cells with apical granular eosinophilic cytoplasm around centroacinar cells with pale eosinophilic cytoplasm.

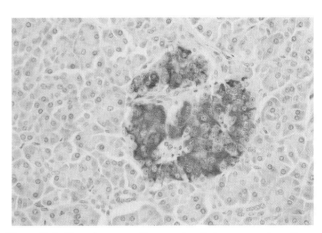

Figure D–5. Normal pancreas. Numerous insulin immunoreactive cells are demonstrated in a B-cell rich islet.

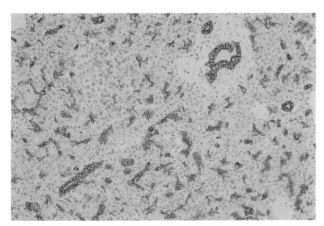

Figure D–3. Normal pancreas. Keratin immunoreactivity of the centroacinar cells and ductules.

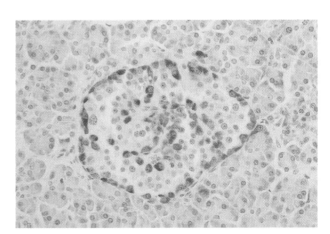

Figure D–6. Normal pancreas. Glucagon-immunoreactive cells showing their normal distribution at the periphery of the islet, as well as nearby capillaries in the center of the islet.

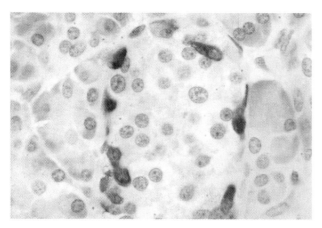

Figure D–7. Normal pancreas. Somatostatin immunoreactive cells appearing as irregularly shaped cells with cytoplasmic processes at the periphery of the islet.

- The main pancreatic duct traverses the pancreas from left to right. It begins in the tail, receiving tributary ducts from the lobules composing the gland, joining the main duct at right angles, reaches the neck where it increases in size, and comes into relation with the bile duct.
- Together, the main pancreatic duct and the bile duct open into the major papilla in the duodenum, 10 cm distal to the pylorus.
- The accessory duct, which receives tributary ducts from the lower part of the head, opens in the duodenum through the minor duodenal papilla.

Innervation

- The pancreas is innervated by autonomic sympathetic and parasympathetic fibers.
- Its nerves are derived from the vagus and the splanchnic nerves and reach the pancreas through the splenic plexus.
- The afferent vagus fibers regulate capillary blood flow as well as endosecretory and exosecretory activity of the pancreas.

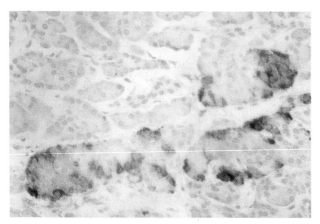

Figure D–8. Normal pancreas. Irregularly shaped islets rich in human pancreatic polypeptide immunoreactive cells.

- The efferent sympathetic fibers that originated in the pancreas pass into the splanchnic nerves, leaving the sympathetic trunk to reach the posterior nerve root.

Arteries and Veins

- The pancreas receives the blood supply from six groups of arteries.
  - The anterior arcade, formed by the anterior superior pancreaticoduodenal artery (a branch of the gastroduodenal artery) and the anterior inferior pancreaticoduodenal artery (a branch of the mesenteric artery).
  - The posterior arcade, formed by the posterior superior pancreaticoduodenal artery (a distal branch of the gastroduodenal artery) and the posterior inferior pancreaticoduodenal artery (a branch of the superior mesenteric artery).
  - The dorsal pancreatic artery (a branch of the celiac, hepatic, splenic, or superior mesenteric arteries), supplies the uncinate process and the dorsal part of the head of the pancreas.
  - The inferior pancreatic artery, a continuation of the left branch of the dorsal pancreatic artery, runs along the inferior border of the body of the organ.
  - The great pancreatic artery (a large branch of the splenic artery) divides within the gland into two branches: the right and left branches, which run along the main pancreatic duct.
  - The tail of the pancreas is supplied by the caudal pancreatic arteries, small branches of the splenic artery, and anastomotic branches of the inferior and great pancreatic arteries.
- The veins course alongside the arteries. In the head the gastroduodenal and superior pancreaticoduodenal veins empty into the portal vein.
- Venous channels from the body and tail empty into the splenic, inferior mesenteric, and portal veins.

Lymphatics

- Small lymphatic vessels are present next to capillaries closely attached to and surrounding the exocrine acini.
- Small anastomotic perilobular and interlobular lymphatic channels running along the head and body of the pancreas drain into five collecting trunks and lymph nodes.
- The lymphatic of the tail of the gland drains into the splenic lymph nodes.
- The superior trunks collecting from the anterior and posterior half segment of the pancreas drain into the suprapancreatic lymph nodes along the head and body of the organ.
- The inferior trunks collecting from the inferior half of the pancreas drain into the inferior pancreatic lymph nodes along the inferior segment of the head and body of the pancreas.
- The anterior trunk consists of two trunks collecting from the head of the pancreas draining into the infrapyloric and pancreaticoduodenal lymph nodes.
- The posterior trunk collecting from the posterior head of the pancreas drains into the posterior pancreaticoduodenal and common bile duct lymph nodes.

- The splenic trunk collecting from the tail of the pancreas drains into the superior and inferior lymph nodes of the tail of the organ.

Histology

- The pancreas is a compound gland, in which the major exocrine component accounts for 98% of the gland weight and is responsible for the secretion of fluids, electrolytes, and digestive enzymes into the duodenum. The endocrine component, which accounts for 2% of the gland, controls carbohydrate, protein, and lipid metabolism under neurohormonal regulation.
- The exocrine pancreas is organized into small lobules bound together by thin connective tissue stroma extending from its capsule, through which blood vessels, lymphatics, nerves, and interlobular ducts run.
- **Acinar components:**
  - The acini are rounded structural units composed of a single row of epithelial cells resting on a basal lamina around a variably sized central lumen.
  - The acinar cells are large pyramidal-shaped cells with a narrow apex toward the luminal aspect. They are polarized cells characterized by a broad basal homogeneous basophilic cytoplasm and a supranuclear eosinophilic granular cytoplasm filled with zymogen granules. The round nuclei with prominent central nucleoli and dark appearing chromatin are close to the basal one third of the cell.
  - *Electron microscopy:* acinar cells are crowded extensively by rough endoplasmic reticulum basally, whereas zymogen granules, the Golgi complex, and numerous free polyribosomes are in the apical portions of the cells; the apical portion of the cells stores zymogen granules, and the free surface of the acinar cell projects microvilli into the luminal surface.
  - Digestive enzymes are synthesized in the basal cytoplasm of the acinar cells, where they accumulate in the lumen of the endoplasmic reticulum, from where they are channeled in the Golgi complex and concentrated into characteristic zymogen granules, which discharge their contents by exocytosis.
- **Ductal system:**
  - The intercalated ducts or intra-acinus segment of the interlobular ducts are lined by flattened or low cuboidal centroacinar cells with a characteristic pale-staining cytoplasm and elongated nucleus.
  - The intralobular ducts result from the merging of the intercalated ducts. They are of variable size, and the smaller ones are lined by cells similar to the centroacinar cells. The larger ones have larger cuboidal or low columnar cells with rounded nuclei surrounded by a small amount of connective tissue.
  - The interlobular ducts are of a major caliber and formed by low-columnar epithelium with occasional goblet cells interspersed along them and a moderate layer of connective tissue around them.
  - The main pancreatic ducts—the Wirsung and the Santorini—are lined by tall columnar cells with basally located nuclei, with numerous interspersed goblet cells and a prominent connective tissue layer around them. One characteristic of this cell is the process of continuous exfoliation and replacement by new cells that appear at the basal region of the epithelium.
- **Endocrine pancreas:**
  - The adult pancreas has more than 1 million islets that are scattered through the gland but constitute only 1% to 2% of its total volume.
  - Islets are more numerous in the tail than in the body and head of the gland.
  - Islets are compact, lightly stained masses of cells that contain endocrine cells separated from the acini by thin reticulum fibers with a rich capillary network.
  - Islets from the posterior head and uncinate process of the pancreas are irregularly shaped and rich in pancreatic polypeptide cells. These cells are seen not only at the periphery of the islets but also scattered along the pancreatic acini.
  - The **insulin cells,** which are the most numerous of the endocrine cells (60% to 80%), constitute two thirds of the population of the endocrine cells. Located centrally in the islets, these cells are somewhat larger than the rest; they have characteristic crystalline membrane-bound granules of variable configuration, with a size range between 250 to 400 nm. The insulin cells can be identified by histochemical methods, such as the aldehyde fuchsin and aldehyde thionin stains, imparting to the cells a purple to blue color of variable intensity reflecting the granularity of the cells. Specific demonstration of insulin is achieved by the immunohistochemical techniques.
  - The **glucagon cells** are less numerous, representing 15% to 20% of the endocrine cells, and are predominantly located at the periphery of the islets and scattered along the capillaries inside the islets. They are of a smaller size than the insulin cells and are in close association with the somatostatin cells. The cells have eccentric electron-dense core granules measuring from 200 to 300 nm concentrated at the secretory pole of the cell. Histochemically, the cells can be demonstrated by silver stains such as Grimelius and Sevier-Munger and specifically by the immunohistochemical techniques.
  - The **somatostatin cells** (5%) are irregularly shaped cells with cytoplasmic processes located anywhere in the islets, but mostly at the periphery of the islets, interspersed with the insulin and glucagon cells. These cells are heterogeneous according to the size, shape, and density of the granules. The size of the granules varies from 150 to 400 nm. Somatostatin is stored in large granules, which are considerably less dense than the glucagon granules. These cells can be identified by using the silver technique of Hellerström-Hellman and specifically by the immunohistochemical techniques.
  - The **pancreatic polypeptide cells** have granules that distinguish them from the glucagon cells. The granules display round to ovoid electron-dense cores, surrounded by a clear halo, measuring from 90 to 200 nm. These cells are located at the periphery of the islets and are frequently seen in the irregularly shaped islets of the posterior head of the pancreas. The cells are not visualized by histochemical stains, and they are identifiable only by immunohistochemical techniques.

Bibliography

Conklin JL. Cytogenesis of the human fetal pancreas. Am J Anat 1962; 111:81–193.

Cooper MJ, Moossa AR. Cellular composition and physiology of the exocrine pancreas. In: Moossa AR, ed. Tumors of the Pancreas. Baltimore: Williams & Wilkins, 1980, pp. 21–28.

Cubilla Al, Fitzgerald PJ. Tumors of the exocrine pancreas. In: Hartman WH, Sobin LH, eds. Atlas of Tumor Pathology. Second Series. Fascicle 19. Washington, DC: Armed Forces Institute of Pathology, 1986, pp. 5–59.

Fawcett DW. Pancreas. In: Bloom and Fawcett: A Textbook of Histology. 11th edition. Philadelphia: WB Saunders, 1986, pp. 716–730.

Heitz PU, Begingler C, Gyr K. Anatomy and physiology of the exocrine pancreas. In: Klöppel G, Heitz PU, eds. Pancreatic Pathology. Edinburgh: Churchill Livingstone, 1984, pp. 3–21.

Kern HF. Fine structure of the human exocrine pancreas. In: Go VLW, DiMagno EP, Gardner JD, et al, eds. The Exocrine Pancreas: Biology, Pathobiology, and Diseases. New York: Raven Press, 1993, pp. 9–19.

Klöppel G, Lenzen S. Anatomy and physiology of the endocrine pancreas. In: Klöppel G, Heitz PU, eds. Pancreatic Pathology. Edinburgh: Churchill Livingstone, 1984, pp. 133–153.

Laitio M, Lev R, Orlic D. The developing human pancreas: An ultrastructural and histochemical study with special reference to exocrine cells. J Anat 1974; 117:619–634.

Lee PC, Lebenthal E. Prenatal and postnatal development of the human exocrine pancreas. In: Go VLW, DiMagno EP, Gardner JD, et al, eds. The Exocrine Pancreas: Biology, Pathobiology, and Diseases. New York: Raven Press, 1993, pp. 57–73.

Liu HM, Potter EL. Development of the human pancreas. Arch Pathol 1962; 74:439–452.

Lloyd RV. Endocrine pancreas: Development and anatomy. In: Endocrine Pathology. New York: Springer-Verlag, 1990, pp. 85–86.

Moore KL, Persaud TVN. Development of the pancreas. In: Moore KL, Persaud TVN, eds. The Developing Human: Clinically Oriented Embryology. 5th edition. Philadelphia: WB Saunders, 1993, pp. 244–245.

Oertel JE, Heffess CS, Oertel YC. Pancreas. In: Sternberg SS, ed. Histology for Pathologists. New York: Raven Press, 1992, pp. 657–664.

Warwick R, Williams PL. The pancreas. In: Warwick R, Williams PL, eds. Gray's Anatomy. 35th British edition. Philadelphia: WB Saunders, 1975, pp. 1299–1302.

APPENDIX E

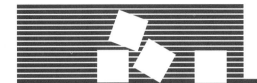

Adrenal Gland

Embryology

- The adrenal glands have dual origin: the adrenal cortex is of mesodermal origin and the adrenal medulla is of ectodermal origin.
- Bilaterally, between the root of the dorsal mesentery and the developing gonad, small aggregates of proliferating mesodermal cells constitute the first indication of the developing adrenals during the 6th week of gestation; the cortex, at the 10-mm stage, becomes enveloped ventrally and dorsally by a capsule of mesonephric origin, which also gives rise to the inner connective tissue framework.
- During the same period, the proliferating cortex is disorganized by invasion of the sympathochromaffin tissue from the adjacent developing sympathetic ganglionic masses to form the medulla; this tissue contributes to the development of the venous sinuses that will be joined by capillaries originated from adjacent mesonephric arteries entering the cortex radially.
- From the rudimentary subcapsular zona glomerulosa, proliferating cords of cells passing in between vessels toward the medulla degenerate, becoming granular and eosinophilic and finally autolyzed. These cells constitute the fetal or provisional cortex, which degenerates rapidly between the first 2 weeks after birth, resulting in the involution of the gland.
- A second proliferation of mesenchymal cells arising from mesothelium takes place in the 14-mm embryo, giving rise to the definitive or permanent cortex.
- After birth, proliferating cells of the glomerular zone form the fasciculata and reticular zones of the adult cortex, which become fully differentiated by about the 12th year. The maturation process of the cells is slower than that of the fetal cortex.
- The adrenal medulla derives from primitive cells (sympathogonia) of the neural crest. The latter also gives origin to the adjacent sympathetic ganglion. Strands of cells and nerve fibers migrate ventrally and penetrate the anlagen of the adrenal cortex on its medial side to take a central position in the primitive gland. While some cells invade the cortex, intra-adrenal chromaffin cells develop independently and slowly.
- The adrenal medulla has three cell types.

- The sympathetic cells or sympathogonia, which is a small cell with hyperchromatic nuclei and scanty cytoplasm.
- The pheochromoblast, which is a larger cell with larger nuclei, one or two prominent nucleoli, and abundant cytoplasm.
- The pheochromocyte, which has a single nucleolus.
- The sympathetic cells and the pheochromoblast give a negative chromaffin reaction, and the pheochromocytes give a positive chromaffin reaction at the 50-mm stage or later. The pheochromocytes increase in number by division, while the primitive cells decrease.
- Most of the chromaffin tissue is extra-adrenal during development and involutes after birth. The fetal adrenal gland is large—it tends to be 10 to 20 times larger than the adult adrenal gland. The large adrenal glands result from the extensive size of the adrenal cortex, and they become smaller during the first year owing to regression of the adrenal cortex.
- The adrenal glands lose one third of their weight during the 3 weeks after birth, regaining the original weight at the end of the 2nd year.

Anatomy

- The adrenal glands are flattened, yellowish glands with a combined weight of 10 g at birth and less than 10 g in adults, the medulla being about one tenth of the total weight.
- The adrenals are situated on each side of the median plane, behind the peritoneum. The glands are surrounded by loose connective tissue and are enclosed with the kidneys in the renal fascia, overlying the superior poles.
- Each adrenal gland measures $50 \times 30 \times 10$ mm.
- Both adrenal glands differ in shape.
  - The right gland has a pyramidal shape and is *posterior* to the vena cava and the right lobe of the liver and *anterior* to the diaphragm and the superior pole of the kidney.
  - The left adrenal gland has a crescentic shape with a prominent groove and is loosely attached to the tail of the pancreas. The concave posterior surface lies in the medial border of the superior pole of the kidney.

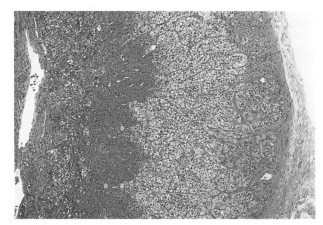

Figure E–1. Normal adrenal gland. Beneath the capsule (extreme right) are clusters of glomerulosa cells, columns of fasciculata cells, and zona reticularis cells lying in the deep cortex adjacent to the medullary cells (left side of the illustration).

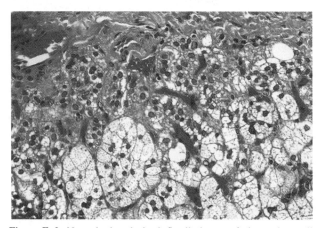

Figure E–2. Normal adrenal gland. Small clusters of glomerulosa cells with an eosinophilic cytoplasm are seen beneath the capsule (top). Cells of the zona fasciculata are also present.

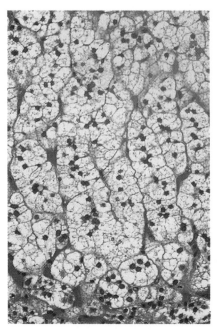

Figure E–3. Normal adrenal gland. Characteristic of the zona fasciculata is the presence of long cords of cells with a clear vacuolated cytoplasm.

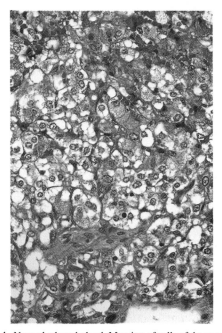

Figure E–4. Normal adrenal gland. Merging of cells of the zona reticularis into the adrenal medulla.

- The adrenal glands have three parts—the head, body and tail—with the head placed medially; the adrenal medulla is concentrated in the head and body.
- Each gland consists of an outer part or external lipid rich cortex measuring 0.5 mm in thickness and an inner grayish central medulla composed of chromaffin cells.

Arteries and Veins

- The adrenal gland is richly vascularized. The arteries that supply each adrenal gland derive from the aorta, the inferior phrenic arteries, and the renal arteries.
- The arteries are divided in three groups, including the superior, inferior, and medial arteries; these vessels cover all aspects of the adrenal glands and divide into numerous small vessels, forming a subcapsular plexus.
- From the subcapsular plexus, capillaries surround the glomerulosa, extend into the fasciculata, and open into interconnecting channels in the zona reticularis, forming a second vascular plexus that ends at the corticomedullary junction and drains into medullary sinusoids.

- Some arterial branches traverse the cortex, giving few or no branches until reaching the medullary region, where they form a rich capillary network around the chromaffin cells.
- The medulla has a dual blood supply: one from the cortical sinusoids and the other via medullary arteries that course from the capsule to the medulla. The capillaries of the medulla empty in the same venous system that drains the cortex.

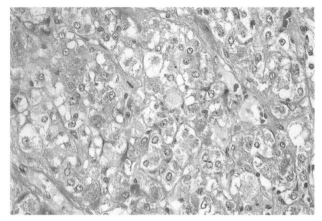

Figure E–5. Normal adrenal medulla. Pheochromocytes with basophilic cytoplasm and delicate vascular stroma.

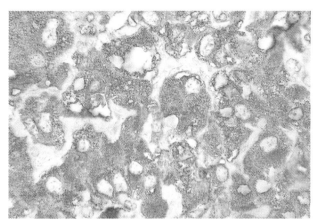

Figure E–7. Normal adrenal medulla. Strong chromogranin immunoreactivity is present in the pheochromocytes.

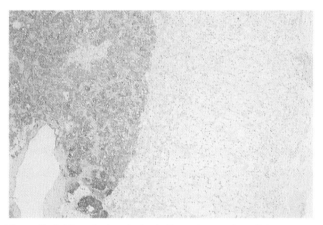

Figure E–6. Normal adrenal gland. Sharp demarcation of the synaptophysin reactive medulla (left) from the non-reactive cortex (right).

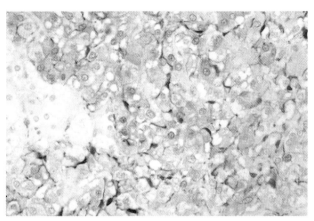

Figure E–8. Normal adrenal medulla. Sustentacular cells, difficult to identify by light microscopy, are readily seen by their strong S-100 protein immunoreactivity around nests of chromaffin cells.

■ The multiple venules form the central veins, which emerge from the hilus of the glands; the right central vein opens into the inferior vena cava, and the left central vein opens into the renal vein.

Nerves

■ The adrenal cortex is not innervated.
■ The medulla is richly innervated.
   • There are preganglionic sympathetic nerve fibers arising from the lower thoracic and lumbar regions of the spinal cord passing through the sympathetic chain and via splanchnic nerves to the adrenal capsule, forming a nerve plexus. From this plexus, preganglionic nerves traverse the cortex, ending in the medulla.
   • Isolated or grouped ganglion cells are seen among pheochromocytes.

Lymphatics

■ The adrenal cortex has no lymphatic supply. Lymphatics are in the adrenal gland capsule and also are distributed in the adventitia of the central vein and tributaries, draining into aortic lymph nodes.

Histology

■ The adrenal glands are surrounded by a connective tissue capsule of variable thickness that carries the blood vessels, nerves, and lymphatics.
■ The cortex of the adrenal gland has three concentric zones: the outer subcapsular zone called the **zona glomerulosa,** a wider middle layer that comprises the **zona fasciculata,** and the innermost zone of the cortex called the **zona reticularis.**
   • The **zona glomerulosa** consists of a discontinuous subcapsular band of cells that merges with the continuous zona fasciculata. It is composed of packed, rounded cell aggregates or short, twisted columns of cells supported by a thin fibrovascular stroma. The cells are polyhedral in shape and have scanty eosinophilic or amphophilic cytoplasm. Small, scattered lipid droplets may be present. The rounded nuclei are deeply stained and contain one or two nucleoli.
   • *Electron microscopy:* characteristic of these cells are the prominent endoplasmic reticulum forming anastomotic branches throughout the cytoplasm. The Golgi

complex is well developed. The rounded mitochondria have lamellar cristae.

- The **zona fasciculata** lies internal to the zona glomerulosa and is composed of large cells arranged in straight two cell columns with parallel sinusoids coursing in between cords. The polyhedral cells have distinct cell borders, eosinophilic cytoplasm, vesicular nuclei, and a single nucleolus. The cells contain numerous lipid droplets in the fresh state and dissolve during fixation, imparting to the cytoplasm a foamy vacuolated appearance.
  - *Electron microscopy:* the cells are characterized as having a round nucleus with a prominent nucleolus and clump heterochromatin at its periphery. The extensive branching and anastomosing tubules of smooth endoplasmic reticulum occupy one half of the cell volume. Cisternae of rough endoplasmic reticulum are present. The Golgi apparatus is well developed. The large elongated or round mitochondria with tubular cristae are numerous. Scattered lysosomes appearing as small dense bodies, lipofuscin granules, and an abundance of lipid droplets are present.
- The deepest area of the cortex is the **zona reticularis,** arranged in cell cords and anastomosing cords of smaller rounded cells separated by capillaries. The cells have a cytoplasm with fewer lipid droplets, and, particularly toward the medulla, they have a darker granular cytoplasm largely due to the accumulation of lipofuscin pigment. The nuclei are vesicular in the light cells and hyperchromatic in the darker cells. The transition from the fasciculata to the reticularis is gradual.
  - *Electron microscopy:* smooth and granular endoplasmic reticulum, lipid droplets, and lysosomes are present. The cells exhibit lipofuscin bodies and glycogen granules, and the mitochondria has tubulovesicular cristae.
- Hormonal secretion includes the following:
  - The zona glomerulosa is the site of aldosterone production
  - The zona fasciculata and reticularis synthesize glucocorticoids and sex hormones.

Medulla

- The medulla measures up to 2 mm in thickness. It is located deeper in the head and body of the adrenal gland, with occasional extension into the tail.
- The medulla is composed of rounded groups of cells, the pheochromocytes, which are in intimate relationship with capillaries and venules. These cell groups are surrounded by a second population of cells, the sustentacular cells, which are not seen routinely in histologic sections but are easily demonstrated by S-100 protein immunostaining.
- The medullary cells have poorly demarcated borders, a fine granular basophilic cytoplasm, and variably sized and shaped nuclei, occasionally placed eccentrically. The nuclei have prominent eosinophilic nucleoli.
- The medullary cells contain catecholamine granules that turn brown in the presence of potassium bichromate solutions, ammoniacal silver nitrate, and osmium tetroxide because of the oxidation and polymerization of epinephrine and norepinephrine granules. The browning of the cells is known as the "chromaffin reaction."
- *Electron microscopy:* medullary cells are characterized by the presence of numerous membrane-bound dense granules that vary from 100 to 300 nm in diameter. Glutaraldehyde-fixed tissue exhibits two types of cells distinguishable by the characteristics of their granules. Cells storing norepinephrine have eccentrically located dense-core granules. Cells storing epinephrine have less electron-dense homogeneous granules.

Bibliography

Carney JA. Adrenal gland. In: Sternberg SS, ed. Histology for Pathologists. New York: Raven Press, 1992, pp. 321–346.

Fawcett DW. Adrenal gland and paraganglia. In: Bloom and Fawcett: A Textbook of Histology. 11th edition. Philadelphia: WB Saunders, 1986, pp. 516–531.

Lack EE. Pathology of the adrenal and extra-adrenal paraganglia. Vol. 29. Major Problems in Pathology. Philadelphia: WB Saunders, 1994, pp. 186–199.

Lack EE, Kozakewich PW. Embryology, developmental anatomy, and selected aspects of non-neoplastic pathology. In: Pathology of the Adrenal Glands. New York: Churchill Livingstone, 1990, pp. 1–19.

Lloyd RV. Adrenal gland. In: Endocrine Pathology. New York: Springer-Verlag, 1990, pp. 141–144.

Moore KL, Persaud TVN. The urogenital system. In: The Developing Human: Clinical Oriented Embryology. 5th edition. Philadelphia: WB Saunders, 1993, pp. 279–281.

Page DL, DeLellis RA, Aubrey JH Jr. Tumors of the adrenal gland. In: Hartman WH, Sobin LH, eds. Atlas of Tumor Pathology. Fascicle 23. Second Series. Washington, DC: Armed Forces Institute of Pathology, 1986, pp. 6–35.

Rittmaster RS, Arab DM. Morphology of the adrenal cortex and medulla. In: Becker KL, ed. Principles and Practice of Endocrinology and Metabolism. 2nd edition. Philadelphia: JB Lippincott, 1995, pp. 641–643.

Sasano N, Sasano H. The adrenal cortex. In: Kovacs K, Asa SL, eds. Functional Endocrine Pathology. Boston: Blackwell Scientific, 1990, pp. 546–549.

Warwick R, Williams PL. The suprarenal glands. In: Gray's Anatomy. 35th British edition. Philadelphia: WB Saunders, 1973, pp. 1377–1381.

INDEX

Note: Page numbers in *italics* refer to illustrations; page numbers followed by t refer to tables.

ATLASES IN DIAGNOSTIC SURGICAL PATHOLOGY

Series Consulting Editor: *Gerald M. Bordin, MD*

THE **ATLASES IN DIAGNOSTIC SURGICAL PATHOLOGY (SXASP) series** provides current, accurate, and detailed visual guidance on specific areas of diagnostic surgical pathology.

The volumes reflect the distilled wisdom of their authors, providing a scholarly review of the topic and practical surgical assistance for the reader. Excellence of text, illustration, and reference are the hallmarks of the series.

Now—you can preview the **Atlases in Diagnostic Surgical Pathology** volumes of your choice **FREE for 30 days!**

Simply indicate your selections on the postage-paid order card...**call toll-free 1-800-545-2522** (8:30 - 7:00 Eastern Time)...or **FAX us FREE at 1-800-874-6418.** Be sure to mention **DM#40110.**

Become an Atlases in Diagnostic Surgical Pathology series subscriber! You'll receive each new volume in the **series** as soon as it's published— 1 to 3 titles per year—and save shipping costs!

If you're not completely satisfied with any volume you order through the mail or the toll-free numbers, just return the book with the invoice within 30 days at no further obligation. You keep only the volumes you want. *Your satisfaction is guaranteed!*

VALUABLE ADDITIONS TO YOUR WORKING LIBRARY!

Available from your bookstore or the publisher.

Complete and mail today for a FREE 30-day preview!

▼

☑ YES! Please send me the **ATLASES IN DIAGNOSTIC SURGICAL PATHOLOGY** titles I've indicated below. If not completely satisfied with any volume, I may return it with the invoice within 30 days at no further obligation.

☐ W2911-3 **Atlas of Orthopedic Pathology** *(Wold, McLeod, Sim & Unni)*

☐ W2893-1 **Atlas of Pulmonary Surgical Pathology** *(Colby, Lombard, Yousem & Kitaichi)*

☐ W2657-2 **Atlas of Liver Pathology** *(Kanel & Korula)*

☐ W6730-9 **Atlas of Gastrointestinal Pathology** *(Owen & Kelly)*

☐ W4032-X **Atlas of Head and Neck Pathology** *(Wenig)*

☐ W4476-7 **Atlas of Cardiovascular Pathology** *(Virmani, Burke & Farb)*

☐ W5284-0 **Atlas of Surgical Pathology of the Male Reproductive Tract** *(Ro, Grignon, Amin & Ayala)*

☐ W5917-9 **Atlas of Endocrine Pathology** *(Wenig, Heffess & Adair)*

☐ Enroll me in the **SXASP Subscriber Plan** so that I may receive future titles immediately upon publication and save shipping costs! I may preview each new volume FREE for 30 days—and keep only the volumes I want.

Name_____

Address _____

City _____ State _____ Zip _____ Telephone (_____) _____

Staple this to your purchase order to expedite delivery.
© W.B. SAUNDERS COMPANY 1997. Printed in USA. Shipping additional outside the USA. Offer valid in USA only.
C#14897   DM#40110

ATLASES IN DIAGNOSTIC SURGICAL PATHOLOGY

- **Atlas of Orthopedic Pathology** *(Wold, McLeod, Sim & Unni)* Order #W2911-3

- **Atlas of Pulmonary Surgical Pathology** *(Colby, Lombard, Yousem & Kitaichi)* Order #W2893-1

- **Atlas of Liver Pathology** *(Kanel & Korula)* Order #W2657-2

- **Atlas of Gastrointestinal Pathology** *(Owen & Kelly)* Order #W6730-9

- **Atlas of Head and Neck Pathology** *(Wenig)* Order #W4032-X

- **Atlas of Cardiovascular Pathology** *(Virmani, Burke & Farb)* Order #W4476-7

- **Atlas of Surgical Pathology of the Male Reproductive Tract** *(Ro, Grignon, Amin & Ayala)* Order #W5284-0

- **Atlas of Endocrine Pathology** *(Wenig, Heffess & Adair)* Order #W5917-9

ENROLL TODAY!
SEE REVERSE SIDE FOR DETAILS.